DATE DUE

MAR 2 5 2004	
NOV 0 2 2004	
NOV 1 6 2004	
NOV 0 2 2005	
JAN 1 7 2006	
NOV 1 3 2009	

Surgery
of the
Cervical
Spine

Surgery
of the
Cervical
Spine

Sanford E. Emery, M.D.
Associate Professor of Orthopaedic Surgery
Department of Surgery
University Hospitals of Cleveland
Case Western Reserve University School of Medicine
Cleveland, Ohio

Scott D. Boden, M.D.
Professor
Department of Orthopaedic Surgery
Emory University School of Medicine
Director, Emory Spine Center
Atlanta, Georgia

Artist: Wendy Beth Jackelow

SAUNDERS
An Imprint of Elsevier Science

SAUNDERS
An Imprint of Elsevier Science

The Curtis Center
Independence Square West
Philadelphia, Pennsylvania 19106

SURGERY OF THE CERVICAL SPINE   ISBN 0-7216-5780-X
Copyright © 2003, Elsevier Science (USA). All rights reserved.

Notice

Surgery is an ever-changing field. Standard safety precautions must be followed, but as new research and clinical experience broaden our knowledge, changes in treatment and drug therapy may become necessary or appropriate. Readers are advised to check the most current product information provided by the manufacturer of each drug to be administered to verify the recommended dose, the method and duration of administration, and the contraindications. It is the responsibility of the treating physician, relying on experience and knowledge of the patient, to determine the dosages and the best treatment for each individual patient. Neither the publisher nor the editor assumes any liability for any injury and/or damage to persons or property arising from this publication.

THE PUBLISHER

Library of Congress Cataloging-in-Publication Data

Surgery of the cervical spine / [edited by] Sanford E. Emery, Scott D. Boden; Wendy Beth Jackelow, artist.
   p. ; cm.
     Includes bibliographical references.
     ISBN 0-7216-5780-X
   1. Cervical vertebrae–Surgery. 2. Cervical vertebrae–Diseases. I. Emery, Sanford E.
   II. Boden, Scott D.
     [DNLM: 1. Cervical Vertebrae–surgery. 2. Spinal Diseases—surgery. WE 725 S96171 2003]
     RD533 .S885 2003
617.5'6059–dc21   2001049785

Editor-in-Chief: Richard Lampert
Project Manager: Mary Anne Folcher

GW/MVY

Printed in the United States of America.

Last digit is the print number: 9 8 7 6 5 4 3 2 1

To residents and fellows involved in the diagnosis and management of disorders of the cervical spine

CONTRIBUTORS

Todd J. Albert, M.D.
Professor and Vice Chairman
Department of Orthopaedics
Jefferson Medical College of Thomas Jefferson University
Rothman Institute
Philadelphia, Pennsylvania
Surgical Approaches to the Cervical Spine

Paul A. Anderson, M.D.
Associate Professor
Department of Orthopaedic Surgery
University of Wisconsin Medical School
Madison, Wisconsin
*Fractures and Dislocations of the Lower Cervical Spine and
Cervicothoracic Junction*

Thomas A. Becherer, M.D.
Division of Neurosurgery
University of Kentucky College of Medicine
University Hospital
Lexington, Kentucky
Spinal Cord Tumors

Deborah A. Blades, M.D.
Division of Neurosurgery
University of Kentucky College of Medicine
University Hospital
Lexington, Kentucky
Spinal Cord Tumors

Laurel C. Blakemore, M.D.
Assistant Professor
Department of Orthopaedic Surgery
University of Michigan Medical School
Ann Arbor, Michigan
Congenital and Pediatric Disorders of the Cervical Spine

Mark H. Blechner, M.D.
Orthopaedics Specialty Group
Fairfield, Connecticut
Posterior Cervical Instrumentation

Scott D. Boden, M.D.
Professor
Department of Orthopaedic Surgery
Emory University School of Medicine
Director, Emory Spine Center
Atlanta, Georgia
*Cervical Radiculopathy, Rheumatoid Arthritis of the Cervical
Spine*

Henry H. Bohlman, M.D.
Professor
Department of Orthopaedic Surgery
University Hospitals of Cleveland
Case Western Reserve University School of Medicine
Cleveland, Ohio
Cervical Spine in Ankylosing Spondylitis

Michael J. Bolesta, M.D.
Associate Professor
Department of Orthopaedic Surgery
University of Texas Southwestern Medical School at
    Dallas
Dallas, Texas
Surgical Complications

Gregory D. Carlson, M.D.
Assistant Clinical Professor
University of California, Irvine, College of Medicine
Orthopaedic Specialty Institute
Orange, California
*Spinal Cord Trauma: Pathophysiology and Medical
Management*

Donald P.K. Chan, M.D.
Professor and Head
Division of Spine Surgery
University of Virginia Medical Center
Charlottesville, Virginia
Cervical Spine Infections

Rick B. Delamarter, M.D.
The Spine Institute at Saint John's Health Center
Santa Monica, California
*Cervical Myelopathy with Ossification of the Posterior
Longitudinal Ligament*

Sanford E. Emery, M.D.
Associate Professor of Orthopaedic Surgery
Department of Surgery
University Hospitals of Cleveland
Case Western Reserve University School of Medicine
Cleveland, Ohio
*Anterior Cervical Reconstruction and Internal Fixation,
Cervical Spondylotic Myelopathy and Cervical Kyphosis,
Primary and Metastatic Bone Tumors of the Cervical Spine,
Rheumatoid Arthritis of the Cervical Spine, Cervical Spine in
Ankylosing Spondylitis*

Mark A. Fye, M.D.
Assistant Professor
Department of Orthopaedic Surgery
Hahnemann-MCP University School of Medicine
Allegheny General Hospital
Pittsburgh, Pennsylvania
Anterior Cervical Reconstruction and Internal Fixation

Alexander J. Ghanayem, M.D.
Associate Professor
Department of Orthopaedic Surgery
Loyola University Medical Center
Maywood, Illinois
Cervical Spine Biomechanics

Robert A. Hart, M.D.
Assistant Professor
Department of Orthopaedics and Rehabilitation
Oregon Health Sciences University School of Medicine
Portland, Oregon
Anatomy of the Cervical Spine

John G. Heller, M.D.
Professor
Department of Orthopaedic Surgery
Emory University School of Medicine
Emory Spine Center
Decatur, Georgia
Posterior Cervical Instrumentation

Muzaffar Hussain, M.D.
University of Virginia School of Medicine
Charlottesville, Virginia
Orthopaedic Surgeon
VA Medical Center
Amarillo, Texas
Cervical Spine Infections

A. Alexander M. Jones, M.D.
Department of Spine Surgery
Kaiser Permanente
Denver, Colorado
Fractures and Dislocations of the Lower Cervical Spine and Cervicothoracic Junction

James D. Kang, M.D.
Associate Professor of Orthopaedic Surgery and Neurosurgery
University of Pittsburgh School of Medicine
Pittsburgh, Pennsylvania
Fractures and Dislocations of the Upper Cervical Spine

John W. Klekamp, M.D.
Piedmont Orthopaedic Associates
Greenville, South Carolina
Posterior Cervical Instrumentation

Odysseas Paxinos, M.D.
Fellow
Department of Orthopaedic Surgery
Loyola University Medical Center
Maywood, Illinois
Cervical Spine Biomechanics

Steven C. Scherping, Jr., M.D.
Assistant Professor
Department of Orthopaedic Surgery
Georgetown University School of Medicine
Washington, D.C.
Fractures and Dislocations of the Upper Cervical Spine

Jeffrey H. Schimandle, M.D.
Emory Clinic Spine Center
Decatur, Georgia
Cervical Radiculopathy

Peter V. Scoles, M.D.
Adjunct Professor of Orthopaedics
Temple University School of Medicine
Attending Surgeon, Shriners Hospital
Senior Vice President, National Board of Medical Examiners
Philadelphia, Pennsylvania
Congenital and Pediatric Disorders of the Cervical Spine

J. Scott Smith, M.D.
The Spine Institute at Saint John's Health Center
Santa Monica, California
Cervical Myelopathy with Ossification of the Posterior Longitudinal Ligament

Robert G. Viere, M.D.
Orthopaedic Surgeon
North Texas Spine Care, LLP
Dallas, Texas
Surgical Complications

Jeffrey C. Wang, M.D.
Chief, Spine Service
Assistant Professor of Orthopaedic Surgery and of Neurosurgery
Department of Orthopaedic Surgery
University of California, Los Angeles, UCLA School of Medicine
Los Angeles, California
Spinal Cord Trauma: Pathophysiology and Medical Management

Jung U. Yoo, M.D.
Associate Professor
Department of Orthopaedic Surgery
University Hospitals of Cleveland
Case Western Reserve University School of Medicine
Cleveland, Ohio
Anatomy of the Cervical Spine

PREFACE

The art of progress is to preserve order amid change and to preserve change amid order.
—Alfred North Whitehead
(English mathematician and philosopher, 1861–1947)

We are born weak, we need strength; helpless, we need aid; foolish, we need reason. All that we lack at birth, all that we need when we come to man's estate, is the gift of education.
—Jean-Jacques Rousseau
(Swiss-born French philosopher and political theorist, 1712–1778)

Things change. Diagnostic methods are refined, disease descriptions are modified, procedures are invented. Some surgical techniques become obsolete, some endure. *Surgery of the Cervical Spine* is focused on a blend of "gold standard" and cutting-edge operative treatments of cervical spine disorders, based on each contributor's experience as well as the orthopaedic and neurosurgical scientific literature. It reflects the rapid changes that have occurred in this arena over the past two decades, when technological changes in spinal imaging fostered a greater understanding of pathoanatomy and subsequent surgical options. Our group of contributors includes some of the best and brightest spine surgeons who have the training and commitment for treating complex conditions of the cervical spine. We thank them for their expertise and effort.

Although it is imperative that medicine and surgery change over time, it is equally imperative to preserve the educational vigor of our graduate training programs. The patient care and research success demonstrated two decades from now will have their foundation in the training of residents and fellows today. *Surgery of the Cervical Spine* should be of value to the practicing spine surgeon, but its birth grew from a desire to assist in the education and training of young surgeons with an interest in the spine.

The text is organized into seven sections including core knowledge, pediatric disorders, degenerative disorders, traumatic injuries, neoplasms, inflammatory disorders, and postoperative considerations. We hope the chapters are concise yet thorough for the designated topics. The historical introductions are designed to provide some perspective, and the quotations may offer insight into the inner psychology of the contributors. Surgical treatment options are emphasized, with further explanation of the preferred method. Our illustrator, Wendy Beth Jackelow, has provided significant skill and labor for the drawings that are fundamental to an operative textbook.

Sanford E. Emery, M.D.
Scott D. Boden, M.D.

ACKNOWLEDGMENTS

Our acknowledgments go to several people who were instrumental in the creation of *Surgery of the Cervical Spine*. Val Schmedlen in our department at University Hospitals of Cleveland/Case Western Reserve School of Medicine put in many hours of editing, typing, and research that was of tremendous assistance. Richard Lampert (Editor-in-Chief) and Mary Anne Folcher (Project Manager) at Saunders provided guidance, expertise, and perseverance in initiating and completing the entire project.

We also thank our teachers for their time and energy devoted to education and for advancing the art and science of spinal surgery. This is particularly true for our mentor, Henry H. Bohlman, M.D., professor of Orthopaedic Surgery at University Hospitals of Cleveland/Case Western Reserve School of Medicine, who trained and inspired us both to pursue a career in academic spine surgery. Most importantly, we thank our wives and children for supporting this project and tolerating the demands of the specialty, of which those of you reading this book are well aware. We sincerely hope it serves as a useful resource in the care and treatment of our collective patients.

TABLE OF CONTENTS

Core Knowledge

1

ANATOMY OF THE CERVICAL SPINE

Jung U. Yoo, M.D.
Robert A. Hart, M.D., M.A.

If a general knows the enemy and himself, his victory will not stand in doubt; if he knows the terrain, he may make his victory complete.

— Sun Tzu (The Art of War, 400 B.C.)

This chapter describes the basic anatomy of the cervical spine, emphasizing clinical and functional details. Structures described include the bony architecture, the articulations, soft tissue structures (including the ligaments and intervertebral disks), neurologic structures, vascular structures, the fascia and musculature, and finally associated cervical structures of significance in spinal surgery.

OSSEOUS AND ARTICULAR STRUCTURES

The cervical spine comprises seven vertebrae, all of which are characterized by the presence of the foramen in the transverse process. The upper two vertebrae were given unique names primarily due to their distinctive morphology and function. The first cervical vertebra (C1) supports the skull and is called the *atlas,* after the Greek god whose duty it was to uphold the heavens. The second cervical vertebra (C2), the *axis,* contains the center of rotation about which the atlas pivots during axial rotation. The third through sixth vertebral bodies (C3 to C6) are considered typical cervical vertebrae, with small, roughly cylindrical bodies and short, bifid spinous processes. The seventh cervical vertebra (C7) is a transitional vertebra that has a large nonbifid spinous process similar to those of the thoracic vertebrae, and is thus known as the *vertebra prominens.*

The atlas has neither a spinous process nor a vertebral body. It is a ring comprised of two lateral masses connected by a short anterior bony bridge and a longer posterior bony bridge. Incomplete formation of the bony ring is not uncommon and most commonly occurs posteriorly. The lateral masses of C1 give rise to paired superior and inferior articular facets. The superior facets articulate with the occipital condyles, and the inferior facets articulate with the superior articular facets of C2. Each transverse process contains a foramen transversarium, through which the vertebral arteries pass before turning posteromedially, around the superior articular process, and entering the foramen magnum, where they join to form the basilar artery (Fig. 1–1).

The axis is characterized by the odontoid process, or dens, which projects superiorly from the C2 vertebral body and articulates with the posterior aspect of the anterior arch of the atlas. The dens measures approximately 14.5 mm high and 10.5 mm in diameter and replaces the vertebral body of the atlas.[12] Lateral to the C2 vertebral body and directly adjacent to the base of the dens are the superior facets. Unlike the lower cervical spine, the superior facets of the axis arise anterior to the pedicles. The pedicles of the axis are large and project superiorly. The inferior facets are located posterior to the pedicles, as in the typical cervical vertebrae. The caudal aspect of the axis is very much like that of a typical cervical vertebra (Fig. 1–2).

The atlanto-axial articulations consist of four synovial joints. The two lateral facet joints are formed by the inferior articular facets of C1 and the superior articular facets of C2. The C2 nerve roots exit posterior to these facet joints, rather than anteriorly as in the subaxial cervical spine.[11] These

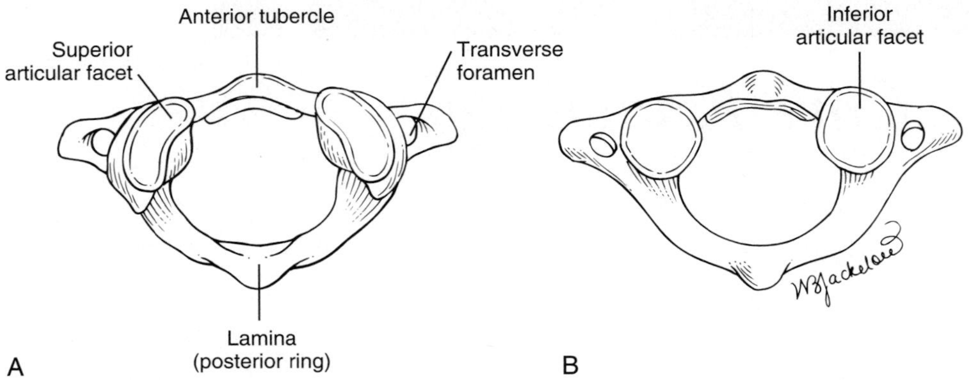

Superior
articular facet

Anterior tubercle

Transverse
foramen

Inferior
articular facet

Lamina
(posterior ring)

A

B

Figure 1–1. *Cranial (A) and caudal (B) views of the C1 vertebra (atlas). Note the absence of a spinous process and vertebral body. The superior and inferior articular facets are oriented in a nearly horizontal plane.*

facet joints are located nearly in the transverse plane, allowing significant axial rotation between C1 and C2 because of their capsular laxity. The anterior aspect of the dens and the posterior aspect of the anterior C1 arch form the third synovial joint; the posterior aspect of the dens and the anterior aspect of the transverse ligament make up the fourth synovial articulation. The orientation of these articulations also allows significant axial rotation. The inferior facets of C2 articulate with the superior facets of C3, as in typical cervical vertebrae.

The more typical cervical vertebrae, from C3 to C6, contain a broad vertebral body connected to the transverse processes laterally and the pedicles posterolaterally (Fig. 1–3). A foramen transversarium is present in each of the transverse processes, serving as a conduit for the vertebral artery. The C6 transverse process has a large anterior tubercle called the carotid tubercle because the common carotid pulse can be felt against it. Also referred to as Chassaignac's tubercle, this is palpable as a landmark in thin patients on manual examination. The superior and inferior articular processes form pillars at the junction of the pedicles and laminae. These pillars are referred to as the lateral masses of the cervical vertebrae.

The roughly cylindrical vertebral bodies of C3 through C6 are composed predominantly of cancellous bone with a thin cortical shell surrounding it circumferentially. Their cranial and caudal surfaces also consist of thin bony endplates. The upper endplates are concave in the coronal plane and convex in the sagittal plane. This surface is matched by the lower surface of the adjacent vertebral body, which is convex in the coronal plane and concave in the sagittal plane. This cupping arrangement of cervical

vertebral bodies, which has been compared to an under-formed ball-and-socket joint, provides some inherent stability between adjacent vertebral segments. Also contributing to this stability are cranial projections at the posterolateral aspects of the superior surface of the caudal vertebra. These projections, called uncinate processes (see Fig. 1–3), articulate with the convex posterolateral inferior surface of the cephalad vertebra in the uncovertebral joints, or joints of Luschka.

The facet joints of the adjacent segments from C2 distally are diarthrodial joints with hyaline articular cartilage and small menisci, surrounded by a tough fibrous capsule and lined by a synovial membrane.[5, 10] The facet joints of the cervical spine are oriented at an approximate 45-degree angle to horizontal in the sagittal plane. These joints provide additional sagittal stability to the cervical spine motion segments; incompetence of these joints is required before listhesis, or slipping, of the cranial relative to the caudal vertebra can develop. The two facet joints and the intervertebral disk have been described as a three-joint complex (Fig. 1–4). The clinical implication of this relationship is that instability and abnormal motion of one component leads to abnormal loading and motion of the other components, with secondary degeneration occurring throughout the entire complex.

As discussed earlier, C7 is a transitional vertebra between the cervical and thoracic spines. It has a prominent spinous process that is not bifid. Its transverse process varies in size with a small foramen transversarium. Occasionally, a small cervical rib can be found anterior to this transverse process. The vertebral artery does not run through the C7 foramen, but rather enters

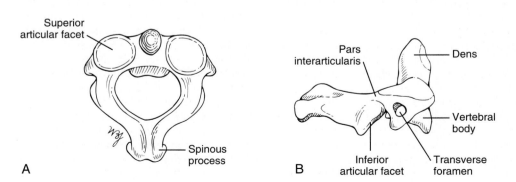

Superior
articular facet

Pars
interarticularis

Dens

Vertebral
body

Transverse
foramen

Spinous
process

Inferior
articular facet

A

B

Figure 1–2. *Cranial (A) and lateral (B) views of the C2 vertebra (axis). Note the upward extension of the odontoid process from the C2 body. The pedicles of C2 are the largest of any cervical vertebra. Note the change in orientation between the superior and inferior facets.*

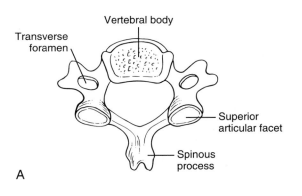

A

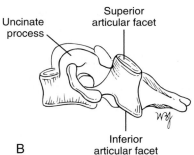

B

Figure 1–3. Cranial (A) and lateral (B) views of a typical subaxial vertebra. Note the location of the foramen transversarium anterior to the posterior edge of the vertebral body and intervertebral foramen. The uncinate processes (arrow) articulate with the posterolateral vertebral bodies of synovial joints at each level.

at the C6 vertebra. Generally, a small accessory vertebral vein runs in the C7 foramen.

The posterior vertebral arch, composed of the paired pedicles, laminae, and transverse processes with a single midline spinous process, completes a bony ring with the anterior vertebral body. The central opening formed by this ring is called the vertebral canal. The vertebral canal houses the spinal cord and the initial segments of the nerve roots. The continuous series of vertebral foramina make up the spinal canal.

Clinically, the most important anatomic dimension of the spinal canal is the sagittal diameter, because canal encroachment and compromise most often occur in this direction. The sagittal dimension averages 23 mm at C1 and decreases to 17 mm at C5 and to 15 mm at C7.[8] The vertebral canal can be narrowed by various pathological conditions, including retropulsed fragments of bone or disk in traumatic injuries and vertebral body osteophytes protruding posteriorly at the disk space because of spinal degeneration. This narrowing of the vertebral canal can lead to acute or chronic impingement of the spinal cord and nerve roots, with secondary neurologic deficits.

A deep, smooth notch is present on the lower edge of each pedicle, with a corresponding, shallower notch on the upper edge. These notches form the superior and inferior margins of the intervertebral foramen, respectively. The posterolateral aspect of the uncovertebral joint and the intervertebral disk forms the anterior border of the foramen, whereas the superior articular facet of the caudal vertebra

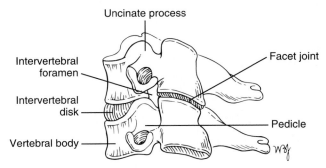

Figure 1–4. The articulation between adjacent subaxial vertebrae. The three-joint complex comprises the intervertebral disk and the paired facet joints. Note the borders of the intervertebral foramen (arrow).

and the facet joint capsule form the posterior border. The spinal nerve roots exit through these foramina, occupying approximately one-third of the available space. The balance of the space is filled with epidural fat and vessels.

The ovoid-shaped cervical intervertebral foramina project in a 45-degree oblique direction from anterocranial to posterocaudal. They average 9 to 12 mm high and 4 to 6 mm wide.[5] These dimensions are not static, but change with the position of the cervical spine. Flexion bilaterally increases the sagittal dimension and extension correspondingly decreases it, whereas axial rotation unilaterally decreases the width of the foramen. Structural abnormalities such as disk protrusion or uncovertebral osteophytes also can significantly narrow foramen size, with resulting compression and irritation of the spinal nerve root.

INTERVERTEBRAL DISK AND LIGAMENTS

Structural integrity across cervical motion segments is highly dependent on the intervertebral disks and ligamentous structures. The osseous structure of the cervical spine provides very little inherent stability. The ligamentous arrangement from occiput to axis is unique, corresponding to the unique structures and articulations of the C1 and C2 vertebrae. From the caudal portion of C2 distally, the ligamentous arrangement is highly uniform.

Two membranous attachments are described between the atlas and the occiput. The anterior and posterior atlanto-occipital membranes connect the anterior and posterior arches of C1 with the corresponding margins of the foramen magnum. The anterior atlanto-occipital membrane is a continuation of the anterior longitudinal ligament. The posterior atlanto-occipital membrane is pierced on either side above the posterior arch of C1 by the vertebral arteries and the first cervical nerve roots. Only minimal bony stability is afforded by the superior facet articulation of atlas with the occipital condyles because of their relatively flat surfaces, and thus the stability of the atlanto-occipital joint is highly dependent on these two membranous attachments and the capsular ligaments.

The atlantoaxial complex comprises C1, C2, and their associated articulations and ligamentous attachments. Posterior stability comes from the ligaments and the facet joint capsules, whereas anterior migration of C2 relative to C1 is prevented by the bony architecture of the odontoid process

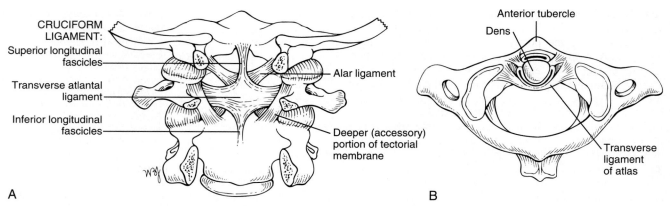

A

B

Figure 1–5. The atlantodental ligamentous complex. The cruciform ligament lies posterior to the apical and alar ligaments.

and the anterior ring of C1. The transverse ligament attaches laterally to the inner aspect of the atlas, adjacent to the lateral masses, and serves as the primary stabilizer to prevent posterior migration of the odontoid into the vertebral canal. The transverse ligament blends with superior and inferior longitudinal bundles from the occiput to the C2 body to form the cruciate ligament.

There are three primary ligamentous connections from the odontoid process to the occiput. The apical ligament extends from the tip of the dens to the anterior edge of the foramen magnum. The two alar ligaments extend on either side of the posterior body of C2 and the posterior longitudinal ligament to the upper surface of the basilar portion of the occipital bone and the anterior aspect of the foramen magnum. They often include connections to the lateral masses of C1 as well. These three ligaments serve as secondary stabilizers to prevent posterior migration of the odontoid (Fig. 1–5).[1]

The anterior longitudinal ligament is broad and thick, extending caudally from the anterior atlanto-occipital membrane and attaching superiorly to the anterior tubercle of the atlas. It continues caudally with relatively constant width, with its longitudinally arranged fibers joining loosely to the periosteum of the anterior vertebral bodies but blending intimately with the annulus fibrosis of the anterior vertebral disk. The posterior longitudinal ligament lies posterior to the vertebral bodies and intervertebral disks. It runs longitudinally, narrowing behind each vertebral body but widening at the intervertebral disk, again densely adherent to the annulus fibrosis. Cranially, the posterior longitudinal ligament blends with the tectorial membrane and inserts onto the anterior aspect of the foramen magnum, supporting the atlantoaxial ligamentous attachments. These ligaments are continuous throughout the thoracic and lumbar spine as well.

The intervertebral disks are fibrocartilaginous structures that join the adjacent vertebrae from C2–C3 and distally. The intervertebral disk has three main components. The tough outer annulus fibrosis derives its strength from a highly organized spiral arrangement of type I collagen. The soft gelatinous inner nucleus pulposus consists of a loose, haphazardly arranged type II collagen matrix. These two components are sandwiched superiorly and inferiorly by

two very thin endplates of hyaline cartilage, which in turn are adherent to the bony vertebral endplates. Most of the nutrition to the nucleus pulposus passes through these cartilaginous endplates by a process of diffusion. In older patients, these cartilaginous endplates may calcify, hampering diffusion of solutes to the nucleus pulposus and possibly contributing to degeneration of the intervertebral disk.

The anterior and posterior boundaries of the intervertebral disk are formed by the anterior and posterior longitudinal ligaments. The cervical disks are bounded posteriorly and laterally by the uncinate processes. There are no other structural restraints on the lateral aspects of the annulus fibrosis.

The posterior ligamentous complex consists primarily of the ligamentum nuchae, the interspinous ligaments, and the ligamentum flavum. The ligamentum nuchae extends from the external occipital protuberance to C7, continuing

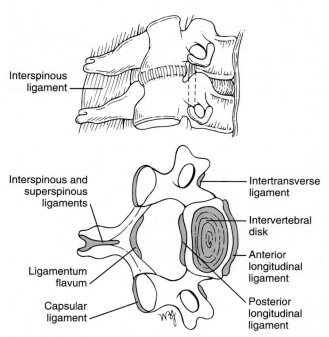

Figure 1–6. Subaxial ligamentous structures.

caudally as the supraspinous ligament of the thoracic spine. This ligament runs sagittally, separating the musculature of the two sides of the posterior cervical spine. Its deeper layers attach to the posterior tubercle of the atlas and the spinous processes of each cervical vertebrae. The interspinous ligament is generally very thin in the cervical spine. It runs in the sagittal plane, extending between the spinous processes from their posterior tips to the ligamentum flavum anteriorly. The ligamentum flavum lies in the semicoronal plane, connecting adjacent laminae. Its lateral expansions blend with the capsules of the facet joints at each level. Along with type 1 collagen, it contains a significant amount of elastin, which imparts the yellowish color from which it derives its name (Fig. 1–6).[11]

NEURAL STRUCTURES

The spinal cord extends from the foramen magnum as a continuation of the medulla oblongata. It lies within the cervical spinal canal and is encased within the dural tube, a continuation of the dura mater surrounding the brain. An epidural venous plexus surrounds the dura, with a layer of epidural fat separating the dural tube posteriorly from the posterior vertebral elements and ligamentum flavum. The arachnoid is a much thinner membrane than the dura and is closely adherent to it. The subarachnoid space lies between the arachnoid and pia mater, which is closely adherent to the cord itself. This space is filled with cerebrospinal fluid, vessels, and cervical spinal nerve rootlets.

The dimension of the spinal cord varies along its length. It is generally ovoid and narrower in the sagittal dimension than in the coronal plane. The cord itself enlarges from C3 to C6, because of the large number of nerve roots that innervate the upper extremities and the corresponding lower motor neuron cell bodies in these segments.[6]

A cross-section of the spinal cord shows a butterfly-shaped inner gray matter comprising neuronal cell bodies surrounded by white matter composed of axons, myelin, and glial cells organized in a number of spinal tracts. The anterior horns of the gray matter contain lower motor neuron cell bodies, and the posterior horns contain the somatosensory neurons. The white matter is in three identifiable columns. The posterior columns lie between the posterior horns of the gray matter and contain ascending sensory tracts that are responsible for proprioceptive, vibratory, and tactile sensations. These fibers carry ipsilateral sensory input and cross at the decussation of the medial lemniscus at the level of the inferior olivary nucleus in the medulla, synapsing in the contralateral thalamus.

The lateral columns are located between the anterior and posterior root entry zones and contain the lateral corticospinal tracts and lateral spinothalamic tracts. The lateral corticospinal tracts are descending pathways that carry ipsilateral motor fibers, which represent 85% of all voluntary motor fibers. These fibers cross in the medulla at the decussation of the pyramids. The lateral spinothalamic tracts transmit ascending impulses of pain and thermal sensation from the contralateral side, as the lower sensory neuronal axon crosses at or near its level of entry.

Finally, the anterior columns lie between the anterior fissure and the anterior root entry zones and contain the anterior corticospinal and anterior spinothalamic tracts. The ascending fibers of the anterior spinothalamic tracts convey contralateral impulses associated with light touch, whereas the anterior corticospinal tracts contain the 15% of uncrossed fibers concerned with fine motor control. All of the aforementioned tracts are laminated in structure, with upper extremity sensory and motor fibers the most medial, followed by the trunk and lower extremities, and perianal sensation and motor control the most lateral (see Chapter 11).

Several patterns of incomplete spinal cord injury are recognized based on the anatomic representation and location of the spinal tracts. These include Brown–Séquard syndrome, with ipsilateral loss of motor function and vibratory and proprioceptive sensation and contralateral loss of pain, temperature, and light touch sensation. Anterior cord syndrome commonly results from retropulsed bone or disk fragments and involves variable loss of motor function and pain, temperature, and light touch sensation, with relative preservation of vibratory and proprioceptive sensation. Central cord syndrome often occurs with hyperextension of a spondylotic cervical spine due to a pinching of the spinal cord between anterior vertebral body osteophytes and posterior buckling of a hypertrophic ligamentum flavum. This syndrome presents with greater loss of motor and sensory function in the upper extremities and relatively greater preservation of lower extremity or sacral function. The rare posterior cord syndrome involves loss of proprioceptive and vibratory sensation because of isolated injury to the posterior columns.

The surface of the spinal cord contains various fissures. Anteriorly, a single median fissure transmits the anterior spinal artery and veins. The ventral rootlets, an average of 20 at each ventral root, exit the cord at the ventral lateral sulci. On the posterior surface, the posterior median sulcus separates the posterior columns and two posterior lateral sulci at the lateral border of these columns. The posterior rootlets enter the spinal cord near the posterior lateral sulci; between 5 and 16 posterior rootlets make up each dorsal root.

The cell bodies of the posterior rootlets are located in the dorsal root ganglion. The dorsal root ganglion is located between the vertebral artery and the superior articular process. The dorsal and ventral roots unite immediately distal to the ganglion to form the corresponding spinal nerve. The spinal nerve then exits the vertebral column through the intervertebral foramen, posterior to the vertebral artery. The nerve root exits at approximately the midpoint of the lateral mass as observed posteriorly, implying that cranial orientation of screws placed in the lateral mass should avoid injury to the nerve root.[15]

The numbering of the cervical spinal nerves relative to their respective foraminal exits differs from the numbering of the nerves of the thoracic and lumbar spine. Because the first cervical spinal nerve exits between the occiput and atlas, subsequent cervical spinal nerves are numbered corresponding to the caudal of the two vertebrae between which it exits. Thus, the third cervical nerve exits between C2 and C3, whereas in the lumbar spine the third lumbar nerve exits between the third and fourth lumbar vertebrae. The eighth cervical nerve exits between C7 and the first thoracic vertebra, accounting for the shift in the thoracic and lumbar spines.

Outside of the intervertebral foramina, the cervical nerves divide into dorsal and ventral primary rami. The sympathetic cervical chain makes up the gray rami, which then joins the primary rami. The three cervical sympathetic ganglia and the sympathetic chain are located between the longus coli and the longus capitis near the carotid sheath. Surgical dissection in this area can cause injury to the sympathetic nerves and may result in Horner syndrome.

The anterior rami of the first through fourth cervical nerves form the cervical plexus, and the anterior rami of the fifth through eighth cervical nerves and the first thoracic nerve form the brachial plexus. The cervical plexus gives off the ansa cervicalis, which innervates all of the strap muscles and infrahyoid muscles except for the thyrohyoid. The cervical plexus also gives off the phrenic nerve, which innervates the diaphragm with some contribution from the fifth cervical nerve.

VASCULAR STRUCTURES

The vertebral arteries arise from the first part of the subclavian arteries bilaterally and enter the cervical spine through the transverse foramina of C6. At C7 they lie just anterior to the transverse process and the seventh and eighth cervical nerves. They then ascend through the transverse foramina from C6 through C2, in front of the ventral rami of the cervical nerves. In this region they lie within a fibro-osseous tunnel. At the atlas, the vertebral arteries pass through the vertebral foramen of C1 and travel posteriorly and medially behind the lateral mass and then superiorly from the posterior arch of the atlas. The arteries then pierce the posterior atlanto-occipital membrane, joining to form the basilar artery (Fig. 1–7).

The location of the vertebral arteries must be constantly kept in mind during anterior cervical diskectomy and corpectomy, because they are vulnerable to injury during these procedures. The vertebral foramen have been shown to converge toward the midline and to move slightly posteriorly in their ascent from C6 to C3; thus the risk of injury is greater in the more cranial vertebrae.[2, 14] The incidence of an anomalous course of a vertebral artery is around 3%.[4] Anomalies of the vertebral artery are generally associated with a medial course of the artery at the midportion of the vertebral body, with a return to the normal lateral position at the disk space level.[4] Because one of the vertebral arteries is hypoplastic or absent in 5% to 10% of individuals, occlusion or ligation of an injured dominant artery can produce cerebellar ischemia, sometimes with clinically observable results.[3]

The vertebral arteries give off segmental branches, which enter the spinal canal through the intervertebral foramina and then join to form a single anterior spinal artery. This

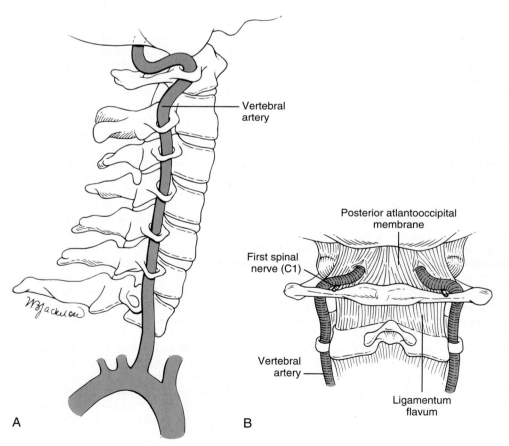

Vertebral artery

Posterior atlantooccipital membrane

First spinal nerve (C1)

Vertebral artery

Ligamentum flavum

A

B

Figure 1–7. Lateral (A) and posterior (B) views of the course of the vertebral arteries. The arteries enter at the C6 vertebra and ascend within a fibro-osseous column. At the C1 vertebra, they wind posteriorly along the superior edge of the lamina and converge to form the basilar artery just inside the foramen magnum.

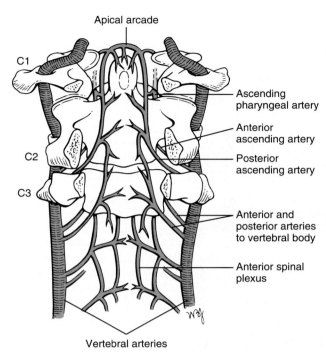

Figure 1–8. *The apical arcade supplying the dens. The anterior and posterior ascending branches from the vertebral arteries anastomose with an apical arcade from the ascending pharyngeal branches of the external carotid arteries.*

Labels in figure:
- Apical arcade
- C1
- C2
- C3
- Ascending pharyngeal artery
- Anterior ascending artery
- Posterior ascending artery
- Anterior and posterior arteries to vertebral body
- Anterior spinal plexus
- Vertebral arteries

artery runs within the anterior median fissure of the spinal cord, providing blood supply to roughly the anterior two-thirds of the spinal cord. The posterior third of the spinal cord is supplied by two posterior spinal arteries, which arise from either the vertebral artery or the posterior inferior cerebellar arteries. The nerve roots are supplied by radicular branches from the spinal arteries.

The blood supply to the cervical vertebral bodies also originates from the vertebral arteries. Anterior and posterior segmental branches from the vertebral arteries traverse ventrally and dorsally around the subaxial vertebral bodies, supplying the bodies and the anterior and posterior longitudinal ligaments along their course. Additional branches pass dorsally at each segment to supply the laminae and posterior elements. The blood supply to the odontoid process consists of a plexus with contributions from anterior and posterior ascending branches of the vertebral arteries as well as anastomoses with the apical arcade from the ascending pharyngeal branches of the external carotids.[9] Whereas the clinically observed problem of nonunion of fractures of the odontoid process has been attributed to a scant blood supply, this does not appear to be the primary causative factor (Fig. 1–8).

Venous drainage of the cervical spine occurs through internal and external venous plexi. The external veins run paired with the arteries described earlier. The internal plexus lies within the spinal canal and consists of a valveless series of epidural sinuses. This complex of veins is continuous from the cerebral sinuses distally to the pelvis. These veins

are most prevalent at the vertebral bodies and thinnest at the disk spaces. They drain through the intervertebral foramina into the caval and azygos systems.[10]

FASCIA AND MUSCULATURE

Understanding the fascial layers of the neck is critical to effective use of the anterior approach to the cervical spine. The superficial cervical fascia surrounds the neck just below the skin layer, enveloping the platysma and the external jugular vein anteriorly. The deep cervical fascia includes all fascial layers deep to the superficial layer. The deep cervical fascia comprises superficial, middle, and deep layers (Fig. 1–9).[11, 13]

The superficial layer of deep cervical fascia also runs circumferentially about the neck, attaching to the sternum, clavicle, acromion, scapular spine, and the cervical spinous processes. It envelops the trapezius and the sternocleidomastoid, as well as the anterior and external jugular veins. It also forms the roof of the anterior and posterior triangles of the neck. The middle layer of the deep cervical fascia encases the infrahyoid and the strap muscles. The pretracheal visceral fascia is also considered part of the middle layer and forms the sheath of the thyroid gland. It also invests the trachea, larynx, esophagus, and pharynx.

The prevertebral or deep layer of the deep cervical fascia surrounds the vertebral column itself as well as the deep musculature applied directly to the bony structures. Anteriorly, it attaches to the anterior longitudinal ligament and covers the longus capitis and coli muscles. Posteriorly, it terminates in the ligamentum nuchae. Laterally, it invests the three scalene muscles as well as the carotid sheaths, and attaches to the transverse processes.

The muscle groups of the neck can be considered according to their location and their actions. Posteriorly located musculature, which tends to produce extension, includes the splenius capitis and cervicis, the semispinalis capitis and cervicis, the longissimus capitis and cervicis, and the interspinalis and the rectus and obliquus capitis groups. The trapezius also assists in extension with paired activity. Anterior musculature, producing flexion of the cervical spine, includes the sternocleidomastoid, the longus colli and capitis, and the rectus capitis anterior. Laterally located muscles, which produce axial rotation and lateral flexion of the cervical spine, include the sternocleidomastoid, the scalenes, the levator scapulae, the iliocostalis cervicis, the multifidi, and the intertransversarii. The splenius capitis and cervicis, the longissimus capitis, the longus colli, the obliquus capitis inferior and superior, and the rectus capitis lateralis also produce lateral movement with unpaired activity.

Posteriorly, the trapezius is the most superficial of the aforementioned muscles. It is innervated by the 11th cranial nerve. Originating from the occipital protuberance, the nuchal ligament of the entire cervical spine, and the spinous processes of the thoracic spines, the trapezius inserts on the scapular spine and acromion process, as well as the clavicle. With the shoulder girdle fixed, it functions to extend the

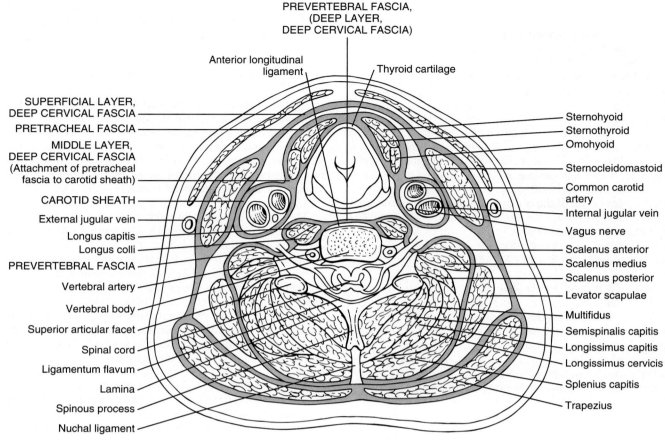

PREVERTEBRAL FASCIA,
(DEEP LAYER,
DEEP CERVICAL FASCIA)

Anterior longitudinal
ligament

Thyroid cartilage

SUPERFICIAL LAYER,
DEEP CERVICAL FASCIA

PRETRACHEAL FASCIA

MIDDLE LAYER,
DEEP CERVICAL FASCIA
(Attachment of pretracheal
fascia to carotid sheath)

CAROTID SHEATH

External jugular vein

Longus capitis

Longus colli

PREVERTEBRAL FASCIA

Vertebral artery

Vertebral body

Superior articular facet

Spinal cord

Ligamentum flavum

Lamina

Spinous process

Nuchal ligament

Sternohyoid

Sternothyroid

Omohyoid

Sternocleidomastoid

Common carotid
artery

Internal jugular vein

Vagus nerve

Scalenus anterior

Scalenus medius

Scalenus posterior

Levator scapulae

Multifidus

Semispinalis capitis

Longissimus capitis

Longissimus cervicis

Splenius capitis

Trapezius

Figure 1–9. Transverse section of the neck showing the layers of the cervical fascia.

cervical spine. The next layer of musculature includes the splenius cervicis and splenius capitis. These muscles originate deep to the trapezius from the spinous processes of the lower cervical and upper thoracic spines. The splenius cervicis inserts into the transverse processes of the upper cervical spine, whereas the splenius capitis inserts onto the mastoid process. Like the other posterior cervical muscles, they are innervated segmentally by the posterior cervical rami.

The next muscular layer includes, from lateral to medial, the iliocostalis cervicis, the longissimus capitis and cervicis, and the semispinalis capitis and cervicis. The iliocostalis extends from the medial angles of the upper six ribs to the transverse processes of the lower cervical vertebrae. The longissimus cervicis extends between the transverse processes of the upper thoracic spine and those of the lower cervical vertebrae, whereas the longissimus capitis, superficial to the cervicis, extends to the mastoid process. Most medially, the semispinalis cervicis extends from the transverse processes of the upper thoracic and lower cervical vertebrae cranially to the spinous processes of the subaxial cervical vertebrae, and the semispinalis capitis extends to the superior nuchal ridge of the occiput.

In the lower cervical spine, the deepest muscular layer comprises the multifidi, which extend across two to five

motion segments from the caudal transverse process to the cranial spinous process. The short and long rotators are arranged similarly but cross only one or two motion segments. In the upper cervical spine, the small head extensors include the rectus capitis posterior major and minor and the obliquus capitis inferior and superior. The spinous process of the atlas is the origin of all of these muscles except the rectus capitis posterior minor, the only muscle originating from the posterior ring of the atlas. These muscles insert onto the occiput. The vertebral artery and the first cervical nerve root emerge between the arch of the atlas and the foramen magnum and supply these muscles.

The anterior muscles of the neck are divided by the hyoid bone, which serves as the origin or insertion of all of the superficial muscles. Cranial to the hyoid, the digastric muscle attaches to the lateral border of the hyoid by a ligamentous sling, whereas the mylohyoid inserts onto the hyoid from the mandible. These muscles lie over the first two cervical vertebrae. Caudal to the hyoid, the sternohyoid and the omohyoid lie superficially, whereas the thyrohyoid and sternothyroid lie deeper. The omohyoid is sometimes divided to assist retraction during the anterior cervical approach, because its fibers cross the field obliquely.

The sternocleidomastoid is the most prominent of the

superficial anterior muscles, and its medial border serves as the landmark for the superficial portion of the anterior cervical (Robinson–Southwick) approach. It arises from two heads, medially from the sternum and laterally from the clavicle, and inserts into the mastoid process. The primary axial rotator in unpaired activity, it also is a strong flexor of the cervical spine during paired activity. It is innervated at its cranial aspect by the spinal accessory nerve (cranial nerve XI).

The deep anterior musculature of the neck is associated with the vertebrae themselves. This includes the longus coli and capitis, which arise along the lateral aspects of the vertebral bodies and the lateral masses. The longus capitis is the deeper muscle, running from C3 to C6 and inserting into the basilar portion of the occiput. The longus coli runs more superficially from C1 to the upper thoracic spine. The sympathetic chain lies between these muscles. Cranially, the rectus capitis anterior and lateral arise from the lateral mass and transverse process of the atlas and insert onto the occiput.

Along with the sternocleidomastoid, the levator scapulae and the anterior, middle, and posterior scalenes are also considered lateral muscles. The scalenes originate from the first two ribs and act along with sternocleidomastoid as either flexors or axial rotators of the cervical spine. They are innervated segmentally by the ventral cervical roots. The levator runs from the posterior transverse processes of the upper cervical vertebrae to the medial border of the scapula; it is covered by the sternocleidomastoid superiorly and by the trapezius posteriorly.

ASSOCIATED CERVICAL STRUCTURES AND ANATOMIC TRIANGLES

Additional structures of importance to the standard anterior cervical approach include the trachea, esophagus, carotid sheath, and recurrent laryngeal nerves. The trachea is prominent superficially in the midline of the neck. The cartilaginous rings are directly palpable and serve as landmarks to the underlying bony anatomy. The cricoid cartilage lies at approximately C6, whereas the larger thyroid cartilage overlies C4 and C5. The cricothyroid membrane extending anteriorly between these rings is the routine site of tracheostomy placement.

The esophagus lies posterior to the trachea and anterior to the vertebral bodies. In a left-sided anterior approach, the trachea and esophagus are mobilized together toward the right. Caution must be maintained during dissection to separate the esophagus from the underlying longus coli and capitis, which are elevated laterally off the vertebral bodies. Excessive retraction of the esophagus against the relatively stiff trachea can also produce injury.

The carotid sheath contains the common carotid artery, the internal jugular vein, and the vagus nerve. Direct palpation of the carotid pulse is performed after the medial border of the sternocleidomastoid is mobilized during the anterior approach. The carotid divides into the internal and external branches in the upper cervical spine, and several vascular branches of the external carotid then cross the field transversely. In ascending order, these include the superior thyroid artery, the lingual artery, the ascending pharyngeal artery, and the facial artery. These branches can be ligated, along with their corresponding venous branches of the internal jugular, if necessary during a high cervical approach.[7] The superior laryngeal and hypoglossal nerves may be similarly visualized during this approach.

The recurrent laryngeal nerve on the right branches from the vagus and loops under the subclavian artery before reentering the neck between the trachea and esophagus. On the left, the recurrent nerve loops under the aortic arch before returning to the larynx by a similar course. Because the anatomy on the left side is more constant, the nerve nearly always crosses to the midline distal to the dissection, and thus the left-sided approach is felt to be safer than an approach from the right.[11, 12]

Finally, a description of the anatomic triangles of the neck is warranted. The sternocleidomastoid divides the neck into the large anterior and posterior triangles. The anterior triangle is completed by the mandible superiorly and the midline anteriorly. The posterior triangle is completed by the clavicle inferiorly and the anterior border or the trapezius posteriorly. The anterior triangle is subdivided by the digastric and omohyoid muscles into three smaller triangles, the digastric, carotid, and muscular triangles. The posterior triangle is divided by the omohyoid into the subclavian and occipital triangles. These subdivisions are used by anatomists to locate various structures of the neck.

REFERENCES

1. Dvorak J, Panjabi, MM: Functional anatomy of the alar ligaments. Spine 12:183–189, 1987.
2. Ebraheim NA, Lu J, Brown JA, et al: Vulnerability of vertebral artery in anterolateral decompression for cervical spondylosis. Clin Orthop 322:146–151, 1996.
3. Golfinos JG, Dickman CA, Zabramski JM, et al: Repair of vertebral artery injury during anterior cervical decompression. Spine 19:2552–2556, 1994.
4. Curylo LJ, Mason HC, Bohlman HH, Yoo JU: Tortuous course of the vertebral artery and anterior cervical decompression: A cadaveric and clinical case study. Spine 15:2860–2864, 2000.
5. Heller JG, Pedlow FX: Anatomy of the cervical spine. In Clark CR (ed): The Cervical Spine, 3rd ed. Philadelphia, Lippincott-Raven, 1998, pp 3–36.
6. Kameyama T, Hashizume Y, Ando T, Takahashi A: Morphometry of the normal cadaveric cervical spinal cord. Spine 19:2077–2081, 1994.
7. McAfee PC, Bohlman HH, Riley LH, et al: The anterior retropharyngeal approach to the upper part of the cervical spine. J Bone Joint Surg 69A:1371–1383, 1987.
8. Panjabi MM, Duranceau J, Goel V, et al: Cervical human vertebrae: Quantitative three-dimensional anatomy of the middle and lower regions. Spine 16:861–869, 1991.
9. Parke WW: The vascular relations of the upper cervical vertebrae. Orthop Clin North Am 9:879–889, 1978.
10. Parke WW, Sherk HH: Normal adult anatomy. In CSRS Editorial Committee (ed): The Cervical Spine, 2nd ed. Philadelphia, JB Lippincott, 1989, pp 11–32.

11. Robinson RA, Southwick WO: Surgical Approaches to the Cervical Spine. Instructional Course Lectures, The American Academy of Orthopaedic Surgeons, vol. 17. St. Louis, CV Mosby, 1960, pp 299–330.
12. Schaffler MB, Alson MD, Heller JG, Garfin SR: Morphometry of the dens: A quantitative study. Spine 17:738–743, 1990.
13. Southwick WO, Robinson RA: Surgical approaches to the vertebral bodies in the cervical and lumbar regions. J Bone Joint Surg 39A:631–643, 1957.
14. Vaccaro AR, Ring D, Scuderi G, Garfin SR: Vertebral artery location in relation to vertebral body as determined by two-dimensional computed tomography evaluation. Spine 19:2637–2641, 1994.
15. Xu R, Ebraheim NA, Nadaud MC, et al: The location of the cervical nerve roots on the posterior aspect of the cervical spine. Spine 20:2267–2271, 1995.

2

CERVICAL SPINE BIOMECHANICS

Alexander J. Ghanayem, M.D.
Odysseas Paxinos, M.D.

*. . . the seven spondyles (vertebrae) of the neck
through which the nerves go from the medulla and
are spread to the arms giving them sensibility . . .*
— Leonardo da Vinci, 1510

The cervical spine must perform several functions simultaneously to provide the necessary two functions of dimensional mobility of the head on the torso and protection of the spinal cord and exiting nerve roots. This is accomplished through a fine mechanical balance between the vertebrae (levers), disks and facet joints (pivots), ligaments (passive restraints), and muscles (action elements). Disturbance of the anatomy or of the physical and mechanical properties of the elements of the cervical spine may lead to various clinical symptoms. The upper cervical spine segment (C0 to C2) and the lower cervical spine (C3 to C7) have distinct anatomic and functional features and are described separately.

FUNCTIONAL ANATOMY
Upper Cervical Spine

The upper cervical spine consists of the occiput (C0), the atlas (C1), and the axis (C2). Major differences from the middle and lower cervical spine include the absence of intervertebral disks, the absence of ligamentum flavum, and the presence of the dens. The occipitoatlantal and atlantoaxial joints are anatomically and functionally two of the most complex joints of the skeleton, and motion is coupled between the two joints.

Kinematics of the C0–C1–C2 complex are defined by the bony shape and the ligamentous attachments that span the two articulations. The complex is uniquely adapted to accommodate the needs of the highly mobile head–neck transitory zone and has a common embryonic origin. Instead of an intervertebral disk in the occiput–C1 level, the developmental process results in the formation of the apical and alar ligaments as well as the cranial portion of the dens. At birth, the atlas has two centers of ossification that correspond to the lateral masses. Ossification proceeds posteriorly and anteriorly. C1 does not form a distinct body, and there is no intervertebral disk between C1 and C2. Instead, the caudal part of the C1 somite and the cranial part of the C2 somite fuse to form the odontoid process. The odontoid process fuses with the body of C2 at age 4 years and is complete at age 7 years. Almost one third of adults will have a remnant of cartilaginous tissue between the odontoid and the body of C2.[33]

C0–C1 Kinematics

The C0–C1 joints have a cup-shaped configuration that is deeper in the frontal plane than in the sagittal plane. Motion in the sagittal plane is the primary function at this junction and is reported to average between 13 degrees[40] and 25 degrees.[24] Flexion of C0–C1 is limited by the tip of the dens impinging on the anterior margin of the foramen magnum, on what Werne[40] called the bursa apicis dentis. The tectorial membrane controls extension. The membrane that inserts at the body of C2 and the anterior rim of the foramen magnum becomes taut and limits extension. Flexion at C0–C1 will make again the membrane taut and will also limit further flexion at the C1–C2 level. Translation at this junction is minimal under normal conditions. Flexion and extension should result in no more than 1 mm of translation between the basion and tip of the dens.[43] Axial rotation and lateral bending in C0–C1 is limited to about 5 degrees in each side and is controlled by the capsules and the alar ligaments.

The alar ligaments are symmetrical on both sides and about 10 to 13 mm long, with one portion connecting the dens to the occiput and the remaining ligament connecting the dens to the atlas. During left lateral bending, the right upper alar ligament (connected to the occiput) and the left lower ligament (connected to the ring of C1) become taut. When the head rotates to the left, both components of the right ligament become taut.[5, 6, 23, 40] The instantaneous center of rotation (IAR) for the C0–C1 articulation has not been defined, although the x-axis is considered to pass through the mastoids and the z-axis 2 to 3 mm above the tip of the dens. Compressive sagittal plane translation (z-axis) is minimal under normal conditions because of the cup-shaped articular anatomy. Distraction is restricted mainly by the tectorial membrane, with minor contribution from the alar ligaments. The apical ligament and the anterior and posterior atlanto-occipital membranes have not been found to contribute against distraction.

C0–C1 Instability

Clinical instability in the C0–C1 level compatible with life is uncommon and most often traumatic in origin. Occipitocervical dislocations can occur in anterior, posterior, or longitudinal directions. The dens–basion distance and Power's ratio are useful in these conditions. The normal distance from the tip of the dens to the basion is <5 mm in

Table 2–1. *Criteria for C0–C1 and C1–C2 Instability*

>8	Axial rotation C0–C1 to one side
>1 mm	C0–C1 translation
>7 mm	Overhang C1–C2 (total right and left)
>45	Axial rotation C1–C2 to one side
>4 mm	C1–C2 translation at the AADI
<13 mm	Posterior atlantodental interval
Avulsed transverse ligament	

(Adapted with permission from White AA, Panjabi MM: Clinical Biomechanics of the Spine, 2nd ed. Philadelphia, JB Lippincott, 1990.)

adults and <10 mm in children. An increase in the distance is indicative of a possible longitudinal dislocation. Power's ratio is the ratio of the distance from the basion (B) to the posterior arch of the atlas (C) divided by the distance from the opisthion (O) to the anterior arch of the atlas (A). A ratio (BC/AO) value >1.0 is indicative of an anterior dislocation; a ratio <0.7, of posterior subluxation. Additional criteria for clinical instability at the occipital–C1 joint include >1 mm of translation between the dens and basion on flexion/extension radiographs[43] and >8 degrees of unilateral axial rotation in axial CT images.[8] Basilar invagination represents vertical or compressive instability at the occiput–C1 joint, and numerous radiographic criteria have been proposed. Vertical instability can be either traumatic (e.g., unstable C1 ring fractures) or degenerative (e.g., rheumatoid) in origin. Various radiographic criteria have been established to evaluate the upper cervical spine for clinical instability (Table 2–1).

C1–C2 Kinematics

The atlantoaxial joint (C1–C2) is composed of two facet joints and the highly specialized atlantodental articulation. The facet joints are relatively unstable because of their horizontal orientation and the small contact area between the biconvex articular surfaces. Stability at this highly mobile junction depends primarily on ligamentous structures. Sagittal plane motion (flexion–extension) at C1–C2 has been reported to be an average of 11 degrees and may be facilitated by a rounded tip of the dens.[9, 40] Unilateral rotation in the upper cervical spine represents 60% of the entire cervical spine rotation and has been reported to be between 39 and 47 degrees. Lateral bending is negligible. The IAR for sagittal plane motion is located in the region of the middle third of the dens, that for axial rotation, in the central axis of the dens. Anterior displacement of the atlas is prevented by the strong transverse part of the cruciate ligament. Fielding et al.[10] have shown that the alar ligaments deform under loads that can rupture the transverse ligament, and they are not expected to prevent displacement. Representative values of ranges of motion for the C0–C1–C2 complex are listed in Table 2–2.[41]

C1–C2 Instability

Instability is more common at the C1–C2 level than at the C0–C1 level and can be the result of trauma, rheumatoid arthritis, or tumor. There can be up to 3 mm of physiologic anterior sagittal translational motion at the C1–C2 level; this distance is called the anterior atlantodental interval (AADI). Translation >3 mm indicates that the transverse ligament must be attenuated; >5 mm, that the ligament has ruptured.[10] A V-shaped predental space is not indicative of instability and can measure 0 to 18 degrees, with a mean value of 6 in neutral and 9 in flexion.[14, 41] In traumatic cases where a V-shaped predental space is discovered, it is possible that the transverse ligament may be attenuated and the anterior ring of the atlas may hinge on the anterior atlantodental ligaments described by Dvorak and Panjabi.[6] Clinical evaluation of the patient will differentiate between a preexisting laxity and a new pathology. With the transverse ligament intact, a complete bilateral dislocation can occur at 65 degrees of rotation. With transverse ligament disruption, dislocation can occur at 45 degrees of rotation.[10] Sagittal plane axial instability is indicative of an underlying pathologic process. Compressive loads are transferred to the lateral mass articulation of the C1–C2 joints.

Fractures of the atlas ring with disruption of the transverse ligament or erosive destruction can result in basilar invagination. Total lateral displacement >6.9 mm of the lateral masses of C1 over the masses of C2 as measured on an anteroposterior radiograph is indicative of a burst fracture of the atlas with insufficiency of the transverse ligament.[35] Distractive forces acting on the C1–C2 junction are resisted mainly by the tectorial membrane.[40] Criteria for C1–C2 instability are outlined in Table 2–1.

Middle and Lower Cervical Spine
Functional Spine Unit

The middle and lower cervical spine segments (C3 to C7) have essential similar anatomic and functional characteristics and can be effectively represented by the functional spinal unit (FSU). The FSU is defined as the smallest segment of the spine that exhibits biomechanical characteristics similar to those of the entire spine.[25] The motion of the upper FSU vertebra can be described in a three-dimensional coordinate system in relation to the lower vertebra. Every FSU has 6 degrees of freedom: three rotations and three translations about the three-axis system.[26, 42] The load deformation curve of the FSU is biphasic. At smaller loads, the spine deforms easily and offers little resistance. At higher loads, the spine provides increased resistance to deformation. Panjabi[27] has termed the first phase of the FSU load-deformation curve the

Table 2–2. *Range of Motion of the Upper Cervical Spine*

	Motion	Degrees
C0–C1	Total flexion-extension	25
	Lateral bending (one side)	5
	Axial rotation (one side)	5
C1–C2	Total flexion-extension	20
	Lateral bending (one side)	5
	Axial rotation (one side)	4

(Adapted with permission from White AA, Panjabi MM: Clinical Biomechanics of the Spine, 2nd ed. Philadelphia, JB Lippincott, 1990.)

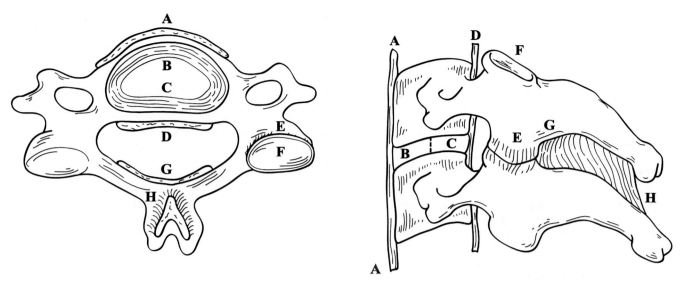

Figure 2–1. *Axial and lateral views of a function spine unit of the middle and lower cervical spine. Detailed anatomic structures are the anterior longitudinal ligament (A), anterior disc and annulus (B), posterior disk and annulus (C), posterior longitudinal ligament (D), facet capsules (E), facet joints (F), ligamentum flavum (G), and interspinous ligament (H).*

neutral zone (NZ) and has termed the second phase the elastic zone (EZ). The range of motion of the FSU is the sum of the NZ and the EZ. Loads that exceed the EZ result in permanent (catastrophic) deformation and represent the phase of plastic deformation. The FSU of the lower cervical spine is composed of two vertebral elements, the intervertebral disk, and associated ligamentous and capsular structures (Fig. 2–1).

Anatomy

The C3 to C7 vertebral bodies have a concave upper and a convex lower surface. The posterolateral projections of the upper endplate, the unci (hooks), form the uncovertebral joints of Luschka with the corresponding convex posterolateral surface of the lower endplate of the superior vertebra. These joints support part of the axial load after disk degeneration. The average vertebral body size increases from C3 to C7, with width ranging from 15.6 to 23.4 mm and depth ranging from 15.6 to 18.1 mm. The average pedicle height is 7 mm, and the average pedicle width is 5 mm. The angle made by the pedicle decreases from 40 degrees at C3 to 29 degrees at C7.[26] The laminae project posteromedially from the pedicles and form the spinous process in the midline and the facets laterally. The articular surfaces of the facets are inclined approximately 45 degrees from the horizontal plane and become steeper in the lower segments. The vertebral artery lies just lateral to the uncovertebral joints. Anterior diskectomy or corpectomy should stay medial to the lateral portion of this joint to avoid injury to the artery. The motion segments are connected and stabilized by the intervertebral disk, the ligaments, and the facet capsules.

Intervertebral Disk

Compressive forces are transferred through the intervertebral disk, the vertebral body, and the facet joints. The intervertebral disk is a viscoelastic material, and its mechanical properties are dependent on the rate of loading. The disk deforms and is more flexible at low load rates, and it becomes stiff at higher loading rates.[27, 41] Degeneration and dehydration of the disk will affect the viscoelastic characteristics (creep and relaxation). The degenerated disk will deform more and faster than the healthy disk, applying more load to the periphery of the endplate through the annulus. The disk is the major compressive component of the spine; its ability to tolerate vertical loading in excess of the failure point of the vertebral body is well documented.[12, 39] The tensile properties of the disk annulus are related to the orientation of the collagen fibers. The annulus is stronger in a direction 15 degrees from horizontal and weakest along the disk axis.[10] The disk responds to loading by dehydrating and becoming stiffer until a new equilibrium is reached. When the applied stress is reduced, the disk rehydrates accordingly.[1]

Vertebral Body

There is an obvious trend toward increased compression strength from the upper cervical to lower lumbar levels. The average value of 1700 N comes from the classic work of Messener.[13] A similar value of 1570 N was found in various studies of vertical impact loading with cadavers.[44] Bell et al.[2] have shown that a 25% decrease in osseous tissue results in a >50% decrease in the strength of a vertebra. In general, vertebral strength decreases with age. The rate of load application (fast or slow) is an important factor in determining the type of fracture. Fast loading rates produce burst-type fractures with gross displacement, and slow loading rates produce wedge-shaped fractures.[3]

Facet Joints

The facet joints aid in resisting compressive loads, depending on the position of the spine. The superior articular facets of C2 to C4 face posteromedially and are circular or oval. Caudal to T1, the facets face posterolaterally and have a more transverse orientation. The transition between the two orientations can be gradual or sudden. The most frequent site of the transition is the C5–C6 segment.[19] Zdeblick has studied the role of the facet capsules and joints in stability.[46, 47] Up to a 50% capsule resection or a 50% facetectomy had minimal effect on sagittal and torsional stability. A 75% resection resulted in a 32% decrease in sagittal stiffness and a 25% decrease in torsional stiffness. Additional torsional stability is provided by the intervertebral disk.[39]

Uncovertebral Joints

The exact role of the uncovertebral joints of Luschka is not known. A finite element model study of the C5–C6 FSU found that the uncovertebral joints are important contributors to the coupled motion of the lower cervical spine.[4] The uncinate processes were found to reduce both the primary and the couple motion, and surgical resection is expected to increase instability of the FSU.[4]

Ligaments

The ligaments of the cervical spine provide passive stability and guide motion. Spinal ligaments are pretensioned but tend to lose some of their mechanical properties with increased age. The ligamentum flavum is the body tissue with the highest percentage of elastic fibers and has the highest preload (18 N in the young spine and 5 N in the older spine).[17] This pretension avoids impingement of the cord from ligament bulking. The ligamentum flavum is relatively constant in width (5 mm). The other spinal ligaments are also pretensioned but with significantly lower loads.[36] The anterior longitudinal ligament (ALL) is attached firmly to the bodies and loosely to the disk. The posterior longitudinal ligament (PLL) is firmly attached to the disk but loosely attached to the body. The ALL and PLL are approximately 7.5 mm wide and 12 mm long, respectively, at levels C3 through T1.[25] The ALL and PLL have similar material properties. The ALL is twice as strong as the PLL because it has twice the cross-sectional area.[31, 36] The supraspinous ligament is more vertically oriented than the interspinous ligament by 15 to 20 degrees. A recent morphometric and biomechanical study found that the ALL and PLL have higher failure stress values (strength) compared to the ligaments of the posterior complex.[45] In contrast, failure strain (elongation to failure) was higher in the posterior ligaments (interspinous ligament, joint capsules, and ligamentum flavum).[45]

The capsule ligaments provide flexion stability to the FSU.[20, 42] The capsular ligaments are oriented posteriorly at approximately 45 degrees to the transverse plane. Zdeblick et al.[46] found that resection of >50% of the facet capsule leads to significant instability. A recent clinical study compared the magnetic resonance imaging findings in patients with unilateral and bilateral facet dislocation. Anterior longitudinal ligament rupture was significantly associated with a bilateral facet dislocation. Damage to the posterior longitudinal ligament was not a consistent finding in unilateral facet dislocations. Disk disruption was a common finding in both injury types.[38] To produce a unilateral facet dislocation in vitro, the ipsilateral facet capsule, annulus fibrosus, and ligamentum flavum had to be disrupted.[34]

Kinematics

The FSU has 6 degrees of freedom about the three-axis system of coordinates (three rotations and three translations). The primary motion at the lower cervical spine is flexion and extension in the sagittal plane. The average IAR for this rotation has been estimated to lie inside the posterior half of the body of the inferior vertebra, and it moves superiorly toward the disk from C2 to C7. As the IAR moves closer to the disk space, the arc of rotation becomes sharper.[9] Rotation and lateral bending are coupled motions in the lower cervical spine, the result of inclination of the facet joints. Panjabi[27] has found that every 1 degree of axial rotation produces 0.75 degree of lateral bending in the same direction. Lateral bending produces also coupled axial rotation in a ratio of 0.67 at C2 and 0.13 at C7. Moroney et al.[15] found that the coupled lateral bending to axial rotation was 0.51 and the coupled axial rotation to lateral bending was 0.32. Representative values for range of rotation in the middle and lower spine are depicted in Table 2–3. Translations are clinically very important in determining instability of the FSU. The maximum value of normal anteroposterior translation has been found to be 2.7 mm, with a reported average of 0.5 mm[15] to 2 mm.[22] Lateral translations (one side) were found to average between 0.14 and 1.5 mm. Vertical translations were negligible. The differences between the values found were attributed to the different moments applied at these experiments (19.6 N vs. 50 N, respectively).

Table 2–3. *Range of Motion (Degrees) of the Middle and Lower Cervical Spine*

Level	Total Flexion-Extension	Lateral Bending (One Side)	Axial Rotation (One Side)
C2–C3	10	10	3
C3–C4	15	11	7
C4–C5	20	11	7
C5–C6	20	8	7
C6–C7	17	7	6

(Adapted with permission from White AA, Panjabi MM: Clinical Biomechanics of the Spine, 2nd ed. Philadelphia, JB Lippincott, 1990.)

Table 2–4. *Checklist for the Diagnosis of Clinical Instability in the Middle and Lower Cervical Spine*

Element	Point Value
Anterior elements destroyed or unable to function	2
Posterior elements destroyed or unable to function	2
Positive stretch test	2
Radiographic criteria	4
A. Flexion/extension x-rays	
1. Sagittal plane translation >3.5 mm or 20% (2 pts)	
2. Sagittal plane rotation >20 (2 pts)	
OR	
B. Resting x-rays	
1. Sagittal plane displacement >3.5 mm or 20% (2 pts)	
2. Relative sagittal plane angulation >11 (2 pts)	
Abnormal disk narrowing	1
Developmentally narrow spinal canal	1
1. Sagittal diameter <13 mm	
OR	
2. Pavlov's ratio <0.8	
Spinal cord damage	2
Nerve root damage	1
Dangerous loading anticipated	1
Total of 5 points or more = unstable	

(Adapted with permission from White AA, Panjabi MM: Clinical Biomechanics of the Spine, 2nd ed. Philadelphia, JB Lippincott, 1990.)

Subaxial Cervical Spine Instability

One widely accepted definition of clinical instability of the spine is that given by White and Panjabi:

> Clinical instability is the loss of the ability of the spine under physiologic loads to maintain relations between vertebrae in such a way that there is neither initial nor subsequent damage to the spinal cord or nerve roots, and in addition, there is neither development of incapacitating deformity nor severe pain.[41]

The upper cervical spine kinematics are highly constrained by bony morphology and ligamentous attachments, making the establishment of radiologic criteria easier. In the subaxial cervical spine, the viscoelastic intervertebral disk and the coupled kinematics make recognition of clinical instability more difficult.

Gross instability can be safely detected with static or dynamic radiographs. Translation and rotation of the FSU can then be compared with the normal values found from kinematic studies in vitro. Considering 2.7 mm the highest reported value of anterior translation in vitro and an average radiographic magnification of 30%, the result is the criterion of 3.5 mm of maximum normal sagittal plane translation proposed by White and Panjabi. Angular deformity in the sagittal plate can also be compared with the normal values found in vitro. Any increase in sagittal rotation of the injured FSU >11 degrees in dynamic radiographs compared with the presumed intact FSU above or below is indicative of instability. An FSU exhibiting >20 degrees of sagittal rotation in dynamic flexion–extension radiographs is above all normal limits found in vivo[7, 30] and in vitro studies[41] and is considered unstable. All of these criteria have been included in the "checklist for the diagnosis of clinical instability" (Table 2–4).

In cases of degenerative painful cervical syndromes, the definition of clinical instability is more difficult. In most of these cases, the range of motion of the FSU is within normal limits, but sometimes lower. Panjabi conducted an in vitro study to measure the effects of the external fixation on the load-deformation curve of the stabilized FSU. He found that the greatest decrease occurred in the neutral zone (69%), with the total range of motion losing only 39% of the intact value. These findings led Panjabi to redefine clinical instability as follows:

> Clinical instability is defined as a significant decrease in the capacity of the stabilizing system of the spine to maintain the intervertebral neutral zones within the physiological limits, so that there is no neurological dysfunction, no major deformity, and no incapacitating pain.[27]

Neural Tissue

Although there is abundant information about the biomechanics of the osseoligamentous structures of the spine, such information is lacking for the physical properties of the spinal cord and nerves. The spinal cord together with the vascular pia has an elastic strain value of about 10% the original length. This deformation is possible with minimal stress (0.01 N). Further strain is opposed with highly increased stress. Failure stress was found to be about 20 to 30 N. The deforming forces acting on the cord produce a combination of compressive, tensile, and shear forces. A bending moment will create tensile forces on the concave and compressive stresses on the convex side of the bent spinal cord. The close relation of the cord to the canal dimensions is more evident in the football spine injuries. Torg et al.[37] reported extensively on neurapraxias in football players with a developmental canal that exposed the flexed cervical spines in axial load. The flexed canal eliminates physiologic cord kinematics and creates high stresses that can result in quadriplegia.[37]

MODELS FOR BIOMECHANICAL RESEARCH

The biomechanical models of the cervical spine have provided valuable information on the functional anatomy, kinematics, injury patterns, instability, and behavior of different reconstruction constructs and spinal instrumentation. Over the past years many new models have been developed. A general description of models classifies them into four types: physical models, in vitro models, in vivo models, and computer models.[28]

Physical Models

Physical models are made of artificial materials. They are used to test a basic hypothesis when anatomy and material properties are not important. The "missing vertebra" model is used extensively as a worst-case scenario to evaluate the mechanical characteristics of different spinal implants. These models are inexpensive and reproducible because the material properties of the model are known, but their use is limited because they cannot address clinical problems. Good examples of this model are fatigue testing of unicortical vertebral body screws and testing the load of the constraining mechanism between an anterior cervical plate and the vertebral body screw to failure. In these tests, the screw or screw–plate construct is inserted into uniform blocks of polymethylmethacrylate and repetitively loaded until a predetermined failure point (e.g., screw breakage or disengagement of the screw–plate junction) is reached.

In Vitro Models

In vitro biomechanical models use human cadaveric or animal specimens to test hypotheses in which anatomy is an important factor. These are very reliable and widely used models for testing the effect of trauma or various surgical procedures on spinal stability. Problems with these models include the availability of specimens and the variability of the mechanical properties between specimens. Most of the human donors are of old age, and thus the specimens are osteopenic with stiffened ligaments and disks. The specimens are usually harvested and then stored in a freezer (fresh-frozen) at −20°C. Specimens can be thawed when ready for testing. Using one freeze-thaw cycle, physical properties of the soft tissues can be preserved.[21] In in vitro experiments, the whole cervical spine or a single FSU can be used. In general, the kinematics are tested by applying pure moments in different directions and measuring displacement, thus creating a load-displacement curve. When testing the entire cervical spine, little or no preload is typically applied, because it has been found that cervical spine in

vitro buckles under only 10 N of load. The unsupported weight of the head will impart a load of 50 N, and the cervical spine in vivo can sustain loads that can reach 1200 N.[16] Panjabi[22] has shown that the major denominator of instability in vitro is the increase in the NZ. Subsequent experiments using single FSUs under physiologic loads have shown that the NZ is effectively reduced under preload. Many in vitro studies have been with single FSUs under nonphysiologic conditions.[22, 27]

Follower Load Model

Patwardhan et al.[29] successfully addressed the problem of preload using the follower load model. Instead of applying the preload vertically, the compressive load was applied along a path that approximated the tangent to the curve of the cervical spine passing through the IAR of the FSUs, minimizing shear and applying almost pure compression at each disk level. This technique offers a novel model for testing multisegmental cervical spine specimens under compressive loads of physiologic magnitude, making possible the study of different clinical scenarios on the NZ and range of motion (Fig. 2–2).

In Vivo Models

Studying the long-term effects of biologic processes such as osteopenia, surgical procedures, fusion techniques, and spinal cord trauma requires the use of animal models. In such an experiment, the animals are sacrificed at different time intervals after the initial procedure and the results of the biologic process are evaluated with radiologic, histologic, and biomechanical tests.

In vivo biomechanical studies in humans are very rare but very important, because they provide valuable information on the real behavior of the spine. In vivo intradiskal pressure measurement is a classical example.

Computer Models

The finite-element method of computing structural mechanical problems was introduced in 1956 and since then has been used extensively to simulate biologic tissues. A finite element is a set of mathematical equations that incorporate the geometry and physical properties of the structure that they represent. The early models of the cervical spine treated the vertebrae as simple rigid masses connected by beam or spring elements. These early models did not produce realistic results. Advances in computing have resulted in three-dimensional models of cervical spine segments that incorporate realistic geometry of the vertebrae taken from computed tomography scans and realistic physical properties of the ligaments and disks from in vitro studies of these tissues. Validation is an important link between the development of the finite-element model and its intended use. Validation ensures that the finite element as a sum of the separate elements behaves the same as an in vitro model under similar conditions. The importance of finite-element models lies in the ability to measure

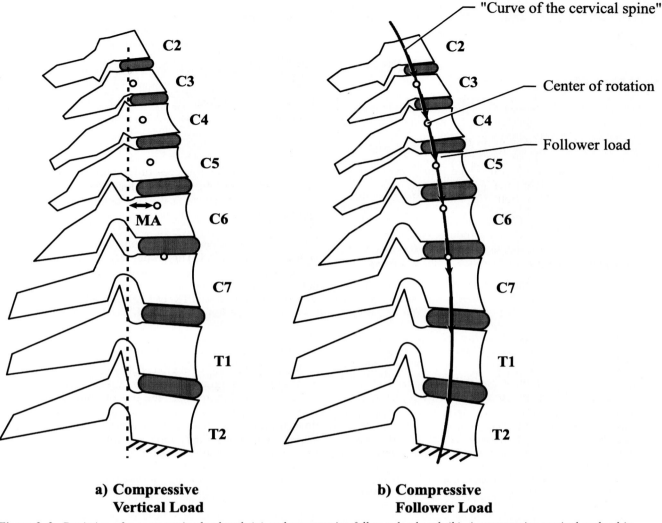

**a) Compressive
Vertical Load**

**b) Compressive
Follower Load**

Figure 2–2. Depiction of a compressive load path (a) and compressive follower load path (b). A compressive vertical preload induces bending moments owing to the moment arm (MA) and causes a large angular change at small loads. Using the compressive follower load path, a compressive preload remains tangential to the spinal curve passing through the instantaneous center of rotation at each level. This action minimizes the bending moments and shear and allows the cervical spine to support large, physiologic preloads while mechanically testing an entire subaxial cervical spine in vitro.

internal stresses and strains. In addition, the researcher can modify any parameter and study the effects. These models are also repeatable and can be used to test a hypothesis before it can be validated with a more expensive in vitro experiment. A good example of a computer model study is the report published by Clausen et al. on the effects of uncovertebral joints.[4] By simulating obliteration of the clefts with disk material, the authors were able to study the effects of loss of the uncovertebral joints on the kinematics of the cervical spine. Such an experiment is not possible in vitro, because the natural clefts of the Luschka joints cannot be eliminated without altering the physical properties of the disk.

Modes of Mechanical Testing

All physical and in vitro models are tested mechanically to determine mechanical properties. There are three basic types of tests: strength tests, fatigue tests, and stability tests. During a strength test, the specimen is loaded to failure, and a load deformation curve is plotted. Failure can either be catastrophic or a predetermined displacement. In fatigue tests, the specimens are cycled up to or at a predetermined maximum load at continuous rate. The test concludes once a predetermined failure point is reached. This can be nondestructive, destructive, or catastrophic. Stability testing is typically nondestructive. To test the stability of different cervical spine constructs, the specimen is fixed to a pot on one side, and a load (flexibility test) or a given displacement (stiffness test) is applied to the other side. A load-displacement curve is plotted, allowing the effects of different procedures to then be compared.[22]

SUMMARY

The cervical spine as a whole is the most mobile portion of the spinal axis, particularly from the occiput to C2. While maintaining a relatively vast range of motion, it protects the cervical cord and nerve roots from both subtle and catastrophic injury. This is accomplished through the sum total of its passive and active components from bone to disk and ligaments to muscle. Understanding the mechanical principles of properties of the cervical spine as a complete unit as well as the basic FSU can aid understanding of the various clinical syndromes that produce symptoms. More importantly, this understanding can lead to successful and safe treatment of a variety of cervical spine disorders.

REFERENCES

1. Adams MA, Hutton WC: The effect of posture on the fluid content of lumbar intervertebral disks. Spine 8:665–671, 1983.
2. Bell GH, Dunbar O, Beck JS, Gibb A: Variation in the strength of vertebrae with age and their relation to osteoporosis. Calcif Tissue Res 1:75, 1967.
3. Carter JW, Mirza SK, Tencer AF, Ching RP: Canal geometry changes associated with axial compressive cervical spine fracture. Spine 25:46–54, 2000.
4. Clausen JD, Goel VK, Traynelis VC, Scifert J: Uncinate processes and Luschka joints influence the biomechanics of the cervical spine: Quantification using a finite element model of the C5–C6 segment. J Orthop Res 15:342–347, 1997.
5. Dvorak J, Panjabi MM, Gerber M: CT–Functional diagnostics of the rotatory instability of the upper cervical spine: An experimental study in cadavers. Spine 12:197, 1987.
6. Dvorak J, Panjabi MM: Functional anatomy of the alar ligaments. Spine 12:183, 1987.
7. Dvorak J, Froehlich D, Penning L, et al: Functional radiographic diagnosis of the cervical spine: Flexion/extension. Spine 13:748, 1988.
8. Dvorak J, Panjabi MM, Gerber M, Wichmann W: CT–Functional diagnostics of the rotatory instability of the upper cervical spine. Spine 12:726, 1987.
9. Dvorak J, Panjabi MM, Novotny JE, Antinnes JA: In vivo flexion–extension of the normal cervical spine. J Orthop Res 9:824–834, 1991.
10. Fielding JW, Cochran GVB, Lawsing JF, Hall M: Tears of the transverse ligament of the atlas: A clinical and biomechanical study. J Bone Joint Surg Am 56A:1681–1691, 1974.
11. Galante JO: Tensile properties of the human annulus fibrosus. Acta Orthop Scand 100(suppl): 1–91, 1967.
12. Hirsch C: The reaction of intervertebral disks to compression forces. J Bone Joint Surg Am 37A:1188, 1955.
13. Messener O: Uber Elasticitat and Fesigkeit der Meuschlichen Knochen. JG Cottaschen Buchhandling, 1880.
14. Monu J, Bohler SP, Howard G: Some upper cervical norms. Spine 12:515–519, 1987.
15. Moroney SP, Schultz AB, Miller JAA, Andersson GBJ: Load-displacement properties of lower cervical spine motion segments. J Biomech 21:767, 1988.
16. Moroney SP, Schultz AB, Miller JAA: Analysis and measurement of neck loads. J Orthop Res 6:713–720, 1988.
17. Nachemson A, Evans J: Some mechanical properties of the third lumbar interlaminar ligament (ligamentum flavum). J Biomech 1:211, 1968.
18. Nightingale RW, McElhaney JH, Richardson WJ, Myers BS: Dynamic responses of the head and cervical spine to axial impact loading. J Biomech 29:307–318, 1996.
19. Pal GP, Routal RV, Saggu SK: The orientation of the articular facets of the zygoapophysial joints at the cervical and upper thoracic region. J Anat 198:431–441, 2001.
20. Panjabi MM, White AA, Johnson RM: Cervical spine mechanics as a function of transection of components. J Biomech 8:327, 1975.
21. Panjabi MM, Krag MH, Summers D, Videman T: Mechanical time-tolerance of human spine specimens. J Orthop Res 3:292–300, 1985.
22. Panjabi MM, Summers DJ, Pelker RR, et al: Three-dimensional load displacement curves of the cervical spine. J Orthop Res 4:152, 1986.
23. Panjabi M, Dvorak J, Crisco JJ 3rd, et al: Effects of alar ligament transection on upper cervical spine rotation. J Orthop Res 9:584–593, 1991.
24. Panjabi MM, Oxland TR, Parks EH: Quantitative anatomy of cervical spine ligaments. Part I. Upper cervical spine. J Spinal Disord 4:270–276, 1991.
25. Panjabi MM, Oxland TR, Parks EH: Quantitative anatomy of cervical spine ligaments. Part II. Middle and lower cervical spine. J Spinal Disord 4:277–285, 1991.
26. Panjabi MM, Duranceau J, Goel V, et al: Cervical human vertebrae. Quantitative three-dimensional anatomy of the middle and lower regions. Spine 16:861–874, 1993.
27. Panjabi MM, Dvorak J, Sandler A, et al: Cervical spine kinematics and clinical instability. In The Cervical Spine, 3rd ed. Philadelphia, Lippincott-Raven, 1998.
28. Panjabi MM: Cervical spine models for biomechanical research. Spine 23:2684–2700, 1998.
29. Patwardhan A, Havey RM, Ghanayem A, et al: Load carrying capacity of the human cervical spine in compression is increased under a follower load. Spine 25:1548–1554, 2000.
30. Penning L: Normal movement of the cervical spine. Am J Roentegenol 130:317–326, 1978.
31. Przybylski GJ, Patel PR, Carlin GJ, Woo SL: Quantitative anthropometry of the subatlantal cervical longitudinal ligaments. Spine 23:893–898, 1998.
32. Saldinger P, Dvorak J, Rahn BA, Perren SM: Histology of the alar and transverse ligaments. Spine 15:257–261, 1990.
33. Sherk HH: Developmental anatomy of the normal cervical spine. In: The Cervical Spine, 3rd ed. Philadelphia, Lippincott-Raven, 1998.
34. Sim E, Vaccaro AR, Berzlanovich A, et al: In vitro genesis of subaxial cervical unilateral facet dislocations through sequential soft tissue ablation. Spine 26:1317–1323, 2001.
35. Spence K, Decker S, Sell K: Bursting atlantal fracture associated with rupture of the transverse ligament. J Bone Joint Surg Am 52:543–549, 1970.
36. Tkaczuk H: Tensile properties of human lumbar longitudinal ligaments. Acta Ortop Scand (suppl):115, 1968.
37. Torg JS, Vegso JJ, O'Neill MJ, Sennett B: The epidemiologic, pathologic, biomechanical, and cinematographic analysis of football-injured cervical spine trauma. Am J Sports Med 18:50–57, 1990.
38. Vaccaro AR, Madigan L, Schweitzer ME, et al: Magnetic resonance imaging analysis of soft tissue disruption after flexion-distraction injuries of the subaxial cervical spine. Spine 26:1866–1872, 2001.

39. Virgin W: Experimental investigations into physical properties of intervertebral disk. J Bone Joint Surg Br 33B:607, 1951.

40. Werne S: Studies on spontaneous atlas dislocation. Acta Orthop Scand 23:1–150, 1957.

41. White AA, Panjabi MM: Clinical Biomechanics of the Spine. Philadelphia, JB Lippincott, 1990.

42. White AA, Johnson RM, Panjabi MM, Southwick WO: Biomechanical analysis of clinical stability in the cervical spine. Clin Orthop 109:85, 1975.

43. Wiesel SW, Rothman RH: Occipito-atlantal hypermobility. Spine 4:187, 1979.

44. Yoganandan N, Sances A, Maiman DJ, et al: Experimental spinal injuries with vertical impact. Spine 11:855–860, 1986.

45. Yoganandan N, Kumaresan S, Pintar FA: Geometric and mechanical properties of human cervical spine ligaments. J Biomech Eng 122:623–629, 2000.

46. Zdeblick TA, Zou D, Warden KE, et al: Cervical stability following foraminotomy: A biomechanical *in-vitro* analysis. J Bone Joint Surg Am 74A:22–27, 1992.

47. Zdeblick TA, Abitbol JJ, Kunz DN, et al: Cervical stability after sequential capsule resection. Spine 18:2005–2008, 1993.

3

SURGICAL APPROACHES TO THE CERVICAL SPINE

Todd J. Albert, M.D.

"God doesn't play dice with the universe."
— Albert Einstein

Form certainly follows function. The anatomy of the neck, whether by design or evolution, is quite orderly. Exploitation of this orderly anatomy for surgical approaches allows for atraumatic and relatively simple access to almost any level of the cervical spine either anteriorly or posteriorly. Thorough knowledge of the anatomical structures at risk during dissection and the fascial layers allows facility and ease of surgical exposure. This chapter focuses on proximal and distal anterior and posterior exposures to the cervical spine and the relevant anatomy that is violated during these exposures.

RELEVANT SURGICAL ANATOMY

The cervical region contains the connecting apparatus from the head to the rest of the body. Blood flow to and from the brain and the neural pathways courses through the neck. Organs vital to speech and deglutition are contained here. The cervical spine, located deep in the neck, brings mobility and stability to the cervical region and protects the spinal cord. Although the anatomy is complex, five fascial layers invest all of its structures and allow compartments that facilitate surgical exposure. The surgeon must understand the one superficial and four deep layers of cervical fascia to understand surgical exposure. The fascial layers consist of:

1. Superficial fascia, which includes the platysma

2. The superficial layer of the deep fascia surrounding the sternocleidomastoid and overlying the anterior and external jugular veins

3. The middle layer of deep cervical fascia, investing the strap muscles and forming the visceral fascia that encloses the trachea, esophagus, and recurrent nerve

4. The alar fascia, which fuses in the midline to the visceral fascia and forms two carotid sheaths

5. The deepest prevertebral fascia covering the spine, longus coli, and scalenus muscles (Fig. 3–1).

The sternocleidomastoid is the most prominent muscle in the cervical region. It courses in a transverse manner from the mastoid tip to the clavicular and sternal areas, where it divides into two heads: the clavicular head and the sternal head. As the sternocleidomastoid muscle is retracted laterally, the carotid sheath is seen just deep and running in a nearly parallel plane. The space immediately deep to the sternocleidomastoid is a potential space known as Burn's space. The omohyoid, one of the superficial layers of the strap muscles of the neck, is commonly encountered during anterior dissection of the spine. The omohyoid is invested by the middle layer of the deep cervical fascia and is found coursing in a posterolateral direction at approximately the C5–C6 level.

The carotid and vertebral arteries carry crucial blood supply to the brain. The carotid artery, through branching, also supplies the visceral compartments of the neck. A number of vessels course transversely through the cervical region. Knowledge of their anatomy is extremely important, because they are commonly encountered during cervical spine surgery and often need to be ligated to improve exposure (Fig. 3–2).

Moving from an inferior to superior direction, the middle thyroid vein is usually seen at the level of C4–C5. With dissection carried more superiorly, the first division of the carotid artery, the superior thyroid artery, is found. The superior thyroid vein and superior laryngeal nerve are in close proximity to this artery as they course from a lateral to medial direction transversely. The lingual artery is usually found one interspace above the superior laryngeal nerve and is deep but proximal to the hypoglossal nerve. The facial artery is superior and more superficial than the lingual artery and is intimately associated posteriorly with the submandibular gland. We often ligate the facial artery during high cervical exposure.

Knowledge of the neural anatomy within the layers of cervical exposure is paramount, because these nerves are often encountered during exposure and are subject to injury. The superficial ansa hypoglossus divides into a superficial branch and a deep branch. These nerves, which supply function to the strap muscles of the larynx, are often sacrificed during exposure of the cervical spine with minimal subsequent morbidity.

The left recurrent laryngeal nerve descends from the skull base with the vagus nerve in the carotid sheath. It leaves the vagus nerve within the thorax as it loops under the aortic arch beneath the ligamentum arteriosum and ascends back into the neck within the tracheoesophageal groove. The right recurrent laryngeal nerve, more commonly nonrecurrent,

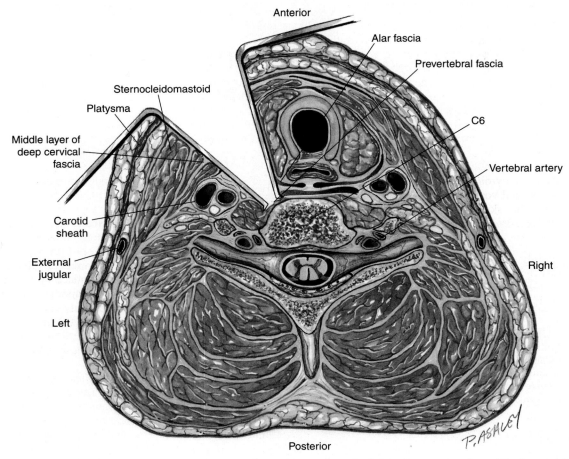

Figure 3–1. *Cross-sectional view at the C6 vertebral body level. (From Albert TJ, Balderston RA, Northrup BE: Surgical Approaches to the Spine. Philadelphia, WB Saunders, 1997.)*

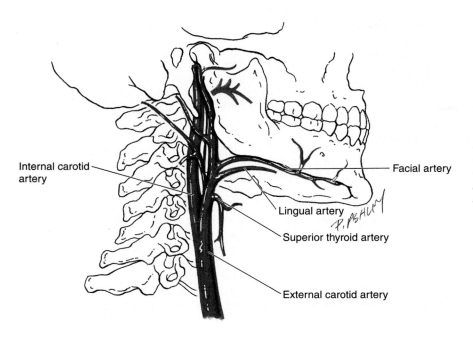

Figure 3–2. *Branches of the carotid system. (From Albert TJ, Balderston RA, Northrup BE: Surgical Approaches to the Spine. Philadelphia, WB Saunders, 1997.)*

usually descends from the skull base with the vagus nerve in the carotid sheath and loops around the subclavian artery as it ascends back into the neck within the tracheoesophageal groove. The usual course of a nonrecurrent laryngeal nerve, almost always occurring on the right side, crosses in a transverse direction at the level of the thyroid gland. It is at risk during a right-sided exposure. For this reason, we attempt to perform all exposures on the left side.

The superior laryngeal nerve passes transversely from the vagus nerve in close proximity to the superior thyroid artery and vein at the level of C3. The nerve then divides into an internal branch and an external branch and innervates the cricothyroid muscle. Injury to this nerve may cause hoarseness and voice fatigue. The hypoglossal nerve descends from the skull base near the carotid sheath, coursing transversely as it crosses the carotid artery near the superior thyroid artery and vein. It then passes deep to the digastric sling at the level of the hyoid bone (Fig. 3–3). Injury to the hypoglossal nerve may result in paralysis of the ipsilateral tongue musculature, creating difficulties with speech and swallowing.

The marginal mandibular nerve is the most superficial and superiorly positioned nerve of the cervical region at risk for injury during cervical spine surgery. A division of the facial nerve, the marginal mandibular nerve extends into the cervical region just below the angle of the mandible and courses in a plane beneath the platysma toward the submandibular triangle.

Careful identification and preservation of the neural structures of the neck is important during cervical spine approaches. Inadvertent clamping or sectioning of the nerves obviously results in permanent injury. Overly aggressive traction produces neuropraxia, which can last for months or years. Maintaining a soft tissue buttress between the nerves and retractors is extremely helpful in avoiding compression injury. Excessive traction is to be avoided.

The cervical sympathetic ganglion passes in a vertical direction near the lateral aspect of vertebral bodies in close proximity to the prevertebral musculature and extends from the thoracic inlet to the second cervical vertebra. Three prominent ganglionic enlargements (superior, middle, and inferior) are found in the cervical region. The superior ganglion is at C2 or C3. The location of the middle ganglion is variable but usually is at the level of C6, whereas the inferior ganglion is located near T1 and forms a stellate ganglion. Injury to any of these structures may result in ipsilateral myosis and lid ptosis, also known as Horner's syndrome.

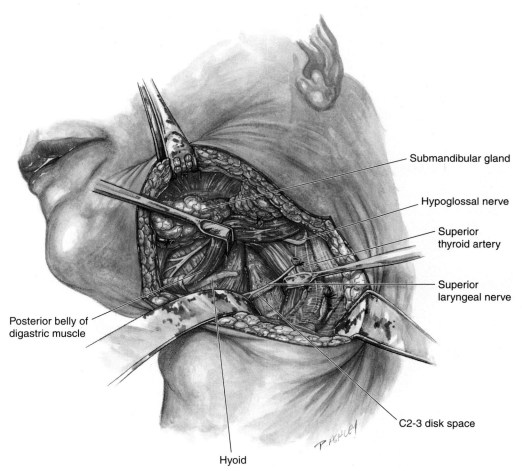

Figure 3–3. High retropharyngeal approach after dissection. *(From Albert TJ, Balderston RA, Northrup BE: Surgical Approaches to the Spine. Philadelphia, WB Saunders, 1997.)*

Thorough knowledge of vertebral artery anatomy is crucial to avoiding injury during cervical exposures. It is not typically identified, but injury can have catastrophic consequences. The first branch of the subclavian artery, the vertebral artery enters the transverse foramen of the C6 and ascends through successive vertebral transverse foramina to the C1. After leaving the transverse foramen of C1, it curves posteromedially over the posterior ring of the atlas and penetrates the posterior atlanto-occipital ligament before ascending through the foramen magnum. Intracranially, it joins the contralateral vertebral artery, forming the basilar artery and communicating with the circle of Willis. The vertebral vein accompanies the artery in close proximity. A portion of the sympathetic chain may be identified in the most superior limits of the arterial course. In 5% to 10% of people, vertebral artery entry is at the usually empty C7 foramen transversarium.

UPPER CERVICAL EXPOSURES

Transoral Approach

The transoral exposure is used as an approach to the odontoid and the anterior arch of C1 for resection of a tumor or rheumatoid pannus. Exposure is relatively straightforward. Fiberoptic nasal intubation is used. If extensive retraction or manipulation of the tongue and pallet is planned, then a tracheotomy may need to be considered. The uvula is retracted with a nasogastric tube, and an oral retractor is inserted (Fig. 3–4). A vertical incision is made in the posterior pharyngeal mucosa and carried through the constrictor muscles to the longus coli. Subperiosteal dissection can be carried out with cautery or periosteal dissectors. If more proximal exposure is needed, then the uvula can be split as can the soft palate in the midline. A portion of the hard palate can also be rongeured or burred away as necessary for exposure (Fig. 3–5).

If more distal exposure is needed, then aggressive takedown of the oral contents can be accomplished with a lip split and mandibulotomy. Beyond this, the tongue can also be split and a high extrapharyngeal exposure combined for extensile exposure between C2 and approximately C5. The details of these exposures are beyond the scope of this chapter, however.

HIGH CERVICAL AND RETROPHARYNGEAL EXPOSURE

Retropharyngeal exposure of the upper cervical spine carries significant risks of morbidity to the cranial motor nerves, which must be mobilized to gain exposure. Adequate exposure often can be gained only by placing a significant amount of traction on these nerves. Although nerve palsy may result, this is usually temporary. However, because mobilization of the trachea and esophagus of the spine are necessary, palsy is often magnified by the resultant edema. A period of swallowing dysfunction may occur, especially in elderly patients.

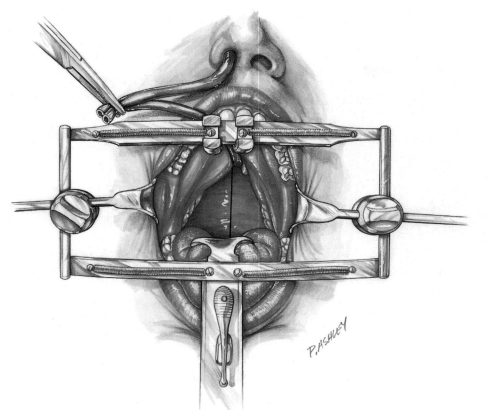

Figure 3–4. Vertical incision through the posterior pharyngeal mucosa. (From Albert TJ, Balderston RA, Northrup BE: Surgical Approaches to the Spine. Philadelphia, WB Saunders, 1997.)

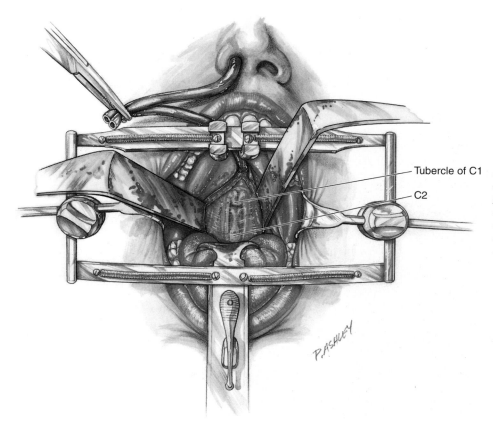

Tubercle of C1

C2

Figure 3–5. Subperiosteal dissection exposing the atlantoaxial process. (From Albert TJ, Balderston RA, Northrup BE: Surgical Approaches to the Spine. Philadelphia, WB Saunders, 1997.)

Patients are usually positioned as for middle and lower cervical exposures, which entails placing a rolled-up towel longitudinally in the interscapular area. We typically do not use cranial traction. If the patient is at all myelopathic or has any evidence of cord compression, then positioning is done after spinal cord monitoring is instituted. The shoulders are routinely taped and typical draping is done.

For upper cervical exposures, after baseline monitoring is obtained, we attempt to avoid anesthetic paralytic agents until exposure of the spine is completed, to facilitate identification of the cranial motor nerves at risk. We prefer an incision in the natural skin crease on the left side placed approximately 4 cm below the angle of the mandible and extending to the midportion of the sternocleidomastoid muscle from the midline (Fig. 3–6).

Although some surgeons place the incision more cranially along the mandible, we believe that the risk of marginal mandibular nerve damage is too great, although access is slightly easier with a more proximal incision. After the subplatysmal flaps are elevated, the greater auricular nerve lying over the sternocleidomastoid muscle is identified and preserved. The facial vein is identified and divided, and dissection is continued deep to this vein to preserve the marginal mandibular nerve. The digastric and omohyoid muscles are identified. These can be divided if necessary to improve exposure. Only the digastric muscle needs to be reapproximated. The majority of the dissection from this point is blunt and takes advantage of the natural fascial planes. We often use a Kittner dissector for blunt dissection. The hypoglossal nerve is identified deep to the digastric muscle lying superiorly and medially. The

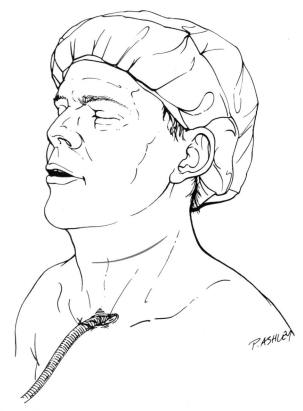

Figure 3–6. Incision for high retropharyngeal approach. (From Albert TJ, Balderston RA, Northrup BE: Surgical Approaches to the Spine. Philadelphia, WB Saunders, 1997.)

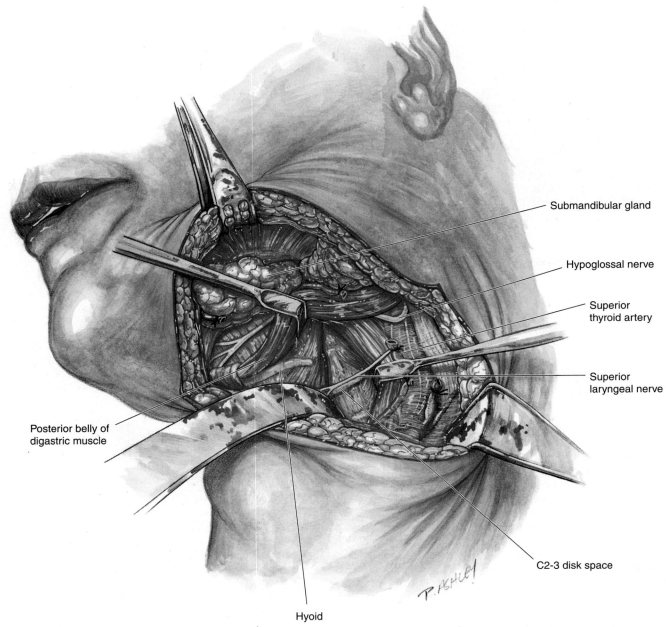

Figure 3–7. *High retropharyngeal approach after dissection. (From Albert TJ, Balderston RA, Northrup BE: Surgical Approaches to the Spine. Philadelphia, WB Saunders, 1997.)*

hypoglossal nerve is retracted superiorly, because less retraction is needed in this direction. The carotid sheath is identified and retracted laterally, and any branches of the internal jugular vein and external carotid artery are divided as necessary to improve exposure. The superior laryngeal vessels are mobilized along with the superior laryngeal nerve. In many cases, the vessels must be divided for exposure and the superior laryngeal nerve mobilized from the vagus nerve at its entry into the larynx through the thyrohyoid membrane. This exposure is more difficult than a lower cervical exposure, because these important nerves course horizontally in the operative field, whereas the

recurrent laryngeal nerve courses vertically in the middle and lower cervical exposures, making it easier to retract. After the superior laryngeal nerve and the hypoglossal nerve are mobilized, blunt dissection easily exposes the prevertebral fascia, the longus coli, and the spine (Fig. 3–7). We elevate the longus coli using a sucker tip for retraction and cautery for subperiosteal dissection. We always begin elevation of longus at the midvertebral body level so the protection of the transverse process allows good lateral exposure while the vertebral artery is protected. After subperiosteal elevation of the longus coli is completed, retractors can be placed both horizontally and vertically.

LATERAL RETROPHARYNGEAL APPROACH TO THE UPPER CERVICAL SPINE (WHITESIDES APPROACH)

This approach, performed lateral to the carotid sheath, was first described by Whitesides and Kelly in 1966. Advantages include a low risk of infection and few neural structures at risk during dissection. Disadvantages are that it places the surgeon more lateral than the medial retropharyngeal approach and is predominantly a unilateral exposure and thus cannot be used for bilateral pathology. Bilateral incisions can be made to treat a bilateral problem using this approach. The Whitesides approach is ideally indicated for excision of tumors at C1–C2, instability problems, failure of earlier C1–C2 fusion attempts, anterior placement of screws, and treatment of infections.

An anatomic appreciation of the carotid sheath and sternocleidomastoid muscle is fundamental to this approach, which requires detachment of the sternocleidomastoid from its insertion on the mastoid tip. The greater auricular nerve is often encountered during this approach just posterior and distal to the base of the ear.

The ideal position in which to perform this approach is with the patient supine with the head turned away from the side of the approach. Nasotracheal intubation opposite the side of the incision is preferred. This is usually possible unless the patient has to be held in a halo ring with a vest attachment and is constrained in this manner. Before the patient is positioned, the earlobe is sewn anteriorly to provide access to the posterior aspect of the ear. The skin inside and outside of the ear is prepped with povidone/iodine (Betadine). The incision begins posterior to the earlobe and runs transversely to below the base of the ear and then is carried longitudinally and distally along the anterior border of the sternocleidomastoid (Fig. 3–8). The plane of dissection is shown in Figure 3–9. High in the neck, the carotid sheath and its contents and the parotid gland are anterior to the dissection. The first palpable bony prominence is the lateral process of the ring of C1.

After the skin incision is made, the greater auricular nerve is identified and dissected in the subcutaneous tissue. It is dissected bidirectionally to allow cranial or caudal retraction. In rare instances, the nerve must be sacrificed, leaving a small patch of sensory deficit. The sternocleidomastoid is obvious after dissection through the subcutaneous levels. It is usually detached from the mastoid process. The spinal accessory nerve enters the sternocleidomastoid 3 cm distal to the mastoid tip. This nerve is identified and protected. Dissection is carried out bluntly posterior to the carotid sheath and sternocleidomastoid as well as the parotid gland. A bent malleable retractor of the appropriate curvature is levered against the contralateral transverse process at the appropriate vertebral body (see Fig. 3–9) if a limited exposure is to be carried out. The spinal accessory nerve can be retracted anteriorly along with the sternocleidomastoid and the contents of the carotid sheath. For a more extensile approach to the subaxial vertebral bodies, the spinal accessory nerve is dissected from the jugular foramen and retracted laterally and posteriorly after the sternocleidomastoid is everted (Fig. 3–10). If more medial dissection is necessary, the surgeon should subperiosteally dissect the ipsilateral longus coli from medial to lateral.

Complications with this approach include injury to the spinal accessory nerve and the vessels in the area (internal jugular vein, carotid artery, and vertebral artery). Injury to the esophagus should be avoided with careful retraction. We check the integrity of the esophagus by flooding it with dilute indigo carmine via a retracted nasogastric or orogastric tube at the end of the procedure.

EXPOSURE TO THE MIDDLE AND LOWER CERVICAL SPINE

The approach from C3 to T1 exploits the interval between the sternocleidomastoid and carotid laterally and the trachea and esophagus medially. Dissection is carried out from superficial to deep through each of the fascial planes described earlier. This approach is useful for excision of herniated disks, corpectomy, excision of tumors, and infection.

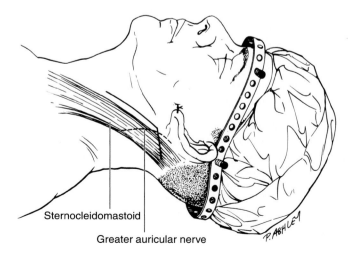

Sternocleidomastoid

Greater auricular nerve

Figure 3–8. *The patient is in supine position with a halo ring in place. A "hockey stick" incision is outlined. The ear is sewn anteriorly. The greater auricular nerve is shadowed in. In rare circumstances, the greater auricular nerve needs to be sacrificed, producing a small insensate area that is not disabling to the patient. (From Albert TJ, Balderston RA, Northrup BE: Surgical Approaches to the Spine. Philadelphia, WB Saunders, 1997.)*

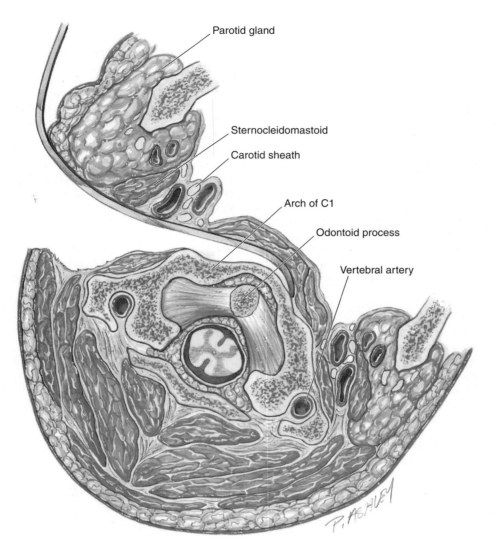

Parotid gland

Sternocleidomastoid

Carotid sheath

Arch of C1

Odontoid process

Vertebral artery

Figure 3–9. Cross-sectional reference at the C1 arch showing the plane of dissection. A bent malleable retractor is levered against the contralateral anterior portion of the atlas to retract the parotid gland, sternocleidomastoid, and contents of the carotid sheath, as well as the esophagus. This plane of dissection does not place the vertebral arteries at risk, because they are posterior and encased in bone at this level. (From Albert TJ, Balderston RA, Northrup BE: *Surgical Approaches to the Spine.* Philadelphia, WB Saunders, 1997.)

For approaches to one, two, or three disk spaces, we prefer a transverse incision because of the cosmetic advantages of using a skin crease. However, if we are using anterior cervical plates across three disk spaces or two vertebral bodies or performing a three-level corpectomy, then we use a longitudinal incision placed along the anterior border of the sternocleidomastoid. The left side is preferred, given the more constant course of the recurrent laryngeal nerve. Traction is rarely used except for three-level or greater corpectomy or in unstable situations. The patient is placed, as described earlier, on a rolled-up towel placed longitudinally in the interscapular area. The shoulder is stabilized with tape to the table, and the neck and iliac crests are prepped and draped in a standard fashion. For a one- or two-level diskectomy, an incision is carried out from the midline to, but not significantly crossing, the medial border of the sterno-cleidomastoid. We identify the site of incision placement by palpating the carotid tubercle; superficial landmarks are generally unreliable (Fig. 3–11). After sectioning the platysma horizontally, we find the superficial layer of the deep cervical fascia. This layer is cut along a "T" with a horizontal incision the length of the incision and the arms of the "T" being the distal and proximal extent of the anterior border of the sternocleidomastoid. Veins sometimes must be ligated at this point. This release is key to gaining extensile exposure through the transverse skin incision. Care must be taken to not dissect deeply into the carotid sheath. At this point, once a release is made, the carotid sheath is palpated with the left index finger and retracted laterally (Fig. 3–12). A Richardson appendiceal retractor is used to pull the tracheoesophageal contents medially, making the middle layer apparent. The omohyoid usually can be delineated at this juncture. A blunt Kittner dissector is used to violate the middle layer of fascia. The esophagus can be more easily retracted laterally as the neck is bluntly opened via the middle layer in a craniocaudal direction. At this point, the pretracheal and prevertebral fascia come into view and can be dissected, either sharply or bluntly, exposing

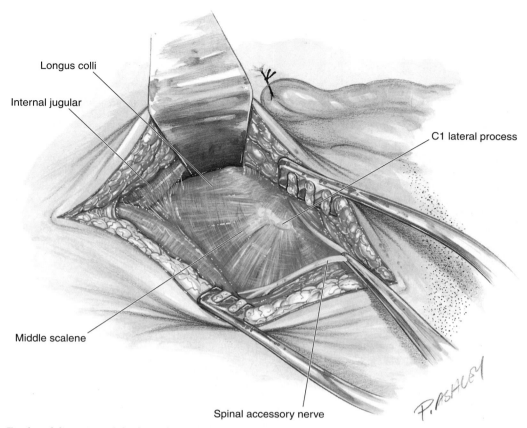

Figure 3–10. Further delineation of the lateral process is carried out. The dissection can be made extensile by dissecting distally the same plane anterior to the vertebral bodies. The longus colli may need to be taken off the lateral aspect of the vertebral body to identify the disk spaces and vertebral bodies. (From Albert TJ, Balderston RA, Northrup BE: Surgical Approaches to the Spine. Philadelphia, WB Saunders, 1997.)

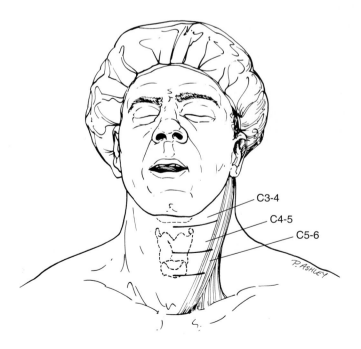

Figure 3–11. Landmarks for transverse incision for the anterolateral exposure to the cervical spine; frontal view. (From Albert TJ, Balderston RA, Northrup BE: Surgical Approaches to the Spine. Philadelphia, WB Saunders, 1997.)

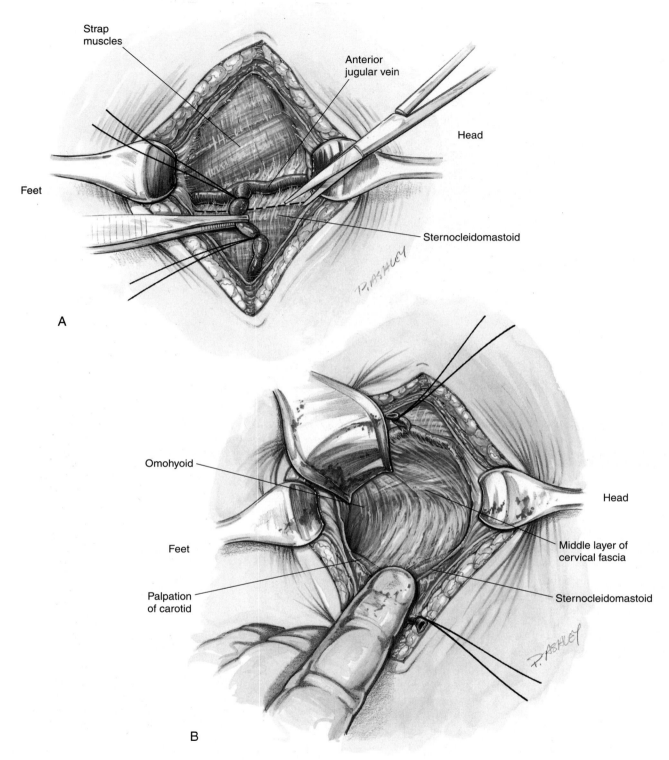

Figure 3–12. *A, Connecting veins between the internal and external jugular vein often need to be ligated. The vertical incision is in the fascia surrounding the sternocleidomastoid. Cushing vein retractors are used for superior and inferior retraction. B, The carotid is palpated after sternocleidomastoid release. An appendiceal retractor exposes the middle layer of the cervical fascia. (From Albert TJ, Balderston RA, Northrup BE: Surgical Approaches to the Spine. Philadelphia, WB Saunders, 1997.)*

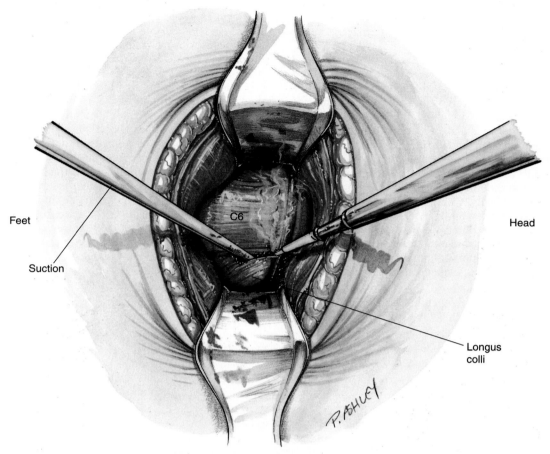

Figure 3–13. *The longus colli being elevated with cautery with hand-held retractors in place. (From Albert TJ, Balderston RA, Northrup BE: Surgical Approaches to the Spine. Philadelphia, WB Saunders, 1997.)*

the levels to be operated on. We palpate for the carotid tubercle to delineate C6 and always obtain an intraoperative x-ray. Once the surgical level is determined and exposed, electrocautery is used to subperiosteally dissect the longus colli, beginning at the vertebral body above and below that disk space and then connecting the dissection so that the longus colli is well elevated (Fig. 3–13). Self-retaining retractors are placed, with care taken to place the teeth under the longus colli in a mediolateral direction. A vertically oriented smooth-bladed retractor is also placed (Fig. 3–14).

This approach can be used for multilevel corpectomy by making an oblique incision along the anterior border of the sternocleidomastoid, dissecting off the fascia close to the sternocleidomastoid, and bluntly dissecting up and down the spine. If the upper thoracic spine must be approached and the clavicle is obstructing access, then a modified cervicothoracic approach is possible. Alternatively, a sternotomy can be performed, but this carries the added morbidity associated with entering the chest cavity.

MODIFIED ANTERIOR APPROACH TO THE CERVICOTHORACIC JUNCTION

This approach requires an understanding of the anatomy of the cervicothoracic junction, which is essentially the anatomy of the thoracic inlet. The top of the sternum (manubrium) articulates with the two clavicular heads. Immediately posterior to this lie the subclavian vein and artery. The sternocleidomastoid inserts onto the sternal manubrium (sternal head) and clavicle (clavicular head) (Fig. 3–15). Posterior to this, at the root of the neck, the junction of the internal jugular vein into the brachiocephalic vein on the left is apparent. The thoracic duct is at the cervicothoracic junction but lateral to the carotid system. Keeping the dissection medial to the carotid system ensures avoidance of injury to the thoracic duct. Identification of the sternocleidomastoid and the space behind it (Burn's space) will lead the surgeon to the thoracic inlet. Finger dissection behind the sternocleidomastoid and in front of the carotid sheath protects the vessels and creates the potential space. The cupula of the lung lies inferior and adjacent to the thoracic inlet bilaterally.

Patient positioning is similar to that for the anterolateral approach to the middle and lower cervical spine, with a longitudinal rolled-up towel placed between the patient's scapulae. The patient's head is turned to the right side opposite the approach. Preparation and draping is lower on the chest than in our standard cervical exposures. We perform this approach on the left side given the consistency of the recurrent laryngeal nerve on that side. An angled skin incision is made with the transverse limb beginning 1 to 2 inches proximal to the left clavicle (Fig. 3–16).

The incision extends from the medial half of the sternocleidomastoid to the midline of the neck. The vertical limb extends distally to point just past the junction of the manubrium and sternum from its starting point at the medial edge of the transverse portion of the incision. After an incision is made into this subcutaneous tissue, the platysma is incised in line with the skin incision, and the subplatysmal flaps are raised. The medial supraclavicular nerve and external jugular vein are apparent at this point. In some

cases, the external jugular vein must be sacrificed for improved exposure. The clavicular and manubrial heads of the sternocleidomastoid are sharply detached off the distal attachments to bone and retracted proximally. The strap muscles are carefully cut deep to the clavicle and elevated proximally and medially (see Fig. 3–15). The remainder of the periosteum is stripped from the medial third of the left clavicle and the left half of the manubrium. A Gigli saw is carefully passed under the clavicle at the junction of the middle and medial third (Fig. 3–17). After the clavicle is cut, the medial third of the clavicle is disarticulated from the manubrium. The interval between the carotid sheath and sternocleidomastoid laterally and the trachea and esophagus medially is now further delineated using blunt dissection. Hand-held Richardson retractors are used to retract the tracheoesophagus medially and the carotid sheath laterally, exposing the spinal column. Self-retaining retractors are not useful in this situation, given the size and depth of the exposure (Fig. 3–18). The longus colli can be elevated subperiosteally as described earlier.

This exposure is extremely useful if an upper thoracic exposure is needed. The resected clavicle acts as a good structural bone graft. Theoretical risks include shoulder

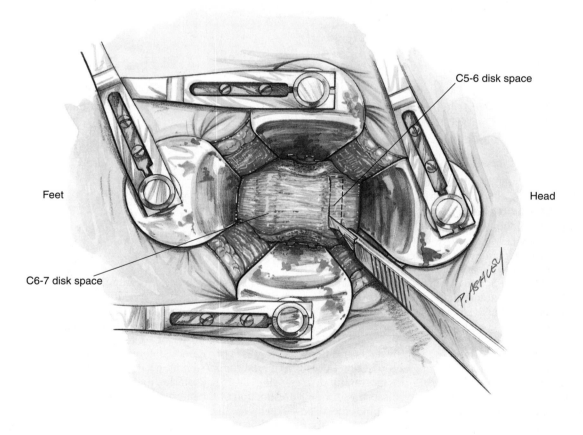

Feet

C5-6 disk space

Head

C6-7 disk space

Figure 3–14. *Self-retaining Cloward retractors in place with toothed retractors under the longus colli in the medial lateral direction. The longitudinal retractors are smooth retractors. The toothed retractors are held down with a Kocher clamp fastened to the drape (out of view of the picture) on the esophageal side (usually the patient's right). (From Albert TJ, Balderston RA, Northrup BE: Surgical Approaches to the Spine. Philadelphia, WB Saunders, 1997.)*

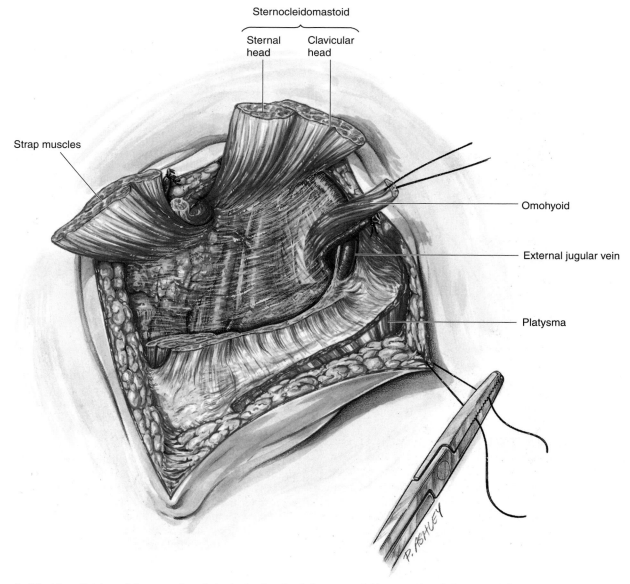

Figure 3–15. *After division of the sternal and clavicular heads of the sternocleidomastoid and division of the strap muscles. The omohyoid is also seen divided. (From Albert TJ, Balderston RA, Northrup BE: Surgical Approaches to the Spine. Philadelphia, WB Saunders, 1997.)*

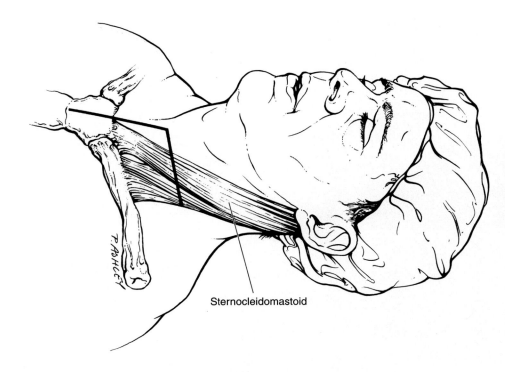

Sternocleidomastoid

Figure 3–16. Incision line for the modified anterior cervicothoracic approach. (From Albert TJ, Balderston RA, Northrup BE: Surgical Approaches to the Spine. Philadelphia, WB Saunders, 1997.)

girdle problems from resection of the proximal clavicle, as well as potential injury to the vessels of the thoracic inlet.

POSTERIOR CERVICAL EXPOSURES

Posterior cervical exposure is quite different than the anterior approach. There are very few vital structures between the skin and the spine, and a midline exposure in a longitudinal fashion through the ligamentum nuchae is performed. This exposure is usually bloodless and truly internervous, thus preventing denervation of the musculature. Bony landmarks are the key to a limited dissection. The spinous processes are most prominent at C2, C7, and T1. The ligamentum nuchae, a fibrous septum with few elastic fibers, inserts on the spinous processes and the cervical paraspinal muscles and provides minimal support. The ligamentum nuchae acts as the primary origin or insertion point for most of the muscles of the posterior neck (Fig. 3–19). Most of the muscles of the upper cervical spine attach to the spinous process of C2. These should be preserved if C2 is not involved with the decompression or fusion procedure, to prevent instability at C2–C3 and/or kyphosis.

The course of the vertebral arteries in the upper cervical spine should be well understood before dissection of the upper cervical spine is undertaken. The course of the artery along the posterior arch of C1 makes it prone to injury if the dissection strays more than 1.5 cm (1 cm in a child) from the midline of the posterior tubercle. Slippage into the interlaminar space along the posterior aspect of the spine can cause a dural tear or neurologic injury (Fig. 3–20).

Positioning for posterior cervical approaches usually involves placing the patient in Mayfield tongs in the prone position (Fig. 3–21) or in a halo vest prone and padded. It is important to stay strictly in the midline through the ligamentum nuchae to keep the dissection bloodless. Strict subperiosteal dissection allows for this. Given the bifid nature of the spinous processes of the cervical spine, the surgeon can err into the paraspinal musculature, causing significant increased bleeding. When dissection is done laterally along the lamina, a "hill" will be encountered that represents the lateral mass. This includes the facet joint. Dissection should be performed very carefully at the lateral edge of the joint, because the nerve root and vertebral artery lie anterior to the spinolamellar membrane of the adjoining transverse process. Overaggressive dissection or lateral stripping may damage the nerve root and/or vertebral artery (Fig. 3–22). Cerebellar retractors are usually adequate for retracting the thickened musculature of the posterior neck.

CONCLUSION

In cervical spine surgery, a thorough knowledge of anatomy is paramount to obtaining safe and atraumatic exposure. The anterior neck contains multiple structures important for swallowing and speech functions. Careful avoidance of these structures and a knowledge of the fascial planes allows for an atraumatic exposure that can be limited or extensive. Although the posterior neck has many less visceral components, dissection in the midline is necessary to maintain a bloodless exposure. Finally, respect for the neural elements during positioning, retraction, and reconstructive surgery is of utmost importance. Attention to these details will allow successful access to the entire anterior and posterior cervical spine as well as to the cervicothoracic junction. *Text continued on page 39*

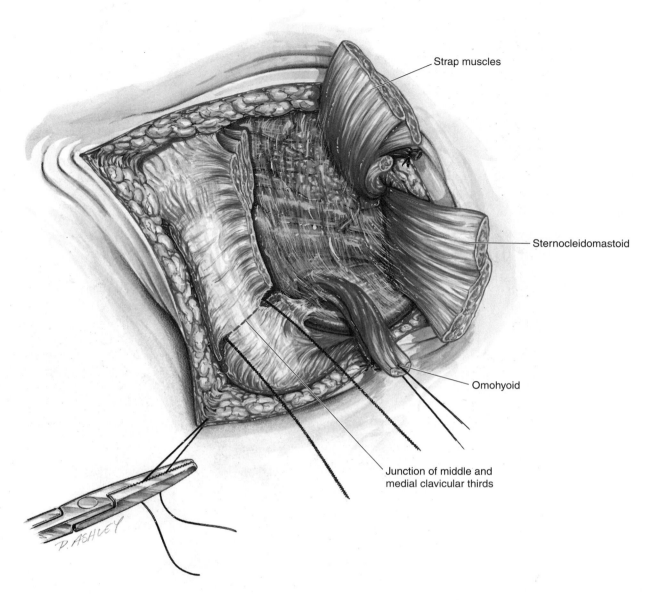

Figure 3–17. *A Gigli saw is used to cut the clavicle at the junction of the middle and medial thirds. Care is taken to avoid injury to the closely apposed subclavian vein. (From Albert TJ, Balderston RA, Northrup BE: Surgical Approaches to the Spine. Philadelphia, WB Saunders, 1997.)*

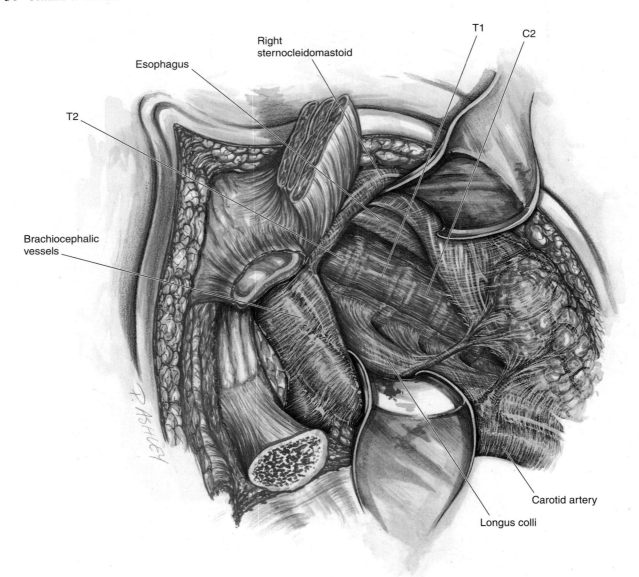

Figure 3–18. *After dissection of the deep layers of the cervical fascia, exposure of the cervicothoracic junction is facilitated with Richardson retractors. Self-retaining retractors should not be used. (From Albert TJ, Balderston RA, Northrup BE: Surgical Approaches to the Spine. Philadelphia, WB Saunders, 1997.)*

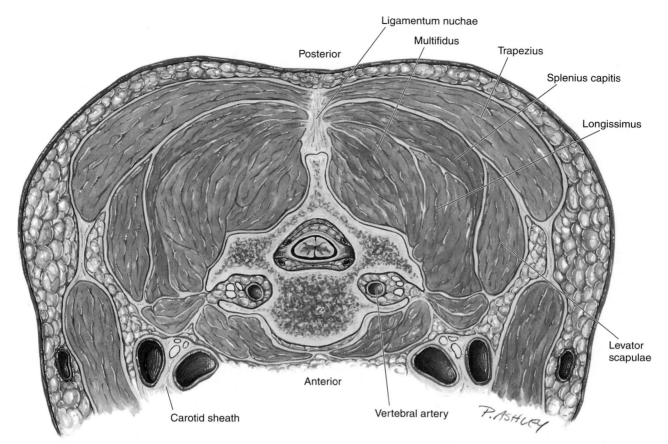

Figure 3–19. *A cross-section of the neck shows the direct midline approach to the cervical spine and the attachments of the paraspinal muscles to the posterior tubercle and ligamentum nuchae. The individual muscle layers are bound by the cervical fascial layers, which all attach to the ligamentum nuchae. Note the paucity of vital structures that are encountered posteriorly. (From Albert TJ, Balderston RA, Northrup BE: Surgical Approaches to the Spine. Philadelphia, WB Saunders, 1997.)*

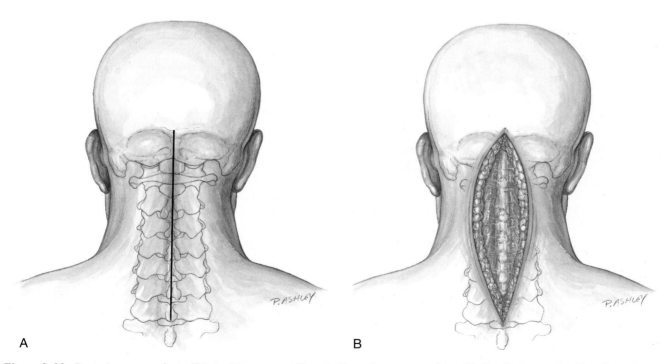

Figure 3–20. *Posterior approach. A, Skin incision over midline. B, Extensive exposure from C2 distally is very dry if performed by splitting the ligamentum nuchae. (From Albert TJ, Balderston RA, Northrup BE: Surgical Approaches to the Spine. Philadelphia, WB Saunders, 1997.)*

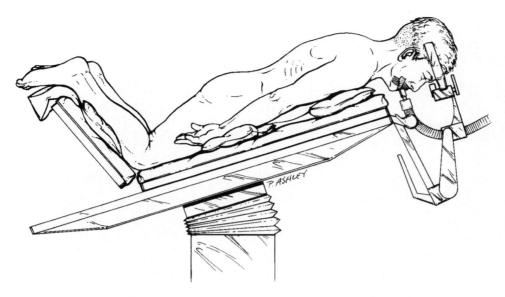

Figure 3–21. *The position for most posterior cervical spine surgery is the reverse Trendelenburg position. Note the head tongs or holder to stabilize the head and neck. The chest should be supported by rolls to allow expansion, and the knees should be bent to relax the sciatic nerve and stabilize the patient. (From Albert TJ, Balderston RA, Northrup BE: Surgical Approaches to the Spine. Philadelphia, WB Saunders, 1997.)*

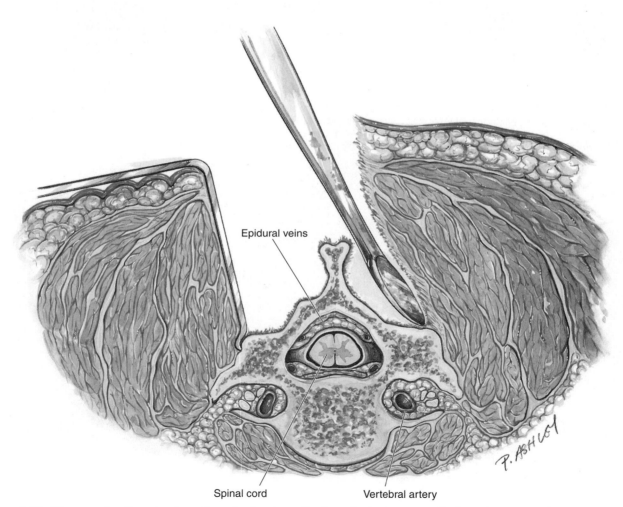

Epidural veins

Spinal cord

Vertebral artery

Figure 3–22. *The posterior dissection is performed subperiosteally along the lamina out to the lateral margin of the lateral masses. The paraspinal muscles are removed unilaterally or bilaterally as needed. Note the single Taylor retractor on the border of the lateral mass for a unilateral approach. (From Albert TJ, Balderston RA, Northrup BE: Surgical Approaches to the Spine. Philadelphia, WB Saunders, 1997.)*

REFERENCES

1. An HS, Gordin R, Renner K: Anatomic considerations for plate-screw fixation of the cervical spine. Spine 16:S548–S551, 1991.
2. Arbit E, Patterson RH Jr: Combined transoral and median labiomandibular glossotomy approach to the upper cervical spine. Neurosurgery 8:672–674, 1981.
3. Ashraf J, Crockard HA: Transoral fusion for high cervical fractures. J Bone Joint Surg Br 72:76–79, 1990.
4. Fielding JW, Buerstein AH, Frankel VH: The nuchal ligament. Spine 1:3–14, 1976.
5. Henry AK: Extensile Exposure. New York, Churchill Livingstone, 1957, pp 53–80.
6. Krespi YP, Har-El G: The transmandibular-transcervical approach to the skull base. In Sekhar LN, Janecka IP (eds): Surgery of Cranial Base Tumors. New York, Raven, 1993, pp 261–265.
7. Kurz LT, Pursel S, Herkowitz HN: Modified anterior approach to the cervicothoracic junction. Spine 16:S542–S547, 1991.
8. McAfee PC, Bohlman HH, Riley LH, et al: The anterior pharyngeal approach to the upper part of the cervical spine. J Bone Joint Surg Am 69:1371–1383, 1987.
9. Robinson RA, Smith GW: Anterolateral cervical disc removal and interbody fusions for cervical disk syndrome. Bull Johns Hopkins Hosp 96:223–224, 1955.
10. Southwick WO, Robinson RA: Recent advances in surgery of the cervical spine. Surg Clin North Am 41:1661–1683, 1961.
11. Stauffer ES: Open-mouth and transmandibular approaches to the cervical spine. In Sherk HH (ed): The Cervical Spine: An Atlas of Surgical Procedures. Philadelphia, JB Lippincott, 1993, pp 79–91.
12. Verbiest H: Anterolateral operations for fractures and dislocations in the middle and lower parts of the cervical spine. J Bone Joint Surg Am 51:1489–1530, 1969.
13. Whitesides TE Jr, Kelly RP: Lateral approach to the upper cervical spine for anterior fusion. South Med J 59:879–883, 1966.
14. Whitesides TE Jr, McDonald P: Lateral retropharyngeal approach to the upper cervical spine. Orthop Clin North Am 9:115–127, 1978.

4

ANTERIOR CERVICAL RECONSTRUCTION AND INTERNAL FIXATION

Mark A. Fye, M.D.
Sanford E. Emery, M.D.

*Every generation laughs at the old fashions, but
follows religiously the new.*
— Henry David Thoreau

HISTORICAL PERSPECTIVE

Although Bailey and Badgley,[4] Smith and Robinson,[50] and Cloward[14] developed interbody fusion techniques for degenerative conditions of the cervical spine in the 1950s, these techniques proved less useful over multiple segments. In 1976, Whitecloud and LaRocca[55] were the first to report the use of a fibular strut graft for reconstructive surgery of the cervical spine after multiple-level corpectomy. This study indicated that fibular cortical bone was acceptable as an alternative for cervical spine fusion for multiple-level disease. Other, later studies have confirmed the use of fibula struts in this patient population.[6, 15] In 1981, Abe et al.[1] described the use of bone graft taken from the ilium for reconstruction of the cervical spine in patients with ossification of the posterior longitudinal ligament (OPLL). Since that time, Boni et al.,[10] Hanai et al.,[24] and Yonenobu et al.[56] have reported on the use of a tricortical iliac strut graft for stabilization after anterior cervical decompression. Because of the morbidity associated with either iliac or fibular graft harvest, in 1991 Fernyhough et al.[18] investigated the success of fusion with allograft versus autograft fibula for cervical spine reconstruction. Although the use of allograft bone eliminated harvest site morbidity, the lower fusion rate continued to be problematic.

Evolution of Anterior Internal Fixation

As internal fixation of long bones developed in the 1960s and 1970s, anterior fixation for spine fractures was described by Böhler in 1965 for vertebral body fractures[8] and by Nakanishi et al. in 1982 for odontoid fractures.[36] These techniques spread to North America in the 1980s, and various authors have reported on the use of screw fixation for treatment of type II odontoid fractures and anterior cervical plates for fractures, tumors, and degenerative conditions.[9, 13, 19–21, 26, 33, 37, 42, 47, 51]

Historically, acute fractures of the axis have been managed by closed reduction and halo vest immobilization.

Surgical treatment for these fractures was first proposed by Mixter and Osgood in 1910.[32] In concert with Nakanishi's description of anterior screw fixation for odontoid fractures, in 1982, Böhler reported good results for this technique for dens fractures.[7] In 1985, Clark and White reported on a multicenter study of anterior screw fixation for odontoid fractures grouped by the Anderson and D'Alonzo classification.[13] Other authors have reported excellent results in patients with acute type II and type III fractures as well as nonunions of the odontoid.[2, 11, 19, 21, 30, 33] Several authors have supported using two cancellous compression screws for the anterior fixation of odontoid fractures.[7, 17, 27, 29] However, others have suggested that one screw is sufficient to stabilize odontoid fractures.[17, 19, 30, 36]

In the 1970s, Herrmann,[26] Orozco and Llovet-Tapies,[37–39] and Senegas and Gauzère[47] reported on the use of small fragment plate and screws for internal fixation of anterior cervical spine fractures. In the 1980s, Böhler and Gaudernak,[9] Caspar,[12] Gassman and Seligson,[20] Morscher et al.,[34] and others[2, 34, 42, 44, 51] reported good results treating patients with cervical fractures using anterior screw plate fixation devices.

The first anterior plate devices included those in which the screw was placed through the plate and secured to either the anterior cortex or both the anterior and posterior cortex. Several authors recommended routinely obtaining purchase of the posterior cortex to prevent screw loosening and potential esophageal dysfunction.[35, 41, 57] Newer plate fixation devices include a locking device to prevent the screws from backing out from the plate; these devices do not require purchase of the posterior cortex of the vertebral body. Unicortical screw techniques have hopefully reduced the possibility of iatrogenic neurologic injury when using bicortical techniques.

Strut Graft Substitutes

Polymethylmethacrylate (PMMA) was initially used for spinal problems by Knight in 1959.[28] In 1984, Asnis et al.[3] reported using PMMA with a bone bolt after anterior decompression of the cervical spine for pathologic fractures. In 1986, McAfee et al.[31] in 1986 reported on the major disadvantages of using PMMA in the anterior cervical spine. In 1993, Shono et al.[48] also showed in a biomechanical study that PMMA loosens at the bone–cement interface.

Recently, carbon fiber–reinforced cages have been added to the armamentarium for reconstruction of the cervical spine after anterior decompression. In 1993, Shono et al.[48] demonstrated in a biomechanical study that these carbon fiber–reinforced cages demonstrated more rigidity in flexion/extension than PMMA or iliac strut grafts. More recently, titanium mesh cages, ceramics and cervical threaded cylinder cages have been developed for reconstruction of the anterior cervical spine. The indications for these devices are presently evolving and require continued biomechanical as well as clinical study to determine their appropriate use in cervical spine reconstruction.

INDICATIONS AND TECHNIQUES

This section focuses on the indications for and techniques of anterior cervical reconstruction after a single-level or multilevel corpectomy. Indications for single-level or multilevel corpectomy include (1) compressive pathology behind the body that cannot be decompressed through the disk space alone, be it osteophytes, OPLL, fracture, or tumor; (2) three- or four-level diskectomy procedures in situations where using multiple Robinson-type grafts has an unacceptable nonunion rate; and (3) correction of cervical kyphosis.

Generally, iliac crest strut grafts are used for single-level corpectomy unless severe osteopenia is present, in which case a fibular strut graft may be used. Iliac crest grafting is acceptable for a two-level corpectomy, though we favor fibula grafting for multilevel corpectomy procedures.

Anterior Plating

Since the early 1980s, many devices have been developed to improve the stabilization of the anterior cervical spine. Surgical indications for internal plate fixation of the anterior cervical spine include trauma, degenerative conditions, and tumors. For patients with a burst fracture or flexion-teardrop injury requiring an anterior corpectomy and reconstruction with a strut graft, a cervical plate will allow stabilization through the same approach (Fig. 4–1). This may obviate the need for postoperative halo vest immobilization or a posterior stabilization procedure.

Recently, several authors have described the use of anterior plate fixation devices for degenerative conditions of the cervical spine.[20, 25, 42, 51] Degenerative conditions such as disk herniation, spondylosis with radiculopathy and/or myelopathy, congenital spinal stenosis, and spondylolisthesis are a few of the conditions of the cervical spine that have traditionally undergone arthrodesis without internal fixation; however, the addition of anterior cervical screw plate fixation devices may be appropriate. The indications for use of internal fixation in these degenerative conditions are still evolving, but some guidelines will be proposed.

Anterior plating of a single-level cervical diskectomy and fusion is not always needed, or recommended, based on the high fusion rate associated with this operation. Wang et al. published a study noting no difference in fusion rates for single-level diskectomy and autogenous bone-grafted patients with or without a plate.[54A] Some clinical studies have shown the efficacy of anterior cervical plates for two-level anterior cervical diskectomy and fusion,[14A, 47A, 54] with the added benefit of decreased bracing requirements. With the increased pseudarthrosis rate associated with three-level anterior cervical diskectomy and fusion, anterior plate fixation is recommended by some investigators[16, 54B] (Fig. 4–2) but not by others.[9A] Anterior cervical plate fixation may also be used to facilitate anterior fusion for the repair of a pseudarthrosis.[51A] Other relative indications for anterior cervical plating in degenerative conditions include patients undergoing corpectomy for spondylotic myelopathy or OPLL. We use anterior plates routinely following single-level corpectomy and strut graft procedures as well as some two-level corpectomy and strut grafting procedures, provided good bone stock is available for screw purchase. For three-level corpectomy and fusion procedures, however, we prefer to avoid anterior plate fixation, as the results to date have been mixed.[40, 52] Anterior plating may also be indicated for reconstruction of the cervical spine following corpectomy for tumors, providing increased stability in potentially very unstable situations.

Another type of anterior device is an anti-kick plate (Fig. 4–3). This is a small T-type plate secured with screws to the inferior vertebral docking site of the strut graft to help prevent graft dislodgment anteriorly without maintaining distraction. Indications for this technique are evolving,[53] although there is some risk of soft tissue or airway impingement if the plate displaces anteriorly.[43]

Odontoid Screws

Halo immobilization continues to be the treatment for most nondisplaced odontoid fractures. Displaced type II and shallow type III fractures (Anderson and D'Alonzo classification) have been problematic, with reported nonunion rates of 15% to 85%.[33] Alternative surgical options have been developed in an attempt to decrease the nonunion rates in these fractures. Several factors have been reported to identify the potential for odontoid fracture nonunion. In 1985 Hadley et al. reported a 67% nonunion rate in odontoid fractures displaced more than 6 mm, but only a 10% rate with displacement less than 4 mm.[23] In 1975 Schatzker et al. reported that patients with posterior displacement of the odontoid are more prone to nonunion than patients with anterior displacement.[46] They also stated that patients over 50 years old have an increased risk of nonunion. In 1985 Clark and White reported that odontoid fractures angulated more than 10 degrees have an increased rate of nonunion.[13]

In 1982 Böhler described using two screws to treat odontoid fractures because of the theoretical biomechanical advantages over one screw.[7] Since that time, Aebi et al.,[2] ElSaghir and Böhm,[14B] Jeanneret et al.,[27] and Knoringer[29] have supported using two small cancellous compression screws for the anterior fixation of odontoid fractures. However, others, including Esses and Bednar,[17] Fujii et al.,[19] Lesoin et al.,[30] and Nakanishi et al.,[36] advocate one screw for anterior fixation of odontoid fractures. In 1993 Graziano et al.[22] and Sasso et al.[45] compared one- and two-screw techniques for odontoid fracture fixation. Results showed no significant differences

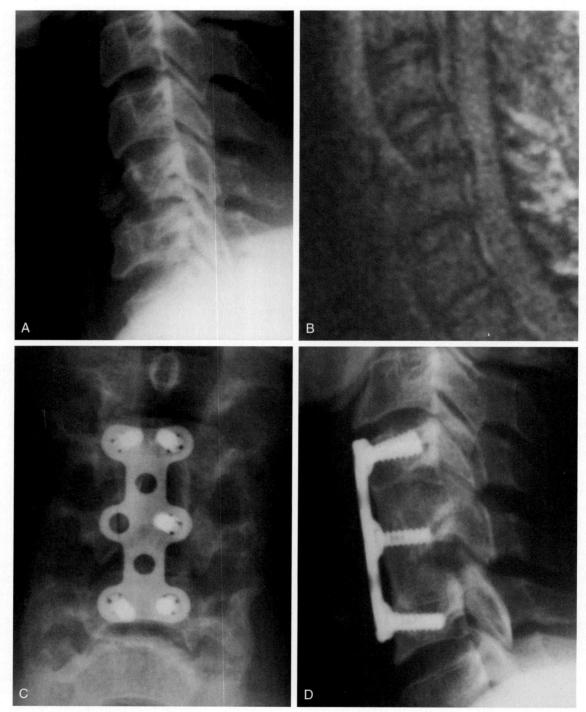

Figure 4–1. *A 22-year-old male sustained a C5 flexion-teardrop fracture with complete quadriplegia after a diving accident. A, The lateral plain film demonstrates the fractured vertebra with retrolisthesis of C5 on C6. B, A sagittal MRI shows spinal cord impingement due to the fracture with retrolisthesis of the C5 body. Anteroposterior (C) and lateral (D) plain films taken 1 year after a C5 corpectomy and iliac strut fusion with anterior plating were performed for decompression and stabilization of the fracture. The patient was treated postoperatively in a Philadelphia collar. Nerve root recovery did occur at the C6 level, but he is still quadriplegic.*

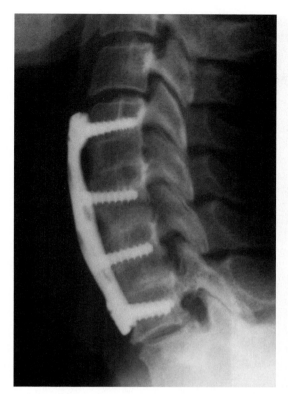

Figure 4–2. Lateral x-ray of a three-level anterior cervical diskectomy and fusion with plating. Segmental fixation has been achieved, and the grafts have progressed to successful arthrodesis.

between using one screw or two screws for anterior fixation of odontoid fractures.

Direct anterior screw fixation of odontoid fractures allows open reduction if needed and internal fixation while preserving C1–C2 rotation. The indications for anterior screw fixation for odontoid fractures have continued to evolve and remain controversial in the literature. Primary fracture patterns for which anterior screw fixation is considered are displaced type II and shallow type III odontoid fractures, because of their greater nonunion rate. Optimal indications for anterior screw fixation for acute odontoid fractures include an unreducible odontoid fracture requiring open reduction, a second fracture requiring anterior decompression and stabilization (see Fig. 4–7), an odontoid fracture associated with a C1 laminar fracture, and fractures in patients for whom use of a halo vest is contraindicated.

For nonunions of odontoid fractures, the indications for direct anterior screw fixation remain controversial. In 1982, Böhler concluded that patients with odontoid nonunion should be treated with anterior and posterior arthrodesis.[7] In 1991, however, Montesano et al. obtained good results treating nonunions using anterior screw fixation and curettage of the nonunion with grafting.[33] Contraindications to anterior screw fixation of odontoid fractures include rupture of the transverse and C1 ligament (rare), fractures from pathologic or osteoporotic bone that prevents solid screw purchase, and os odontoideum. An oblique fracture pattern that does not allow the fracture site to compress with

screw fixation is a relative contraindication, especially if the fracture line parallels the direction of the screw. Finally, anterior screw fixation is not recommended in those patients with nonunions where the fracture site cannot be curetted and bone grafted anteriorly.

Anterior Bilateral C1–C2 Facet Arthrodesis

The typical approach for atlantoaxial arthrodesis has been and continues to be posterior bone grafting with some type of internal fixation. If a posterior approach is less attractive, such as in failed arthrodesis attempts, in postlaminectomy patients with minimal surface to graft, or in patients requiring an anterior approach to address other levels, then an anterior facet fusion of C1 and C2 may be desirable.[30] A high retropharyngeal approach to the upper cervical spine is used, the atlantoaxial facet joints are denuded of cartilage under direct vision, and the joints are packed with cancellous graft. Two screws aimed superiorly and laterally are placed through C2 up into the lateral masses of C1 to provide stability (Fig. 4–4). A 3.5- or 4.0-mm screw approximately 25 mm long is satisfactory.

A related alternative to posterior fusion is lateral atlantoaxial arthrodesis. This method requires separate bilateral incisions to obtain bone grafting and screw fixation aimed posteroinferiorly through the C1 facet into C2.[5, 49] This alternative approach can be considered for unusual salvage situations requiring atlantoaxial fusion.

Alternative Surgical Procedures
Anterior Cervical Reconstruction

Reconstruction alternatives after single-level or multilevel corpectomy include allograft iliac or fibular strut grafts, PMMA, and titanium cages filled with bone graft. In patients with multilevel diskectomies and vertebrectomies

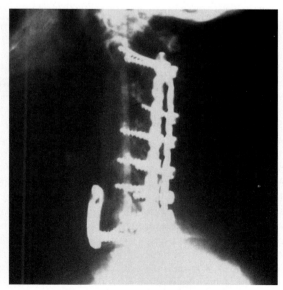

Figure 4–3. A lateral plain film example of an anterior anti–kick plate device. (Courtesy of Dr. Todd Albert.)

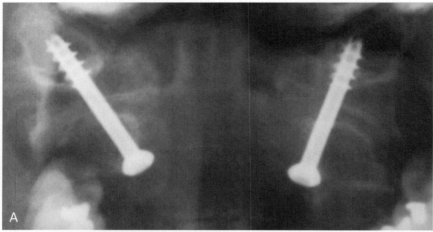

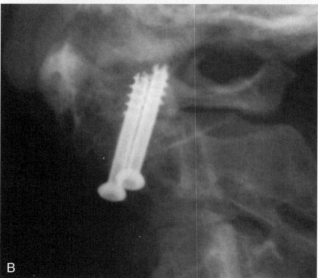

Figure 4–4. A 57-year-old male with postlaminectomy kyphosis requiring anterior corpectomy and strut grafting also had C1–C2 instability. Anteroposterior (A) and lateral (B) postoperative radiographs demonstrates anterior screw fixation with cancellous bone grafting for atlantoaxial arthrodesis.

for spondylosis, Fernyhough et al. reported a 41% nonunion rate using allograft fibular strut graft compared to a 27% nonunion rate using autografts.[18] Their technique uses a notched fibula resting on the anterior lip of the vertebra, rather than centralized as in our recommended technique. Fernyhough et al. also noted that the nonunion rate increases as more motion segments are fused.[18] Zdeblick et al. studied the fusion rate of autogenous bone versus allograft bone for three-level anterior cervical diskectomy and fusion in a goat model.[58] Their results supported an increased fusion rate of autogenous bone graft for cervical spine fusions.

PMMA and, recently, titanium cages filled with either PMMA or autogenous bone graft have been used to reconstruct the cervical spine after corpectomy for tumor. Generally, we prefer to use autogenous strut grafts for these procedures; however, in tumor patients, if the prognosis is poor with expected survival of less than 6 months, then PMMA as well as titanium cages may be appropriate and generally have had good success. More long-term data are needed to support the use of these surgical treatment alternatives following corpectomy in various patient populations.

Internal Fixation

Surgical treatment alternatives for anterior cervical plating include using no plate if the spine is not unstable, as in routine degenerative conditions; increasing the rigidity of postoperative immobilization devices (such as a halo vest); and performing posterior stabilization procedures (e.g., triple wire technique, posterior lateral mass plating) after anterior cervical strut graft placement.[16A] Excellent stability can be achieved with posterior fixation, but the obvious drawback is the need for a second approach to the spine.

Odontoid Screw Fixation

Alternative treatments for odontoid fracture include techniques of cervical orthoses, including use of a halo vest, and posterior atlantoaxial arthrodesis. Gallie and Brooks wiring techniques are commonly used, as is the more recently developed transarticular screw fixation. More unusual anterior or lateral atlantoaxial facet grafting with screw fixation as described earlier may also be considered.

PREFERRED TECHNIQUES

Single-Level and Multilevel Strut Grafting

Iliac strut grafting is generally used with single-level corpectomy, and fibular strut grafting is used with multilevel corpectomy. The decompression technique for single-level and multilevel corpectomy is described in Chapter 9. For all patients, intraoperative monitoring of the cervical spinal cord is highly recommended. We prefer a left-sided surgical approach, using a transverse incision. Intraoperative traction is used and generally is increased to 15 or 20 lb after successful anterior decompression. Once the spinal cord has been decompressed anteriorly, the neck may be extended to correct kyphosis.

The bone grafting technique is critical for success in multilevel strut fusions. The cephalad and caudal endplates of the inferior and superior vertebral bodies must be removed to expose bleeding subchondral bone. Using a burr, the body is sculpted into a flat surface centrally where the graft will seat. Anterior and posterior lips are constructed to prevent graft dislodgement. The graft must be measured precisely and the ends of the graft contoured to fit the endplate docking sites. The superior end of the strut graft is inserted first, the traction is manually increased by the anesthesiologist, and, finally, the graft is tapped in inferiorly until it is seated posterior to the anterior lip of the vertebral body (Fig. 4–5). The ideal position of the lower pole of the graft is adjacent to the posterior lip; this centralizes axial load stress and minimizes the risk of fracture of the anterior aspect of the body. An intraoperative lateral x-ray is needed to check the position of the graft before wound closure. Caspar screw post distractors may be used for single-level corpectomy to distract and thus facilitate graft placement.

Whether the anterior cortex of an iliac tricortical strut graft should be placed anterior or posterior remains controversial; we have used both methods successfully. If plate fixation is used, the cortical face of the iliac strut allows for screw purchase into the graft. Although the fibula does not pose the same issues as an iliac crest strut graft, generally the flat surface of the fibula is placed posteriorly to allow maximum room for the decompressed spinal canal.

Anterior Plate Fixation

We generally prefer to use anterior cervical plate fixation in cases of multilevel anterior cervical diskectomy and fusion, single-level corpectomy with iliac strut graft, and some two-level corpectomy and fibula strut graft cases. The cervical plate generally extends from the midbody of the superior and inferior noninvolved vertebral bodies, and it must be contoured to the anterior spine

to allow maximum contact. Care should be taken to maintain proper orientation of the plate to stay midline. Identification of the lateral borders of the vertebral bodies and the strut graft will help keep the plate midline. An intraoperative anteroposterior x-ray may be taken if necessary but is not done routinely. Before plate fixation, the traction must be removed to avoid locking the graft in a distracted construct. Screws generally are not used to secure a fibular graft to the plate, because of the risk of weakening the graft; however, one screw can be safely added in the cortical face of an iliac strut after a single-level corpectomy. In multilevel diskectomy and fusion with plating, it is ideal to obtain segmental fixation of as many vertebral bodies as is allowed by screw hole placement for maximum stability.

When placing the screws into the vertebral bodies, care should be taken not to penetrate the endplate into the adjacent disk above or below the strut graft. This is particularly important to note at the lower level, because of the angle of the disk spaces (Fig. 4–6). Before drilling and tapping the screws, an x-ray can be done to determine optimum plate length before final fixation. A second x-ray is certainly done to check the final position of the instrumentation.

Many anterior plate fixation systems are available for use after cervical reconstruction procedures. Generally, 4.0-mm to 4.35-mm screws are used to fix the plate to the vertebral bodies. Screw length should be determined from the preoperative lateral radiograph of the cervical spine, but usually 14- to 16-mm screws are used. Locking mechanisms are recommended for plates that use unicortical screws.

Odontoid Screw Fixation

Treatment for acute odontoid fractures begins with prompt reduction and halo vest immobilization. If the fracture fails to reduce or if it fails to maintain reduction with halo traction, then operative stabilization is required. Before surgical stabilization, a computed tomography (CT) scan is obtained for thorough preoperative planning (Fig. 4–7). The size of the dens is measured to determine whether one screw or (preferably) two screws can be placed. The patient is placed supine with a halo or Gardner-Wells tongs with approximately 10 to 20 lb of longitudinal traction. Before surgical stabilization, nasotracheal intubation is performed by the anesthesiologist to decrease manipulation of the cervical spine. Reduction of the odontoid process may be indirect (by providing halo traction) or direct (by mobilizing the odontoid process) and should be performed using x-ray. The head should be held anterior and extended in the so-called "sniff" position to maintain reduction. A radiolucent head holder helps visualize the reduction and screw placement. A standard transverse incision is made at the C5 level to allow an adequate angle for screw insertion. The atlas and axis are identified with x-ray, and the anterior tubercle of C2 is palpated. The body of C2, the C2–C3 disk space, and the fracture site of the odontoid (if open reduction is necessary) are dissected of all soft tissues. Appendiceal-

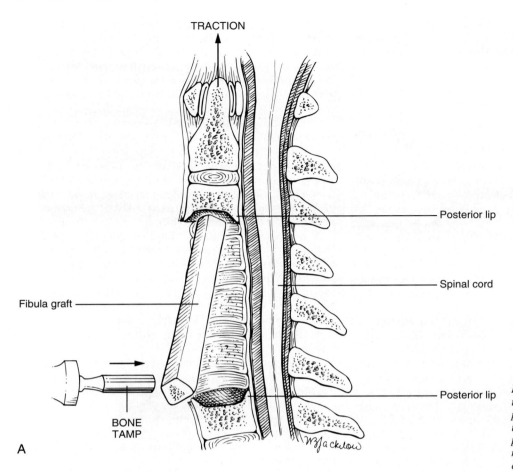

A

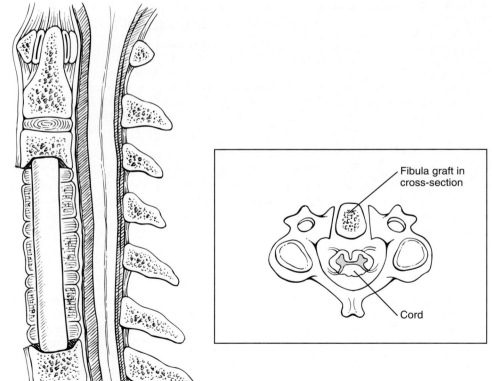

B

Figure 4–5. *A and B, Illustrations of fibular strut graft placement. Note that the docking sites have anterior and posterior lips to prevent graft migration. The fibula is centered in the vertebrae above and below.*

Figure continued on following page

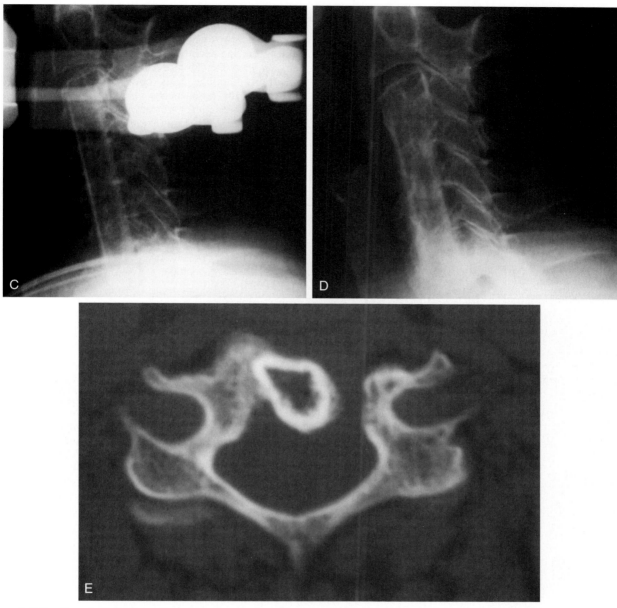

Figure 4–5 Continued. *C, An immediate postoperative lateral x-ray of a fibular strut graft from C3 to C7. The patient is in a rigid two-poster brace. D, The same patient's lateral x-ray taken 2 years postoperatively shows solid union, bone remodeling, and maintenance of sagittal alignment. E, A postoperative CT scan shows spinal canal decompression, position of the fibula strut in cross-section, and healing of the graft to the wall of the vertebral body.*

type retractors are used for cephalad retraction. The anterior-inferior edge of the C2 body is the starting point for screw insertion.

Under biplanar (anteroposterior and lateral) x-ray (see Fig. 4–7), a 2.0-mm K-wire is inserted 3 mm from the midline, at the anterior-inferior edge of C2. The wire is advanced across the fracture site to the tip of the odontoid process. Two wires are placed to obtain rotational stability of the fracture. The K-wire should angle toward the midline and penetrate the posterior apex of the odontoid process. K-wire alignment should be checked in both anteroposterior and lateral planes with x-ray. The K-wire is measured, with the typical screw length approximately 40 mm. A cannulated 3.5-mm drill bit may be used over the K-wire to make a screw start hole. The hole is tapped,

and a 3.5- or 4.0-mm cannulated cancellous screw is placed over each K-wire, obtaining purchase of the far cortex. Screw threads should not cross the fracture site unless the lag technique is used. Care must be taken to ensure that the K-wire does not advance with screw insertion. Flexible drills and taps are useful in some patients with large necks. Under biplanar x-ray, each screw is checked for correct position and length. If the preoperative CT scan suggests inadequate size for placement of two screws, then one-screw fixation is used for stabilization. Postoperatively, depending on the stability of the screw fixation, a halo vest or cervicothoracic orthosis is used for approximately 2 months, or until bony union occurs. A nonunion occurring after this method should be treated with posterior atlantoaxial arthrodesis.

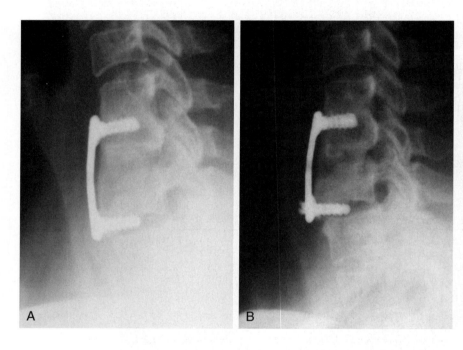

Figure 4–6. A, Lateral x-ray showing an inferior screw penetrating the adjacent endplate into the inferior disk. B, The patient went on to successful arthrodesis, but by 1 year postoperatively the screw had begun to migrate toward the esophagus. It was operatively removed shortly thereafter.

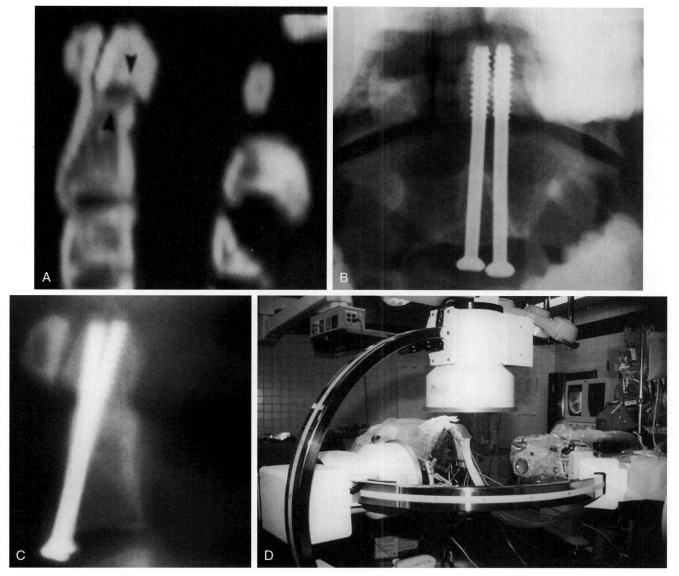

Figure 4–7. *A, A sagittal CT scan showing a moderately displaced odontoid fracture. This patient also had a C5 fracture requiring an anterior approach, so the surgeon elected to use screws to internally fix the dens during the same approach. A postoperative anteroposterior x-ray (B) and lateral CT scan (C) show the position of the odontoid screws and a healed fracture. Note the entry point at the anteroinferior edge of the C2 body, which allows the proper cephalad direction of the screws. D, Intraoperative setup for odontoid screw placement. Two x-ray machines provide anteroposterior and lateral spot views. This greatly facilitates safe and accurate positioning of the K-wires and cannulated screws.*

REFERENCES

1. Abe H, Tsuru M, Ito T, et al: Anterior decompression for ossification of the posterior longitudinal ligament of the cervical spine. J Neurosurg 55:108–116, 1981.
2. Aebi M, Zuber K, Marchesi D: Treatment of cervical spine injuries with anterior plating: Indications, techniques, and results. Spine 16:S38–S45, 1991.
3. Asnis SE, Lesniewski P, Dowling T Jr: Anterior decompression and stabilization with methylmethacrylate and a bone bolt for treatment of pathologic fractures of the cervical spine: A report of two cases. Clin Orthop 187:139–143, 1984.
4. Bailey RW, Badgley CE: Stabilization of the cervical spine by anterior fusion. J Bone Joint Surg Am 42A:565–594, 1960.
5. Barbour JR: Screw fixation and fractures of the odontoid process. S Aust Clin 5:20–24, 1971.
6. Bernard TN Jr, Whitecloud TS III: Cervical spondylotic myelopathy and myeloradiculopathy: Anterior decompression and stabilization with autogenous fibula strut graft. Clin Orthop 221:149–160, 1987.
7. Böhler J: Anterior stabilization for acute fractures and non-unions of the dens. J Bone Joint Surg Am 64A:18–27, 1982.
8. Böhler J: Fractures of the odontoid process. J Trauma 5:386–391, 1965.

9. Böhler J, Gaudernak T: Anterior plate stabilization for fracture-dislocations of the lower cervical spine. J Trauma 20:203–205, 1980.

9A. Bolesta MJ, Rechtine GR, Chrin AM: Three- and four-level anterior cervical diskectomy and fusion with plate fixation: A prospective study. Spine 25:2040–2044, 2000.

10. Boni M, Cherubino P, Denaro V, Benazzo F: Multiple subtotal somatectomy: Technique and evaluation of a series of 39 cases. Spine 9:358–362, 1984.

11. Borne GM, Bedou GL, Pinaudeau M, et al: Odontoid process fracture osteosynthesis with a direct screw fixation technique in nine consecutive cases. J Neurosurg 68:223–226, 1988.

12. Caspar W: Anterior cervical fusion and interbody stabilization with the trapezial osteosynthetic plate technique. Aesculap Scientific Information Leaflet S-039, Ed VII. Burlingame, CA, Aesculap Instruments Corp., 1986, p 36.

13. Clark CR, White AA III: Fractures of the dens. A multicenter study. J Bone Joint Surg 67A:1340–1348, 1985.

14. Cloward RB: The anterior approach for removal of ruptured cervical disks. J Neurosurg 15:602–617, 1958.

14A. Connolly PJ, Esses SI, Kostuik JP: Anterior cervical fusion: Outcome analysis of patients fused with and without anterior cervical plates. J Spinal Disord 9:202–206, 1996.

14B. ElSaghir H, Böhm H: Anderson type II fracture of the odontoid process: Results of anterior screw fixation. J Spinal Disord 13:527–530, 2000.

15. Emery SE, Bohlman HH, Bolesta MJ, Jones PK: Anterior cervical decompression and arthrodesis for the treatment of cervical spondylotic myelopathy. Two to seventeen-year follow-up. J Bone Joint Surg Am 80A:941–951, 1998.

16. Emery SE, Fisher R, Bohlman HH: Three-level anterior cervical diskectomy and fusion: Radiographic and clinical results. Spine 22:2622–2624, 1997.

16A. Epstein NE: The value of anterior cervical plating in preventing vertebral fracture and graft extrusion after multilevel anterior cervical corpectomy with posterior wiring and fusion: Indications, results and complications. J Spinal Disord 13:9–15, 2000.

17. Esses SI, Bednar DA: Screw fixation of odontoid fractures and nonunions. Spine 16:S483–S485, 1991.

18. Fernyhough JC, White JI, LaRocca H: Fusion rates in multilevel cervical spondylosis comparing allograft fibula with autograft fibula in 126 patients. Spine 16:S561–S564, 1991.

19. Fujii E, Kobayashi K, Hirabayashi K: Treatment in fractures of the odontoid process. Spine 13:604–609, 1988.

20. Gassman J, Seligson D: The anterior cervical plate. Spine 8:700–707, 1983.

21. Geisler FH, Cheng C, Poka A, Brumback RJ: Anterior screw fixation of posteriorly displaced type II odontoid fractures. Neurosurgery 25:30–38, 1989.

22. Graziano G, Jaggers C, Lee M, Lynch W: A comparative study of fixation techniques for type II fractures of the odontoid process. Spine 16:2383–2387, 1993.

23. Hadley MN, Browner C, Sonntag VKH: Axis fractures: A comprehensive review of management and treatment in 107 cases. Neurosurgery 17:281–290, 1985.

24. Hanai K, Fujiyoshi F, Kamei K: Subtotal vertebrectomy and spinal fusion for cervical spondylotic myelopathy. Spine 11:310–315, 1986.

25. Herkowitz H: Internal fixation for degenerative cervical spine disorders. Semin Spine Surg 7:57–60, 1995.

26. Herrmann HD: Metal plate fixation after anterior fusion of unstable fracture dislocations of the cervical spine. Acta Neurochir 32:101–111, 1975.

27. Jeanneret B, Vernet O, Frei S, Magerl F: Atlantoaxial mobility after screw fixation of the odontoid: A computed tomographic study. J Spinal Disord 4:203–211, 1991.

28. Knight G: Paraspinal acrylic inlays in the treatment of cervical and lumbar spondylosis and other conditions. Lancet 2:147–149, 1959.

29. Knoringer P: Double threaded compression screws in osteosynthesis of acute fractures of the odontoid process. In Voth D, Glees O (eds): Disease in the Craniocervical Junction, Vol 217. Berlin, de Gruyter, 1987.

30. Lesoin F, Autricque A, Franz K, et al: Transcervical approach and screw fixation for upper cervical spine pathology. Surg Neurol 27:459–465, 1987.

31. McAfee PC, Bohlman HH, Ducker T, Eismont FJ: Failure of stabilization of the spine with methylmethacrylate. J Bone Joint Surg Am 68A:1145–1157, 1986.

32. Mixter SJ, Osgood RB: Traumatic lesions of the atlas and axis. Ann Surg 51:193–207, 1910.

33. Montesano PX, Anderson PA, Schlehr F, et al: Odontoid fractures treated by anterior odontoid screw fixation. Spine 16:S33–S37, 1991.

34. Morscher E, Sutter F, Jenny H, Olerud S: Die vordere verplattung der halswirbelsaule mit dem hohlschrauben plattensystem aus titanium. Chirug 57:702–707, 1986.

35. Naito M, Kurose S, Oyama M, Sugioka Y: Anterior cervical fusion with the Caspar instrumentation system. Int Orthop 17:73–76, 1993.

36. Nakanishi T, Sasaki T, Tokita N, Hirabayashi K: Internal fixation for the odontoid fracture. Orthop Trans 6:176, 1982.

37. Orozco Delclos R, Llovet-Tapies J: Osteointesis en las fracturas de raquis cervical not de tecnica. Revista de Ortopedia y Traumatologica 14:285, 1970.

38. Orozco Delclos R, Llovet Tapies J: Osteosintesis en las lesiones traumaticas y degenerativas de la columna cervical. Revista Traumatol Cirurg Rehabil 1:45–52, 1971.

39. Orozco R: La artrodesis de la columna cervical. Presented at Congreso Torremolinos Hispano, Argentino, 1975.

40. Paramore CG, Dickman CA, Sonntag VK: Radiographic and clinical follow-up review of Caspar plates in 49 patients. J Neurosurg 84:957–961, 1996.

41. Randle MJ, Wolf A, Levi L, et al: The use of anterior Caspar plate fixation in acute cervical spine injury. Surg Neurol 36:181–189, 1991.

42. Rechtine GR, Cahill DW, Gruenberg M, Chrin AM: The Synthes cervical spine locking plate and screw system in anterior cervical fusion. Tech Orthop 9:86–91, 1994.

43. Riew KD, Sethi NS, Devney J, et al: Complications of buttress plate stabilization of cervical corpectomy. Spine 24:2404–2410, 1999.

44. Ripa DR, Kowall MG, Meyer PR Jr, Rusin JJ: Series of ninety-two traumatic cervical spine injuries stabilized with anterior ASIF plate fusion technique. Spine 16:S46–S55, 1991.

45. Sasso R, Doherty BJ, Crawford MJ, Heggeness MH: Biomechanics of odontoid fracture fixation: Comparison of the one- and two-screw technique. Spine 18:1950–1953, 1993.

46. Schatzker J, Rorabeck CH, Waddell JP: Non-union of the odontoid process: An experimental investigation. Clin Orthop 108:127–137, 1975.

47. Senegas J, Gauzère JM: Traitement des lésions cervicales par voie antérieure. Rev Chir Orthop 63:466–469, 1977.

47A. Shapiro S: Banked fibula and the locking anterior cervical plate in anterior cervical fusions following cervical discectomy. J Neurosurg 84:161–165, 1996.

48. Shono Y, McAfee PC, Cunningham BW, Brantigan JW: A biomechanical analysis of decompression and reconstruction

methods in the cervical spine. J Bone Joint Surg Am 75A:1674–1684, 1993.

49. Simmons EH, duToit G Jr: Lateral atlantoaxial arthrodesis. Orthop Clin North Am 9:1101–1114, 1978.

50. Smith GW, Robinson RA: The treatment of certain cervical spine disorders by anterior removal of the intervertebral disc and interbody fusion. J Bone Joint Surg Am 40A:607–624, 1958.

51. Tippets RH, Apfelbaum RI: Anterior cervical fusion with the Caspar instrumentation system. Neurosurgery 22:1008–1013, 1988.

51A. Tribus CB, Corteen DP, Zdeblick TA: The efficacy of anterior cervical plating in the management of symptomatic pseudarthrosis of the cervical spine. Spine 24:860–864, 1999.

52. Vaccaro AR, Falatyn SP, Scuderi GJ, et al: Early failure of long segment anterior cervical plate fixation. J Spinal Disord 11:410–415, 1998.

53. Vanichkachorn JS, Vaccaro AR, Silveri CP, Albert TJ: Anterior junctional plate in the cervical spine. Spine 23:2462–2467, 1998.

54. Wang JC, McDonough PW, Endow KK, Delamarter RB: Increased fusion rates with cervical plating for two-level anterior cervical discectomy and fusion. Spine 25:41–45, 2000.

54A. Wang JC, McDonough PW, Endow K, et al: The effect of cervical plating on single-level anterior cervical discectomy and fusion. J Spinal Disord 12:467–471, 1999.

54B. Wang JC, McDonough PW, Kanim LE, et al: Increased fusion rates with cervical plating for three-level anterior cervical discectomy and fusion. Spine 26:643–647, 2001.

55. Whitecloud TS III, LaRocca H: Fibular strut graft in reconstructive surgery of the cervical spine. Spine 1:33–43, 1976.

56. Yonenobu K, Fuji T, Ono K, et al: Choice of surgical treatment for multisegmental cervical spondylotic myelopathy. Spine 10:710–716, 1985.

57. Zdeblick TA: Complications of anterior spinal instrumentation. Semin Spine Surg 5:101–107, 1993.

58. Zdeblick TA, Cooke ME, Wilson D, et al: Anterior cervical discectomy, fusion, and plating: A comparative animal study. Spine 14:1974–1983, 1993.

5

POSTERIOR CERVICAL INSTRUMENTATION

John G. Heller, M.D.
John W. Klekamp, M.D.
Mark H. Blechner, M.D.

A man has got to know his limitations.
– Clint Eastwood

Cervical stabilization procedures have been used in the treatment of spinal stability since 1881, when posterior wiring was performed by Hadra for Pott's disease. Though effective in their original forms, wiring techniques have evolved considerably during the latter half of this century to enhance their effectiveness in various pathological conditions. As acute care for the injured and medical therapy for infections and tumors have improved, spinal surgeons have been presented with increasingly complex reconstructive challenges in the cervical spine. Over time, these technical challenges have fostered more detailed and quantitative anatomic and biomechanical investigations of the cervical region. In parallel with this, more sophisticated methods of osteosynthesis have been adapted from long bone fixation to the cervical spine. Thus, the contemporary spine surgeon must master a larger and more detailed body of knowledge that will enable him or her to select the appropriate surgical techniques to apply to a given patient's unique circumstances.

This chapter is divided into two sections. The first section addresses the principles of quantitative anatomy, which are important for critically evaluating clinical problems and choosing appropriate treatment methods. The second section describes the spectrum of posterior internal fixation options available for the cervicocranial, atlantoaxial, subaxial, and cervicothoracic regions and discusses their relative success rates.

APPLIED ANATOMY

The anatomy of the occiput and posterior cervical spine presents surgical challenges in both dissection and fixation. The angles are unusual, the contours are irregular, and the bone is relatively thin and small with alternating areas of primarily cortical and cancellous bone. Perhaps more than in any other region, anatomical details in the posterior cervical spine must be fully considered during preoperative planning and intraoperative execution.

Traditionally the cervical spine has been divided into two qualitatively distinct regions: the upper and lower cervical spine. Though descriptively useful, this distinction is of minimal use to the contemporary surgeon. The proliferation of quantitative cervical anatomical data during the 1990s, along with the concomitant evolution in surgical methods, invites us to reconsider this dichotomy. From a surgical perspective it appears more useful to classify the cervical spine into three distinct regions based on their functional anatomy and implications for spinal instrumentation: The cervicocranium (occiput–C2), the true subaxial region (C3–C6), and the cervicothoracic junction (C7 to T2). This regional description of the cervical spine is based on qualitative descriptions of anatomical and functional differences and underlies general principles for treatment of instability patterns in which fixation can be achieved. Different techniques can, therefore, be combined in hybrid constructions for the best results in more complex cases.

Cervicocranium

Occiput

The anatomy of the occiput has only recently been studied in detail, and the information compiled has already begun to influence treatment. Identification of external landmarks and knowledge of the underlying bone morphology and intracranial anatomy are critical to optimizing fixation while minimizing risk (Fig. 5–1). The occipital bone is a pentagonal, convex plate bordered superiorly by the lambdoid sutures, which mark its junction with the paired parietal bones; laterally by the occipitomastoid suture, joining it to the petrous portion of the temporal bones; and inferiorly by the foramen magnum. The upper half is the thicker triangular portion with the upper two sides formed by the lambdoid sutures joined at a 120-degree angle apex. The inferior border of this triangle is delineated by the thickened superior nuchal line. A useful surgical landmark, this line is the attachment of the trapezial and sternocleidomastoid tendons externally and the tentorium cerebelli internally. The thickest bone of the occiput is in the midline of the superior nuchal line between the external occipital protuberance (EOP) and the internal occipital protuberance. The lower half of the occipital bone is the thinner trapezoidal portion, which tapers inferiorly from the superior nuchal line toward the foramen magnum as well as

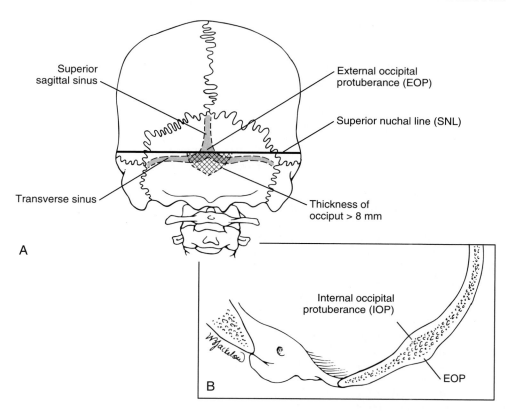

Superior
sagittal sinus

External occipital
protuberance (EOP)

Superior nuchal line (SNL)

Transverse sinus

Thickness of
occiput > 8 mm

A

Internal occipital
protuberance (IOP)

B

EOP

Figure 5–1. *A, Schematic view of the occiput illustrating important external and internal anatomic landmarks. EOP = external occipital protuberance, IOP = internal occipital protuberance, SNL = superior nuchal line. B, Sagittal cross-section of the occipital bone along the midline illustrating the relative thickness of the bone.*

laterally from the midline external and internal occipital crest into the cerebellar fossa on each side.

Detailed maps of the tangential and oblique occipital bone thicknesses as well as intracranial anatomy have guided recent recommendations regarding the type, location, length, depth, and angulation of fixation elements.[27, 110] Along the parasagittal lines 1 cm from the midline below the superior nuchal line, where plate fixation normally occurs, the thickness tapers forming a triangular topographic map. The critical thickness of 8 mm is only present laterally within 23.3 mm at the level of the EOP, 8.6 mm at 1 cm inferior, and 4.5 mm at 2 cm inferior. The bone off the midline below the superior nuchal line can occasionally be so thin as to be translucent.

Fortunately, the cortical bone of the occiput is very dense providing good purchase for cortical screws. Thus, plate fixation is more likely to fail at the cervical end of the plate, where there is less cortical fixation, or by fatigue of the plate without loss of fixation. The greater concern during occipital fixation is intracranial penetration. The dura mater is adherent to the internal cranial surface in all regions and is the only layer protecting the closely approximated venous sinuses along the cerebellar hemispheres. The confluence of the sinuses lies beneath the intersection of bony prominences at the inion and may be associated with a depression or thinning beside the IOP. The center of the confluence actually lies slightly above the inion extending 12.6 mm superior and only 4.7 mm inferior to the EOP leaving a safe zone for fixation within the triangular region of the thickest bone. The occipital bone above the superior nuchal line is approximately 25% thicker than below it, but has more of its inside area covered with venous sinuses. In addition, the

soft tissue coverage is marginal superior to the inion and hardware tends to be prominent.

Atlantoaxial Complex

The atlantoaxial articulation is unique in that there is no intervertebral disk, and the facet joints are oriented horizontally to allow greater rotational motion while increasing vertical stability. This rotational freedom occurs about the odontoid process, which is strapped against the anterior arch of C1 by the transverse ligament complex and provides most of its stability, especially in translation.[24] The posterior elements of the atlantoaxial level have a wide interlaminar space spanned by the posterior atlanto-occipital membrane. The space available for the spinal cord is greatest at this level of the cervical spine.

Subaxial Spine

Vertebral Body. All vertebral body transverse dimensions in the cervical and thoracic spine, including endplate width, depth, and cross-sectional area, increase from rostral to caudal.[81] The most significant increases occur at the cervicothoracic transition levels (C6 to T1). The width is greater and increases more rapidly than the depth in the cervical and upper thoracic levels, causing a steady flattening of the vertebral body as measured by the width to depth ratio. The vertebral height remains constant from C3 to C5 and then decreases slightly at C6 before increasing rapidly at C7. The normal lordosis from C2 to C7 is 35 degrees, divided in equal 7-degree segments.[52] At T1, the lower endplate inclination suddenly reverses. This results in a slightly kyphotic bony wedge at each level, which forms the normal thoracic curve.

The spinal canal width, determined by the bordering pedicles and lateral masses, remains fairly constant throughout the cervical spine because as the vertebral body widens, the pedicle angles narrow. The canal depth and cross-sectional area are greatest at C1 and C2, but decrease precipitously at C3.[103]

Posterior Elements. The posterior elements of the subaxial cervical levels include the pedicles, articular lateral masses, laminae, and spinous processes.

Recently the anatomy of the posterior elements has been described more accurately with respect to anatomic landmarks, fixation points, and structures at risk during instrumentation. The difference between the upper and lower subaxial spine is primarily in the size of the pedicles and facet complexes, which may influence the choice of fixation. There can be significant asymmetry in certain values between the right and left sides; these individual variations must be considered at each level in any given patient.

Pedicle. The pedicle is surrounded by essential structures on all sides. The vertebral artery and its associated venous plexus abut laterally. The thecal sac lies medially. The nerve roots abut superiorly and are separated only slightly inferiorly. Panjabi showed that the outer pedicle dimensions (height, width, and cross-sectional area) are largest at C2 and decrease significantly from C3 to C6; then the height stays fairly constant while the width slowly increases to C7. The pedicle width is the limiting dimension for pedicle screw fixation, because it is almost always smaller than the corresponding height. Panjabi reported that pedicle dimensions consistently exceed 4.0 mm.[81] However, subsequent studies have demonstrated that the outer pedicle width is frequently 4 mm or less, particularly at C3 or C4.[64] The inner pedicle width, the important determinant of safe pedicle fixation, is usually adequate at C2 and C7 but often less than 2 mm at C3 through C6, with the thinnest cortex along the lateral wall throughout the cervical spine.[64] The pedicle at T1 is larger in both dimensions than that of C7 and similar in size to that of C2.

Pedicle shape can be represented by the height to width (H/W) ratio. The vertical oval shape in the upper cervical pedicles (average ratio 1.29) becomes more rounded at the cervicothoracic junction and then elongates again, becoming an even taller oval with a rapid increase in H/W ratio from 1.1 at T1 to 1.9 at T5 and below.

The axial or transverse plane (medial) angle of the pedicle is lowest (i.e., has the most sagittal orientation) at C2 (10 to 15 degrees), then increases significantly at C3 (44 degrees) and slowly decreases to C7 (37°).[94] Ebraheim and Xu have described fixation points using pedicle angles with respect to the plane of the posterior lateral mass wall that are surgically applicable but not very reliable clinically. They show a constant angle from C3 to C6 (average 95.8°) but a sudden significant increase at C7 (107.0°), which may represent flattening of the lateral mass posterior wall in the face of the continued decreased angle with respect to the frontal plane.[106] Similar measurements by Stanescu showed a slower increase without abrupt transition.[94]

The projection of the pedicle on the dorsal surface of the lateral mass can be localized with respect to vertical and horizontal reference lines. The inferior edge of the superior facet is the standard horizontal reference line, but some studies have used the inferior facet or the midline of the transverse process. The outermost margin of the articular mass provides the most reproducible vertical line. For clinical purposes, the horizontal pedicle offset at C2 is best measured from the lateral extent of the spinal canal at the junction of the lateral mass and lamina (7.2 mm) so as to avoid excessive lateral dissection.[28] When measured from the lateral wall of the articular process, the horizontal offset increases from 4.9 mm at C3 to 6.2 mm at C6 corresponding to the changes in transverse plane angle described above.[29] At C7 the horizontal offset is only 2.7 mm corresponding to the decrease in transverse plane angle reported by Xu.[106] At the cervicothoracic junction An described the more horizontal projection plane at the middle of the facet;[3] however, Stanescu reported an inferior medial migration of the projection point from a superior and lateral position at both C5 and T1 with a sharp transition at C7 to T1.

These quantitative observations of pedicle dimensions serve a number of purposes. First, they alert us to the narrow tolerance for error when attempting to insert a pedicle screw in the cervical region. Second, in raising such awareness, they strengthen the need to scrutinize each side of each level to be instrumented in the preoperative planning process. Third, they provide some assistance intraoperatively as one attempts to correlate the visible anatomy with imaging studies. The various rules of thumb proposed by investigators, in the authors' opinion, remain just that—rules of thumb. The dimensions and angles of each pedicle must be accounted for individually as screw paths are prepared. Lastly, these data provide a design envelope, which we must respect as we develop newer instruments and techniques in the future.

Nerve Root. Each cervical nerve exits the spinal canal through an intervertebral foramen and lies in a nerve root groove that extends from the superior edge of the subjacent pedicle along the superior surface of the transverse process to its tip.[26] The ventral and dorsal cervical nerve rootlets branch from the spinal cord's anterior and posterior paramedian sulci leaving the central canal in distinct bundles that are collectively surrounded by a dural root sleeve. They pass along the inferomedial border of the upper pedicle to enter the intervertebral foramen.

The foraminal dimensions steadily increase in size from C3–C4 to C7–T1. As it enters the foramen, the root runs posterior to the inferolateral corner of the upper vertebral body, which forms the upper half of the anterior foraminal wall. The rootlets then cross the midportion of the foramen at the level of the intervertebral disk to the superior lateral border of the lower pedicle. Here they come to lie in the medial zone of the nerve root groove, which comprises the narrower inferior half of the foramen with its edges defined by the underlying pedicle and its length corresponding to the pedicle width. The width of the groove is proportionally smaller than that of the foramen and smallest at C4, similar to patterns of foraminal dimensions. The medial zone, the narrowest portion of the intervertebral foramen, is bordered anteriorly by the uncinate process and posteriorly by the anterior anteromedial edge of the superior articular process. Spondylosis can cause symptoms of nerve root compression here. Foraminal stenosis may result from any combination of disk height loss, osteophyte formation, and degenerative subluxation.[35, 109]

In the middle zone, the dorsal rootlets coalesce into the dorsal root ganglion (DRG), which lies in the posterior and caudal aspects of the groove in a sulcus that crosses the anterior surface of the superior articular process at the inferior third of the articular mass. The ventral rootlets join to form the more anterior and cranial ventral root lying directly posterior to the vertebral artery and its transverse foramen, which defines this zone.[108]

The dorsal root emerges from the DRG and then combines with the ventral root to form the spinal root in the lateral zone. The lateral zone is quite variable, with dimensions of an average width of 6.0 mm and average length of 4.8 mm. It is bordered by anterior and posterior ridges that expand to form tubercles at the end of the transverse process. Finally, the nerve exits the groove at the anterolateral portion of the superior facet and branches into ventral dorsal and communicating rami. The ventral ramus is referred to as the spinal nerve.[3]

Vertebral Artery. The vertebral artery enters the cervical spine above the transverse sulcus at C7 and ascends in a slightly posteromedial course from C6 to C3 within the foramina transversaria of the transverse processes in the middle zone of the nerve root groove. The vertebral artery foramen is circular, and its dimensions are uniform from C6 up to C3 with an average diameter of 5.2 mm.[30] The vertebral artery position is slightly more lateral at C6 than in the upper levels, whereas the apex of the lateral mass is slightly more medial.[105] The transverse foramen becomes more medial with decreasing interforaminal distance as it ascends to C3. With rare exceptions, the foramen lies lateral to the vertebral body at its posterior third and is adjacent to the lateral wall of the pedicle at all levels. From C6 to C3, the foramen moves progressively more posterior with respect to the vertebral body.[99] Depending on arterial dominance patterns, there may be a significant difference in the size of the foramen from right to left. This should be noted on the preoperative imaging studies, because the consequences of inadvertent injury to the dominant vessel may have devastating consequences.

The artery continues in its posteromedial ascent from C3 to the base of C2, where it passes the anteromedial corner of the C2–C3 facet and enters an oblique and slightly enlarged vertebral artery foramen. This foramen continues to lie even more posterior with respect to the vertebral body than at the subaxial levels, with its margin overlapping the posterior vertebral body cortex.[99] In contrast, the C2 foramen reverses the medial migration of the C3–C5 foramina to lie more laterally with an interforaminal distance similar to C6. The artery assumes the path of the foramen, which is angled 45 degrees laterally and slightly anterior, crossing the inferior aspect of the anterolateral mass wall. On exiting the foramen, it turns rostral and continues slightly ventral, crossing the anterolateral border of the C2 isthmus. As it crosses the C1–C2 facet joint, the artery turns from a slightly anterolateral course to a posteromedial angle into

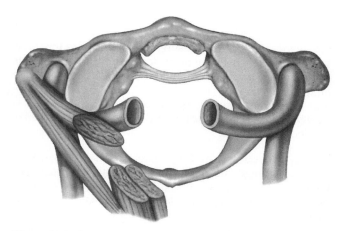

Figure 5–2. *Superior axial cutaway view looking down onto the course of the vertebral arteries as they loop back over the posterior arch of the atlas and penetrate the dura. The location of the arteries defines the practical limit of lateral dissection during posterior fusion procedures.*

the C1 foramen, which is angled in this direction. This vertebral foramen lies directly lateral to the lateral mass of C1. However, because this articular process is more anterior than in the lower levels, the transverse foramen is still more anterior than at C2. The artery exits the foramen and turns sharply to a horizontal posterolateral path. After passing the lateral mass, the artery continues posteromedially in a shallow extension of the same groove that lies along the superior surface of the C1 arch halfway to the midline (Fig. 5–2). Here it turns anteromedially, sometimes through an accessory foramen, and ascends along the clivus to merge with the artery from the contralateral side, forming the basilar artery. The size and location of the vertebral artery in relation to the base of the pedicle at C2 are crucial determinants of the advisability of atlantoaxial transarticular screw fixation.

Transverse Process. The transverse process, which projects anterolaterally from the pedicle, decreases in length from C2 to C6 while the vertebral body width increases, keeping the transverse process band constant. At C7, the transverse process length increases significantly along the vertebral body, causing an increase in the overall width. It is most important clinically as a convenient radiographic reference point on the lateral projection.[83]

Lateral Mass. The dimensions of the facet joint surfaces remain constant throughout the cervical and upper thoracic spine with the exception of the C2 superior articular facet, which is approximately 50% larger.[82] There is a slight increase in width more than height in the cervicothoracic transitional region. The C2 superior facet transverse and sagittal plane angles are 37.1 and 116 degrees, respectively. This makes it nearly horizontal in comparison with the remaining joints. The facets become less coronal and more vertical in orientation from C6 to T4, with the most rapid changes seen in the cervicothoracic transition zone.[12]

The depth of the lateral mass as measured from the midpoint of its posterior surface to its junction with the transverse process at the nerve root groove decreases slowly from C3 (8.9 mm) to C6 (8.0 mm) and then drops suddenly at C7 (6.4 mm).[26] This variation has implications for screw length and strength of purchase. It is also the reason that we consider the "true subaxial region" to be C3 to C6, because the geometry of the lateral masses is rather uniform. The transitional anatomy at the cervicothoracic junction is worthy of separate designation and often calls for alternative methods of fixation.

Lamina. The lamina of C2 is large, reflecting the forces imparted through its many muscular attachments.[23] The laminae from C3 to C6 are taller and shingled, with the inferior edge of the upper lamina often overlapping the superior edge of the lower lamina. They are more uniform and rather thin. The lamina at C7 is large, with a rapid increase in height and especially thickness because of the smaller area and angulation of the lateral mass.[80, 94] In the upper thoracic region, the laminar height and thickness remain constant while the length of the lamina decreases, corresponding to the more sagittal pedicle angle.[10, 94]

Spinous Process. The spinous processes at C2 and C7 are uniformly stout and well developed. They are important points of insertion for the extensor muscles, and their size no doubt reflects the magnitude of forces that they bear. The other subaxial spinous processes are far more variable in their development. They are generally larger as one moves caudally. Their individual size and strength determine whether they are amenable to interspinous wire fixation methods.

POSTERIOR INSTRUMENTATION TECHNIQUES

Cervicocranium

The cervicocranium (occipitoatlantoaxial complex) presents unique challenges for surgical stabilization. Fusion of the upper cervical spine can be subdivided into occipitoatlantoaxial, occipitocervical, and atlantoaxial arthrodeses, depending on the extent of instability and the availability of suitable fixation points. Isolated, significant atlanto-occipital instability is unlikely without concomitant subluxation or instability of C1–C2, because the alar ligaments span both joints. Rare cases of survival from atlanto-occipital dislocation, congenital deficiencies, or inflammatory arthropathy can primarily affect this level, but they are generally associated with at least some C1–C2 hypermobility. Even in the rare case of isolated atlanto-occipital arthritis, isolated occiput–C1 fusion is impractical. Fixation is difficult without extension to C2. Any advantages of preserved rotation at C1–C2 are probably outweighed by the additional stability of fixation and increased likelihood of fusion provided by incorporating C2.

Occipitoatlantoaxial Fusion

Occipitoatlantoaxial fusions are more difficult to achieve than atlantoaxial fusions because of the greater range and multidirectional nature of motion at the cervicocranium. The moments to be resisted by the instrumentation are considerably greater when fixation is extended up to the occiput. Various techniques are available. The specific procedure should be tailored to the needs of the patient, as well as to the skill and experience of the surgeon.

The most straightforward method uses only external fixation with a halo vest. Onlay grafts are used after decortication as a simple, safe, and effective treatment for this region without the risk of internal fixation. A modification of this technique using an osteoperiosteal turndown flap from the occiput has been described by Hensinger for young children.[58] Elia reported an 89% fusion rate with few complications, but treatment requiring 3 months of external immobilization (longer in patients with rheumatoid arthritis), which necessitates frequent adjustments, is associated with many minor difficulties and is frequently undesirable for the patient.[31] This method can be considered in isolated circumstances for adults in which an intrinsically stable occiput–C2 region is being fused for painful arthritis or pseudarthrosis. It cannot be recommended for routine use because of the inherent instability, potential for pseudarthrosis, and frustrations inherent in prolonged use of halo devices. This method is most desirable in children, who have more predictable and rapid healing potential. It may also be useful for unique congenital deficiencies when the posterior elements are not suitable for fixation.

The normal resting occipitocervical angulation of 105 degrees is important in determining level gaze. Internal occipitocervical fixation constructs must be contoured or designed to maintain this normal resting angle.[11] Fixing the cervicocranium in too great an extension will result in a "swan neck" deformity of the cervical spine. Conversely, fusing in flexion requires the patient to assume a hyperextended posture of the subaxial spine. Either has unpleasant cosmetic and functional consequences. Therefore, considerable attention to detail is needed while

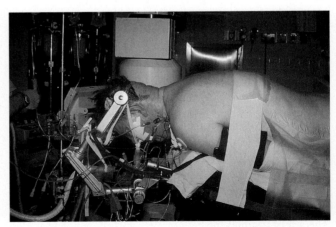

Figure 5–3. Photographic view of our preferred method of positioning patients for most posterior cervical spine procedures. A good view of the brow–chin angle and head–trunk relationship is provided to confirm proper positioning. Pressure on the face and eyes is avoided. Lateral x-ray views are easily obtained, and the proper position of the head and neck is ensured throughout the procedure.

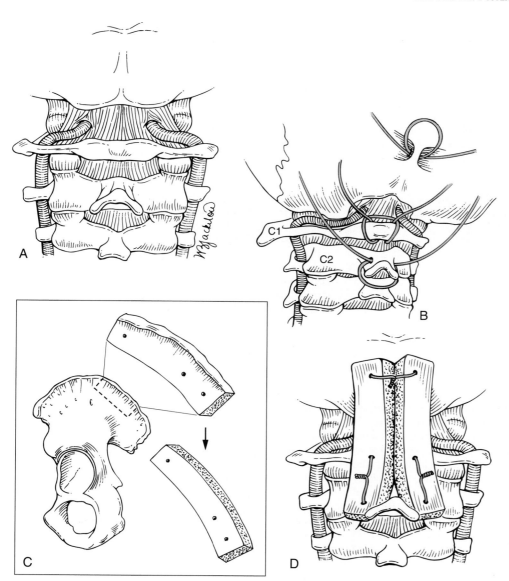

Figure 5–4. Technique of posterior occipitocervical fusion. *A, A burr hole is made in the nuchal bony ridge, staying between the cortical tables. B, 20-gauge wires are passed down; looping the wire through a second time improves the grip and distributes the stress. C, Near–full-thickness corticocancellous grafts are harvested from the ilium. D, The grafts are wired in place as shown. Cancellous bone is also packed in the crevices. (Modified from Werthein SB, Bohlman HH: Occipitocervical fusion: Indications, technique, and long-term results in thirteen patients. J Bone Joint Surg Am 69A:833–836, 1987.)*

positioning the patient for surgery. We prefer to use either a Mayfield three-pin head holder or a halo ring anchored with a special adapter to the Mayfield apparatus. This allows precise positioning of the head with visual and x-ray confirmation of occipitocervical alignment, the brow–chin angle, and the head–trunk relationship. Once the correct position is verified, prepping and draping of the surgical field may proceed (Fig. 5–3).

Meyer's technique of posterior C1–C2 fusion was extended to the occiput by Wertheim and Bohlman using an additional wire passed through a drill hole in the external occipital protuberance and an upper drill hole in each of the two longer strips of corticocancellous graft[102] (Fig. 5–4A,B,C). As with C2 spinous process fixation, a drill hole loop technique can be used to enhance fixation at the external occipital protuberance. In this technique, the C1 and C2 wire ends are tightened over the bone graft on each side, while the two ends of the occipital wire are connected to each other across the midline (Fig. 5–4D). With this technique, they achieved 100% fusion and 77% satisfactory outcomes in 13 patients.[102] McAfee reported an 85% fusion rate in 37 patients with more severe conditions using a similar technique despite the addition of prolonged postoperative halo immobilization.[72] Unicortical wires passed through burr holes in the suboccipital plate provide secure graft fixation. Short lag screws with washers also may be used to fix the upper end of the graft to the occiput.

More rigid fixation is needed for multilevel or severe multidirectional instability. This additional stability can be achieved by using occipital, spinous process, sublaminar, or facet wires connected to more rigid bridging elements, such as rods, to form a buttressed wire construct. These buttresses can be contoured to better conform to the occipitocervical angle, minimizing the posterior translation forces of the wire at C1. When bent into a rectangle or cross-linked, they provide enhanced bending and torsional stiffness (Fig. 5–5). The stability of these constructs depends primarily on the wire–bone interface.

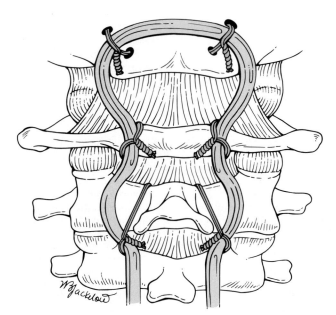

Figure 5–5. *Schematic of a posterior occipitocervical fusion technique using a Ransford loop construct. Although this construct is stiffer than the one illustrated in Figure 5–4, it is not as stable as an occipitocervical plate–screw construct.*

Angular motion in the sagittal plane must be resisted by the bending stiffness of the buttress element, especially if anterior bone deficiencies exist. Various configurations have been used, each yielding reasonable results with 80% to 100% fusion rates. Sliding of the fixation wires along the rods can lead to undesirable axial shortening, especially when trying to maintain reduction in rheumatoid cranial settling or pathologic fractures of the atlas or axis. Buttress configurations that are open at the lower end of the rods, especially those using smooth rods, are particularly prone to this. A threaded or knurled rod can limit the amount of vertical motion; however, lateral bending and some "scissoring" in axial rotation may still occur. Adding cross-links to create a rectangle will strengthen the construct and limit (though not eliminate) these motions.[37] Apostolides reported on the use of a custom-made titanium groove rod to provide interference wire rod fixation and limit sliding.[7] He observed a 92% osseous and a 5% stable fibrous union rate with excellent control of vertical stability.

The use of a prefabricated Luque ring or Heartshal-Ransford rectangle, fashioned in a continuous loop without an open corner, significantly increases bending and torsional stiffness.[32] To achieve maximal stability, the rectangular rods must be sublaminarly fixated at their lowest levels to provide maximum vertical stability. Unfortunately, this may necessitate extension of the fusion to a normal segment. Perhaps more importantly, the risk of multiple sublaminar wire passes increases as the vertebral canal narrows in the lower cervical spine. Because the subarachnoid space is smallest in the subaxial region, and this is the area most commonly narrowed by spondylosis and other conditions, the surgeon should carefully evaluate whether sublaminar wire passage is appropriate for each level. For these and other reasons, plate fixation is our treatment of choice in

cases of profound instability, poor bone quality, or inappropriate posterior element or spinal canal anatomy.

The screw placement for all occipitocervical plating techniques must balance fixation strength versus the risk of injury from intracranial penetration. Unicortical fixation minimizes the risk of sinus penetration and dural penetration associated with cerebrospinal fluid (CSF) leak, meningitis, and possible cerebellar injury. This fixation is often sufficient in patients with normal bone density and a thick outer cortical plate demonstrated on computed tomography (CT) scan. In cases necessitating additional purchase, such as severe rheumatoid arthritis, renal osteodystrophy, or multiple myeloma, the use of more hazardous bicortical fixation can provide a twofold increase in pullout strength over unicortical screw or wire fixation.[15] When bicortical fixation is used, the drill hole may be sealed with bone wax before screw placement if sinus bleeding or cerebral spinal leaks are evident.[47] Although CSF leakage is commonly seen after bicortical holes are drilled, it rarely persists after screws are inserted. Note that the occipital bone can be unicortical and extremely thin in some people, especially lateral to the midline.

Intracranial penetration can be minimized by using a drill stop set at a controlled depth. Roy-Camille advocated the use of 12- to 14-mm-long screws in the occipital region; however, anatomic studies have suggested that this is possible only at the external occipital protuberance along a 45-degree axis. Plate width dictates screw placement approximately 0.5 to 1.0 cm lateral to the midline, where thickness is already decreasing. Consequently, a maximal screw length of 10 to 12 mm should be used in the terminal holes near the superior nuchal line, with shorter screws used inferiorly within the critical triangle. The length of each screw should be determined with a depth gauge. If the plates are sufficiently close to the midline, then screw length can be increased by angling toward the areas of maximal bone thickness at the occipital ridge and superior nuchal line; however, drilling in this direction endangers the venous sinuses.

Heywood first used a contoured, small-fragment T-plate from the C2 spinous process to the occiput with an 86% fusion rate.[59] Other authors have shown excellent results (100% fusion in 14 patients) with contoured pelvic reconstruction plates, which had the advantage of being inexpensive and adaptable for variations in anatomy or longer constructs if needed (Fig. 5–6).[60, 91] Using paramedian AO plates and C1–C2 transarticular screws, Sasso and associates[89] achieved 100% union in 23 patients at an average of 13 weeks, with stable or improved neurologic status evident at 4-year follow-up. In comparison with midline bone grafting and wiring, the plate fixation techniques in patients with rheumatoid arthritis yielded better reduction of deformity and maintenance of alignment with more frequent neurologic improvement and higher fusion rates.[48] The single occipital arm of the Y-plate gains optimal purchase in the strongest bone at the midline ridge and external occipital protuberance.

Bilateral paramedian plating below the level of the superior nuchal line using unicortical screw fixation is recommended for severe multidirectional instability. Plates designed for this fixation have a 105-degree reinforced bend. Augmentation using the midline structural bone graft technique described for the Wertheim and Bohlman method can be added with increased safety when plates are in place, because there is less risk of failure in extension and migration of the graft (Fig. 5–7). Spanning across the atlantoaxial joint without fixation can be effective in stable circumstances, but when C1–C2 subluxation is present, additional sublaminar wiring or transarticular screw fixation through the plates should be considered. Isolated screw fixation of C2 should be placed in the large oblique pedicle, because the lateral masses are shallow and provide limited purchase.

Atlantoaxial Fusion

Atlantoaxial instrumentation and fusion methods can be thought of as midline and bilateral constructs using wires, hooks, or transarticular screws. The stability of the construct depends on its method of fixation to bone, the distance between fixation points, the rigidity of the construct elements, and the integrity of the dens and ring of C1.[61] Traditionally, atlantoaxial fusions use wiring techniques when the posterior elements are intact. The wiring configuration selected may be influenced by the pattern of instability. Interspinous wiring techniques cannot be used in the atlantoaxial region because the C1 lacks a spinous process. Consequently, at least one sublaminar passage is necessary at this level. On rare occasions we have successfully passed an intramedullary wire within a well-developed C1 arch when insufficient room was available beneath the arch for safe sublaminar wire insertion, but this maneuver is rarely used. The Gallie fusion and its variants require only a single sublaminar passage, decreasing the risks but also providing less stability. In multidirectional instability, it provides less resistance to axial rotation, translation, and lateral bending because of the

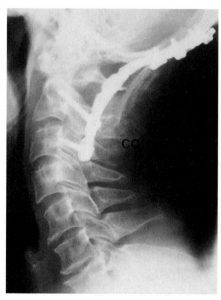

Figure 5–6. *Lateral x-ray taken 1 year after successful occipitocervical plating and fusion for treatment of a pathological fracture of C1 due to lymphoma.*

closely spaced fixation points.[46] The surgeon also must take care to avoid producing hyperextension from overtightening the wires, which can cause a swan-neck deformity.

Wiring with morcellized autograft can be used in intrinsically stable circumstances, but structural grafts should be used whenever possible.[74] The two ends of a single 18- or 20-gauge wire or a braided cable are passed rostrally to caudally beneath the lamina of C1, and then the free ends are passed through the loop to form a hitch around the C1 arch. This is more difficult than passage from below but provides a more direct line of pull in the wire with less tendency to bend and concentrate stress. The free wire ends are then fixed to the C2 spinous process by looping either beneath it or through a transspinous burr hole. Without an intervening buttress, the rigidity of this construct and much of its fusion potential is based on hyperextension of C1 such that its posterior arch contacts and even locks posteriorly to the superior edge of the lamina of C2. When limited by an intact dens, this is a relatively stable construct. However, when the dens is fractured or an os odontoideum exists, posterior translation may lead to spinal cord injury or occipital neuralgia. A structural graft can be of some help in limiting posterior translation, but the surgeon is wise to consider other options in such circumstances.

The Gallie fusion is a midline spinolaminar configuration that uses a structural interlaminar bone graft within the tension band wire construct.[40] This provides some extension stability while avoiding the hyperextended position and increases flexion stability by providing a tension band. It also increases graft–host contact area with compression, widens the distance between fixation points to improve rotational stability, and allows somewhat easier wire passage from below. The original Gallie fusion was identical to midline wiring with onlay graft position between the wire and the posterior elements. In the more widely used modified Gallie technique, a loop of 18- or 20-gauge wire or cable is passed caudally to rostrally beneath the laminar of C1 with the ends separated so that a single strand of wire lies beneath each half of the C1 arch. After both levels are decorticated, a corticocancellous bone graft is carefully contoured to form an interference fit between the C1 laminar edge and C2. The wire loops backward over the superior edge of the C1 lamina and the posterior surface of the interposed graft and hooks beneath the C2 spinous process. The two free ends of the wire are then passed over the lateral edges of the graft, joined at the midline, and tightened, thus fixing the graft in place. Like other posterior wiring constructs, the Gallie configuration is quite stable in flexion. However, it remains biomechanically inferior to the Brooks, Halifax, and Magerl techniques for all motions, with correspondingly greater nonunion rates.[38, 46, 73]

To increase bone purchase, add stability against the posterior translation and avoid disengagement through the C2 spinous process; the wire can be passed around a Kirschner wire or threaded Steinmann pin inserted through the base of the C2 spinous process.[8] This pin is difficult to insert, and its relative contribution is unclear. The spinous process fixation can also be passed through a drill hole at its base before it is passed sublaminarly, but then the two free wire ends must be passed rostrally to caudally to perform a classic Gallie fusion. Finally, Meyer described a modifica-

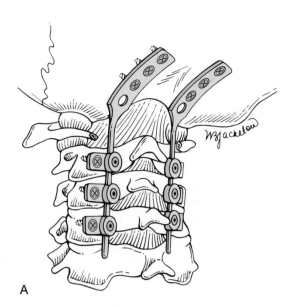

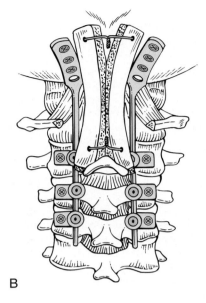

Figure 5–7. Bilateral occipitocervical plating for rigid internal fixation (A) with iliac crest corticocancellous struts wired in place (B).

tion using two separate wires: one sublaminar passage around C1–C2 to form a hitch, similar to the simple midline method described earlier, and a second using open or looped drill hole fixation to the spinous process of C2.[75] The four wire ends that come from the midportion of the lamina and this technique lend themselves to fixation through the bone graft (Fig. 5–8). Because there is a separate fixation of the graft to each lamina, this technique has the advantage of providing some neutralization effect and can resist extension as long as the grafts are rigid. Passage of a second hitch between the arch of C1 as described by Weiland adds two C1 wire ends that can be tightened beneath the C2 spinous process, adding direct spinal laminar stability to structural graft fixation with any modified triple-wire configuration.[101] This should increase flexion stiffness and decrease shear force on the wire at the graft drill holes under flexion loads compared with Meyer's method. Unlike Bohlman's technique in the subaxial spine, however, this modification actually adds a sublaminar passage, thus doubling the potential risk of neurologic injury. We favor a modified Gallie fusion wiring method for cases of minimal or purely flexional instability, in which the anterior intrinsic stabilizing structures are intact and can prevent extension or posterior translation.

The Brooks fusion technique is a sublaminar construct that also uses structural corticocancellous bone grafts for a posterior buttress.[13] Dual twisted strands of 20-gauge wire or titanium cable are passed rostrally to caudally beneath the C1 and C2 lamina and reflected rostrally around the inferior margin of C2 to join with themselves (Fig. 5–9). Using a single sublaminar pass, the loop can be cut and one wire loop passed on each side of the midline. To limit the volume in the canal to a single thickness, we prefer to use an initial thin wire loop to pass two suture loops back through and use the two sublaminar sutures to pull two separate double-ended titanium cables back rostrally to caudally. This yields a pair of fixation cables for each of the two grafts. The wires are then joined over the grafts and tightened. Alternatively, Clark's modification can be used, in which a single large bone graft crosses the midline with a notch in its inferior border to accommodate the spinous process.[16, 17] Although this graft is more difficult to contour between the laminae, it is also less likely to dislodge. The Brooks fusion and Clark's modification yield greater extension and torsional stiffness than the Gallie or midline wiring methods.[50] Flexion stiffnesses are comparable.[92]

Variations of sublaminar fixation also include laminar hook devices, such as the Halifax interlaminar clamp and adaptations of modular pediatric hook-rod systems. These devices can be applied without full sublaminar passage, but

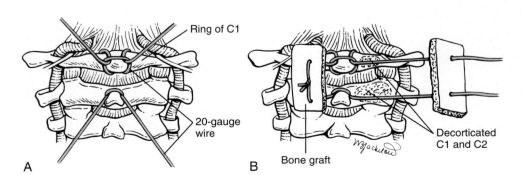

Figure 5–8. Modified Gallie type wiring (A) and bone grafting (B) for atlantoaxial arthrodesis.

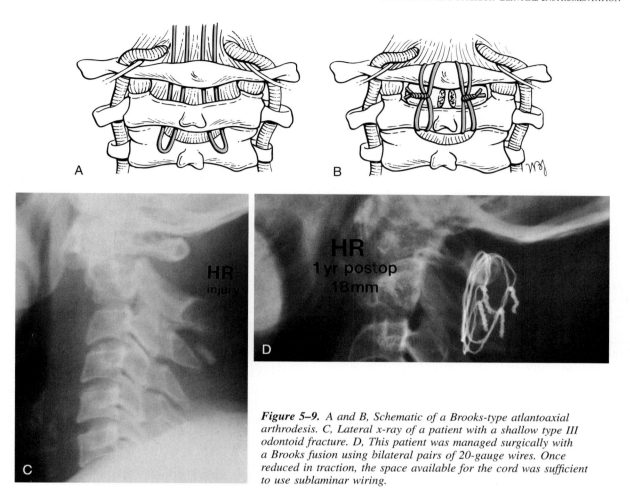

Figure 5–9. *A and B, Schematic of a Brooks-type atlantoaxial arthrodesis. C, Lateral x-ray of a patient with a shallow type III odontoid fracture. D, This patient was managed surgically with a Brooks fusion using bilateral pairs of 20-gauge wires. Once reduced in traction, the space available for the cord was sufficient to use sublaminar wiring.*

they can encroach on the space available for the cord. Although they are simple in concept, assembling them within the depth of the wound can be problematic. They have a larger surface area of fixation, providing less risk of failure at the implant–bone interface. By the same token, they reduce the exposed bone surface for grafting (Fig.

5–10). Like other sublaminar techniques, they impart extension and thus are best used in conjunction with a buttress graft to block extension. These methods have the same indications as those for other bilateral laminar fusions but are best reserved for situations in which sublaminar wires would be difficult or dangerous to pass or broader

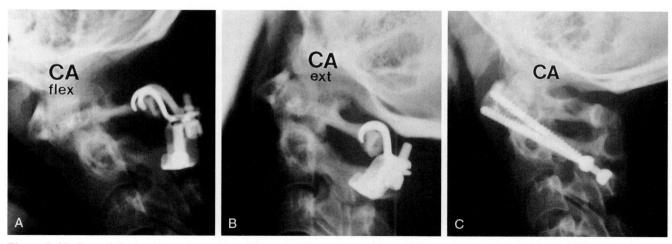

Figure 5–10. *Lateral flexion (A) and extension (B) x-rays illustrating a failed atlantoaxial fusion attempted with a Halifax clamp. Successful salvage arthrodesis was achieved with Magerl transarticular screw fixation (C).*

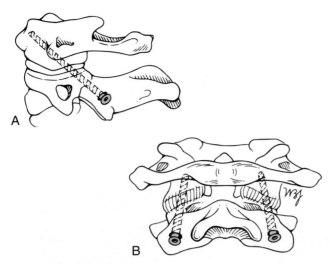

Figure 5–11. *Magerl's C1–C2 transarticular screw technique; lateral (A) and anteroposterior (B) views.*

laminar fixation is needed. All interlaminar techniques have a higher nonunion rate in rheumatoid patients because of their greater instability and poor bone quality.[17] Transarticular screw or occiput–C2 fixation should be considered for these patients.

Magerl's transarticular screw fixation can be applied across both C1–C2 facet joints under x-ray guidance (Fig. 5–11).[70] This is the only posterior atlantoaxial instrumentation technique that can be used with an incompetent C1 arch. It is also useful when the space available for the cord is reduced such that sublaminar wire passage is unwise. With the C2 roots retracted cephalad, the posterior half of the C1–C2 joints can be exposed and decorticated and the joints directly bone grafted, although some authors believe this step to be optional. Whereas fixed C1–C2 subluxation generally presents problems for wiring methods, it can actually facilitate Magerl screw insertion, because a lower screw insertion angle is required.[41] A reminder regarding the vertebral arteries is warranted: Their position relative to the intended screw path must be evaluated, especially with advanced rheumatoid destruction. Routine preoperative sagittal CT reconstructions are recommended to look for a narrow C2 isthmus or anomalous vertebral artery. Consideration might also be given to either magnetic resonance imaging (MRI) or conventional angiography in unusual circumstances. Effective preoperative planning and attention to detail intraoperatively can minimize the risk of vertebral artery injury. Cannulated 3.5- or 4.0-mm screws are useful, allowing the guidewire to remain in place until the screws are in the desired location.

Several of the aforementioned constructs have been studied biomechanically using bovine and human cadaver injury models for odontoid fractures and ligamentous injuries.[46, 92] Each technique significantly restricted unstable motion of the injured spine and returned spinal rigidity back to physiologic levels for flexion, extension, torsion, and anterior shear. The Magerl technique was the only one that could restore posterior shear rigidity back to physiologic levels in the injured spine.[77, 92] It provided the

strongest fixation under all loading conditions.[51, 92] Depending on the stability of the screw fixation, the quality of bone, and the need to minimize external immobilization, the Magerl screws can be augmented with a posterior wiring or suture technique. Bone grafting is performed much like a modified Gallie graft plus additional morcels of autograft. Recently, however, supplemental posterior wire fixation has proven to be unnecessary.[68]

Magerl screws were significantly stiffer after cyclic loading than any of the wire constructs, which all showed loosening independent of whether stainless steel wire or cables were used.[21, 92] This loosening rapidly negated any significant difference between wiring techniques and often approached the instability of the injured spine model.

A retrospective review of 161 patients from 4 centers revealed that transarticular screw fixation resulted in 99.4% fusion with a 5.9% complication rate directly related to the screws.[49] Another study reported a fusion rate of 93% using the Magerl technique and a soft collar, compared with a rate of 58% using a modified Gallie fusion and a halo vest.[34] Though technically exacting, transarticular screw fixation is our preferred method for atlantoaxial fusions provided that the anatomy is suitable.

Subaxial Spine

In the subaxial spine, wiring and plating techniques are available for fastening any combination of posterior arch components to one another. Interspinous fixation is most commonly performed. The advantages of interspinous methods are lower cost, decreased operative time, and decreased risk of neurovascular injury. However, they require intact posterior structures and attention to detail.

Interspinous Wiring

Posterior wire constructs act as tethers to resist distraction and flexion around an anterior axis of rotation. But overtightening must be avoided, because the induced hyperextension can lead to spinal canal or neuroforaminal stenosis. Use of a properly fashioned posterior interspinous buttress, such as a corticocancellous graft of proper height, can resist such hyperextension and posterior translation. Resistance of shear and torsion forces in most of the wiring methods depends on facet joint integrity.

Several alternatives to single-strand stainless steel wire are widely used today. Twisted strands of stainless steel monofilament can be fashioned in the operating room. They have greater tensile strength per unit area than single wires with better resistance to bending, but they may be too bulky for sublaminar use.

Commercially available braided stainless steel or titanium cables with a crimped link obviate the need for twist fastening. The twisted ends of monofilament wires can exhibit rapid initial loosening because of unwinding, and the twists are the primary point of wire failure from stress concentration. Cables also fail at their fastening sites, which are the points of maximal stress but at much higher loads. Cables are three times stronger than single wire and six times stronger than double wire in yield and fatigue tests.[93] Songer[93] noted significantly decreased somatosensory evoked potentials (SSEP) fluctuations with the use of cables. Titanium cables allow postoperative MRI but have tensile strength equivalent to that of double wire and fatigue strength similar to that of single wire with a lower yield point.

Polyethylene cables have recently been developed with tensile strength similar to that of stainless steel and much higher fatigue strength.[22] Polymer tape has been advocated for use in children, patients with tight spinal canals, and patients with osteoporotic bone because of its high tensile strength and low profile. However, tension cannot be maximized because conventional suture knots must be used, and these tend to stretch slightly over time.[39]

Interspinous wiring remains the mainstay of treatment for subaxial posterior ligamentous instability. Several more stable variations have been developed for use in diskoligamentous and fracture instability patterns. The original technique described by Rogers involved extraosseous open-loop fixation around adjacent spinous processes with onlay bone grafting.[85, 86] But this method could not block extension, and wire slippage was possible. Even passing wires through transspinous burr holes, which prevents dislodgement, cannot prevent extension.[84] Such extension, or even hyperextension from excessive wire tightening, can be prevented by inserting a tailored interspinous buttress graft. Safe preparation of transspinous burr holes requires awareness of the location of the spinal canal in relation to the laminae and spinous processes. Spinal cord injury may result from incorrect hole placement or errant wire passage (Fig. 5–12).

The Bohlman triple-wire technique involves a double loop through the burr hole at each level to increase wire pullout resistance, reinforced with two structural corticocancellous bone graft buttresses. The latter are fastened across the midline using separate upper and lower wires through the same spinous process drill holes (Fig. 5–13). The Bohlman technique avoids sublaminar wire passage, provides biomechanically stronger fixation, and yields higher fusion rates. In this method, 18- or 20-gauge

interspinous wires are applied using the open-loop technique as described earlier. The two ends are then fastened together to provide posterior compression. Upper and lower 22- to 24-gauge wires are then passed through the respective drill holes of the corticocancellous graft, through the spinous process, and through the other strut. The upper and lower wires are fastened to one another over the top of each graft. This technique should probably not be used for more than three levels of fixation to avoid the risk of hyperlordosis or inadequate fixation. Although triple wiring provides only marginal improvement in flexion/extension stability, the bilateral bone grafts significantly increase the resistance to axial and coronal rotation by widening the construct. The triple-wire technique is biomechanically equal or superior to other tensioned wire constructs while eliminating the risk of sublaminar passage and enhancing fusion with the corticocancellous graft compressed against the lamina.[71, 95]

Spinous process fixation can be modified by using a Kirschner wire as described by Davey.[20] In this technique, the pin is placed through the base of each spinous process alone or through contoured bone graft struts on each side. This construct is conceptually similar to the triple-wire method, with the added extension stiffness of a midline strut. However, its technical difficulty has limited its practical utility.

Sublaminar wiring is rarely used in this region because of the decreased space available for the spinal cord below C2. It can provide more stable fixation but is also associated with greater risks, including dural tears and neurologic injury.[13, 18, 104] These complications can occur during wire passage, long-term implantation, or removal.[44, 79, 90] The risk is lowest in the occipitocervical region, where the subarachnoid space is largest, but the complications associated with spinal cord contusion at the craniocervical junction are also greater. The surgeon must verify that adequate space remains for safe wire passage. In the subaxial spine, the narrow canal is associated with greater risk of injury with sublaminar wires; this risk is further increased by any pathologic process that narrows the spinal canal. Cervical spinal stenosis caused by spondylosis, ossified posterior longitudinal ligament, subluxation, or kyphosis is considered a relative contraindication to sublaminar wiring. However, in certain circumstances, sublaminar purchase may afford the best trade-off between the quality of fixation and risk of iatrogenic injury. Hook placement in the cervical spine carries similar potential hazards.

Rotational ligamentous instability from facet dislocation with or without articular process fractures can be treated using an oblique wiring configuration.[14] Before midline interspinous wiring is performed, a separate strand is passed through a drill hole in the inferior articular process of the damaged facet. The wire is threaded through a burr hole in the base of the subjacent spinous process. Separate wires are then used to complete the midline wiring.

Multilevel facet buttress wiring can be performed using the techniques of facet wiring and the principles of buttress stabilization as described for occipitocervical constructs. The wires are fastened around a Luque rod, a rib graft (Fig. 5–14), or a threaded Steinmann pin. Southwick reported a fourfold increase in stiffness and 80% decrease in motion

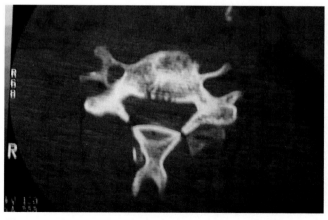

Figure 5–12. *Preparation of spinous process burr holes and safe passage of transspinous wires requires an appreciation of the transition from the spinous process to the lamina. In this instance, the surgeon placed the burr holes too far ventrally, resulting in incomplete quadriplegia.*

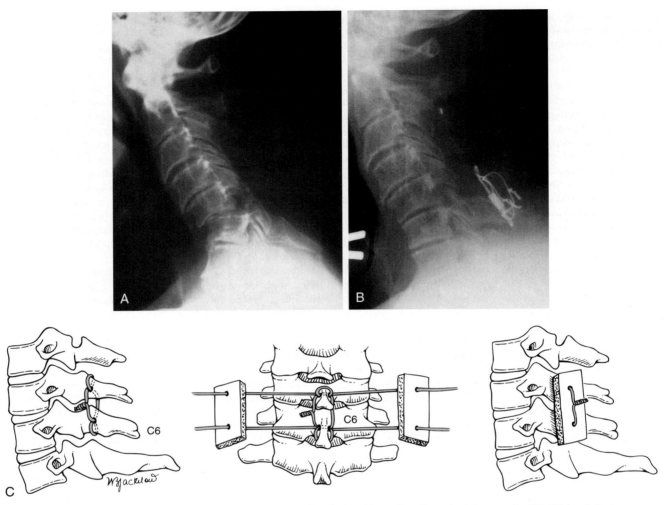

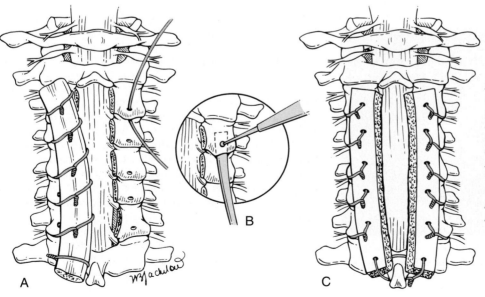

Figure 5–13. *Lateral x-ray of an elderly female who sustained a flexion-distraction ligament injury at the C5–C6 level during a motor vehicle accident (A). Her perched facets reduced spontaneously. A posterior triple-wire fusion procedure was performed with a combination of surgical cable and 22-gauge monofilament wire (B). C, Schematic of the Bohlman triple-wire technique.*

Figure 5–14. *Schematic view (A) of a lateral mass fusion technique as described by Southwick. A rib graft has been used in this instance, but rectangular rods may also be used. A Penfield type of instrument is placed in the facet joint when making the bur holes for wire placement (B); the completed construct (C).*

with the use of spinous process and facet wires.[42, 43] Axial rotation can be eliminated by using rectangular loops or cross-linked rods. When both anterior and posterior osseous deficiencies are present, a cervical level cannot be adequately immobilized by any of the posterior wiring constructs, because they do not provide sufficient resistance to posterior translation, torsion, or axial shortening.[19, 98] Wire fixation for these severe injuries must be augmented with anterior surgery, external immobilization, and/or more rigid posterior internal fixation.

Screw–Plate Fixation

Rigid internal fixation of the posterior cervical spine can be achieved with lateral mass, transpedicular, or transarticular screws through various types of plates to provide single-level or multilevel stabilization. Cervical plating can be applied in the presence of posterior element deficiencies without including normal motion segments. Lateral mass screw fixation methods are differentiated first by the method of screw insertion and second by the type of plating. Most recently, rod–plate combinations provide additional hybrid fixation options. Originally, two conceptually distinct techniques of lateral mass screw fixation for the lower cervical spine were described by Roy-Camille and Magerl. Several variations on this theme have since been described. Each method has its advantages and disadvantages, yet is relatively safe if the surgeon is aware of the anatomic limitations.

Roy-Camille pioneered lateral mass screw fixation techniques using an anterior/posterior trajectory that trades intraosseous screw working length for safety.[88] The entry point is at the center of the rectangular posterior face of the lateral mass or can be measured 5 mm medial to the lateral edge and midway between the facet joints. This starting point is midway between the projections of the exiting nerve roots.[105] The drill is directed perpendicular to the posterior wall of the vertebral body with a 10-degree lateral angle (Fig. 5–15). This trajectory is reproducibly achieved and yields an exit point slightly lateral to the vertebral artery and below the exiting nerve root.[30, 105] The lateral mass depth from C3 to C6 ranges from 6 to 14 mm in males (average 8.7 mm) and 6 to 11 mm in females (average 7.9 mm). An adjustable drill guide set to a depth of 10 to 12 mm is used to prevent penetration beyond the anterior cortex. The depth can then be gradually and safely increased as the local anatomy permits. Roy-Camille recommended use of a 16- or 19-mm screw through his plate to ensure bicortical purchase. If the additional 20% of pullout strength with bicortical fixation is desired, then the exit point should be at the junction of the lateral mass and transverse process.[3] Lateral fluoroscopic imaging makes it easier to choose the optimum trajectory and avoid penetration of the facet joint (Fig. 5–16).

The Magerl technique uses an entry point which is 1 mm medial and rostral to the center point of the posterior surface of the lateral mass.[55] It is oriented at a 45° to 60° rostral angle, parallel to the adjacent facet joint articular surface, and at a 25° lateral angle. This path yields a potential exit point lateral to the vertebral artery and above the exiting

nerve root while engaging the lateral portion of the ventral cortex of the superior articular facet. The proper trajectory for this technique is more difficult to achieve than the Roy-Camille technique. At this inclination the lateral mass working depth is approximately 20 mm compared with 14 mm for the Roy-Camille technique,[78] which probably contributes to its enhanced load to failure.[78] The proper sagittal angle may be obstructed by the prominence of the cervicothoracic junction. The incision may have to be extended and some of the spinous processes may need to be trimmed to gain the proper angle with the drill.

The Roy-Camille trajectory maximizes bone strength per unit length along the path of the screw, but the Magerl trajectory maximizes screw length and yields theoretically greater pullout strength.[33, 78] In either case bicortical fixation is nearly 20% stronger than unicortical.[56] The added purchase strength must be balanced against the increased risk of morbidity associated with anterior cortical penetration. The cranial and caudal levels should be considered for bicortical fixation, particularly in the osteopenic patient. Heller et al demonstrated that the pullout strength of lateral mass screws is maximal in the mid cervical region and then tapers significantly in either direction.[56]

The Roy-Camille trajectory is more likely to result in violation of the inferior facet joint, while the path of the Magerl screw places the nerve root at greater risk and is more frequently misplaced because of obstructive anatomy (Fig. 5–17). A learning curve is evident regardless of the overall surgical experience. But after sufficient practice with either technique, the statistical differences in morbidity risk disappear. The greater technical difficulty of the Magerl technique was demonstrated by a persistently increased malposition rate despite increasing experience.[55]

An et al. demonstrated the optimal position at C3–C6 to be an even greater lateral trajectory requiring an entry point 1 mm medial to the center of the lateral mass with a 33° lateral angle and a compromise between the previously described techniques with a 17° cephalad angle.[3] Anderson proposed another compromise trajectory with a starting point 1 mm medial to the midpoint of the lateral mass angled 30° to 40° cranial and 10° lateral.[5] This orients the screw for the safest anterior cortical fixation point at the lateral ventral surface of the superior articular facet lateral to the vertebral artery and above the exiting nerve root. This can be used for bicortical fixation and may be the most appropriate in the upper levels or in cases where the vertebral foramen is more medial as documented on CT scan. These modifications have similar screw depth and probably similar pullout strength to the Roy-Camille and Magerl techniques, respectively. Using quantitative anatomy based on CT measurements, Arthur determined the optimal entry point in orientation of each cervical level to avoid neurovascular structures and maximize fixation of lateral mass screws.[9] He recommended that the most exacting levels, C6 and C7, be instrumented first followed by the C3 to C5 where fixation parameters, particularly entry points, are more forgiving.

Another potentially useful technique is that of subaxial transfacet screw fixation. Originally proposed by Roy-

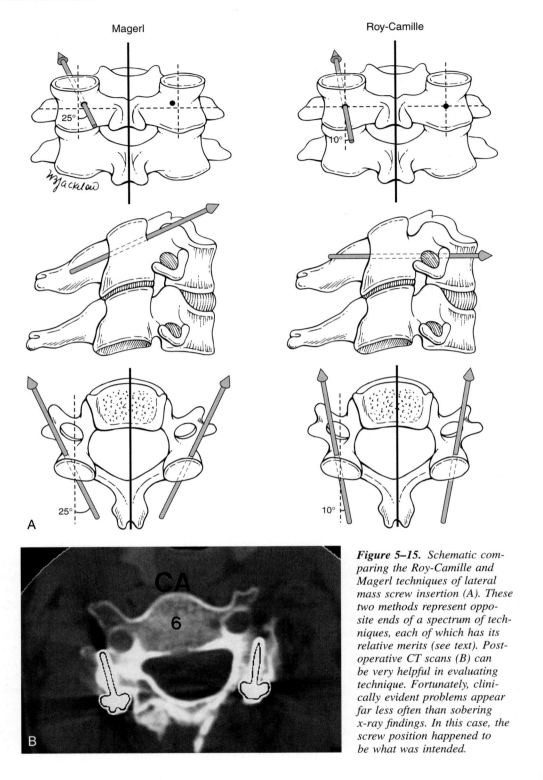

Magerl   Roy-Camille

A

Figure 5–15. Schematic comparing the Roy-Camille and Magerl techniques of lateral mass screw insertion (A). These two methods represent opposite ends of a spectrum of techniques, each of which has its relative merits (see text). Postoperative CT scans (B) can be very helpful in evaluating technique. Fortunately, clinically evident problems appear far less often than sobering x-ray findings. In this case, the screw position happened to be what was intended.

Camille and Saillant[87] in 1972, the screw is angled inferiorly and laterally, traversing both cortices of the inferior articular process and at least one cortex of the superior articular process (Fig. 5–18). The incremental pullout strength of the additional cortex purchased was demonstrated by Klekamp et al.[65] When such a screw is inserted through a lateral mass plate, it theoretically enhances segmental stiffness by transfixing the facet joint. The technique may be used at all but the lowest instrumented level, since one would not want to violate the subjacent normal facet joint.

Hook-plates use a combination of sublaminar and interference fixation to form an articulolaminar construct that increases flexion and torsional stiffness, prevents

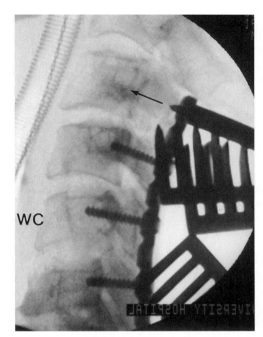

Figure 5–16. True lateral intraoperative x-ray images can be very helpful in selecting the correct sagittal trajectory for lateral mass screws. This is of particular value when performing multilevel procedures, because the holes within a plate will often dictate starting points that are atypical. The arrow points to the transverse process of C3, which is the landmark for insertion by An's method.

anterior translation, and provides compression. This procedure requires intact inferior laminae (Fig. 5–19). Axial compression is also provided by the upward angle of the Magerl screw used in this construct, which pulls the hook cephalad. This screw can also be inserted sufficiently rostrally in the lateral mass to exert dynamic compression effect as it is tightened. This serves to lock the facet and reduce dislocations, but may increase the risk of foraminal impingement. Similar to wiring, this tension band is behind the axis of rotation and causes extension and posterior translation of the upper vertebral level, which can result in hyperlordosis unless blocked by an interspinous buttress graft.

Lateral mass plating is indicated in cases of posterior element fracture, facet fracture with rotational instability, burst fractures, postlaminectomy instability or kyphosis, certain tumors, and fixation to the cervicothoracic junction. It is better suited to multilevel fusions than wire because it provides translation stability without hyperextension, provides enhanced torsional stiffness, and resists axial shortening. As long as the facets remain intact to act as a buttress, even moderate anterior osteoligamentous injuries, such as burst fractures and flexible kyphotic deformities, can be stabilized by lateral mass plates. However, because only the posterior elements are engaged by the technique, it still shares a common limitation of other forms of posterior element fixation, albeit to a lesser degree.

The ideal plate must be able to accommodate the variable anatomy of the region and the different techniques of screw insertion and be stiff enough to promote fusion, yet narrow enough to allow adequate graft–host contact area. The fixed hole position of many plating systems dictates the screw entry point. Plating systems more adaptable to differences in interfacet distances and screw starting points are more easily applied. Modular rod and rod–plate devices that theoretically address some of these issues are under development.

The method of screw insertion to use at any given level of a construct may depend on circumstances. The size and shape of the lateral masses and pedicles, as well as the position along the plate, may influence the choice. Generally, screws with maximum purchase strength at the ends of the plates are desired. Pullout strength is theoretically less critical for intermediate screws. Therefore, using bicortical screws at the ends of a plate may be justified. Because Magerl constructs tend to fail from plate bending, whereas Roy-Camille constructs tend to fail from screw pullout,[78] one could argue that this method is preferable at the ends of plates. This proposition is further supported by the knowledge that a Roy-Camille technique has enhanced risk of violating the normal subjacent facet joint. However, intermediate screws are well suited to the easier Roy-Camille method. Transfacet screws might even further enhance intersegmental stiffness when used in the intermediate or rostral position. Just how all of this applies to the other methods of lateral mass screw insertion is a matter of conjecture, because the other methods represent points on a continuum between the Magerl and Roy-Camille methods.

Just how effective are posterior plating methods in comparison with more traditional posterior or anterior instrumentation options? Data are available from a number of biomechanical studies. Roy-Camille demonstrated in a diskoligamentous injury model that plate fixation provided only marginal increase in stability under flexion load, but a significant increase under extension load in comparison with interspinous and facet wiring. Lateral mass plating provides greater stability, especially in diskoligamentous injuries in translation, rotation, and cyclic flexion loading, but may be slightly less effective in reducing anterior strain

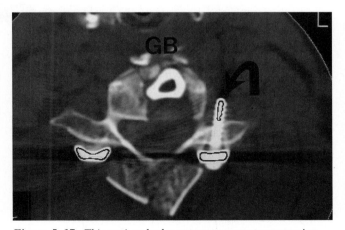

Figure 5–17. This patient had a very narrow anteroposterior lateral mass dimension at C7. A C8 radiculopathy resulted from insertion of an overly long screw.

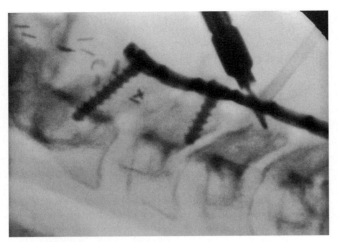

Figure 5–18. *Lateral x-ray of insertion of a cervical trans-facet screw. At least three cortices are engaged in this method (see text).*

because it provides less compression and facet engagement than wiring.[19] Lateral mass plates failed by screw pullout with the proximal end failing more in flexion and the distal end failing more frequently in torsion.

In a calf spine model of posterior wiring, plating, and circumferential constructs, all three methods were found to be equivalent but significantly stiffer than anterior plates under compression loads for single-level posterior and circumferential ligamentous injuries.[66] In multilevel instability, the posterior plate allowed less sagittal rotation than the triple-wire technique, but these differences were not statistically significant. In injury models with intact vertebral bodies and facet joints, no clear differences between posterior plating and wiring have been demonstrated. Because the safety and effectiveness of the triple-wire method are well established, we prefer to keep the procedures as straightforward as possible. We use lateral mass plating for ligamentous instability complicated by loss of bone integrity, such as fractures of the spinous processes, facet joints, or vertebral bodies; laminectomy; or problems involving more than two motion segments.

As for the clinical success of others, Roy-Camille reported 100% fusion in 221 subjects with 8.8% angulation of less than 5 degrees and 3% angulation of 5 to 10 degrees with no plate or screw failure.[88] Using the same technique for posttraumatic instability, Fehlings reported fusion rates of 93% (39 of 42 subjects) with loosening in only 3.8% of screws at 4-year follow-up.[36] For instability of various causes, Ebraheim reported 100% fusion (13 of 13 subjects) with only a 2% rate of screw loosening.[25] When a modified Magerl technique was used with atlanto-occipital reconstruction plates, facet decortication, and bone grafting, a 100% fusion rate was achieved with no neurovascular complications.[5] Magerl plating using the AXIS™ fixation system (Sofamor Danek, Inc., Memphis, TN) in 17 patients resulted in 100% bone union, but some loss of lordosis seen on 2-year follow-up.[96]

In cases of facet fracture subluxation associated with superior articular process fractures, Roy-Camille devised a unique "porte manteau" technique. By combining a "roof tile" plate (plaque en tuile), which simulated the function of the broken articular process, with a lateral mass plate, he was able to reconstruct and stabilize such injuries. This technique involves cutting a 1/3 tubular bone plate to the proper length and then bending it at a 45-degree angle to match the inclination of the facet joint. The bent plate restores the deficient buttress of the facet joint and prevents anterior subluxation of the superior vertebral body. A lateral mass plate is placed over the tile plate spanning the injured motion segment. The inferior lateral mass screw passes through both plates and fixes them to the inferior lateral mass on the injured side. Because the superior articular process is fractured, a Roy-Camille screw technique must be used in this case. The opposite side is instrumented with a lateral mass plate using whatever screw method deemed appropriate.

Pedicle Screw Fixation

At C2, no true lateral mass is available for fixation. The steeply angled inferior facet, elongated and narrow isthmus, horizontal superior facet, and inferior and lateral position of the vertebral artery necessitate an alternate screw position. In contrast, a medial or superior trajectory is available into the relatively spacious pedicles (probably more precisely termed the pars interarticularis) at this level, providing a longer and safer path for improved fixation. C2 pedicle screws can be used with a lag technique to reduce and fix traumatic spondylolisthesis of the axis. When such a C2 traumatic spondylolisthesis is associated with an inferior facet fracture, facet dislocation, C2 teardrop fracture, or C2–C3 instability, segmental fixation can be achieved with a two-hole plate using a C2 pedicle and C3 lateral mass screws.

To guide screw placement, Roy-Camille described direct visualization and palpation of the medial and superior walls of the C2 pedicle through the C1–C2 interlaminar interval, where the space available for the cord is greatest. He

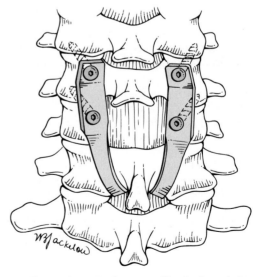

Figure 5–19. *A schematic drawing of hook plates being used to fuse two motion segments after laminectomy. The method is equally useful with fractured laminae or spinous processes.*

recommended using the superomedial quadrant of the C2 lateral mass for the entry point to keep the screw rostral and medial within the pedicle. The screw should follow as close to the superomedial cortex as possible, with a 10- to 15-degree upward inclination and medial angulation. This avoids a lateral or inferior trajectory into the path of the vertebral artery or inferomedial penetration at the exit of the C3 root. The screw length is usually 20 to 30 mm. Magerl recommended a more lateral and caudal entry point 2 mm below the midpoint with a shallow and inward trajectory 25 degrees cranial and medial. This path traverses the medial and cranial part of the isthmus and stops in the subchondral bone beneath the superior articular surface. This steeper path risks violating the C2 superior facet, but the more medial angle may avoid an enlarged or tortuous vertebral artery. Regardless of the method chosen, direct observation of the relevant landmarks combined with intraoperative x-ray guidance makes screw insertion at C2 relatively predictable and safe.

Xu and Ebraheim evaluated transpedicular C2 fixation and defined the entry point as 5 mm inferior to the superior border of the C2 lamina and 7 mm lateral to the lateral border of the spinal canal at the junction of the lamina and lateral mass.[107] They initially used a trajectory of 30 degrees medial and 20 degrees cephalad, but found that this resulted in an unacceptable risk of lateral perforation and potential for vertebral artery injury. They subsequently modified their placement technique and now recommend, as the most accurate and safest method, a nerve retractor to palpate the superomedial wall of the pedicle through the C1–C2 interlaminar space.

Subaxial pedicle fixation may be indicated in the face of bone deficiencies such as hypoplastic or malformed lateral masses, facet fracture, partial facetectomy, bilateral C2 pedicle fracture with traumatic spondylolisthesis of the axis, or articular mass fracture separation. Pedicle fixation is the only posterior technique that can provide three-column fixation of the cervical spine. This added stability might be desirable in extremely unstable situations, such as osteo-ligamentous injuries, or insufficiency with loss of axial stability, such as rheumatoid arthritis, kyphotic deformity, severe fracture, or diffuse tumor infiltration. Pedicle fixation is also recommended at levels with insufficient lateral mass size or bone density for strong fixation, especially at C2 and the cervicothoracic junction, where the pedicles are larger. Greater pullout strength than that obtained with lateral mass screws makes this technique desirable for long constructs with greater moments at their upper and lower ends.[63, 66A]

In single-level posterior ligamentous and circumferential diskoligamentous injuries, pedicle screws provide no significant advantage over lateral mass plating, triple wiring, or a combination of the two techniques.[66] In multilevel involvement of these same instability patterns, pedicle fixation produces a significant increase in torsional and extensional stiffness over the three other techniques. Because pedicle screws have greater pullout strength, they may resist toggling from cyclic axial loading and also improve long-term fixation in cases of anterior injury where the vertebral buttress is destroyed, such as burst fractures or tumor erosion.[63] In some cases, this sort of rigid posterior segmental fixation may eliminate the need for combined

anterior/posterior procedures. Screw loosening with pseudarthrosis or loss of deformity reduction can be expected in some patients instrumented with lateral mass screws, but it has not been reported with pedicle fixation.[5, 36, 57]

The risks of pedicle screw placement, as mentioned earlier, are significant because of the surrounding anatomic structures.[1B] Cervical pedicle screws placed in a laboratory setting using only surface anatomic landmarks for standardized starting point locations and trajectory angles resulted in only 12.5% accurate containment within the pedicle, with a 21.9% rate of noncritical cortical breeches and a 65.5% rate of critical cortical breeches.[67] When a 3.0-mm screw was used, the percentage of contained screws was greater (52.6%), but protruding, impinging, and potentially damaging penetrations were still quite common, occurring at rates of 21.1%, 10.5%, and 15.8%, respectively.[76] When laminoforaminotomy and direct palpation were used to guide placement, the accuracy of a 3.5-mm screw increased to only 45%, with 15.4% noncritical and 39.6% critical breeches.[67] Even the use of frameless stereotactic guidance techniques resulted in only 76% accurate placement of the larger screws, with 13.4% noncritical and 16.6% critical breeches with this technological enhancement.[67] In a critical breech, the vertebral artery and exiting nerve root were considered at risk in 73.9% and 41.5% of the cases, depending on whether the breeches occurred laterally or superiorly.[67, 69] The greatest improvements in accuracy occurred in the larger C6 and C7 pedicles, leaving C3 through C5 at the highest risk for complications. When inserting subaxial pedicle screws, as with those inserted at C2, direct visualization and palpation of the superior, medial, and inferior pedicle walls using a small nerve retractor (e.g., Penfield) through a laminoforaminotomy are recommended.

In contrast, Abumi has pointed out the hazards associated with laminotomy or laminectomy before pedicle screw insertion related to working with instrumentation over the exposure cord and possible weakening of the medial wall of the pedicle, causing fracture.[1, 2] In his technique, the ability of the pedicle to accommodate a screw is ensured by scrutinizing preoperative radiographs and CT scans. Intraoperatively, the starting point on the surface of the lateral mass is estimated by correlating the bone landmarks with preoperative imaging and intraoperative x-ray views. The posterior cortex and cancellous bone of the lateral mass are removed with a small burr so that the red "bull's-eye" of the cancellous bone within the pedicle is directly visualized. A narrow blunt probe is then inserted down into the pedicle, with progress observed by lateral x-ray views (Fig. 5–20). This method has proven safe and reliable in Abumi's hands. The bone sacrificed in preparing the entrance point must compromise purchase to some extent, but the enhanced clinical safety appears to more than justify this method.

Abumi has used transpedicular screw plate fixation in the subaxial spine for both traumatic and nontraumatic lesions.[1, 1A, 1B, 1C, 2] Among trauma victims, he reported 100% solid fusion with no loss of reduction and no implant or skeletal failure. All radicular symptoms resolved, and motor deficits resolved in 63% of cases. No complications involving the spinal cord, nerve root, or vertebral artery were clinically evident. Three medial and one inferior

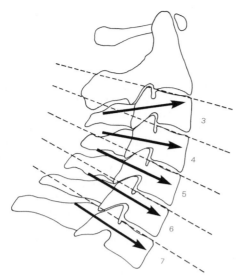

Figure 5–20. *Schematic provided by Abumi illustrating the variable trajectories of pedicle screws in the subaxial spine. These angles are mapped preoperatively and correlated with an intraoperative x-ray as the pedicle holes are sounded with a thin, blunt probe. (From Abumi K, Itoh H, Taneichi H, Kaneda K: Transpedicular screw fixation for traumatic lesions of the middle and lower cervical spine: Description of the techniques and preliminary report. J Spinal Disord 7:19–28, 1994.)*

cortical penetrations were documented. In 45 cases of nontraumatic lesions, Abumi achieved 100% fusion with good correction and maintenance of alignment. Postoperative MRI and CT scan documented no malposition in the 24 C2 pedicle screws and 6.9% penetration in the subaxial pedicles. One of these penetrations was superior and was associated with transient radiculopathy. Of the other malpositioned screws, more than half were medial perforations, but no other neurologic or vascular complications were clinically evident. The predominance of medial

pedicle wall violation is in contrast to the experimental studies discussed earlier, which demonstrated that the vertebral artery was at risk because of lateral penetrations. The differences may well be inherent in the method of screw insertion used.

With widely differing data regarding the accuracy of cervical pedicle screws emerging from laboratory studies and clinical experience, as well as the alleged enhanced safety of frameless stereotactic surgical navigation, Ludwig et al.[68A] sought to compare the best known in vitro method of screw insertion with the clinical method used by Abumi. Under simulated operating room conditions, they compared stereotactic guidance with the x-ray–assisted method used by Abumi. The rates of anatomic accuracy did not differ between the two methods. Significantly, screws were scored as critical breeches in 12% of the Abumi-style screws and in 18% of the stereotactically inserted screws. More importantly, the authors also observed that the likelihood of malposition increased substantially when pedicle diameters were less than 4.5 mm. It is also likely that the low frequency of clinically significant screw malposition reported by Abumi and others[1B, 67, 68A] is linked to local tissue tolerance for error rather than to some uniquely accurate intraoperative execution of a technique. Ludwig et al.[68A] offered tangible parameters to be respected when contemplating the use of cervical pedicle fixation.

Jeanneret recommended pedicle fixation using progressively increasing screw lengths at more caudal levels.[62] He measured the distance from the lateral mass posterior cortex to the vertebral body and anterior cortex and subtracted 6 mm to calculate the optimal screw length as 26 mm for C3–C4, 28 mm for C5, and 30 mm for C6. At C7, the total depth measured was 41 mm, with the increase primarily in the vertebral body segment of the screw path, which is not used for fixation.[29] At this level, Jeanneret recommended a 32-mm screw; however, other anatomic studies suggest that a 30-mm screw may be safer.[106] Although 3.5- to 4.0-mm screws are most commonly used in the cervical spine, smaller screws (2.7 mm) should be

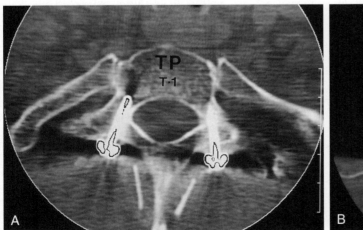
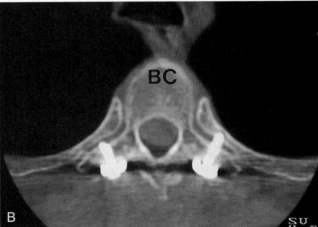

Figure 5–21. *Postoperative CT scan illustrating 3.5-mm screws within the pedicles of T1 in one patient (A) and in the bicortical transverse process position at T1 in another patient (B). Note how the rib heads act to protect the pleura and lung.*

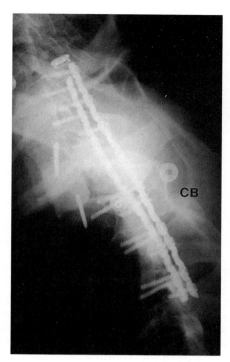

Figure 5–22. *A combined anterior and posterior approach included posterior segmental instrumentation from C5 to T4 for this patient with metastatic melanoma. Lateral mass screws were used in the cervical spine, whereas pedicle screws were inserted in the upper thoracic spine.*

considered if indicated by preoperative CT scan findings, especially at the upper subaxial cervical levels.

The upper thoracic spine is usually well suited to pedicle screw fixation. As pointed out by An and others,[3, 4, 53, 54, 94, 97, 100] the size and orientation of the pedicles can typically accommodate 3.5- to 4.5-mm screws (Fig. 5–21). After the dimensions and orientation of the pedicles have been confirmed, x-ray, laminotomy with palpation of the pedicle, or a combination of the two will provide a reasonable degree of accuracy. This technique works well when bridging the cervicothoracic junction with plates anchored by lateral mass screws in the cervical spine (Fig. 5–22).[2A] Alternatively, if the pedicles are too small or the appropriate starting point and trajectory cannot be achieved through the plate, then placing bicortical screws into the base of the upper thoracic transverse processes could be considered. The neurologic risk is nil, and the rib head usually protects the pleura (see Fig. 5–21B). Shuster et al. found that the mean pullout strength of pedicle screws inserted from T1 to T4 is greater than that of those inserted into the transverse processes.[54] However, the loads to failure for the transverse process screws were comparable to those measured by Heller et al. for lateral mass screws in the subaxial region.[56] Therefore, the transverse process technique remains a safe, albeit biomechanically inferior, alternative to thoracic pedicle screw fixation.

COMPLICATIONS OF POSTERIOR CERVICAL FIXATION

Injuries during fixation differ for the various techniques and can involve the spinal cord, nerve root, vertebral arteries, or facet joints.[1B, 6] Transarticular or C2 pedicle screws can injure the vertebral artery if the trajectory is too low or too lateral, especially when the artery lies in a deep groove or is abnormally large. This can be a mortal event. When too steep a trajectory is chosen or too long a screw is used, undesirable penetration of the occiput–C1 or C1–C2 articulations may occur with these respective techniques (Fig. 5–23). Hypoglossal nerve palsy may occur if the screw tip passes the inner cortex.

Injuries to the spinal cord during fixation are rare but can occur with passage of sublaminar wires, especially below C2, which has the smallest space available for the cord. Failure to account for local anatomic variation can result in erroneous placement of fixation devices, leading to neural or vascular injury. Excessive distraction of an atlanto-occipital instability or disassociation by the application of halo ring traction could cause a stretch injury to the spinal cord. Aggressive posterior wire tightening can result in excessive compression of the facets, causing pain in foraminal height loss. These types of complications can be minimized with scrupulous planning and attention to detail during the procedure.

Experimental studies suggest that facet joint violation and nerve root impingement are the most common complications of lateral mass screws and that the risk of injury to the vertebral artery and spinal cord is low. In a clinical study of multilevel lateral mass screw fixation in 78 patients, Heller et al. reported complication rates using a

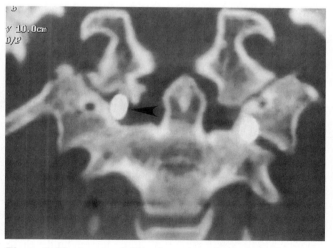

Figure 5–23. *A coronal CT reformation of a patient who presented with acute right-sided head and upper cervical pain 2 years after undergoing transarticular screw fixation and fusion for his combined atlas nonunion and transverse ligament rupture. Note the penetration of the screw tip into the right atlanto-occipital joint (arrow). His symptoms were relieved by screw removal.*

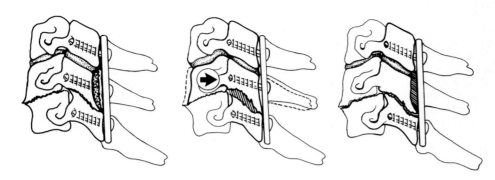

Figure 5-24. In some cases, a lateral mass screw may impart a lag effect, thereby reducing a subluxed lateral mass against the plate. Heller and colleagues reported iatrogenic foraminal stenosis, which they believed was due to this effect. They suggested placing a bone graft "shim" beneath the plate in such instances to block the lag effect. (From Heller JG, Silcox DH III, Sutterlin CE: Complications of posterior cervical plating. Spine 20:2442–2448, 1995.)

modified bicortical Roy-Camille technique.[57] Each lateral mass screw had a composite risk of 1.4%, including a 0.8% risk of malposition, a 0.06% risk of nerve root impingement, and a 0.2% risk of facet violation. But facet violations are clinically significant only at the caudal screws, where acute pain, loss of fixation, or late arthritis can occur. At the intermediate levels, transfacet screws may actually be beneficial. Each case of multilevel lateral mass fixation had a total complication risk of 15.6%. This composite rate included both short-term and long-term problems, such as a 2.6% risk of spinal cord injury, a 2.6% risk of foraminal stenosis (Fig. 5–24), a 1.3% risk of plate fracture, a 2.6% risk of loss of reduction, and a 3.8% risk of adjacent segment degeneration. These complication rates agree with those found in other studies, except for the high loosening rate associated with the loss of reduction reported by Roy-Camille.[88] The rates should also be interpreted in light of the complexity of the cases, as a mean of four motion segments were fused in the patients described by Heller et al.[57]

Higher complication rates were associated with the use of bicortical Magerl lateral mass fixation, as documented by Graham.[45] He reported a 6.1% incidence of screw malposition without placement under x-ray guidance and a 14% reoperation rate for iatrogenic radiculopathy. The rate of screw loosening for 3.5-mm self-tapping bicortical screws was 3.6%.

Complications of cervical pedicle screw malposition depend on the direction of cortical breech. Lateral perforation, the most common complication, can injure the vertebral artery with a starting point of as small as 5 mm and an angular misalignment of as little as 10 degrees. Superior pedicle perforation can injure the exiting nerve root, which lies in the base of the nerve root groove, and/or the screw may enter the intervertebral disk space above the level of fixation. Medial perforation may injure the epidural venous plexus, resulting in bleeding that is difficult to control. Inferior perforations are the least dangerous, because the exiting root lies in the inferior portion of the foramen. Excessively long screws could theoretically penetrate the anterior vertebral body wall and irritate, puncture, or erode the esophagus or pharynx.

CONCLUSION

Recent quantitative advances in anatomical study of the cervical spine have paralleled the evolution of increasingly sophisticated surgical techniques. The contemporary spine surgeon has increasingly better tools available to address more complex problems. However, to optimize outcomes and minimize complications, the surgeon must correctly appreciate the pathoanatomy affecting the cervical spine. Only then can the surgeon infer the biomechanical deficiencies that must be addressed through spinal instrumentation. Familiarity with the various ways of using wire, cables, hooks, and screws to purchase or transfix each level of the cervical spine, along with knowledge of the various ways of interconnecting these points of purchase, enables the surgeon to tailor an operation to the needs of a particular patient with due respect for the potential pitfalls.

REFERENCES

1. Abumi K, Itoh H, Taneichi H, Kaneda K: Transpedicular screw fixation for traumatic lesions of the middle and lower cervical spine: Description of the techniques and preliminary report. J Spinal Disord 7:19–28, 1994.

1a. Abumi K, Kaneda K, Shono Y, Fujiya M: One-stage posterior decompression and reconstruction of the cervical spine by using pedicle screw fixation systems. J Neurosurg 90:19–26, 1999.

1b. Abumi K, Shono Y, Ito M, et al: Complications of pedicle screw fixation in reconstructive surgery of the cervical spine. Spine 25:962–969, 2000.

1c. Abumi K, Takada T, Shono Y, et al: Posterior occipitocervical reconstruction using cervical pedicle screws and plate-rod systems. Spine 24:1425–1434, 1999.

2. Abumi K, Kaneda K: Pedicle screw fixation for nontraumatic lesions of the cervical spine. Presented in part at the 62nd Annual Meeting of the American Academy of Orthopaedic Surgeons, February 16–21, 1995.

2a. Albert TJ, Klein GR, Joffe D, Vaccaro AR: Use of cervicothoracic junction pedicle screws for reconstruction of complex cervical spine pathology. Spine 23:1596–1599, 1998.

3. An HS, Gordin R, Renner K: Anatomic considerations for

plate-screw fixation of the cervical spine. Spine 16:S548–S551, 1991.

4. An HS, Vaccaro AR, Cotler J, Lin S: Spinal disorders at the cervicothoracic junction. Spine 19:2257–2264, 1994.

5. Anderson PA, Henley MB, Grady MS, et al: Posterior cervical arthrodesis with AO reconstruction plates and bone graft. Spine 16:S72–S79, 1991.

6. Andreshak TG, An HS: Complications of cervical spine surgery. In An HS, Simpson JM (eds): Surgery of the Cervical Spine. Baltimore, Williams and Wilkins, 1994, pp 401–426.

7. Apostolides PJ, Dickman CA, Golfinos JG, et al: Threaded Steinmann pin fusion of the craniovertebral junction. Spine 21:1630–1637, 1996.

8. Aprin H, Harf R: Stabilization of atlantoaxial instability. Orthopedics 11:1687–1693, 1988.

9. Arthur DJ, Gundel J, Gregory D, et al: A calibrated CT evaluation of the subaxial cervical lateral mass and current fixation recommendations. Presented at the Twenty-Fourth Annual Meeting of the Cervical Spine Research Society, Palm Beach, FL, 1996.

10. Bailey AS, Stanescu S, Yeasting RA, et al: Anatomic relationships of the cervicothoracic junction. Spine 20:1431–1439, 1995.

11. Boden SD, McCowin PR, Davis DO, et al: Abnormal magnetic-resonance scans of the cervical spine in asymptomatic subjects: A prospective investigation. J Bone Joint Surg Am 72A:1178–1184, 1990.

12. Boyle JJ, Singer KP, Milne N: Morphological survey of the cervicothoracic junctional region. Spine 21:544–548, 1996.

13. Brooks AL, Jenkins EB: Atlanto-axial arthrodesis by the wedge compression method. J Bone Joint Surg Am 60A:279–284, 1978.

14. Cahill DW, Bellegarrigue R, Ducker TB: Bilateral facet to spinous process fusion: A new technique for posterior spinal fusion after trauma. Neurosurgery 13:1–4, 1983.

15. Caruso S, Haher TR, Yeung A, et al: Occipital screw pullout strength: A biomechanical investigation of occipital morphology. Presented at the Twenty-Fourth Annual Meeting of the Cervical Spine Research Society, Palm Beach, FL, 1996.

16. Clark CR, Goetz DD, Menezes AH: Arthrodesis of the cervical spine in rheumatoid arthritis. J Bone Joint Surg Am 71A:381–392, 1989.

17. Clark CR: Trauma and rheumatoid arthritis of the upper cervical spine. In Sherk HH (ed): The Cervical Spine: An Atlas of Surgical Procedures. Philadelphia, JB Lippincott, 1994, pp 127–144.

18. Coe JD, Becker PS, McAfee PC, Gurr KR: Neuropathology with spinal instrumentation. J Orthop Res 7:359–370, 1989.

19. Coe JD, Warden KE, Sutterlin CE III, McAfee PC: Biomechanical evaluation of cervical spinal stabilization methods in a human cadaveric model. Spine 14:1122–1131, 1989.

20. Davey JR, Rorabeck CH, Bailey SI, et al: A technique of posterior cervical fusion for instability of the cervical spine. Spine 10:722–728, 1985.

21. Dickman CA, Crawford NR: Biomechanical characteristics of C1–C2 cable fixations. Presented at the Twenty-Fourth Annual Meeting of the Cervical Spine Research Society, Palm Beach, FL, 1996.

22. Dickman CA, Papadopoulos SM: Comparative mechanical properties of spinal cable and wire fixation systems. Spine 22:596–604, 1997.

23. Doherty BJ, Heggeness MH: Quantitative anatomy of the second cervical vertebra. Spine 20:513–517, 1995.

24. Dvorak J, Schneider E, Saldinger P, Rahn B: Biomechanics of the craniocervical region: The alar and transverse ligaments. J Orthop Res 6:452–461, 1988.

25. Ebraheim NA, An HS, Jackson WT, Brown JA: Internal fixation of the unstable cervical spine using posterior Roy-Camille plates: Preliminary report. J Orthop Trauma 3:23–28, 1989.

26. Ebraheim NA, An HS, Xu R, et al: The quantitative anatomy of the cervical nerve root groove and the intervertebral foramen. Spine 21:1619–1923, 1996.

27. Ebraheim NA, Lu J, Biyani A, et al: An anatomic study of the thickness of the occipital bone: Implications for occipitocervical instrumentation. Spine 21:1725–1730, 1996.

28. Ebraheim N, Rollins JR Jr, Xu R, Jackson WT: Anatomic consideration of C2 pedicle screw placement. Spine 21:691–695, 1996.

29. Ebraheim NA, Xu R, Knight T, Yeasting RA: Morphometric evaluation of lower cervical pedicle and its projections. Spine 22:1–6, 1997.

30. Ebraheim NA, Xu R, Yeasting RA: The location of the vertebral artery foramen and its relation to posterior lateral mass screw fixation. Spine 21:1291–1295, 1996.

31. Elia M, Mazzara JT, Fielding JW: Onlay technique for occipitocervical fusion. Clin Orthop 280:170–174, 1992.

32. Ellis PM, Findlay JM: Craniocervical fusion with contoured Luque rod and autogeneic bone graft. Can J Surg 37:50–54, 1994.

33. Errico T, Uhl R, Cooper P, et al: Pullout strength comparison of two methods of orienting screw insertion in the lateral masses of the bovine cervical spine. J Spinal Disord 5:459–463, 1992.

34. Farey ID, Green J, Smith N: C1–C2 fusion: Magerl technique versus modified Gallie technique. Presented at the Twenty-Fourth Annual Meeting of the Cervical Spine Research Society, The Breakers, Palm Beach, FL, 1996.

35. Farmer JC, Wisneski RJ: Cervical spine nerve root compression. An analysis of neuroforaminal pressures with varying head and arm positions. Spine 19:1850–1855, 1994.

36. Fehlings MG, Cooper PR, Errico TJ: Posterior plates in the management of cervical instability: Long-term results in 44 patients. J Neurosurg 81:341–349, 1994.

37. Fehlings MG, Errico T, Cooper P, et al: Technical reports: Occipitocervical fusion with a five-millimeter malleable rod and segmental fixation. Neurosurgery 32:198–207; comments 207–208, 1993.

38. Fried LC: Atlanto-axial fracture-dislocations: Failure of posterior C1 to C2 fusion. J Bone Joint Surg Br 55B:490–496, 1973.

39. Gaines RW Jr, Abernathie DL: Mersilene tapes as a substitute for wire in segmental spinal instrumentation for children. Spine 11:907–913, 1986.

40. Gallie WE: Fractures and dislocations of the cervical spine. Am J Surg 46:495–499, 1939.

41. Girasole GJ, Spivak JM, Moskovich R, Chen D: C1–C2 lateral mass anatomy: Implications for transarticular screw fixation with varying subluxation. Presented at the Twenty-Fourth Annual Meeting, Palm Beach, FL, 1996.

42. Goel VK, Clark CR, Harris KG, et al: Evaluation of effectiveness of a facet wiring technique: An in vitro biomechanical investigation. Ann Biomed Eng 17:115–126, 1989.

43. Goel VK, Clark CR, Harris KG, Schulte KR: Kinematics of the cervical spine: Effects of multiple total laminectomy and facet wiring. J Orthop Res 6:611–619, 1988.

44. Goll SR, Balderston RA, Stambough JL, et al: Depth of intraspinal wire penetration during passage of sublaminar wires. Spine 13:503–509, 1988.

45. Graham AW, Swank ML, Kinard RE, et al: Posterior cervical arthrodesis and stabilization with a lateral mass plate: Clinical and computed tomographic evaluation of lateral mass screw placement and associated complications [discussion]. Spine 21:323–329, 1996.

46. Grob D, Crisco JJ III, Panjabi MM, et al: Biomechanical evaluation of four different posterior atlantoaxial fixation techniques. Spine 17:480–490, 1992.

47. Grob D, Dvorak J, Panjabi M, et al: Posterior occipitocervical fusion: A preliminary report of a new technique. Spine 16:S17–S24, 1991.

48. Grob D, Dvorak J, Panjabi MM, Antinnes JA: The role of plate and screw fixation in occipitocervical fusion in rheumatoid arthritis. Spine 19:2545–2551, 1994.

49. Grob D, Jeanneret B, Aebi M, Marcwalder TM: Atlanto-axial fusion with transarticular screw fixation. J Bone Joint Surg Br 73B:972–976, 1991.

50. Hanley EN Jr, Harvell JC Jr: Immediate postoperative stability of the atlantoaxial articulation: A biomechanical study comparing simple midline wiring, and the Gallie and Brooks procedures. J Spinal Disord 5:306–310, 1992.

51. Hanson PB, Montesano PX, Sharkey NA, Rauschning W: Anatomic and biomechanical assessment of transarticular screw fixation for atlantoaxial instability. Spine 16:1141–1145, 1991.

52. Harrison DD, Janik TJ, Troyanovich SJ, Holland B: Comparisons of lordotic cervical spine curvatures to a theoretical ideal model of the static sagittal cervical spine. Spine 21:667–675, 1996.

53. Heller JG, Estes BT: Biomechanical comparison of posterior screw fixation techniques at the cervicothoracic junction [abstract]. Presented at the 61st Annual AAOS Meeting, New Orleans, LA, February 26, 1994.

54. Heller JG, Shuster JK, Hutton WC: Pedicle and transverse process screws of the upper thoracic spine: Biomechanical comparison of loads to failure. Spine 24:654–658, 1999.

55. Heller JG, Carlson GD, Abitbol JJ, Garfin SR: Anatomic comparison of the Roy-Camille and Magerl techniques for screw placement in the lower cervical spine. Spine 16:S552–S557, 1991.

56. Heller JG, Estes BT, Zaouali M, Diop A: Biomechanical study of screws in the lateral masses: Variables affecting pullout resistance. J Bone Joint Surg Am 78A:1315–1321, 1996.

57. Heller JG, Silcox DH III, Sutterlin CE: Complications of posterior cervical plating. Spine 20:2442–2448, 1995.

58. Hensinger RN: Congenital anomalies of the cervical spine. Clin Orthop 264:16–38, 1991.

59. Heywood AW, Learmonth ID, Thomas M: Internal fixation for occipito-cervical fusion. J Bone Joint Surg Br 70B:708–711, 1988.

60. Huckell CB, Buchowski J, Richardson WJ, et al: Functional outcome of plate fusions for disorders of the occipitocervical junction. Clin Orthop 359:136–145, 1999.

61. Jeanneret B: Simultaneous rotation and lateral inclination of the head: A clinical sign of limitation of rotation at the atlantoaxial joint. In Louis R, Weidner A (eds): Cervical Spine II. New York, Springer-Verlag, 1990.

62. Jeanneret B, Gebhard JS, Magerl F: Transpedicular screw fixation of articular mass fracture-separation: Results of an anatomical study and operative technique. J Spinal Disord 7:222–229, 1994.

63. Jones E, Heller JG, Silcox DH III, Hutton WC: Cervical pedicle screws versus lateral mass screws: Anatomic feasibility and biomechanical comparison. Spine 22:977–982, 1997.

64. Karaikovic EE, Daubs MD, Madsen RW, Gaines RW Jr: Morphological characteristics of human cervical pedicles. Spine 22:493–500, 1997.

64a. Karaikovic EE, Kunakornsawat S, Daubs MD, et al: Surgical anatomy of the cervical pedicles: Landmarks for posterior cervical pedicle entrance localization. J Spinal Disord 13:63–72, 2000.

65. Klekamp JW, Ugbo JL, Heller JG: Cervical transfacet versus lateral mass screws: A biomechanical comparison. J Spinal Disord 13:515–518, 2000.

66. Kotani Y, Cunningham BW, Abumi K, McAfee PC: Biomechanical analysis of cervical stabilization systems: An assessment of transpedicular screw fixation in the cervical spine. Spine 19:2529–2539, 1994.

66a. Kowalski JM, Ludwig SC, Hutton WC, Heller JG: Cervical spine pedicle screws: A biomechanical comparison of two insertion techniques. Spine 25:2865–2867, 2000.

67. Ludwig SC, Kramer DL, Balderston RA, et al: Placement of pedicle screws in the human cadaveric cervical spine: Comparative accuracy of three techniques. Spine 25:1655–1667, 2000.

68. Lamb DJ, Silcox DH III, Heller JG, Hutton WC: Different methods of fixation for atlantoaxial instability. Presented at the 65th Annual Meeting of the American Academy of Orthopaedic Surgeons, New Orleans, LA, March 23, 1998.

68a. Ludwig SC, Kowalski JM, Edwards CC, Heller JG: Cervical pedicle screws: Comparative accuracy of two insertion techniques. Spine 25:2675–2681, 2000.

69. Ludwig SC, Kramer DL, Vaccaro AR, Albert TJ: Transpedicle screw fixation of the cervical spine. Clin Orthop 359:77–88, 1999.

70. Magerl F, Seemann P: Stable posterior fusion of the atlas and axis by transarticular screw fixation. In Kehr IP, Weidner A (eds): Cervical Spine I. New York, Springer-Verlag, 1987, p 322.

71. McAfee P, Bohlman HH, Wilson WL: The triple wire fixation technique for stabilization of acute cervical fracture-dislocations: A biomechanical analysis. J Bone Joint Surg/Orthop Trans 9A:142, 1985.

72. McAfee PC, Cassidy JR, Davis RF, et al: Fusion of the occiput to the upper cervical spine: A review of 37 cases. Spine 16:S490–S494, 1991.

73. McGraw RW, Rusch RM: Atlanto-axial arthrodesis. J Bone Joint Surg Br 55B:482–489, 1973.

74. McLaurin R, Vernal R, Salmon JH: Treatment of fractures of the atlas and axis by wiring without fusion. J Neurosurg 36:773–780, 1972.

75. Meyer P Jr: Surgical stabilization of the cervical spine. In Meyer P Jr (ed): Surgery of Spine Trauma. New York, Churchill Livingstone, 1989, pp 11–49.

76. Miller RM, Ebraheim NA, Xu R, Yeasting RA: Anatomic consideration of transpedicular screw placement in the cervical spine: An analysis of two approaches. Spine 21:2317–2322, 1996.

77. Montesano PX, Juach EC, Anderson PA, et al: Biomechanics of cervical spine internal fixation. Spine 16:S10–S16, 1991.

78. Montesano PX, Juach E, Jonsson H Jr: Anatomic and biomechanical study of posterior cervical spine plate arthrodesis: An evaluation of two different techniques of screw placement. J Spinal Disord 5:301–305, 1992.

79. Nicastro JF, Hartjen CA, Traina J, Lancaster JM: Intraspinal pathways taken by sublaminar wires during removal: An experimental study. J Bone Joint Surg Am 68A:1206–1209, 1986.

80. Pal GP, Sherk HH: The vertical stability of the cervical spine. Spine 13:447–449, 1988.

81. Panjabi MM, Duranceau J, Goel V, et al: Cervical human vertebrae: Quantitative three-dimensional anatomy of the middle and lower regions. Spine 16:861–869, 1991.

82. Panjabi MM, Oxland T, Takata K, et al: Articular facets of the human spine: Quantitative three-dimensional anatomy. Spine 18:1298–1310, 1993.

83. Panjabi MM, Takata K, Goel V, et al: Thoracic human vertebrae: Quantitative three-dimensional anatomy. Spine 16:888–901, 1991.

84. Pelker RR, Duranceau JS, Panjabi MM: Cervical spine stabilization: A three-dimensional, biomechanical evaluation of rotational stability, strength, and failure mechanisms. Spine 16:117–122, 1991.

85. Rogers WA: Treatment of fracture-dislocation of the cervical spine. J Bone Joint Surg 24:245–258, 1942.

86. Rogers WA: Fractures and dislocations of the cervical spine. J Bone Joint Surg Am 39A:341–375, 1957.

87. Roy-Camille R, Saillant G: Chirurgie du raichis cervical: Luxation-fractures des articulaires. Nouvelle Presses Medicale 1:2484–2485, 1972.

88. Roy-Camille R, Saillant G, Mazel C: Internal fixation of the unstable cervical spine by a posterior osteosynthesis with plates and screws. In Sherk HH (ed): The Cervical Spine, 2nd ed. Philadelphia, JB Lippincott, 1989, pp 390–403.

89. Sasso RC, Jeanneret B, Fischer K, Magerl F: Occipitocervical fusion with posterior plate and screw instrumentation: A long-term follow-up study. Spine 19:2364–2368, 1994.

90. Schrader WC, Bethem D, Scerbin V: The chronic local effects of sublaminar wires: An animal model. Spine 13:499–502, 1988.

91. Smith MD, Anderson P, Grady MS: Occipitocervical arthrodesis using contoured plate fixation: An early report on a versatile fixation technique. Spine 18:1984–1990, 1993.

92. Smith MD, Kotzar G, Yoo J, Bohlman H: A biomechanical analysis of atlantoaxial stabilization methods using a bovine model: C1/C2 fixation analysis. Clin Orthop 290:283–295, 1993.

93. Songer MN, Spencer DL, Meyer PR Jr, Jayaraman G: The use of sublaminar cables to replace Luque wires. Spine 16:S418–S421, 1991.

94. Stanescu S, Ebraheim NA, Yeasting R, et al: Morphometric evaluation of the cervico-thoracic junction: Practical considerations for posterior fixation of the spine. Spine 19:2082–2088, 1994.

95. Sutterlin CE III, McAfee PC, Warden KE, et al: A biomechanical evaluation of cervical spinal stabilization methods in a bovine model: Static and cyclical loading. Spine 13:795–802, 1988.

96. Swank ML, Sutterlin CE III, Bossons CR, Dials BE: Rigid internal fixation with lateral mass plates in multilevel anterior and posterior reconstruction of the cervical spine. Spine 22:274–282, 1997.

97. Thanapipatsiri S, Chan DP: Safety of thoracic transverse process fixation: An anatomical study. J Spinal Disord 9:294–298, 1996.

98. Ulrich C, Woersdoerfer O, Kalff R, et al: Biomechanics of fixation systems to the cervical spine. Spine 16:S4–S9, 1991.

99. Vaccaro AR, Ring D, Scuderi G, Garfin SR: Vertebral artery location in relation to the vertebral body as determined by two-dimensional computed tomography evaluation. Spine 19:2637–2641, 1994.

100. Vaccaro AR, Rizzolo SJ, Allardyce TJ, et al: Placement of pedicle screws in the thoracic spine. J Bone Joint Surg Am 77A:1193–1206, 1995.

101. Weiland DJ, McAfee PC: Posterior cervical fusion with triple-wire strut graft technique: One hundred consecutive patients. J Spinal Disord 4:15–21, 1991.

102. Wertheim SB, Bohlman HH: Occipitocervical fusion: Indications, technique, and long-term results in thirteen patients. J Bone Joint Surg Am 69A:833–836, 1987.

103. White AA III: Clinical biomechanics of cervical spine implants. Spine 14:1040–1045, 1989.

104. Wilber RG, Thompson GH, Shaffer JW, et al: Postoperative neurological deficits in segmental spinal instrumentation: A study using spinal cord monitoring. J Bone Joint Surg Am 66A:1178–1187, 1984.

105. Xu R, Ebraheim NA, Nadaud MC, et al: The location of the cervical nerve roots on the posterior aspect of the cervical spine. Spine 20:2267–2271, 1995.

106. Xu R, Ebraheim NA, Yeasting R, et al: Anatomy of C7 lateral mass and projection of pedicle axis on its posterior aspect. J Spinal Disord 8:116–120, 1995.

107. Xu R, Nadaud MC, Ebraheim NA, Yeasting RA: Morphology of the second cervical vertebra and the posterior projection of the C2 pedicle axis. Spine 20:259–263, 1995.

108. Yabuki S, Kikuchi S: Positions of dorsal root ganglia in the cervical spine: An anatomic and clinical study. Spine 21:1513–1517, 1996.

109. Yoo JU: Effect of cervical spine motion on the neuroforaminal dimensions of human cervical spine. Spine 17:1131–1136, 1992.

110. Zipnick RI, Merola AA, Gorup J, et al: Occipital morphology: An anatomic guide to internal fixation. Spine 21:1719–1724, 1996.

Pediatric Disorders

6

CONGENITAL AND PEDIATRIC DISORDERS OF THE CERVICAL SPINE

Peter V. Scoles, M.D.
Laurel C. Blakemore, M.D.

Grown-ups never understand anything for themselves, and it is tiresome for children to be always and forever explaining things to them.

Antoine De Saint-Exupéry
Author of *The Little Prince,* 1943

Few areas in the care of pediatric orthopedic patients produce as much anxiety for patients, parents, and physicians as the cervical spine. As in the interpretation of developmental variations and injuries around the growing elbow, radiographic images of the immature cervical spine may confound those not well versed in pediatric osteology; overinterpretation and underinterpretation errors are common and may lead to inappropriate treatment. The development of computed tomography (CT) and magnetic resonance imaging (MRI) has greatly increased diagnostic accuracy, but proper interpretation of these tests demands a thorough knowledge of the normal and abnormal developmental anatomy of the cervical spine.

EMBRYOLOGY OF THE CERVICAL SPINE

Development of the vertebral column begins during the third week of gestation, as primitive mesenchymal tissues differentiate in a segmental manner on the sides of the invaginating neural plate. By the end of the fifth embryonic week, a series of bead-like somites are visible on the dorsal aspect of the embryo. The vertebral column arises from the ventral and medial cells of these somites. For many years, fetal development of the spine has been presumed to involve a sequential process of mesenchymal coalescence, transverse segmentation, and secondary recombination into definitive vertebral centra. Late studies invite reconsideration of this concept. The work of Verbout, as summarized by Lonstein,[17] suggests that the process may be more complex, resembling a tube-within-a-tube matrix of more dense peripheral cells and less dense central cells arranged around the notochord. Segmental differentiation of these tubes occurs in an eccentric and asynchronous manner, creating furrows for migration of the spinal nerve and giving rise to the vertebral centrum, neural arch, and intervertebral disc. Late molecular research has identified a family of genes known as homeobox (Hox) that regulate segmentation of the axial skeleton.[30] Mutations in this gene family may play a role in congenital anomalies of the cervical spine.

The evolution of the occiput and C1 and C2 is unique. The first four occipital somites give rise to the basioccipital region; the caudal portion of the fourth occipital somite forms the atlas and is presumed to give rise to the tip of the odontoid. In a sense, the odontoid process of C2 represents the absent body of C1. Fielding and coworkers,[6] drawing on their own experience and summarizing the work of MacAlister, Shapiro, and others, reported that the odontoid process is derived from the sclerotome of C1, which separates from the remainder of the first cervical centrum early in fetal development and coalesces with the second cervical centrum. Two longitudinally oriented ossification centers in the odontoid process appear by the fourth fetal month and unite to form a single ossification center separated from the body of C2 by a physeal plate. This physis lies well below the lateral masses of C2 and persists radiographically until the sixth year (Fig. 6–1).

A V-shaped cleft, representing the site of the terminal ossification center of the odontoid, is often seen on coronal views of the immature cervical spine (Fig. 6–2). The ossiculum terminale, which forms the tip of the odontoid process and fills the cleft at maturity, most probably arises from the fourth occipital somite. The ossification center is present in approximately 26% of normal children and is distinct from the larger, more distal, and much less common ossicle known as the os odontoideum.

Ossification centers are present at birth in the cervical vertebral centra and in each side of the posterior elements of the neural arch. A cartilaginous synchondrosis lies at the junction of the neural arch and centrum, at the anterior end of the vertebral pedicle.

The diameter of the cervical spinal canal at birth approximates that of the mature spine; longitudinal studies from the Brush–Bolton Collection of the Cleveland Study of Growth and Development indicate that the diameter increases slightly until the time of closure of the synchondrosis between the vertebral pedicles and the centrum, but the eventual diameter of the cervical canal appears to be fixed by age 5 years (Fig. 6–3). Children under age 8 years with traumatic cervical spine injury have a higher risk of upper cervical spine injury and associated

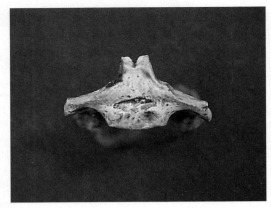

Figure 6–2. Anterior view of C2, age 3 years. The outer surfaces of the synchondroses between the lateral masses and the vertebral centrum have ossified, although the synchondrosis may still be visible radiographically. Note the V-shaped cleft at the tip of the odontoid process. The ossiculum terminale will fill this cleft at maturity.

fatality, whereas those over age 8 years have an adult injury pattern and a low associated fatality rate.[22]

Radiographic assessment of the immature cervical spine must take into account the stage of ossific development and inherent variation of mobility and alignment. Pseudosubluxation of up to 4 mm, most commonly seen at C2–C3 but occasionally at C3–C4, can persist until adolescence. Synchondroses can be mistaken for fractures, and the incomplete ossification gives the vertebral bodies an oval or wedge-shaped appearance until approximately age 8 years. The atlanto–dens interval in this age group should be 5 mm or smaller, which is larger than the 3 mm accepted in patients older than 8 years.[23]

CONGENITAL AND ACQUIRED ABNORMALITIES OF THE CERVICAL SPINE

Abnormalities of the Odontoid Process

During the first half of the 20th century, most presumed that the absence of hypoplasia of the odontoid process was a congenital rather than an acquired lesion, based on the lack of clear history of injury in many patients and the surprisingly low incidence of serious neurologic findings in many affected patients. Gillman[9] credited the first reports to Roberts in 1933 and noted that before his own case report, 21 cases of congenital abnormality of the odontoid had been reported. Gillman classified these cases as total absence of the odontoid, partial absence of the odontoid, and failure of fusion of the tip or a separate tip ossicle (os odontoideum). Noting that in the cases that he reviewed, "the resultant joint instability appears to present less serious clinical problems than the anatomical possibility suggests," Gillman speculated that the absence of the dens decreased the likelihood of brain stem compression.

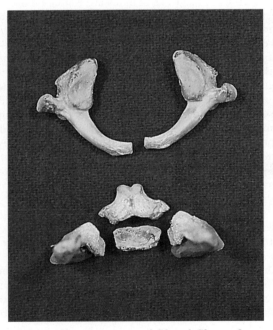

Figure 6–1. Ossification centers of C1 and C2, age 9 months. Note that the anterior ring of C1 has not yet ossified; the anterior arch of C1 is not consistently visible on standard lateral radiographs until age 12 months. The body of C2 is separated from the lateral masses and from the odontoid by cartilaginous synchondroses, which remain visible on radiographs well into childhood.

Hypoplasia and Absence of the Odontoid Process

Rudimentary formation or absence of the odontoid process is well documented in patients with such disorders as Morquio's syndrome, but has also been reported in children with no demonstrable genetic or metabolic disorders.[8, 19, 27] Although in some cases absence of the odontoid may be a result of resorption after fracture,[32] the virtual lack of history of trauma in other patients suggests true congenital absence. In such patients the proximal pole of the odontoid is absent, and the superior surface of the body of C2 is rounded off below the arch of the C1 segment.

In some cases a rudimentary proximal terminal ossification center may be present at the level of the clivus, but it is typically smaller than that found in patients with os odontoideum and may represent the ossiculum terminale rather than the proximal pole of the odontoid process.

Symptoms may vary depending on the degree of C1–C2 instability. It has been suggested that such patients are at less risk for cervical cord compromise than patients with fractures of the odontoid process, because the odontoid process is not present to compress the anterior portion of the cervical cord. In asymptomatic patients with no radiographic evidence of instability, a case can be made for treatment comprising restriction of contact sports and observation. In

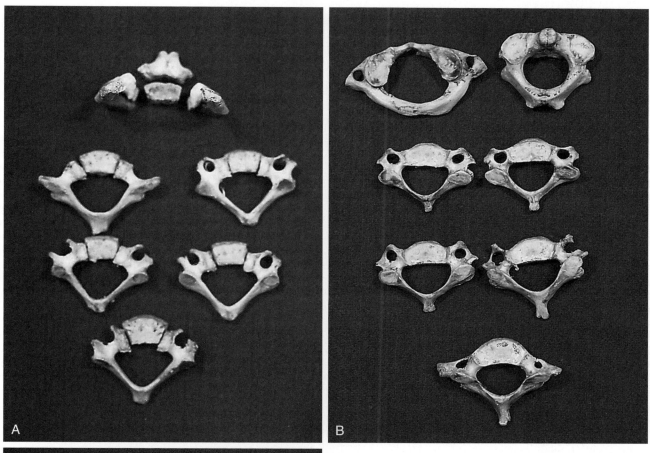

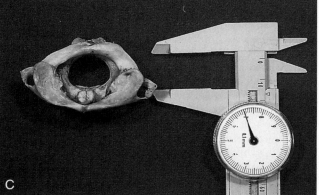

Figure 6–3. *A, Anterior view of C2 and vertical views of C3–C7, age 9 months. Note the synchondrosis between the vertebral body and the posterior elements. A slight increase in the transverse diameter of the canal is possible until these synchondroses close. (B) Vertical views of C2–C7, age 4 years. The synchondroses have closed; no further increase in canal diameter will occur. (C) Vertical view of the articulation of C1 and C2, age 3½ years. The space available for the spinal cord is 1.7 cm.*

comparison, the high incidence of later neurologic complications in patients with Morquio's syndrome is a strong indication for cervical stabilization even when they are asymptomatic and have little instability.[11]

In patients with cervical instability or abnormal neurologic findings, cervical spine stabilization is clearly indicated.[12] The preliminary workup should include controlled flexion and extension radiographs. MRI of the cervical spine performed in the neutral, flexed, and extended positions provides precise information on the size of the cervical canal, the position of the cord within the canal, and the presence of the cervical cord impingement. Anteroposterior plus lateral CT is an excellent technique for identifying small proximal ossicles. Transverse CT and sagittal reconstruction provide detailed information about the craniovertebral junction.

In patients with odontoid hypoplasia and instability limited to the C1–C2 level with a competent posterior C1 arch and no clinical or radiographic evidence of brain stem compression at the foramen magnum, posterior fusion at the C1–C2 level is sufficient. A cranial halo is applied at the beginning of treatment. Meticulous attention to detail when turning and positioning the patient for posterior fusion is essential. Evoked potential monitoring is used, if available, and the position of the spine is verified radiographically after the patient is turned. While the arthrodesis is being performed, care must be taken to avoid exposing the base of the skull or the adjacent lamina of C3 to prevent undesired extension of the arthrodesis. Autologous iliac crest bone is the graft material of choice. The graft is fixed in position with spinous process or sublaminar wiring when safe and feasible.

Postoperative immobilization in a halo vest or halo cast is recommended until radiographic evidence of graft incorporation is seen. This may take 10 to 14 weeks. A cervical brace is less satisfactory in children than in adults and is not recommended as an alternative to immobilization in a halo vest or halo cast.

Os Odontoideum

In 1963, Wollin[32] commented on the difficulty of explaining the os odontoideum on a congenital basis. He suggested that in some patients, a transversely oriented plate of mesenchyme at the junction of the odontoid and the body of C2 might weaken the junction enough to cause it to separate with routine movements of the head. In 1965, Frieberger and coworkers[7] demonstrated resorption of the odontoid process in a 2-year-old girl over a 1-year period after relatively minor trauma to the neck. They suggested that, in at least some cases, the absence, hypoplasia, or separate odontoid ossicle results from trauma and nonunion rather than from congenital lesions.

The subsequent work of Fielding and coworkers[4, 6] strongly suggests that in most patients, os odontoideum is an acquired lesion. They contend that after injury to the immature odontoid process, the alar ligaments pull the proximal odontoid fracture fragment cranially, displacing the fracture and disrupting blood flow to the caudal portion of the proximal fragment. The proximal portion continues to

receive anastomotic flow from the vessels at the base of the skull and may continue to ossify. Fielding also proposed that the size of the proximal fragment is a function of the patient's age at the time of injury.

Although true congenital absence of the odontoid process probably occurs in some instances, current opinion holds that in most cases, absence of the odontoid process in os odontoideum is the result of previous and often unrecognized injury to the immature odontoid process, with subsequent nonunion and variable resorption of the proximal fragment.

Symptoms in such patients vary widely. In some patients, the abnormality appears as an incidental finding on radiographs taken for other reasons. In others, neck pain prompts the radiographic studies that disclose the lesion. In still others, intermittent signs and symptoms of upper cervical spinal cord compression are present. When this lesion was initially described, patients treated surgically had a high incidence of complications, leading some to suggest that even if instability was documented radiographically, patients without symptoms should be treated by observation.[17] Although in some cases the defect appears to be compatible with normal life, the disastrous consequences of upper cervical spinal injury, coupled with improved surgical techniques and postoperative care, have led many surgeons to recommend arthrodesis for treating patients with os odontoideum and cervical instability[27] (Fig. 6–4). Restriction from contact sports and activities that can generate great acceleration forces at the craniovertebral junction, such as diving, parachute jumping, and roller coaster riding, remains an option for asymptomatic patients without radiographic evidence of cervical instability in whom the space available for the spinal cord is not narrowed by the os.

In patients with os odontoideum and cervical instability with no signs and symptoms of myelopathy, no radiographic or clinical evidence of compression of the brain stem at the foramen magnum, and intact neural arches of C1 and C2, we recommend application of a cranial halo followed by posterior fusion of C1–C2 with autologous iliac crest graft and sublaminar or spinous process fixation. The introduction of braided steel and titanium cables has diminished the risk of excessive protrusion of wire loops in the posterior aspect of the cervical canal. Although more costly than single-stranded wire, braided cable offers advantages in some cervical spinal wiring techniques. Postoperative immobilization in a halo vest or halo cast is continued until the fusion is mature.

In patients with long-standing dissociation of the odontoid process from the centrum of C2, ligament contractures and fibrocartilage formation at the base of the odontoid may block reduction. In the absence of myelopathy, if reduction is not achieved on preoperative extension films, it should not be attempted at the time of surgery. In the patient with a history of transient neurologic symptoms in whom reduction does not occur on cervical spine extension, a preliminary period of halo traction may be attempted before surgery. In such cases, application of a halo vest under radiographic control and MRI of the cervical spine are useful before definitive surgery. In the absence of myelopathy, in situ posterior fusion is recom-

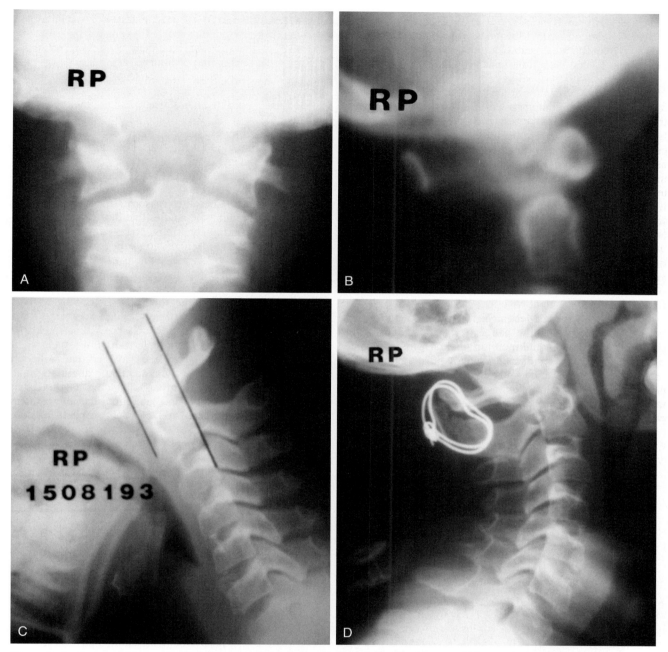

Figure 6–4. *Os odontoideum. (A, B) Anteroposterior and lateral tomograms of a 14-year-old boy with os odontoideum; he had symptoms of neck pain and stiffness, but no signs of spinal cord compression. Three years before presentation he had fallen from a bunk bed and complained of neck pain for 2 days after the fall. No workup was done at that time. (C) Flexion radiographs show marked instability of the upper cervical spine. (D) Posterior arthrodesis was performed to stabilize the C1–C2 articulation.*

mended even if partial reduction has not occurred in traction, except in the presence of significant anterior cervical cord impingement by the os odontoideum and associated fibrocartilage. If myelopathy persists, or if anterior impingement is significant, anterior decompression and posterior fusion must be considered.

In the patient with an incompetent posterior arch of C1 or

a need for posterior decompression of the foramen magnum or atlas, craniovertebral arthrodesis is necessary. The periosteal flap technique of Koop and Winter is useful, and it should be supplemented with a large volume of iliac crest graft.[12] In some older patients, it may be possible to pass cables through burr holes at the base of the skull to enhance graft fixation. During this procedure, great care must be taken to avoid damage to the dura or dural sinuses. Prolonged postoperative immobilization in a halo vest or cast is essential.

Basilar Impression

Basilar impression describes the indentation or encroachment of the skull base by the upper cervical spine on the brain stem and spinal cord. Primary basilar impression is a congenital anomaly associated with other anomalies, such as Klippel–Feil syndrome, odontoid or atlas abnormalities, and atlas occipitalization. Secondary basilar impression is caused by bone-softening disorders, such as osteogenesis imperfecta, Paget's disease, renal osteodystrophy, rheumatoid arthritis, Morquio's syndrome, and skeletal dysplasia.[16] Neurologic impairment is common. The patient may present with purely pyramidal symptoms, cranial nerve symptoms, or, in cases associated with Arnold–Chiari malformation, cerebellar symptoms and ataxia. Hydrocephalus also may occur from obstruction of cerebrospinal fluid flow at the foramen magnum.[16]

Various radiographic parameters are used to assess basilar impression. CT and MRI are helpful in defining the osseous anatomy and degree of neural impingement. Management requires a multidisciplinary effort between the orthopedic surgeon and neurosurgeon, because anterior excision of the odontoid, posterior decompression, or release of dural bands may be needed in addition to posterior stabilization.[31]

Occipitalization of the Atlas

Occipitalization of the atlas, or *occipitocervical synostosis*, has been reported by numerous authors.[1, 18] Clinical findings may include short neck, low posterior hairline, and limited range of motion. Instability has been reported in 50% of patients; symptoms may include neck and occipital pain, pyramidal findings, and cranial nerve dysfunction.[21] Occipitocervical synostosis may occur as an isolated finding in asymptomatic patients or may be associated with anomalies of the axis or lower cervical spine. When it exists as an isolated finding without clinical myelopathy or radiographic signs of instability, no treatment is necessary. When associated with myelopathy or craniovertebral instability, or with a potentially dangerous lesion of the lower cervical spine, stabilization is indicated. Fusion includes the occiput–C1 complex to C2 using autogenous iliac crest bone as the graft material of choice. Decompression may be necessary in cases of neurologic impairment. Immobilization in a halo vest or cast is continued until the fusion mass is mature.[15]

Unilateral Absence of C1

Dubosset[3] described a series of 17 children with torticollis and unilateral absence of C1 (hemiatlas). Clinical findings may be noted at birth and include torticollis, lateral shift of the head relative to the trunk, and aplasia of the ipsilateral neck musculature. Approximately 25% of pa-

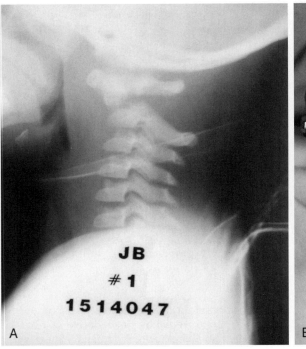 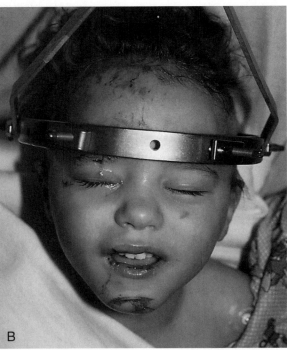

Figure 6–5. *Physeal fracture of the odontoid process. Contusions and abrasions on the chin and forehead signal the likelihood of underlying cervical spine injury in this 3-year-old boy. (A) Radiographs show a physeal fracture at the base of the odontoid process. (B) Reduction was achieved by halotraction, and the patient was immobilized in a halo vest until healing occurred.*

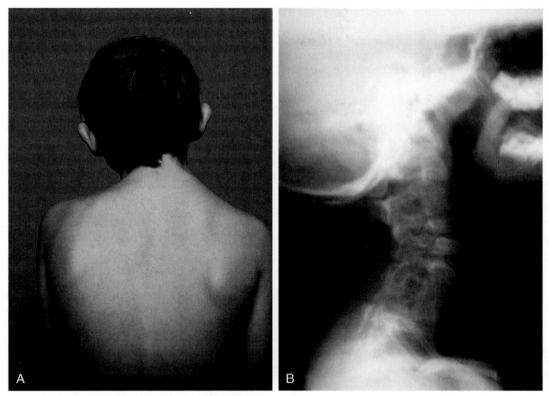

Figure 6–6. Klippel-Feil syndrome. (A) Note the association of low hairline and short neck in this patient with limited neck motion. Congenital elevation of the left scapula (Sprengel's anomaly) is present as well. (B) Radiographs of the cervical spine show multiple areas of coalition.

tients present with neurologic signs or headache.[16] Although plain radiographs may suggest the diagnosis, CT scan is the imaging procedure of choice. Anomalies are divided into three types: type I, isolated hemiatlas; type II, associated congenital anomalies in the lower cervical spine; and type III, partial or complete atlanto-occipital fusion of the incomplete hemiatlas with or without other cervical abnormalities.[16] In the absence of severe deformity, management involves observation for progression. If surgery is needed, preoperative MRI and angiography are required to rule out foraminal stenosis or arterial malformation. Surgical intervention is preceded by halo correction and may include posterior decompression if MRI suggests limited space available for the cord (SAC).

PHYSEAL FRACTURES OF THE BASE OF THE ODONTOID

As noted earlier, the dens is separated from the body of the C2 vertebra by a zone of cartilage known as the *dentocentral synchondrosis,* which closes between the fifth and seventh years.[20] The synchondrosis lies below the articular facets of C2, contiguous with the neurocentral synchondroses and within the region that eventually becomes the centrum of C2. Fractures through this region are uncommon, but they may result from flexion-extension

forces.[14] The injuries resemble physeal fractures elsewhere and have a high likelihood of healing. Minimally displaced fractures may be immobilized and allowed to heal in situ. More severely displaced fractures are reduced in traction and immobilized (Fig. 6–5). A halo vest provides more secure and predictable immobilization than hard collars or cervicothoracic braces. Nonunion of fractures through the dentocentral sychondrosis is apparently uncommon. The paradox involved with current theories about the etiology of os odontoideum is obvious but difficult to explain.

KLIPPEL-FEIL SYNDROME

In 1912, Klippel and Feil reported the clinical triad of short neck, low hairline, and restricted neck motion in a patient with multiple coalitions of the cervical vertebrae. Since their report, others have noted the association of this triad with other congenital and developmental abnormalities of the musculoskeletal system, as well as with congenital abnormalities of the genitourinary tract, auditory system, spinal cord, and cardiovascular system.[10] In patients with coalitions involving two or three vertebral segments, facial abnormalities and cervical motion restrictions may be barely detectable. In patients with involvement of multiple long sections of the cervical spine, severe restriction of motion, webbing of the neck, and torticollis may be present (Fig. 6–6). Sprengel's anomaly, congenital elevation of the scapula thought to result from defective embryonic scapular differentiation or migration, is a common finding and may be severe enough to warrant surgical correction. Patients with Klippel-Feil syndrome have a higher than expected incidence of scoliosis in the apparently normal section of the spine distal to the cervical anomaly. Hensinger reported an incidence above 60% in his series of patients, 18 of whom required treatment at the time of his report.[10] Although some of the curves may have been idiopathic, others may have been associated with internal derangements of the spinal cord or brain stem now detectable by MRI.

Many have noted the high incidence of renal abnormalities in patients with Klippel-Feil syndrome. Hensinger and coworkers[10] reported a 35% incidence of genitourinary tract abnormalities in 45 of 50 patients who underwent intravenous pyelography. In their group of patients, lesions included double collecting systems, renal aplasia, hydronephrosis, horseshoe kidneys, and pyelonephritis. They noted that Klippel and Feil's patient died of uremia, not from the effects of cervical vertebral anomalies.[10] It has been our experience that the severity of the renal abnormality has little relation to the extent of the cervical deformity. Careful evaluation of the genitourinary tract with intravenous pyelography, renal ultrasonography, or MRI is advisable in all affected patients. Rouvreau[26] described 19 children with Klippel-Feil syndrome followed for an average of 12.5 years. Five had neurologic abnormalities associated with occiput–C1 anomalies.

Increased atlanto-occipital and atlantoaxial motion may be present in patients with complete coalitions of the lower cervical vertebrae. At a minimum, such patients should be restricted from activities that put the cervical spine at risk. Surgical stabilization may be necessary for patients with signs and symptoms of cervical cord compression.

Sherk and coworkers[29] described three patients with Klippel-Feil abnormality, Sprengel's anomaly, and iniencephaly, a severe anomaly of the upper cervical spine and base of the skull in which the brain stem and medulla appear to be located in a bifid upper cervical spine below the level of the foramen magnum. They speculated on the relationship of the embryonic events responsible for the associations of the lesions and noted the potential for intracranial ventricular obstruction and syringomyelia. Subsequent studies of patients with other types of congenital vertebral abnormalities have indicated a high rate of internal abnormalities of the brain stem and spinal cord, and thus it is reasonable to assume that patients with Klippel–Feil syndrome also may be so affected. MRI is recommended for patients with abnormal neurologic findings and for patients who require surgical correction of progressive spinal deformity, fixed torticollis, or cervical instability.

CERVICAL SPINE IN DOWN SYNDROME

The association of trisomy 21 (Down syndrome) with abnormalities of the upper cervical spine is well known. Reported abnormalities include atlantoaxial instability,

occipitalization of the atlas, hypoplasia of the posterior arch of C1, and os odontoideum. Instability can occur at multiple levels. If a normal upper limit of the atlanto–dens interval is considered to be 4 mm in children and 3 mm in adults, the overall estimates of the incidence of instability in patients with Down syndrome range from 10% to 25%. The percentage of patients with symptoms related to C1–C2 instability or other cervical spine anomalies is much lower. Burke and coworkers[2] reported no associated symptoms in 32 patients with atlantoaxial instability. Pueschel and coworkers[25] noted symptoms in only 7 of 40 patients with C1–C2 instability. Unfortunately, both of these groups noted cases of significant neurologic injury, including quadriparesis and death, in previously asymptomatic patients. Burke's study was prompted by a case of acute paraplegia resulting from atlanto-occipital dislocation.

A review of reported series of patients with Down syndrome and upper cervical instability indicates that abnormal neurologic signs, when present, are highly variable. The associated intellectual impairment hinders accurate assessment. In some patients, obvious abnormalities, such as incontinence, gait disturbances, and seizures, may be the presenting signs, whereas others may have more subtle signs, such as intermittent balance problems or decreased exercise tolerance. The incidence of instability appears to increase with age. Burke and coworkers[2] documented cervical instability and development of os odontoideum in patients known to have had normal cervical spine radiographs on earlier screening.

The Special Olympics requires screening of participants with Down syndrome using neurologic examination and cervical radiographs taken in the neutral, flexed, and extended positions. Those with no neurologic abnormalities but with radiographic evidence of instability require further evaluation. Flexion–extension MRI can determine the extent of cord compression.

Patients with myelopathy and those with marked instability without myelopathy are candidates for cervical spinal fusion. Decision making is complicated by the lack of knowledge of the long-term outcomes of patients with myelopathy treated without surgery and by the variable outcomes in patients treated with surgery. Unfortunately, the results of surgical treatment of instability in Down syndrome are less predictable than those of instability in other conditions. Failure of fusion and graft resorption may occur. The incidence of complications is high, and preexisting myelopathic changes are not likely to improve. Based on these findings, Segal and coworkers[28] have recommended that patients with instability and no neurologic abnormalities be treated nonoperatively. When operative intervention is necessary, all parties must be aware of the high risk of serious complications.

The occurrence of sudden death in previously normal patients with Down syndrome and the documented development of instability with increasing age raise the issue of whether all patients with Down syndrome should be restricted from potentially dangerous activities. Given the incomplete state of knowledge at this time, this judgment appears best made on a case-by-case basis.

ROTATIONAL DISORDERS OF THE ATLANTOAXIAL JOINT

The principal motion of the C1–C2 articulation is lateral rotation. Various developmental, inflammatory, and traumatic processes may interfere with this motion and produce obvious and often symptomatic torticollis. Fielding and Hawkins[5] termed this process *atlantoaxial rotary fixation* and described the associated clinical and radiographic features.

Rotational translations between C1 and C2 are constrained by several anatomic structures. In addition to limitations imposed by the anatomic structure of the C1–C2 facet joints, the transverse and apical alar ligaments provide critical support to the joint. Anatomic studies indicate that the transverse ligament is the primary stabilizer of the C1–C2 articulation, preventing forward shifting of C1 on C2. When the transverse ligament is competent, rotation between the first and second segments occurs without anterior translation of C1 on C2. When the transverse ligament is deficient, combinations of rotational displacement and forward shift are possible. In such circumstances, the alar ligaments serve both as accessory stabilizers of forward translation and as regulators of rotation of C1 on C2. In the absence of cervical trauma, developmental anomalies of the odontoid process, or deficiency of the atlantoaxial ligaments, rotation of C1 on C2 probably occurs within the constraints imposed by the facet joints and capsular ligaments. When the transverse ligament is intact, dislocation of the articular facets of C1–C2 occurs at 65 degrees of rotation; when the transverse ligament is disrupted, dislocation may occur at 45 degrees of rotation.[5]

The normal range of rotation at the atlantoaxial joint is not clearly established. CT studies of normal subjects have shown that horizontal alignment of the articular facets at the C1–C2 junction permits approximately 30 to 40 degrees of motion at the joint.[13] Unfortunately, the terminology of upper cervical malalignment is often loosely applied. "Rotary dislocation" should be reserved for the relatively uncommon circumstance of complete unilateral or bilateral dissociation of the C1–C2 articular facets. "Rotary fixation" is the appropriate term for the more common finding of restricted atlantoaxial motion malalignment within the anatomic confines of the articular facets.

Rotational malalignment of the cervical spine is a physical finding, not a disease. Various traumatic and inflammatory conditions may produce rotational malalignment of the atlantoaxial joint. Injury to the bones of the spine or the supporting ligaments may be the precipitating factor. It may follow upper respiratory illness, Grisel syndrome, cervical adenitis, or ear infection. It has been reported after dental procedures and oropharyngeal surgery. Lesions of the central nervous system, cranial nerves, or spinal cord that produce secondary torticollis may lead to C1–C2 rotary fixation. Rotational malalignment may be associated with Arnold-Chiari malformation or syrinx formation in the cervical spinal cord. Tumors of the neural or osseous structures of the cervical spine may produce rotational malalignment. They must be considered in the differential diagnosis of torticollis.

Transient torticollis in childhood is common, but few cases result in rotary fixation. The diagnosis of rotary fixation is usually delayed; by the time most patients are seen by a cervical spine specialist, torticollis has been present for some time. The usual clinical presentation is acute-onset torticollis in a previously healthy patient that has persisted longer than predicted by the patient's primary physician. The patient's head is typically rotated away from and tilted toward the affected side in what Fielding and Hawkins[5] termed the "cock robin" position. In contrast to congenital muscular torticollis, sternomastoid spasm occurs on the contralateral side in an effort to correct the deformity. The patient can only experience a worsening, not a correction, of the deformity. The head can be brought to the neutral position but not beyond. Initial physical examination must include a careful neurologic evaluation.

Initial radiographic evaluation includes anteroposterior, lateral, and open-mouth views of the cervical spine, as well as supervised flexion-extension lateral views of the C1–C2 joint. Adequate standard radiographs may be difficult to obtain when the patient has neck pain and is unable to hold the head in a neutral position. Interpretation may be difficult because of the superimposition of the mandible on the upper cervical spine. When adequate plain films can be obtained, malalignment of C1 and C2 is manifested by:

- Apparent asymmetry in the size of the lateral masses of C1.

- Asymmetry in the lateral masses of C1 relative to the odontoid process.

- Tilting of the spinous process of the axis in one direction and rotation in the opposite direction, with the chin and spinous process on the same side of the midline.

Definitive diagnosis of rotary fixation depends on the demonstration of transverse plane malalignment of C1 with respect to C2 that persists on attempts at joint rotation. This is best documented by CT scans done with the head in neutral, left, and right rotation (Fig. 6–7). Three-dimensional reconstruction, if available, is an excellent adjunct to the imaging procedure.

Treatment is directed toward reducing deformity and preventing recurrence. The ability to achieve reduction is related to the duration of symptoms before initiation of treatment. Successful reduction is more likely in patients with torticollis and fixation of less than 1 month's duration than in those with a longer-standing problem. We concur with the protocol outlined by Phillips and Hensinger[24] for the treatment of patients with acute-onset torticollis with no evidence of underlying neoplasia, central nervous system or spinal cord lesions, or spinal fracture. These recommendations are summarized as follows:

1. For patients with signs and symptoms of less than 1 week's duration in whom CT scans do not demonstrate C1–C2 malalignment or fixation, a trial of a soft collar and rest is appropriate.

2. For patients with signs and symptoms of 1 to 4 weeks' duration in whom CT scans show C1–C2 fixation without dislocation, a trial of head halter traction is warranted. If

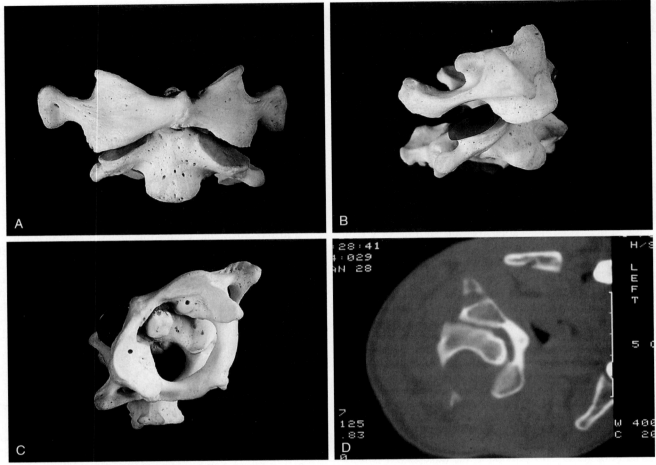

Figure 6–7. *Rotary subluxation of the atlantoaxial joint. (A, B, C) In these cadaver specimens, the first cervical segment has been rotated with respect to the second segment to simulate subluxation of the C1–C2 facet joints. (D) Axial CT scanning demonstrates subluxation of the C1 and C2 facet joints in this patient with torticollis of 4 months' duration following a fall from a horse. If the displacement between the segment does not change when CT views are made with the head in left and right rotation, then fixation can be said to be present.*

realignment is achieved within 24 to 48 hours, then immobilization in a firm collar for 4 to 6 weeks is appropriate.

3. For patients with signs and symptoms of more than 1 month's duration in whom fixation is present, a trial of halo traction is indicated. If reduction is achieved, then a further period of immobilization in a halo vest for a total of 6 to 8 weeks is used.

4. For patients with C1–C2 rotary fixation in whom reduction cannot be achieved, or in whom rotary malalignment recurs after initial reduction, C1–C2 arthrodesis is appropriate. This typically consists of a posterior bone-block arthrodesis and wiring, followed by immobilization in a halo vest for 8 to 12 weeks.

5. For patients in whom C1–C2 dislocation is present on initial evaluation, regardless of the duration of signs and symptoms, a trial of halo traction followed by C1–C2 arthrodesis is performed.

REFERENCES

1. Bharucha EP, Dastur HM: Craniovertebral anomalies. Brain 87:469–480, 1964.
2. Burke SW, French HG, Roberts JM, et al: Chronic atlanto-axial instability in Down syndrome. J Bone Joint Surg Am 67A:1356–1360, 1985.
3. Dubosset J: Torticollis in children caused by congenital anomalies of the atlas. J Bone Joint Surg Am 68A:178–188, 1986.
4. Fielding JW, Griffin PP: Os odontoideum: An acquired lesion. J Bone Joint Surg Am 56A:187–190, 1974.
5. Fielding JW, Hawkins RJ: Atlanto-axial rotary fixation. J Bone Joint Surg Am 59A:37–44, 1977.
6. Fielding JW, Hensinger RN, Hawkins RJ: Os odontoideum. J Bone Joint Surg Am 62A:376–383, 1980.
7. Frieberger RH, Wilson PD, Nicholas JA: Acquired absence of the odontoid process. J Bone Joint Surg Am 47A:1231–1236, 1965.
8. Giannestras NJ, Mayfield FH, Provencio FP, Maurer J:

Congenital absence of the odontoid process. J Bone Joint Surg Am 46A:839–841, 1964.

9. Gillman EL: Congenital absence of the odontoid process of the axis. J Bone Joint Surg Am 41A:345–348, 1959.

10. Hensinger RN, Lang JE, MacEwen GD: Klippel-Feil syndrome. J Bone Joint Surg Am 56A:1246–1252, 1974.

11. Karlen A: Congenital hypoplasia of the odontoid process. J Bone Joint Surg Am 44A:567–570, 1962.

12. Koop SE, Winter RB, Lonstein JE: The surgical treatment of instability of the upper part of the cervical spine in children and adolescents. J Bone Joint Surg Am 66A:403–411, 1984.

13. Kowalski HM, Cohen W, Cooper P, Wisoff JH: Pitfalls in the diagnosis of atlantoaxial rotary subluxation. Am J Neuroradiol 8:697–702, 1987.

14. Lawson JP, Ogden JA, Bucholz RW, Hughes SA: Physeal injuries of the cervical spine. J Pediatr Orthop 7:428–435, 1987.

15. Letts M, Slutsky D: Occipitocervical arthrodesis in children. J Bone Joint Surg Am 72A:1166–1170, 1990.

16. Loder RT, Hensinger RN: Developmental abnormalities of the cervical spine. In Weinstein SL (ed): The Pediatric Spine: Principles and Practice. Philadelphia, Lippincott Williams & Wilkins, 2001, pp 303–319.

17. Lonstein JE: Embryology and spinal growth. In (ed): Moe's Textbook of Scoliosis and Other Spinal Deformities, 3rd ed. Philadelphia, WB Saunders, 1995, pp 23–38.

18. McRae DL, Barnum AS: Occipitalization of the atlas. Am J Roentgenol 70:23–46, 1952.

19. Menezes AH, Ryken TC: Craniovertebral junction abnormalities in the pediatric spine. In Weinstein SL (ed): The Pediatric Spine: Principles and Practice. Philadelphia, Lippincott Williams & Wilkins, 2001, pp 219–237.

20. Murphy MJ, Ogden JA, Bucholz RW: Cervical spine injury in the child. Contemp Orthop 3:615–623, 1981.

21. Nicholson JT, Sherk HH: Anomalies of the occipitocervical articulation. J Bone Joint Surg Am 50:295–304, 1968.

22. Nitecki S, Moir CR: Predictive factors of the outcome of traumatic cervical spine injury in children. J Pediatr Surg 29:1409–1411, 1994.

23. Ogden JA: Radiology of postnatal skeletal development. XII. The second cervical vertebra. Skeletal Radiol 12:169–177, 1984.

24. Phillips WA, Hensinger RN: The management of rotary atlanto-axial subluxation in children. J Bone Joint Surg Am 71A:664–668, 1989.

25. Pueschel SM, Herndon JH, Gelch MM, et al: Symptomatic atlantoaxial subluxation in persons with Down syndrome. J Pediatr Orthop 4:682–688, 1984.

26. Rouvreau P, Glorion C, Langlais J, et al: Assessment and neurologic involvement of patients with cervical spine synostosis as in Klippel-Feil syndrome: Study of 19 cases. J Pediatr Orthop 7:179–185, 1998.

27. Sarwark JF, Diraimmondo C: Mucopolysaccharidoses, mucolipidoses, and homocystinuria. In Weinstein SL (ed): The Pediatric Spine: Principles and Practice. Philadelphia, Lippincott Williams & Wilkins, 2001, pp 771–786.

28. Segal LS, Drummond DS, Zanotti RM, et al: Complications of posterior arthrodesis of the cervical spine in patients who have Down syndrome. J Bone Joint Surg Am 73A:1547–1554, 1991.

29. Sherk HH, Shut L, Chung S: Iniencephalic deformity of the cervical spine with Klippel-Feil anomalies and congenital elevation of the scapula. J Bone Joint Surg Am 56A:1254–1259, 1974.

30. Subramanian V, Meyer BI, Gruss P: Disruption of the murine homeobox gene CDX1 affects axial skeletal identities by altering the mesodermal expression domain of Hox genes. Cell 53:641–653, 1995.

31. Van Gilder JC, Menezes AH: Craniovertebral junction anomalies. In Wilkins RH, Rengachary SS (eds): Neurosurgery. New York, McGraw-Hill, 1985, pp 2097–2102.

32. Wollin DG: The os odontoideum: Separate odontoid process. J Bone Joint Surg Am 45A:1459–1471, 1963.

Degenerative Disorders of the Cervical Spine

7

CERVICAL RADICULOPATHY

Jeffrey H. Schimandle, M.D.
Scott D. Boden, M.D.

*The more original a discovery, the more
obvious it seems afterward.*
— Arthur Koestler

*It doesn't matter how new an idea is,
it matters how new it becomes.*
— Elias Canetti

HISTORICAL PERSPECTIVE

The intervertebral disk was described by Vesalius more than 4 centuries ago, but its role as a cause of various clinical symptoms and syndromes has been realized only for the last 70 years. In 1928, Stookey reported a number of clinical syndromes resulting from cervical disk herniations, but he incorrectly identified these herniations as chondromas or neoplasms of notochord origin.[90] Subsequent investigations by Schmorl[80] in Europe and Keyes and Compere[54] in the United States provided a more detailed comprehension of the pathophysiology of the intervertebral disk. In 1934, Mixter and Barr clearly correlated lumbar disk herniations with the signs and symptoms of nerve root compression.[66] Soon after, injury to the cervical disks became recognized as an important cause of neck and referred pain, myelopathy, and radicular signs and symptoms in the upper extremities.

Historically, the routine surgical approach for symptoms produced by cervical disk disease was posterior. Over the last half century, it became recognized that the primary difficulty with this approach was the technical challenge encountered in attempting to expose and remove compressive structures that lie primarily anterior to the spinal cord and nerve roots. The necessity for easier access to anterior compressive structures led to development of the anterior surgical approach to the cervical spine. In 1952, Bailey and Badgley performed an anterior cervical stabilization procedure for a patient suffering from a lytic lesion of C4 and C5 and in 1960 reported their technique.[5] In 1955, Robinson and Smith described an anterior operative technique for stabilizing a pathologic cervical segment using a horseshoe-shaped graft.[77] Cloward, with no knowledge of the work done by others, first published his technique of anterior disk excision and direct removal of compressive structures in 1958.[24] Numerous refinements have since been made in the anterior approach to the cervical spine for the surgical treatment of cervical radiculopathy including variations in graft configuration, as well as in the source of graft material.

PATHOPHYSIOLOGY

With aging and accumulated wear, the cervical spine undergoes a predictable sequence of degenerative changes. This wear and tear in the intervertebral disks, facet joints, and vertebrae exhibit radiographic features collectively termed cervical *spondylosis* (Fig. 7–1).[58, 74] These features are an inevitable consequence of longevity, being apparent in up to 85% of individuals by the seventh

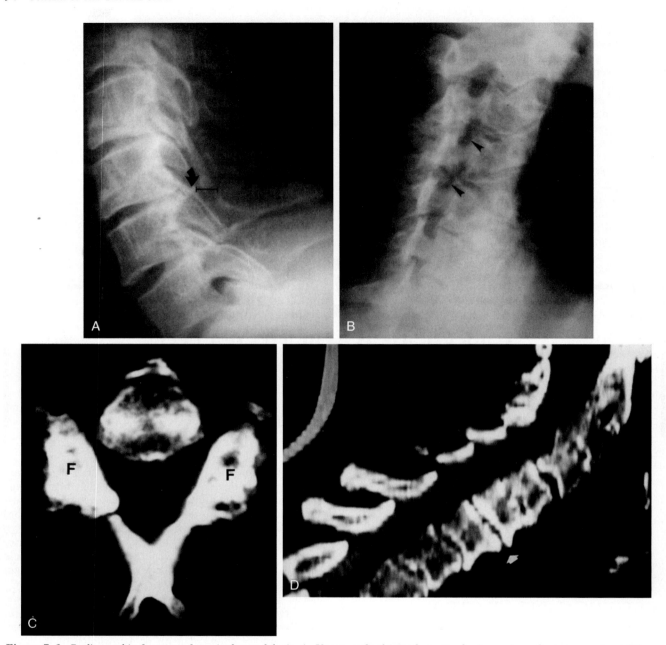

Figure 7–1. *Radiographic features of cervical spondylosis. A, Uncovertebral joint hypertrophy (arrow) results in narrowing of the space available for the cord (SAC) to 7 mm at the C4–C5 level. B, Foraminal encroachment (arrowheads) and facet arthrosis (arrows) at the C3–C4 and C4–C5 levels. C, Axial CT image showing advanced bilateral facet joint arthrosis (F). D, CT sagittal reconstruction showing multilevel disk space narrowing and anterior rim osteophytes (arrow).*

decade of life.[37, 72] Although the degenerative process is inescapable, in most cases the changes are asymptomatic.[4, 9, 16, 17, 37, 64, 99] A subset of people, however, develop clinical manifestations of these changes, called *degenerative cervical disk disease.* Whether the symptoms are truly the result of a "disease" is a matter of semantics. Nonetheless, for some, these morphologic changes result in recognizable symptom patterns related to the neural structure or structures compressed as well as to the cause and duration of compression.

The cervical spinal column serves a dual role. It supports the head and permits a high degree of mobility while protecting the spinal cord from injury.[46] The intervertebral disks and facet joints are the key features of this marvelous design. Unfortunately, degenerative changes of the cervical spine are the price we pay for its inherent degrees of freedom. Most clinically significant spondylosis occurs in the subaxial (C3 to C7) cervical spine. The relevant pathoanatomy is found within the intervertebral disks, facet joints, and the entheses where their associated ligaments attach to bone.[26, 58]

The annulus fibrosus attaches circumferentially to the

vertebral margin. A specialized region of attachment at the posterolateral corner and lateral vertebral margin is known as the uncovertebral joint. Pathologic changes along the posterior vertebral body, which defines the floor of the spinal canal, and at the uncovertebral joint, which forms the ventral limit of the neuroforamen, may compromise the neural structures anteriorly (Fig. 7–2). These are the most common areas in which degenerative cervical pathology creates neurologic compromise. Pathologic changes in the facet joint may compromise the neuroforamen and its contents dorsally (Fig. 7–3). Although less common, clinically relevant arthrosis may also affect these diarthrodial joints. Osteophyte formation, synovitis, and/or subluxation may underlie the onset of symptoms.

Cervical disk disease occurs in order of decreasing frequency at the C5–C6, C6–C7, C4–C5, C3–C4, and C7–T1 motion segments[37, 41] with 94% of spondylotic changes found at the lower three cervical segments (C4 to C7).[102] The predilection for these levels reflects the increased stress and strain seen in these motion segments as compared to other levels. The facet joints, on the other hand, are more commonly affected at the C2–C3 and C3–C4 levels.[60] From skeletal maturity to age 30, few morphologic changes occur in the cervical spine. The incompressible, load-bearing intervertebral disk acts as a shock absorber. The nucleus pulposus converts axial load into well-distributed hoop stresses that strain the annulus and vertebral end plates evenly. The disks maintain normal cervical lordosis and height, and the foraminal area is more than sufficient for the passage of neural elements. A thin ligamentum flavum permits adequate space within the spinal canal. Soft disk herniation through regions of annular attenuation is the most common degenerative cervical affliction in the young adult cervical spine, whereas traumatic, infectious, and neoplastic conditions account for the remainder of clinically significant pathologic conditions.

The progression of normal aging in the cervical spine contributes to and is difficult to differentiate from the pathophysiologic changes. The challenge is to identify where on the continuum of physiologic age-related changes

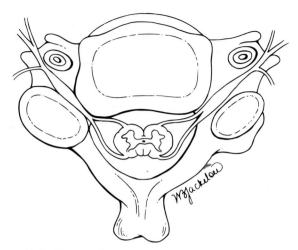

Figure 7–3. *Foraminal stenosis produced by a hypertrophic uncus anteriorly and articular process posteriorly with resultant nerve root compression.*

the processes become pathologic.[26] From the fourth decade onward, the water content of the intervertebral disk, particularly the nucleus pulposus, undergoes progressive desiccation. In patients younger than age 30, the disk approaches 90% water by weight; by the eighth decade of life, this percentage decreases to less than 70%. With aging, the large hydrophilic proteoglycans diminish in size and number. Degenerated disks, with fewer proteoglycans and less water capacity, become more compressible and less elastic.[7] A higher collagen content replaces the previously gelatinous nucleus, and the boundary distinguishing nucleus from annulus, at one time clearly defined, becomes less distinct. The annulus fibrosus also loses proteoglycans, and the number and activity of fibroblasts decreases measurably. The tightly woven meshwork of type I collagen is replaced by larger collagen fibrils that are less densely packed. Concomitantly, associated changes in the vertebral endplates occur.[74] Sclerosis, fissures, and a reduced number of vascular communications between the vertebral body and the intervertebral disk are observed. As a result, changes in oxygen delivery, waste removal, and usable energy sources contribute to the degenerative changes observed in the disk. The final common pathway is a more compressible and less elastic nucleus, an annulus that is predisposed to tearing,[18] and vertebral endplates that are less supportive.

An attenuated or torn annulus will permit herniation of nuclear material. If this occurs when the nucleus pulposus is still relatively well hydrated, a *soft disk herniation* occurs that may compress the nerve roots or spinal cord (Fig. 7–4). Patients with smaller cervical canal diameters are more likely to develop neurologic symptoms.[29a] Soft disk herniations are progressively less common with advancing age. Older patients tend to experience neural compromise resulting from the loss of intervertebral height associated with the pathophysiology described earlier. As this happens, the annulus bulges outward circumferentially, and the associated enthesopathy leads to the formation of traction osteophytes. These osteophytes, in combination with the more prominent annulus, may then cause neurologic

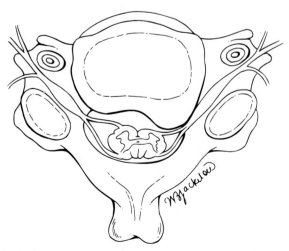

Figure 7–2. *Anterior nerve root compression from a hypertrophic uncus.*

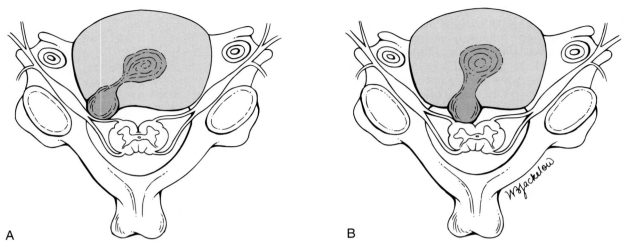

A   B

Figure 7–4. *Soft disk herniations compressing exiting nerve root (A) and spinal cord (B).*

compromise (Fig. 7–5). Additionally, the neuroforamina become narrowed in their vertical dimension, and the thickened ligamentum flavum becomes foreshortened, encroaching dorsally on the space available for the cord. These changes are secondary to the geometric influences of decreased disk height.

In summary, predictable age-related phenomena affect the cervical spine. The principal region of interest is the intervertebral disk because of the biochemical and mechanical changes that occur and their pathoanatomic sequelae. Whether by herniation of nuclear material, intervertebral settling, annular bulging with osteophyte formation, thickening and infolding of the ligamentum flavum, or any combination of these mechanisms, the neural elements are susceptible to compromise. The most remarkable aspect of these progressive changes is their universal presence and yet the relative rarity of clinically significant symptoms. This is testimony to the remarkable adaptive potential of neural tissue.

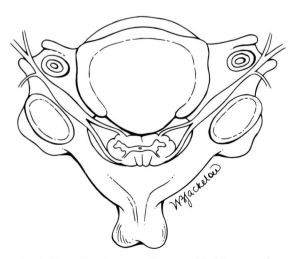

Figure 7–5. *Posterior rim osteophytes and bulging annulus, producing central stenosis.*

CLINICAL SYNDROMES

Any and all of the tissues, hard or soft, that define the spinal canal or intervertebral foramen can be involved in the production of symptoms and development of the various clinical syndromes seen in cervical disk degeneration. The mechanisms of pain production are varied and include direct neural compression, inflammatory changes of the soft tissues, mechanical instability, vascular compromise, and sympathetic dysfunction. The physician should be familiar with the spectrum of clinical symptoms produced by cervical pathology, as well as with those problems commonly confused with them.[26, 46, 58, 59, 63, 67, 83, 102] The clinical syndromes of cervical disk degeneration can be classified as (1) neck and referred pain, (2) radiculopathy, (3) myelopathy, or (4) miscellaneous syndromes (e.g., cephalgia, vertebrobasilar insufficiency, sympathetic dysfunction, dysphagia). The etiology of symptoms may be multifactorial, and thus the patterns of signs and symptoms can and often do overlap.

Neck and Referred Pain

Axial complaints—most commonly neck and referred pain—in the absence of neurologic signs are the most common symptoms of cervical disk degeneration. Patients generally complain of aching, stiffness, and limited motion. The pain is commonly posterior and paracentral but may be referred into the trapezius, rhomboids, and interscapular area. Associated pain commonly occurs in one or both shoulders (71% of cases), arm (44%), forearm (31%), and hand (28%).[42] Headaches, typically suboccipital or temporal, are reported by one-third of patients.

The origin of axial neck pain has been the basis of much speculation and limited study. Branches from the dorsal and ventral rami of the spinal nerves innervate surrounding structures such as the annulus fibrosus, anterior and posterior longitudinal ligaments, periosteum, and facet capsules (Fig. 7–6). Primary muscle afferents also travel with motor nerves to the paraspinal, shoulder girdle, and scapular muscles. It seems reasonable to assume that axial and referred pain may be produced either by direct compression of the nerve, its branches, or by focal stimulation of peripheral nociceptive fibers distributed among the aforementioned structures. Numerous investigators have reported reproduction of axial pain during provocative procedures such as diskography or direct stimulation of the facet joints or annulus fibrosus.[2, 33, 98] In an uncontrolled clinical series, Bogduk and Marsland reported successful transient relief of certain cervical pain patterns by blocking either the medial branches of the dorsal ramus or the facet joint itself.[12]

The neck pain of cervical disk degeneration is frequently precipitated, aggravated, and perpetuated by motion, especially neck extension. The pain is relieved by rest. Most patients are not aware of the common daily activities that stress the neck until specifically asked. Mundane activities such as shaving, putting on socks and shoes, reading with bifocals, vacuuming, reaching for high shelves, and maintaining incorrect posture while driving or using the telephone can all precipitate or aggravate degenerative symptoms. The pain also can be exacerbated by fatigue, anxiety, or stress.

The patient commonly assumes a slightly flexed position to maximize comfort. Neck motion is restricted to varying degrees. Mild loss of motion in all planes is expected after age 45 and usually is not associated with pain at the limits of movement. In cervical disk degeneration, extension is the first movement lost. Although lateral flexion may be markedly decreased in the erect position, when the patient lies down with the head resting on the bed, the range of movement is increased. This is because of reduced static

loads from the weight of the head and lower dynamic loads as the cervical muscles relax.

The patient may report discomfort when pressure is applied to the spinous processes; this tenderness is rarely severe, however. When overly dramatic tenderness is elicited, an emotional or functional component to the patient's disability should be considered. Anterior cervical tenderness should be sought and may be of specific and localizing value. With the patient relaxed and the head supported on a pillow, the examiner's fingers are gently placed into the sulcus between the sternocleidomastoid muscle and trachea. The trachea is displaced medially, and the anterior surface of the vertebral bodies is palpated. Although uncomfortable, pressure over the involved cervical segment in the patient suffering from cervical disk degeneration may reproduce the reported pattern of complained of clinically.

Plain x-rays are inexpensive, readily available, and useful in defining the changes seen in patients with neck pain secondary to cervical disk degeneration. They can provide important information when physical findings are present.[73] Occasionally, they will uncover previously unsuspected rheumatologic, infectious, or neoplastic lesions of the cervical spine as the source of neck pain. Disk space narrowing may be seen on the lateral view of the subaxial cervical spine and is the first and most constant feature of cervical spondylosis. Cervical instability may be present and can be demonstrated on lateral flexion/extension x-rays. Anteroposterior (AP) canal diameter and the degree of foraminal encroachment can be measured from good-quality lateral and oblique x-rays, respectively. Morphologic imaging studies, including myelography, computed

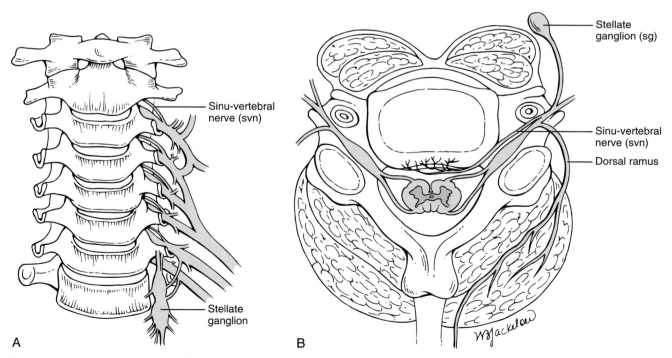

Figure 7–6. *Innervation of surrounding cervical structures. Coronal (A) and axial (B) schematics showing the relationship of the stellate ganglion (sg), sinuvertebral nerve (svn), and dorsal ramus to anterior and posterior structures of the cervical spine.*

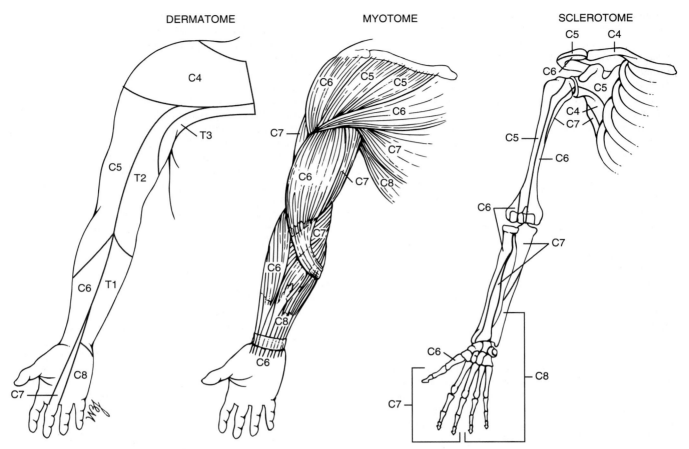

Figure 7–7. *Dermatomal, myotomal, and sclerotomal maps of the upper extremity.*

tomography (CT), and magnetic resonance imaging (MRI), are rarely helpful. These expensive tests should be ordered selectively. Although the clinical symptoms of patients with neck or referred pain correlate poorly with plain x-rays of the degenerative cervical spine,[37, 41, 42] the use of x-rays still represents the best initial screening study in the evaluation of the patient with a symptomatic cervical spine condition.

Radiculopathy

Cervical radiculopathy is a clinical diagnosis based on a sclerotomal distribution of motor and/or sensory changes or complaints. Any process in the cervical spine that causes impingement of exiting nerve roots can lead to a radiculopathy. Impingement may be brought about by acute pathologic changes or by progressive degenerative changes, as seen with cervical spondylosis. Radiculopathy due to chemical irritation of the nerve root from neurohumoral factors (e.g., phospholipase A_2) has also been described.

Nerve root compression due to a *soft disk herniation* is the most common cause of cervical radiculopathy in young adults. The herniation is usually posterolateral, near the entrance zone of the foramen. In older patients, spondylosis, manifested by annular bulging and *uncovertebral osteophytes,* compresses the nerve root anteriorly, causing a radicular syndrome. Less commonly, osteophytes arising

from the ventral portion of the superior articular process may cause foraminal narrowing and radiculopathy. Loss of disk height leads to reduced neuroforaminal volume, making the nerve root more susceptible to compression. In addition, degenerative spondylolisthesis in the cervical spine may cause radicular pain.

Classically, reflex, sensory, and motor deficits are found within the distribution of the affected nerve root. However, despite the detailed mapping shown on dermatomal charts, the degree of functional overlap among spinal nerve roots provides variable findings from patient to patient. For example, a C6 radiculopathy generally causes pain in the neck, shoulder, medial border of the scapula, lateral arm, and radial forearm. But the distribution of pain is often less extensive and more proximal, whereas paresthesias predominate distally. Some patients have only paresthesias in the limb, whereas their pain is axial, particularly in the paracervical musculature or medial scapular border. Furthermore, it is not unusual to see patients whose distribution of pain or paresthesias in the arm are sufficiently vague and nondescript as to defy delineation. The fact that the symptoms do not follow the dermatome map does not exclude the existence of a symptomatic nerve root. The pattern may conform to a *myotomal* or *sclerotomal* pattern instead (Fig. 7–7).

The reflex and motor deficits accompanying a particular

radiculopathy will vary depending on the relative contribution of the nerve root to the musculotendinous unit being tested. In some individuals, a C6 lesion will manifest as a depressed or absent biceps reflex. In others, an abnormal brachioradialis or wrist extensor reflex will be found. Motor weakness must be sought carefully and is subject to similar variability. Given the known variations in brachial plexus anatomy,[49] as well as the numerous intradural and extradural anastomoses between nerves,[11, 43, 62] such variability is hardly surprising.

Other clinical signs suggestive of radiculopathy have been described. Davidson et al.[29] described the shoulder *abduction relief sign.* When the patient puts the hand of the affected limb on top of the head (shoulder abduction), significant relief of arm pain is noted. Beatty et al.[6] believed that this sign was highly suggestive of disk herniation, whereas the sign was unlikely to be present in those patients with radicular symptoms caused by spondylosis. *Spurling's sign* is the provocation of the patient's arm pain with induced narrowing of the neuroforamen. Oblique cervical extension augments nerve root compression and increases symptoms. Finally, direct palpation or percussion over the exiting nerve root may provoke limb or axial pain. If the tenderness or Tinel's sign is elicited more laterally, such as in the supraclavicular fossa, the diagnosis of a radicular syndrome should be questioned. In the absence of confirmatory neurologic findings, a detailed examination of the shoulder, thoracic outlet, and peripheral nerves must be done to exclude those conditions often mistakenly attributed to cervical pathology. The possibility of a Pancoast tumor may be considered if the patient has a significant history of smoking.

In patients with signs and symptoms of nerve root compression, it should be possible to rule out other conditions and arrive at a clinical diagnosis of radiculopathy. The anatomical level of involvement is not always obvious, but this does not obviate a trial of conservative therapy. Extensive testing to determine root level, using electromyography (EMG), CT/myelography, or MRI, is expensive and usually unnecessary, and should be done only if surgery is contemplated.

Plain x-rays are an inexpensive and reasonable first step in evaluating the patient with radiculopathy. As discussed in the section on neck and referred pain, they will show the changes associated with disk degeneration, but more importantly, can exclude infectious and neoplastic lesions.

When the diagnosis of radiculopathy is in doubt and the differential diagnosis includes other neurologic syndromes, EMG examination of the arm and paraspinal muscles may be the study of choice. Electrophysiologic studies will usually help differentiate between root, plexus, and peripheral nerve disorders as well as intrinsic muscle disease. Because of the tremendous variation in innervation in the cervical spine, however, EMG will not necessarily reveal the anatomic level for surgical decompression and thus is of limited help in preoperative planning. Recent refinements, including somatosensory evoked potentials (SSEPs) and motor evoked potentials (MEPs), can be used to diagnose a radiculopathy and may help determine the level of involvement. When a radiculopathy is known to be

present, but the level is unclear or confirmation is required, anatomic imaging is necessary to define the level and anatomy of the problem. These technologies, the merits of which are discussed later in this chapter, usually are not used until conservative therapy has failed and surgery is contemplated.

Although the natural history of cervical radiculopathy has not been as well studied as that of lumbar radiculopathy, it is estimated that more than half of the adult population will experience neck pain with radicular symptoms at some time during their lifetime.[31, 51] A review of the natural history of cervical radiculopathy by Lees and Turner[57] found that the condition rarely progressed to myelopathy. In patients treated nonoperatively, however, long-term follow-up revealed persistent symptoms in 66% of the affected population. In two other studies, 23% of the patients with persistent neck pain or radicular symptoms were unable to return to their original occupation.[30, 38]

Myelopathy

Although cervical myelopathy is the focus of another chapter (Chapter 9), it is part of a continuum of syndromes and may be present with radiculopathy (i.e., myeloradiculopathy). Cervical spondylosis is the most common cause of myelopathy in middle-aged and elderly patients. A combination of several factors contributes to the development of the myelopathy.[15, 59] When cervical spondylosis (which includes annular bulging, osteophyte formation, facet hypertrophy, and ligamentum flavum infolding) is superimposed on a developmentally narrow cervical canal, myelopathy is most likely to develop.[96] The excessive reduction in cross-sectional area available for the spinal cord causes clinically significant compression of the spinal cord and production of the signs and symptoms of myelopathy.

Miscellaneous Syndromes

Numerous other syndromes are attributable to cervical disk degeneration; a detailed discussion of these atypical entities is beyond the scope of this chapter, however. Four miscellaneous syndromes of interest are discussed briefly to alert the reader to their existence.

Headaches of varying frequency and severity can be associated with cervical disk degeneration in one-third of patients. These may occur as the sole manifestation or as part of a more typical symptom pattern. Such headaches are usually suboccipital, but may radiate to the base of the neck or vertex of the skull. It is not clear why cervical disk degeneration causes headaches. Jackson specifically noted headaches frequently associated with cervical disk disease due to compression and irritation of nerve roots in the upper cervical segments.[52] Calliet has suggested that they were caused by greater occipital nerve compression through "tension myositis" from either direct traction or induced ischemia.[20] This theory remains controversial. Such pain is usually relieved with immobilization, nonsteroidal anti-inflammatory drugs (NSAIDs), and rest, although the supine position may exacerbate the neck pain because of the awkward neck position assumed during sleep. Pathology of the cervicocranium is rare, but may present with a chief complaint of headaches. Primary atlanto-occipital or atlantoaxial arthritis will cause headaches with varying patterns of pain. We have encountered at least one individual with occipital pain and brachialgia due to unilateral atlantoaxial arthritis following minor trauma. In these situations the symptoms are clearly exacerbated by motion of the affected joint. The physical examination will support the diagnosis. Selective passive motion of the joint while applying a load to the vertex will increase the pain. Conversely, manual traction during the same motion will markedly reduce the pain. Plain x-rays and selected imaging studies will confirm the pathology.

Osteophytes protruding laterally from the uncovertebral joint or anteriorly from the inferior articular process can compress the vertebral artery as it passes through the foramen transversarium. This occurs most commonly at the C5–C6 and C6–C7 levels, the area of the cervical spine most frequently afflicted by spondylosis. In most situations, the natural flexibility of the arterial wall, particularly in accommodating slowly developing compression, and the collateral circulation in the vertebrobasilar system make this condition only rarely symptomatic. When symptomatic, patients may complain of vertigo, visual symptoms (e.g., diplopia), ataxia, and syncope. These symptoms can sometimes be profoundly aggravated by extremes in neck position,[44, 70] sudden and violent neck movements (such as in aggressive cervical manipulation),[55, 65, 71, 79, 84] or when the vessel is compressed by osteophytic spurs.[23, 39, 45, 69, 82, 92] Complete occlusion of the artery will lead to Wallenberg's syndrome with sequelae of dysphagia, vocal cord paralysis, sensory loss to the fifth cranial nerve, Horner's syndrome, palatal weakness, cerebellar dysfunction, and potential death. The diagnosis is made by history and dynamic angiography with the patient's head in the most symptomatic position during contrast injection.

Various patterns of autonomic dysfunction can be caused by cervical disk degeneration. Patients may present with bizarre vasomotor symptoms consisting of facial flushing, visual blurring, tinnitus, and facial pain or numbness. Such symptoms may be mediated by the sympathetic contributions to the sinuvertebral nerves from the stellate ganglion, rami communicantes, or perivascular cervical plexus. The perivascular plexus is closely approximated to the vertebral artery throughout its course through the foramina transversaria and can be irritated by the same osteophytes that may compress the artery. It is possible that vertebrobasilar symptoms might be caused by reflex vasospasm of the vertebral artery through this pathway. Successful treatment by decompression of the affected cervical sympathetic nerves in such patients has been reported.[20]

Some individuals with cervical disk degeneration experience difficulty swallowing. In many instances, the cause of dysphagia is unknown; in others, large anterior osteophytes from advanced cervical spondylosis or diffuse idiopathic skeletal hyperostosis (DISH) produce a mechanical obstruction to the pharynx or upper esophagus.[48, 61] A cine-esophagram should establish the cause when due to external compression. For extremely large symptomatic osteophytes, surgical treatment may be necessary.

DIAGNOSTIC EVALUATION

Physical examination links the patient's complaints to the underlying pathophysiology and is critical in the evaluation of patients who present with the signs and symptoms of cervical disk degeneration. The number and pattern of symptoms is often confusing and requires that the physician perform an orderly and sequential evaluation and carefully organize his findings enabling him to clearly identify the specific etiology of neurologic compromise. The time-proven method of obtaining a history, inspection, physical examination, and finally arriving at an impression and formulating a plan is the only sure way to categorize the numerous complex symptoms and findings of the individual with cervical disk degeneration.

The single most important element of physical diagnosis is spending adequate time listening to the patient's problem. A thorough history not only provides valuable subjective information, but also affords the physician a sense of the patient's psychological character. Inquiring about the causation, duration, or progression of symptoms is helpful in categorizing possible diagnoses. If the symptoms are chronic, then previous successful and unsuccessful treatments should be discussed. The detailed history will direct the physician toward further examination, with specific emphasis on the physical findings.

Inspection is a too-often ignored aspect of the physical examination and begins with the first encounter with the patient. Inspection is best performed both during the initial history taking, when the patient is less apprehensive and guarded, and as a separate aspect of the physical examination. Significant information can be obtained by observing the patient's posture, gait, neck position, generalized movements, arm motion, and pain behavior. Inspection of the neck should include observing the overall symmetry of the head, neck, and shoulder complex and evaluating for muscle atrophy or hypertrophy and skin lesions or discoloration. The overall relationship of the back musculature and scapulae with alignment of the spine, rib prominence, thoracic rotation, or curvature should be noted.

The physician is obliged to perform a complete neurologic examination in the symptomatic patient. A systematic evaluation of the cranial nerves and brachial plexus must be part of this examination. The patient's lower extremities should also be examined for evidence of long-tract signs, the sine qua non of myelopathy. The physician must be able to differentiate a history of peripheral nerve entrapment from cervical radiculopathy. Entrapment syndromes include thoracic outlet syndrome, cubital tunnel syndrome, radial tunnel syndrome, anterior interosseous syndrome, pronator syndrome, carpal tunnel syndrome, and Guyon's canal syndrome. A C6 radiculopathy is often confused with carpal tunnel syndrome, anterior interosseous syndrome, or pronator syndrome, and a C7 radiculopathy may present similarly to radial tunnel syndrome. Thoracic outlet syndrome, cubital tunnel syndrome, and Guyon's canal syndrome should be ruled out in patients with a suspected C8 radiculopathy. Peripheral nerve entrapment can sometimes present with cervical radiculopathy and is known as the "double crush" phenomenon.

Assessment of the cranial nerves is performed to rule out the possibility that the patient's symptoms are due to a central lesion such as a cerebrovascular accident (CVA) or intracranial mass. Active and passive cervical range motion is evaluated and signs of nerve root compression are sought. Several radicular and compression signs exist as discussed earlier. These include the neck compression test (radicular symptoms produced by lateral neck flexion, slight rotation, and axial compression), Spurling's sign (radicular symptoms produced with oblique neck extension and compression of the head and neck), Lhermitte's sign (axial shock-like discomfort or extremity tingling with neck flexion or axial compression), the finger escape sign (deficient adduction and/or extension of the ulnar two to three digits of the affected hand), Valsalva's test (radicular symptoms produced with increased intra-abdominal pressure), and the shoulder abduction test (relief of radicular symptoms with arm abduction over the patient's head). Deep tendon reflexes in the upper extremities are tested and the left and right sides compared. The inverted radial reflex and Hoffmann's sign are abnormal reflexes thought to reflect spinal cord irritability. Finally, manual motor, two-point discrimination, and posterior column (proprioception, vibration sense) testing is performed. After completing the neurologic examination, the physician should then attempt to classify the patient's symptoms in terms of the aforementioned cervical syndromes and determine which diagnostic studies should be performed.

The diagnosis of cervical nerve root or spinal cord compression requires careful correlation of the history, physical examination, and imaging results. Demonstration of unequivocal neural compression that correlates with the signs and symptoms is the cornerstone of a successful operative plan. Other than plain x-rays, spinal imaging is unusual unless conservative treatment has failed and operative intervention is anticipated. An exception to this rule occurs when the history raises the possibility of spinal infection or tumor. The cost of screening laboratory studies and selective imaging is then justifiable. CT/myelography, MRI, and radionuclide scans are expensive and should not be used to conduct a "fishing expedition" when the diagnosis and the need for conservative treatment are apparent on clinical grounds.

Plain Radiography

The standard radiographic examination is a valuable first step in the evaluation of cervical disk degeneration. The series may include AP, neutral/flexion/extension lateral, oblique, and open-mouth views. The AP and neutral lateral x-rays are obtained initially. They display the disk height and overall bony alignment of the spine and reveal any congenital abnormalities that may be present. Congenital block vertebrae and posterior element fusions are common and may lead to abnormal motion and stress patterns at levels above and below the anomaly. The disk space height and sagittal diameter of the spinal canal can be assessed on the lateral view. The normal sagittal diameter of the lower cervical spinal canal (C3–T1) is 17 ± 5 mm[19, 72, 101]; if the diameter is < 12 mm, significant spinal stenosis is present. Flexion/extension lateral views are used to identify abnormal motion and instability within a spinal segment. Oblique x-rays view the neuroforamina and reveal early degenerative changes within the uncovertebral or facet joints that can cause nerve root impingement. Plain x-rays can also identify previously unknown rheumatologic, infectious, or neoplastic pathology as the source of the patient's complaints.

Computed Tomography/ Myelography

At this time, myelography and postmyelography CT scans are an inseparable pair. To do either alone substantially reduces the value of the technology. CT scans performed without intrathecal contrast in the cervical spine rarely play a role in the management of patients with cervical disk degeneration. Noncontrasted CT may be used to complement an MRI when greater definition of bone detail is required independent of the neuroanatomy.

CT/myelography has a number of clinical advantages. Bone anatomy is rendered in exquisite detail, as is intradural and extradural pathology. This is especially important in patients with spondylotic myelopathy, because the neuroforamina, lateral recesses, and spinal canal are often compromised by osteophytes (Fig. 7–8A). CT/myelography readily distinguishes neural compression by soft tissue from bony compression, which may strongly influence surgical planning (Fig. 7–8B). The neuroanatomy is seen in clear silhouette against the water-soluble contrast medium and bone. The region under study may be rapidly assessed with the myelographic views to exclude previously unsuspected pathology. Finally, the technology is widely available and is usually used on an outpatient basis.

The disadvantages of CT/myelography are few but important. Ionizing radiation is required to generate the images. Dural puncture for the introduction of water-soluble contrast material is invasive and carries a relative risk of complications. Although allergic reactions are uncommon, patients can experience headaches, nausea, and vomiting. The current generation of contrast agents has drastically reduced the risk of arachnoiditis, meningitis, and seizures. Assessment of the postoperative spine can be impaired by excessive metal artifact from spinal implants, and the inability to distinguish scar from disk material. Finally, CT/myelography lacks specificity for intramedullary processes because it renders this anatomy only indirectly.

The surgeon requesting these studies should insist on slice thicknesses of 3 mm or less in the cervical spine. Bone and soft tissue windows must be provided. It is also the responsibility of the ordering physician to communicate any special concerns about pathology or regions of interest directly to the radiologist so that the study can be tailored to the needs of the patient and surgeon.

Magnetic Resonance Imaging

The advent of MRI has significantly advanced the neuroradiographic study of cervical disk degeneration. MRI not only demonstrates the high contrast between cerebrospinal fluid and disk material or osteophyte, but also is capable of providing multiplanar images and reconstruc-

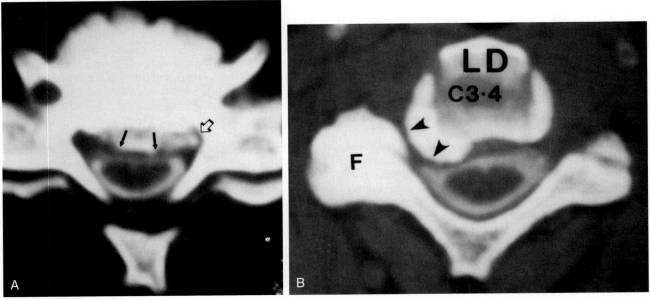

Figure 7–8. Postmyelography axial CT images. A, A broad posterior osteophyte (arrows) produces effacement of the anterior thecal sac and left lateral recess stenosis (open arrow). B, Significant right lateral recess and foraminal stenosis is seen, due to hypertrophy of the uncus (arrowheads) and advanced arthrosis of the right facet complex (F).

tions, including three-dimensional reformations. Anatomic information is available for the entire region of interest, but with a higher degree of specificity than provided by CT/myelography. MRI also provides information regarding the pathophysiologic and biochemical changes occurring within the bony and soft tissues and does so without ionizing radiation or the invasiveness of myelography. The administration of intravenous paramagnetic contrast agents can allow scar to be differentiated from disk material in a patient who has undergone earlier spinal surgery. Additionally, the total acquisition time for imaging is shorter than that for CT/myelography (Fig. 7–9).

The relative disadvantages of MRI include its inability to clearly delineate certain sources of cord and root compression. This lack of specificity may leave uncertain whether a patient's canal is compromised by cervical spondylosis, a thickened posterior longitudinal ligament, ossification of the posterior longitudinal ligament (OPLL), hematoma, or simply congenital stenosis. CT/myelography may be necessary to make these distinctions. The neuroforamen may also be difficult to accurately assess with MRI. Patients with magnetic or electronic implants (e.g., certain aneurysm clips, pacemakers) cannot be imaged. Finally, the noninvasive nature of MRI has lowered the barrier to spinal imaging that once existed when CT/myelography was the only alternative. This has led to overuse of this technology and increased costs of care.

Radionuclide Imaging

Technetium, gallium, and indium scans play a limited role in evaluating degenerative cervical pathology. Technetium bone scans are a cost-effective way to exclude primary or metastatic bone tumors or infections as a cause of persistent neck pain. All radionuclide studies suffer from the

lengthy acquisition times and poor specificity. Their sensitivity may also be degraded by ongoing treatment, such as antibiotic administration for infections in the case of gallium and indium scans.

Imaging Recommendations

If the goal is to provide high-quality, cost-effective patient care, then some thought must be given to the timing and choice of imaging. Plain x-rays represent the first line of defense. They are not usually necessary during an initial visit unless there is a history of trauma or unless compelling historical information exists for consideration of tumor,

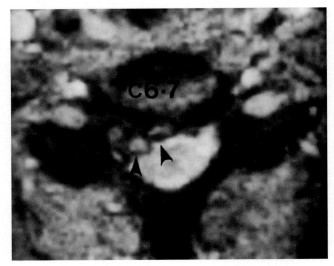

Figure 7–9. Axial MRI showing extruded disk fragments (arrowheads).

infection, or instability. If the patient has not responded to treatment or is worsening clinically and surgery is being considered, then the diagnosis must be refined. It should be noted that most patients would have improved before this point is reached. Whether to choose MRI or CT/myelography depends on the suspected pathology, the patient's age, availability, and the existence of any relative contraindications to the studies.

Given that the costs of MRI and CT/myelography are similar, MRI is favored because of its noninvasive nature, regional anatomic visualization, and superior ability to image neoplasms, infection, and intramedullary pathology. However, in older patients who are prone to spondylotic myelopathy, OPLL, foraminal stenosis, and similar problems, the superior bone imaging capabilities of CT/myelography make it more desirable. Occasionally both studies are necessary to provide complementary information essential to refining the operative plan, as with metastatic lesions or osteomyelitis.

Finally, the high incidence of morphologic false-positive results seen on these images cannot be overstated. Spondylosis correlates with age; it is ubiquitous by the seventh decade of life. Also, the incidence of asymptomatic disk herniation correlates positively with age.[8] The physician must not jump to the conclusion that any identified pathology is responsible for the patient's symptoms. The triad of corresponding symptoms, signs, and correlative anatomical imaging must be present for responsible and effective treatment.

Electrodiagnostic Studies

Nerve root compression may lead to motor, sensory, reflex, and/or autonomic changes. In cases of multilevel radiculopathies or complex clinical diagnoses, electrodiagnostic modalities may be necessary to help differentiate radiculopathy from peripheral neuropathy.

EMG has historically been the modality of choice for differentiating cervical radiculopathies from more peripheral nerve pathology. Electomyographic changes represent a continuum that begins with a decrease in motor-unit potentials and progresses to fibrillation potentials of multiple muscles. Many of the changes occurring in chronic radiculopathies are not unique to radiculopathy and require careful interpretation. EMG has been shown to correlate better with clinical symptoms than plain x-ray. In a review of 108 patients, disk height and neuroforaminal size were of little use in predicting clinical findings, in contrast to EMG findings.[50]

The usefulness of EMG depends on its ability to detect motor changes occurring as a result of nerve compression. In radiculopathy, abnormalities in sensory nerve action potentials are uncommon. Typically, compression that leads to cervical radiculopathy occurs proximal to the dorsal root (sensory) ganglion, and unless the dorsal root ganglion at the distal most aspect of the neuroforamen is involved, the sensory nerve action potentials will remain normal. Bilateral sensory nerve action potential changes are suggestive of peripheral polyneuropathy. Compound muscle action potentials show a decrease in amplitude proportional to muscle atrophy. Significant alterations in potentials

may be seen in polyradiculopathies with multiple muscle involvement. Dramatic changes are more commonly seen in lumbar stenosis but may occur in cases of severe cervical spondylosis.

Nerve conduction velocity (NCV) and latency changes are not typically found in cervical radiculopathies unless there is extreme demyelination of axons. Because the lesion is proximal to the region tested, peripherally oriented studies are of limited use.

Another alternative for electrically evaluating cervical radiculopathies is cervical root stimulation (CRS). With this technique, cervical roots are stimulated by placing monopolar needles in the paraspinal muscles, and compound muscle action potentials are recorded in the biceps, triceps, and abductor digiti minimi muscles. The literature currently favors CRS over EMG for accurate differentiation of cervical radiculopathy. Tsai et al. compared NCV, CRS, and EMG findings in 32 patients with clinical signs and symptoms suggestive of cervical radiculopathy.[95] Conventional EMG was positive in more than 50% of the patients, whereas CRS was abnormal in more than 75%. The CRS study was positive in 25 patients. Thirteen of the 25 patients subsequently underwent surgery, which documented intraoperative findings consistent with radiculopathy. Only 10 of these 13 had a positive EMG study.

The overall role of electrodiagnostic testing is to assist in difficult diagnostic situations and to rule out peripheral neuropathies. It is not to be an additional test for confirmation of a clear monoradiculopathy. Whether the physician chooses EMG or CRS, the temporal sequence remains constant. These studies should follow plain x-ray, and a period of conservative management and should precede more complex imaging studies. In clinical practice, electrodiagnostic testing is reserved for patients with unusual presentations, in those with polyneuropathy (such as in diabetes), or to rule out peripheral compression neuropathy.

INDICATIONS FOR SURGERY

The treatment of cervical radiculopathy is based on a clear understanding of the natural history of acute inflammatory processes. The anatomic lesion that has given rise to the symptoms is virtually irrelevant at the time of presentation. As long as myelopathic, infectious, or neoplastic conditions are excluded, patience and restraint should guide treatment recommendations. Acute inflammation is the final common pathway through which pain is mediated. The type of lesion usually does not alter the natural tendency for acute inflammatory processes to resolve. Given adequate time, the vast majority of these problems will resolve spontaneously. Nonoperative treatment should involve patient education, reassurance, and modalities that facilitate the resolution of inflammation and that tend to reduce the probability of recurrence.

Rest and immobilization are the mainstays of therapy for both acute episodes and exacerbations in patients with cervical radiculopathy.[10, 83] Recumbent rest unloads the cervical structures. The static weight of the head is eliminated, as are the dynamic loads imparted by the cervical musculature as they work to balance the head on top of the spine. A few days of such rest may be necessary, but it should not be continued beyond 48 to 72 hours. A well-fitted cervical collar holding the head in a neutral or slightly flexed position will usually provide sufficient comfort for the symptomatic patient. The choice of soft or hard collar depends on fit and preference. At first, the patient should wear the collar day and night for 3 weeks, removing it only to bathe and to perform isometric exercises. An additional 3 weeks of nighttime-only wear may be helpful for persistent symptoms. The patient must understand that the neck is particularly unprotected from awkward positions and movements during sleep and thus that wearing the collar during sleep is important. This initial period of rest and immobilization can significantly relieve acute pain and allow progression to other modalities.

Medications also play a role in the treatment of acute cervical pain.[32] Anti-inflammatory drugs, muscle relaxants, and analgesics will usually improve patient comfort and should be used as a supplement to neck immobilization, not a substitute. NSAIDs are most commonly prescribed because of their relative safety and lack of addiction potential. Tapering courses of oral steroids may also provide relief. We use systemic steroids sparingly, however, because of the rare but devastating complication of avascular necrosis. Selective nerve root blocks with local anesthetics/steroids may be used in lieu of systemic steroids and have the added benefit of providing diagnostic information regarding the specific level of root involvement. If muscle spasm is a prominent feature of the presentation, muscle relaxants may be effective. Because these drugs are central nervous system depressants, they should be used cautiously in patients with active psychological issues, especially depression. Narcotic analgesics are only occasionally necessary in the acute treatment of cervical pain syndromes; reliance on these medications may cause problems later because of their addictive potential. Finally, in chronic pain syndromes, antidepressants may be of value in treating the physical complaints, particularly if depression and/or sleep disturbance are components of the patient's problem.

Most patients will respond to this approach within 2 to 3 weeks, as the acute inflammation resolves. Those patients who do not improve should begin a program of physical therapy. The collar is then weaned over the next 2 to 3 weeks as symptoms permit, allowing increased daytime removal with continued use at night. Those who are slow to improve should continue with immobilization, NSAIDs, and physical therapy.

Physical therapy is a useful treatment modality for cervical spine disorders.[93] The program must be tailored to address the patient's specific needs. Exercises or modalities that provide relief in one patient may exacerbate the symptoms in another, and thus a "cookbook" approach will fail. The physician must consult with a knowledgeable therapist who is willing to individualize treatment protocols for each patient.

A patient with acute neck pain can have difficulty participating in active physical therapy programs. A short course of passive modalities, such as heat, ultrasound, or massage, may allow the patient to advance to the active phase of therapy. Active therapeutic modalities are then introduced with the goal of establishing a useful, painless range of motion and prohibiting extremes of motion. These modalities include isometric exercises and cervical stabilization techniques. The objective is to recondition the cervical musculature and to increase the patient's general aerobic conditioning and exercise tolerance. If manual traction applied to the cervical spine during physical examination provides pain relief, then this can be added to the therapy regimen. Traction may exacerbate the symptoms and typically does not significantly alter the natural history of the recovery process. If relief is afforded, it may allow the patient to take advantage of the exercise plan. The patient should understand that he or she will have to expend significant time and effort to achieve adequate reconditioning of the neck. It is especially important that the patient appreciate that recovery is an active process in which he or she must participate. Without the patient's dedication to the effort, treatment will fail.

If no significant improvement in symptoms is seen after 3 to 4 weeks of treatment, then some form of invasive therapy may be indicated. Various types of injection may help provide short-term relief, thus enabling the patient to participate more fully in the recovery program. Variable success has been described with trigger point injections, facet blocks, dorsal ramus blocks, and cervical epidural steroid injections. One should remember that they are not a substitute for the patient's full and active participation in getting well.

The patient should be treated conservatively for up to 6 weeks. Most patients will be improving at this point. If this initial treatment regimen fails, then further studies, including plain x-rays with lateral flexion/extension views, a bone scan (i.e., single photon emission computed tomography [SPECT]), and a medical evaluation must be considered to assess the cervical spine for arthrosis, instability, tumor, and infection. X-rays taken before this 6-week point are not usually helpful, because of the similar degenerative findings in both symptomatic and asymptomatic patients.[37, 41] A thorough medical examination may reveal problems missed earlier during the initial stages of the evaluation. If at any time during the conservative treatment plan the patient's symptoms evolve and suggest an alternative diagnosis, the physician should not hesitate to reconsider the original diagnosis. If the medical evaluation is negative, the patient should undergo a complete psychosocial assessment including evaluation of secondary gain, underlying emotional or environmental stresses, and coping skills. If the psychosocial evaluation is unremarkable, then the patient is considered to have chronic neck pain.

The outlook for chronic degenerative neck pain is fair with a tendency toward slow improvement over time. However, about one-third of these patients tend to have moderate to severe neck pain on long-term follow-up (Table 7-1).[42]

These patients need patience, encouragement, and education. They and their physicians must know that surgery will generally not benefit them unless a specific cause for their pain can be proven. These patients need to

Table 7–1. *Change in Neck Pain Severity Noted After 10 or More Years of Nonoperative Treatment*

Change in Pain	Percentage
Completely gone	43
Less but still present	36
Same	13
Worse	8

Adapted from Gore DR, Sepic SB, Gardner GM, Murray MP: Neck pain: A long-term follow-up of 205 patients. Spine 12:1–5, 1987.

steer clear of narcotics and remain on a daily exercise regimen. Aerobic fitness will improve their pain tolerance, and many will respond to an antidepressant drug such as amitriptyline (Elavil). Finally, these patients deserve periodic reevaluation to determine if either their symptom complex or medical insight has evolved such that a treatable cause for their complaints can be identified.

Occasionally, it is difficult to distinguish patients who have a true neck problem from those individuals using neck pain as an excuse to stay out of work and collect compensation or because of pending litigation. The outcome of treatment of cervical disk degeneration has been shown to be adversely affected by litigation.[31] Frequently with hyperextension (whiplash) neck injuries, there are no objective findings to substantiate the subjective complaints. This does not mean that all such patients are malingering. If it is not certain whether secondary gain is a significant factor in the compensation setting, then an independent medical examination and psychological assessment is recommended early in the course of treatment.

Finally, comment must be made with reference to neurologic deficits. All too often patients are referred "for surgery." They have been told that there is weakness, numbness, or a reflex change, and that "surgery must be done to prevent paralysis." On the contrary, most neurologic deficits tend to resolve with nonoperative treatment, and many patients are not aware that reflex, sensory, and motor deficits can persist even after surgery. Their presence is not a sufficient rationale for proceeding with diagnostic imaging and surgery. Only documented progression of weakness, or lack of recovery of functionally significant weakness, warrants aggressive intervention. Too often, patients are robbed of the opportunity to benefit from the natural history of their symptoms. The wise and scrupulous physician should depend on the propensity for spontaneous improvement among the syndromes of degenerative cervical disk disease.

The therapeutic goal in treating patients with degenerative neck pain is prompt return to normal activity with the least diagnostic and therapeutic expense. Although many noninvasive treatment modalities exist, most are based on empiricism and tradition and lack scientific validation. With few exceptions, patients with degenerative cervical pain syndromes are treated with an initial period of conservative therapy, because the natural history favors spontaneous resolution. Those with a clinical history suggesting progressive myelopathy, infection, or malignancy warrant more aggressive initial assessment and treatment.

SURGICAL TREATMENT ALTERNATIVES

Most patients with symptoms of cervical disk degeneration may be effectively treated with a conscientious program of nonoperative therapy. However, there are no data to suggest that any of the conservative modalities influence the natural history of cervical disk degeneration other than alleviating the acute symptoms.[42] When the degenerative process progresses to produce a neurologic deficit or symptom complex that is persistent, increasing despite adequate conservative management, or disabling, then surgical intervention may be considered. Surgical options are available for any neurocompressive lesion, and the operative strategy and tactics (posterior, anterior, or both) must take into account the specific etiology of the segmental pathology and neurologic compression.

Indications for surgery to remove the cervical intervertebral disk and provide fusion of the motion segment in patients with radiculopathy were first outlined by Smith and Robinson.[86] These indications include failure of conservative treatment to relieve upper extremity radicular pain or pain that became excessively debilitating. Current surgical indications for cervical radiculopathy include (1) persistent or recurrent disabling upper extremity pain unresponsive to an adequate trial of conservative management (6 to 12 weeks), (2) progressive neurologic deficit, (3) stable neurologic deficit associated with radicular pain, and (4) confirmatory neuroradiographic study consistent with the clinical examination (e.g., MRI, CT, and/or myelography).

Various operative approaches have been used to relieve compression of the cervical spinal cord and nerve roots. In most cases, either the anterior or posterior approach can be used with satisfactory results. There is no statistical difference in clinical results between the two approaches to the management of cervical radiculopathy, although more long-term follow-up is available for the anterior approach.[15a, 100a] We prefer anterior approaches for most degenerative cervical problems. These exposures have practical limitations, however. Certainly, the visualization of the cervical roots is limited. Multilevel pathology may be quite difficult to manage with the anterior approach, particularly if more than three motion segments are involved. A further problem with anterior fusion is the potential problem of progressive adjacent level instability. Finally, when the spine is approached anteriorly, several visceral structures are at risk for injury.[94] Surgeons unfamiliar with long extensile exposures of the anterior cervical spine may not feel comfortable with this approach. In addition, the issues of strut graft extrusion, collapse, or nonunion must be considered. Despite these limitations, however, anterior approaches predominate, because they allow direct decompression of the spinal cord and axillae of the nerve roots, as most degenerative pathology is anterior.

Reports of successful treatment of cervical radiculopathy using the posterior approach antedate anterior surgery by almost 2 decades. In 1944, Spurling and Scoville described the posterior approach to treat primarily laterally displaced disk fragments.[89] Before the advent of anterior cervical surgery, posterior decompression was performed for all cervical spinal pathology, ranging from posterolateral soft disk herniations to midline spondylosis with myelopathy. With the description of the anterior approach in 1955,[77] the pendulum has swung distinctly away from posterior decompression. Nevertheless, posterior cervical procedures are still an alternative weapon in the surgeon's arsenal.

The posterior approach affords exposure for a wide variety of procedures in the treatment of degenerative cervical disorders, ranging from single-level foraminotomy to multilevel decompressions with segmental instrumentation and fusion. The posterior approach for lateral disk herniations allows immediate mobilization of the neck, preserves the disk structure, and allows two or more roots to be explored without additional diskectomy. Though it might seem that posterior approaches are reserved for pathology that compromises the neural elements from their dorsal aspect, this is not always the case. Our indications for posterior cervical surgery include (1) foraminal stenosis due to facet arthropathy, (2) persistent symptomatic foraminal stenosis following anterior cervical decompression and fusion, (3) anterior cervical nonunions, (4) anterior cervical cord compression involving more than three motion segments in lordotic cervical spines, and (5) supplemental posterior fusion in patients at high risk for nonunion after extensive anterior procedures.

Preparation for a successful posterior procedure involves the same precautions for intubation and positioning as are taken with anterior procedures. One notable exception is that the patient must be turned from supine to prone for final positioning on the operating table. In the presence of high-grade cord compression or instability, the surgeon may wish to keep the patient awake after intubation for final positioning on the operating table; this allows the patient to use his or her musculature to protect himself or herself. After final positioning, neurologic function is confirmed and general anesthesia induced. Under most circumstances, the patient's head and neck are supported by a Mayfield horseshoe headrest. However, if the cervical spine is highly unstable, if screw fixation is undertaken, or if protracted operating time is expected, we are inclined to use Mayfield skull tongs for enhanced control of the head and neck and relief of pressure about the face.

SSEPs are monitored in any cases where the patient has significant myelopathy or instability or when screw fixation is anticipated. It is important that one monitor the appropriate peripheral nerves that are associated with the segments to be operated. For example, lateral mass plating extending down to C7 must include SSEPs of the ulnar nerve as well as the median nerve so that inadvertent nerve root injury in the lower cervical spine can be identified. Perhaps one of the greatest benefits of monitoring is the ability to record potentials before and after positioning of the neck before surgery. Monitoring of evoked potentials ensures that the neck position chosen before performing several hours of surgery does not result in decreased cord conduction; if it does, then it is clearly due to neck positioning, and adjustments can be made.

The surgeon must be sure to prepare a large enough surgical site to allow for extensile exposure if this becomes necessary intraoperatively. When harvesting a posterior iliac crest autograft is anticipated, we routinely prepare both posterior iliac crests generously so that the option to obtain additional grafts is available. Blood loss can be minimized if a dilute solution of epinephrine (1:500,000 in normal saline solution) is used to inject the dermis and paracervical musculature. Meticulous attention to dissection along the median raphe further minimizes blood loss. Any deviation into the paracervical musculature significantly increases bleeding. Finally, the surgeon is cautioned to limit the exposure to the operative levels. Subperiosteal dissection of the muscles beyond the necessary levels or damage to the facet capsules at adjacent levels should be avoided.

Foraminotomy

Unilateral or bilateral posterior cervical foraminotomy may be performed at one or more levels to relieve nerve root compression due to foraminal stenosis or to decompress lateral soft disk herniations. This operation is not commonly indicated, because in most degenerative cervical disorders, foraminal stenosis is due to uncovertebral joint osteophytes compressing the nerve root from its anterior aspect. Occasionally, facet arthropathy will cause dorsal encroachment of the nerve root. In this case, foraminotomy may be appropriate. Foraminotomy is also indicated for failed nerve root decompression after healed anterior cervical diskectomy with fusion. In this situation, if the fusion is known to be healed, then the surgeon may take the liberty of unroofing the entire foramen to ensure complete nerve root decompression. However, if an anterior nonunion exists, then a portion of the facet joint must be preserved and a supplemental posterior fusion performed.

When performing a posterior foraminotomy, the surgeon should be familiar with the relationship between the nerve root, the facet joint, and the pedicle above and below the exiting root. The keyhole foraminotomy is initiated using a high-speed burr with cutting, then diamond, tips. The overlying ligamentum flavum and facet capsule are carefully removed to identify the lateral dura and the take-off of the cervical nerve root. Control of the epidural vessels can be problematic, and hemostatic agents and bipolar coagulation should be used judiciously. Retraction of the nerve root and spinal cord is ill advised.

The nerve root is then followed along its course as the foraminotomy is performed (Fig. 7-10). Biomechanical studies have indicated that at least 50% of the facet joint and its capsule must be preserved if foraminotomy is being performed in the absence of fusion. Excessive facetectomy contributes to clinical instability.[28, 75, 103, 104] We prefer to monitor SSEPs in such procedures.

Many clinical studies have reported good to excellent results in as many as 96% of patients treated with posterior foraminotomy.[1, 35, 42a, 47, 56, 68, 81, 89, 100, 100b, 105] Risks include transient increased root deficits, particularly when

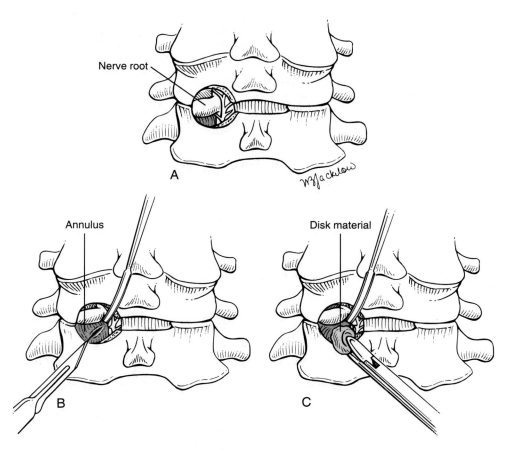

A

B

C

Figure 7–10. Posterior foraminotomy. A, Keyhole foraminotomy is created with a high-speed burr. The overlying ligamentum flavum and medial facet capsule have been removed, exposing the lateral dura and root take-off. B, Coagulation of epidural vessels and annulotomy is performed. C, Disk material is extracted, decompressing the nerve root.

Nerve root

Annulus

Disk material

more than one root is exposed, in addition to cord injury secondary to cord retraction, particularly during transdural approaches to a herniated disk. Recently, a microendoscopic approach has been described that may minimize the posterior muscle pain following foraminotomy.[18a]

OUR PREFERRED METHOD

Since the first observations on neurologic disturbances caused by cervical spondylosis were written, various surgical strategies have been described. Initially, the posterior approach to decompression was favored. However, difficulty in both exposing and safely removing compressive structures lying anterior to the spinal cord and nerve roots fostered the evolution of an alternative surgical approach.

In 1955, Robinson and Smith[77] described an anterior surgical procedure in which the cervical intervertebral disk was removed and a horseshoe-shaped tricortical iliac crest graft was inserted into the disk space to achieve fusion. They suggested the following benefits of this approach:

1. The anterior approach minimizes manipulation within the spinal canal, avoiding the consequences of surgical trauma to its contents.

2. Further osteophyte formation is arrested.

3. Osteophytes already present will eventually regress.

4. Infolding of the ligamentum flavum and posterior longitudinal ligament is reduced by distracting the disk space, thus increasing the space available for the cord and nerve roots.

Some surgeons still advocate anterior cervical diskectomy without fusion. Although many of these patients achieve spontaneous fusion, kyphosis often occurs, and long-term clinical outcomes are not as favorable.[94a] We do not advocate anterior cervical diskectomy without fusion.

Anterior Cervical Diskectomy and Fusion

The anterior approach to cervical diskectomy and fusion (ACDF) is popular and performed widely. The classic indication for using the anterior approach is for decompression of focal root or cord compression caused by soft disk herniations or osteophytes. Although the approach remains essentially the same as that described by Southwick and Robinson in 1957,[88] the basic procedure has been refined. Several different cervical graft configurations have been reported and include the dowel graft described by Cloward,[24] the iliac strut graft reported by Bailey and Badgley,[5] and the keystone graft introduced by Simmons and Bhalla.[85] The horseshoe-shaped graft has been shown to be the strongest[97] graft and is the one that we prefer. The use of specific anesthetic protocols to minimize the unique perioperative risks associated with intubation and positioning, monitoring intraoperative SSEPs, and using improved instruments (e.g., Caspar retractors,[21, 22] diamond burrs, microinstruments) have all enhanced the safety and efficacy of this procedure.

In the patient with a stable cervical spine who does not develop neurologic symptoms during preoperative neck extension, routine endotracheal intubation is safe. In those patients with short necks, cervical instability, or paresthesias with neck extension, an awake fiberoptic nasotracheal intubation should be performed. After the neck is positioned, but before draping, the arms are padded and secured at the patient's sides. Wide adhesive tape is applied over the shoulders, depressing them for better visualization on localizing x-rays. This is particularly useful in patients with short necks and those undergoing decompression at C5–C6 or C6–C7 (Fig. 7–11). Oral intubation should be avoided when operating on higher cervical levels, because this precludes normal occlusion of the teeth and does not allow retraction of the mandible.

The anterior approach can be performed from the patient's left or right side. The advantage of the left-sided approach is decreased risk of injury to the recurrent laryngeal nerve, especially when decompressing the lower cervical levels. The one potential disadvantage is injury to the thoracic duct when operating at the cervicothoracic junction, where the duct loops over the subclavian artery at T1 before entering the subclavian vein. Such injuries are quite rare. We usually use a transverse incision made in a skin crease to minimize the scar. The level of incision is based on anatomical landmarks; generally, the hyoid bone is at C3, the thyroid cartilage is at C4–C5, and the cricoid cartilage is at C6 (Fig. 7–12). The transverse incision allows adequate exposure of two, and sometimes three, levels; when greater exposure is needed, a longitudinal incision along the medial border of the sternocleidomastoid muscle may be used. A longitudinal incision may also be preferred when operating for pathology at the cervicothoracic junction, because inadvertent injury to the inferior thyroid

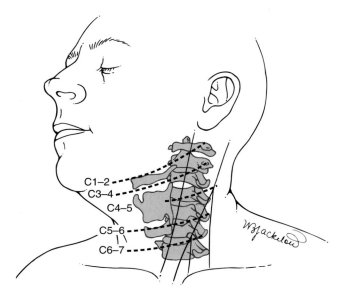

Figure 7–12. *Placement of skin incisions for the anterior approach to the cervical spine. Various landmarks are helpful but serve only as approximations. A lateral x-ray will provide a more accurate determination of level if needed.*

vessels at this level can be managed more readily through an extensile longitudinal approach.

Either loupe magnification (2.5 to 3.5×) and fiberoptic headlamp illumination or an operating microscope is used. The subcutaneous tissue is incised, and a plane is dissected both cephalad and caudally for 1 to 2 cm between the superficial layer of the deep cervical fascia and the platysma muscle to facilitate exposure. We prefer to cut the platysma perpendicular to its fibers, although it may also be split parallel to its fibers. The latter technique is said to produce a cosmetically superior result; however, better exposure is obtained by cutting the muscle, and there is a negligible difference in cosmesis (Fig. 7–13A). Using a combination

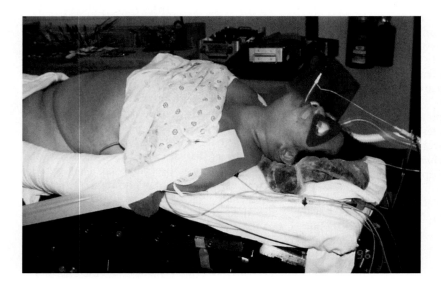

Figure 7–11. *Operative positioning for a patient undergoing anterior cervical diskectomy and fusion using a left-sided approach. The neck is slightly extended, the arms are well padded and secured at the sides, and the shoulders are depressed with wide cloth tape.*

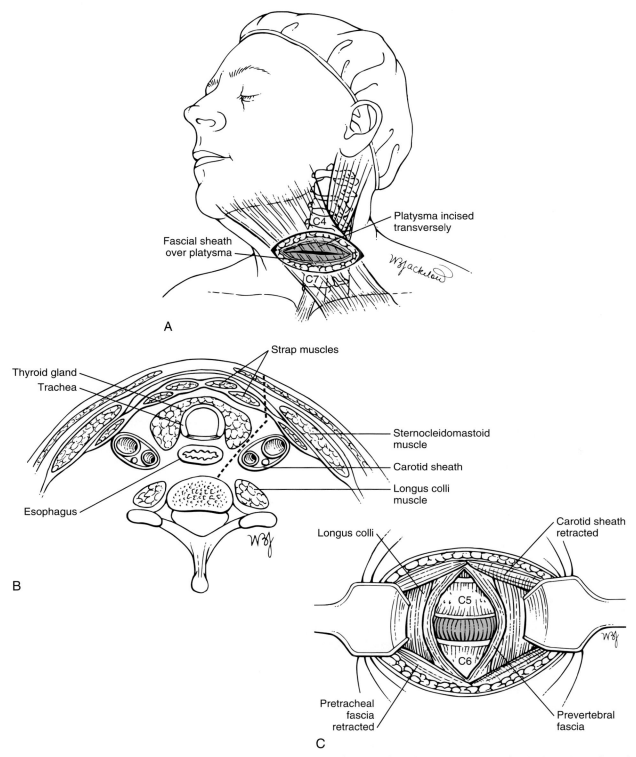

Figure 7–13. Anterior approach for cervical diskectomy and fusion at the C5–C6 level. A, A transverse skin incision is made and carried down through subcutaneous tissue to the platysma muscle, which is incised transversely. B, Cross-section of the surgical approach to the anterior cervical spine. The dissection proceeds between the sternocleidomastoid muscle (SCM) and carotid sheath (CS) laterally and the thyroid gland (TG), strap muscles (SM), trachea (T), and esophagus (E) medially. The disk space is marked with a bent spinal needle. C, The prevertebral fascia is incised, and the anterior longitudinal ligament and longus colli muscles are elevated cephalad and caudal to the disk space. Figure continued on following page

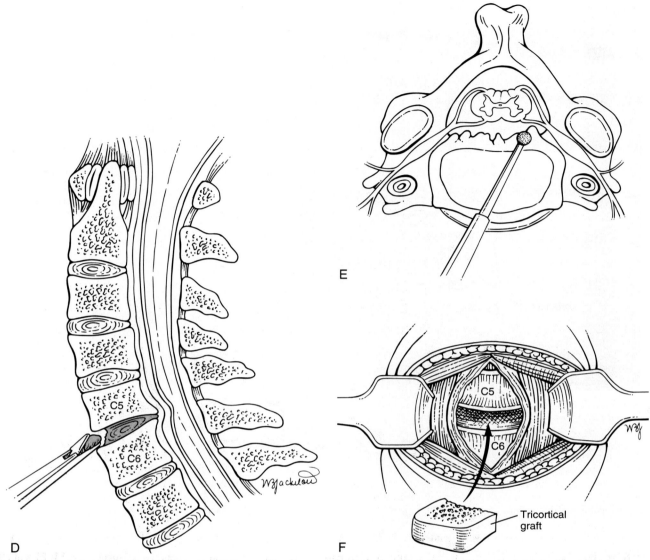

D

E

F

Tricortical
graft

Figure 17–13 *Continued. D, Curettes and pituitary rongeurs are used to excise disk material and the cartilaginous endplates. E, Posterior osteophytes are thinned with a cutting, then a diamond burr. Resection is completed with small Kerrison rongeurs and microcurettes. F, The disk space dimensions are determined, and a tricortical graft is harvested from the iliac crest. The vertebral endplates are decorticated down to punctate bleeding bone, and biconcave recipient beds are fashioned. The graft is tailored to fit the disk space and is gently tamped into place, with the graft recessed 1 to 2 mm from the anterior vertebral cortex.*

Figure continued on following page

of blunt and sharp dissection, a plane is developed between the sternocleidomastoid muscle and carotid sheath laterally and the trachea and esophagus medially. The superficial layer of the deep cervical fascia is released proximally and distally along the sternocleidomastoid muscle to permit adequate exposure (Fig. 7–13B). The carotid artery should be palpated beneath the surgeon's fingers and the sheath, then retracted laterally with a hand-held retractor. A second hand-held retractor is used to hold the esophagus medially. Both retractors are held with posteriorly directed pressure, which has the effect of clearing the midline of soft tissue and preventing the retracted structures from slipping underneath the retractors. The prevertebral fascia is opened sharply. Midline orientation is gained by observing the

longus colli muscles on each side of the midline. The midline is marked, a bent spinal needle is inserted into the disk space, and the level confirmed radiographically. The medial borders of the longus colli muscles are then elevated and freed from their vertebral attachments for a distance of one-half a vertebral body above and below the area of intended disk and bone resection (Fig. 7–13C). Electrocautery is required for hemostasis. Hand-held or self-retaining retractors are used beneath the muscle edges to gain mediolateral exposure. When better vertical exposure is needed, a second set of retractors may be positioned perpendicular to the first. Only after satisfactory exposure is attained and hemostasis achieved can disk, bone, and osteophyte resection begin.

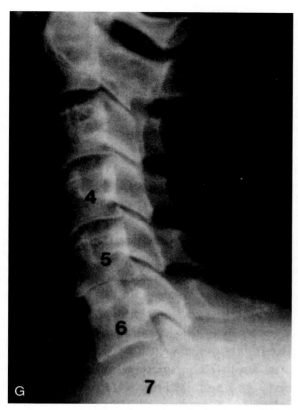

Figure 7–13 Continued. *G, Lateral x-ray showing a well-positioned intervertebral graft at C5–C6.*

The anterior longitudinal ligament and annulus are incised. Straight and angled curettes and pituitary rongeurs are used to excise the disk and cartilaginous endplates laterally to the uncovertebral joints and posteriorly to the posterior longitudinal ligament (Fig. 7–13D). Full visualization of the uncovertebral joints ensures proper midline orientation, thus minimizing the risk of injury to the vertebral arteries.[87] After sufficient disk material is removed, an intervertebral spreader is placed to distract the disk space and allow greater visualization for posterior decompression. We prefer the Caspar intervertebral distractor using the 14-mm threaded pins (Aesculap).[21, 22] In straightforward soft disk herniations, the offending disk material must be found and removed. If it is not located readily, the posterior longitudinal ligament must be resected and the fragments sought. In soft disk herniations with significant posterior uncovertebral osteophytes, anterior foraminotomy should be performed. This is done by initially thinning the posterior uncus, inferior vertebral lip, and osteophytes bilaterally using a cutting burr. The resection is then completed using a diamond burr, small Kerrison rongeurs (1 to 2 mm), and microcurettes (Fig. 7–13E). When the intended bone removal is complete, the surgeon should reconnoiter and ensure that adequate decompression has been achieved. Several authors have stated that osteophyte removal and spinal cord decompression are not necessary, because fusion of the disk space will result in resorption of the osteophytes.[77] Because there is no valid radiographic evidence of this, we recommend that the offending osteophytes be removed and the roots or cord decompressed before bone grafting is done.[53] In a small canal, this must be done cautiously to avoid iatrogenic neurologic deficits. Surgeons unfamiliar with these operative techniques should probably not attempt the procedure, because improper attempts to resect the osteophytes carry a significant risk of spinal cord injury.[13]

The ideal bone graft should have structural integrity, be easy to shape, and incorporate rapidly and reliably with a negligible nonunion rate. The autogenous tricortical iliac crest graft is used for these reasons, although some authors report comparable results when freeze-dried allograft fibula is used for one-level fusions. Before the graft is harvested, the endplates are burred down to bleeding subchondral bone[34] to create slightly biconcave recipient beds. Be advised that the Caspar distraction device is powerful, and it is easy to overdistract the vertebrae, a maneuver that may produce increased neck pain in the postoperative period. The depth and height of the graft bed are measured and an autogenous tricortical iliac crest graft is harvested.

The graft is then tailored to the precise size and shape using a cutting burr or rongeur. A small amount of the cortex (0.5 to 1.0 mm) is removed from the superior and inferior surfaces to render the cancellous bone in a biconvex shape. The prominent cancellous surfaces should mate exactly with the recipient site, producing better load distribution across the graft and a secure interference fit. After final contouring, the vertical cortical height of the graft must be ≥ 5 mm, to decrease the risk of graft fracture and collapse.[14] The Caspar distraction allows the graft to be placed without excessive force. The tricortical graft may be inserted with its cancellous side facing anteriorly. Thus, a cortical surface faces the spinal canal floor. This has two advantages. First, because greater loads are transmitted through the posterior vertebral body in the cervical spine, the strongest part of the graft bears the higher loads. Second, it is easier to identify the posterior aspect of the graft radiographically relative to the spinal canal. Alternatively, the graft may be inserted with its cortical side facing anteriorly (Fig. 7–13F). This method allows easier tamping of the graft into position. Before the vertebral distractor is released, the graft fit should be slightly loose. After release, it should be firmly locked in place (Fig. 7–13G).

If interbody grafts are to be placed at more than one level, then a few cautions are in order. First, care must be taken to avoid placing an oversized graft in the first space. This will risk pain production from overdistraction as well as make inserting the next graft more difficult. It is also likely to result in the insertion of an adjacent graft that is undersized and has a greater risk of collapse and failure. Second, if the patient has either small cervical vertebrae or significant osteopenia, or if significant amounts of vertebral bone have been removed to excise osteophytes, then corpectomy and a strut graft should be considered rather than adjacent interbody grafts. This creates a more mechanically sound reconstruction with a lower failure rate.

Once the graft position is confirmed radiographically, closure is performed over a closed-section drain. We prefer to use interrupted sutures for the platysma muscle and a subcuticular suture for skin. The patient wears a well-fitted cervical orthosis (type and size determined preoperatively) for 6 to 8 weeks. Static anteroposterior and lateral x-rays are obtained before discharge and again 6 weeks postoperatively. Lateral flexion/extension views are taken at 12 weeks or later postoperatively to confirm graft healing.

Complications

Although anterior cervical diskectomy and fusion for radiculopathy is highly effective in treating cervical nerve root and cord compression, it carries a number of potential complications. Transient dysphagia secondary to soft tissue swelling is a common postoperative complaint and can be quite disabling. Direct esophageal injury was reported by Cloward[24] and Connolly and coworkers,[27] but with no long-term sequelae. This is in contrast to the cases reported in the series by Flynn,[36] in which some patients with esophageal injury ultimately died. With the anterior approach at the C7–T1 level, injury to the dome of the parietal pleura of the lung with secondary pneumothorax is a particular risk.

Problems may occur at the outset from improper patient positioning. The procedure, done with the neck extended, may be hazardous in a patient with a congenitally narrowed canal or in a patient with osteophytes projecting into the canal, thereby compromising the space available for the cord. Cloward[25] reported hoarseness as being transient in 8% and permanent in 2% of patients. Riley and coworkers[76] reported a 4% incidence of hoarseness. The sympathetic ganglia located on the anterior surface of the longus colli muscle can be injured, resulting in ipsilateral pupillary miosis, ptosis, and anhidrosis. Such an injury is rare but represented 4.2% of the neurologic complications in Flynn's series.[36] Injury to the cord and/or nerve roots can be just as catastrophic,[91] the risk to these structures being greater with decompression of hard disks. Graft extrusion or angulation following collapse, a recognized risk of anterior interbody fusion in this procedure, is seen in 2% to 8% of cases.[30, 40, 85, 86] Aronson reported a 5.5% incidence of slipped grafts, which were reoperated for reinsertion, although these patients were not necessarily symptomatic.[3] The necessity of reoperation for extruded grafts may be questioned, because Robinson noted satisfactory fusion and a good clinical result without reoperation.[78]

Graft Site Complications

Autogenous bone is considered the most suitable bone graft material for cervical fusion. Complications may occur in a significant number of patients, however. Graft harvest complications include increased surgical morbidity from an additional operative site, chronic donor site pain, increased operative time, increased blood loss and risk of transfusion, and additional cost. Potential complications of harvesting autogenous fibula include stress fracture of the tibia at the level of the ostectomy and peroneal nerve injury from extensive proximal dissection.

SUMMARY

Successful treatment of cervical radiculopathy rests on a thorough understanding of the pathophysiology of cervical disk disease and clear identification of the specific etiology of neurologic compromise. A careful analysis of the symptom complex, physical signs, and appropriate imaging studies will help to isolate the source of most, but not all, complaints referable to the cervical spine. When the pathoanatomy is established, treatment is adapted to address the specific problem. Consideration of the pathogenesis and natural history of the degenerative process, as well as knowledge of the available medical and surgical treatment options, is essential to instituting rational treatment recommendations.

Surgical treatment of cervical radiculopathy should be considered only after an adequate trial of conservative management has failed. When surgery is contemplated, the decision must be based on sound indications, and the operative strategy and approach must address the specific pathology responsible for the patient's symptom complex. Both anterior and posterior procedures have roles in the operative treatment of cervical radiculopathy. Regardless of the approach taken, when the appropriate patient is selected, the surgery is performed based on a rational assessment of the anatomic and clinical factors present, and attention is directed to the technical aspects of exposure, neural decompression, and fusion, a satisfactory outcome can be expected.

REFERENCES

1. Aldrich F: Posterolateral microdiscectomy for cervical monoradiculopathy caused by posterolateral soft cervical disk sequestration. J Neurosurg 72:370–377, 1990.
2. Aprill C, Dwyer A, Bogduk N: Cervical zygapophyseal joint pain patterns II: A clinical evaluation. Spine 15:458–461, 1990.
3. Aronson NI: The management of soft cervical disc protrusions using the Smith-Robinson approach. Clin Neurosurg 20:253–258, 1973.
4. Bailey P, Casamajor L: Osteo-arthritis of the spine as a cause of compression of the spinal cord and its roots: With reports of five cases. J Nerv Ment Dis 38:588–609, 1911.
5. Bailey RW, Badgley CE: Stabilization of the cervical spine by anterior fusion. J Bone Joint Surg 42:565–594, 1960.
6. Beatty RM, Fowler FD, Hanson EJ Jr: The abducted arm as a sign of ruptured cervical disk. Neurosurg 21:731–732, 1987.
7. Blumenkrantz N, Sylvest J, Asboe-Hansen G: Local low-collagen content may allow herniation of intervertebral disk: Biochemical studies. Biochem Med 18:283–290, 1977.
8. Boden SD, McCowin PR, Davis DO, et al: Abnormal magnetic resonance scans of the cervical spine in asymptomatic subjects: A prospective investigation. J Bone Joint Surg 72:1178–1184, 1990.
9. Boden SD, McCowin PR, Davis DO, et al: Abnormal magnetic resonance scans of the cervical spine in asymptomatic subjects: A prospective investigation. J Bone Joint Surg 72:1178–1184, 1990.
10. Boden SD, Wiesel SW: Nonoperative management of cervical disk disease. In Camins MB, O'Leary PF (eds):

Disorders of the Cervical Spine. Baltimore, Williams & Wilkins, 1992, pp 157–164.

11. Bogduk N: The clinical anatomy of the cervical dorsal rami. Spine 7:319–330, 1982.

12. Bogduk N, Marsland A: The cervical zygapophysial joints as a source of neck pain. Spine 13:610–617, 1988.

13. Bohlman HH: Cervical spondylosis with moderate to severe myelopathy: A report of seventeen cases treated by Robinson anterior cervical diskectomy and fusion. Spine 2:151–162, 1977.

14. Bohlman HH: Degenerative arthritis of the lower cervical spine. In Evarts CM (ed): Surgery of the Musculoskeletal System, vol 2, 2nd ed. New York, Churchill Livingstone, 1990, pp 1857–1886.

15. Bohlman HH, Emery SE: The pathophysiology of cervical spondylosis and myelopathy. Spine 13:843–846, 1988.

15a. Bohlman HH, Emery SE, Goodfellow DB, Jones PK: Robinson anterior cervical discectomy and arthrodesis for cervical radiculopathy: Long term follow-up of one hundred twenty-two patients. J Bone Joint Surg Am 75:1298–1307, 1993.

16. Brain L: Some unsolved problems of cervical spondylosis. Br Med J 1:771–777, 1963.

17. Brain WR, Northfield D, Wilkinson M: The neurological manifestations of cervical spondylosis. Brain 75:187–225, 1952.

18. Brown MD: The pathophysiology of disc disease. Orthop Clin North Am 2:359–370, 1971.

18a. Burke TG, Caputy A: Microendoscopic posterior cervical foraminotomy: A cadaveric model and clinical application for cervical radiculopathy. J Neurosurg 93:126–129, 2000.

19. Burrows EH: The sagittal diameter of the spinal canal in cervical spondylosis. Clin Radiol 17:77–86, 1963.

20. Calliet R: Neck and Arm Pain. Philadelphia, FA Davis, 1964, pp 37–41.

21. Caspar W, Barbier DD, Klara PM: Anterior cervical fusion and Caspar plate stabilization for cervical trauma. Neurosurg 25:491–502, 1989.

22. Caspar W, Harkey HL: Anterior cervical fusion: Caspar osteosynthetic stabilization. In Young P (ed): Microsurgery of the Cervical Spine. New York, Raven, 1991, pp 109–142.

23. Chin JH: Recurrent stroke caused by spondylotic compression of the vertebral artery. Ann Neurol 33:558–559, 1993.

24. Cloward RB: The anterior approach for removal of ruptured cervical disc. J Neurosurg 15:602–614, 1958.

25. Cloward RB: New method of diagnosis and treatment of cervical disc disease. Clin Neurosurg 8:93–132, 1962.

26. Connell MD, Wiesel SW: Natural history and pathogenesis of cervical disc disease. Orthop Clin North Am 23:369–380, 1992.

27. Connolly ES, Seymour RJ, Adams JE: Clinical evaluation of anterior cervical fusion for degenerative cervical disc disease. J Neurosurg 23:431–437, 1965.

28. Cusick JF, Yoganandan N, Pintar F, et al: Biomechanics of cervical spine facetectomy and fixation techniques. Spine 13:808–812, 1988.

29. Davidson RI, Dunn EJ, Metzmaker JN: The shoulder abduction test in the diagnosis of radicular pain in cervical extradural compressive monoradiculopathies. Spine 6:441–446, 1981.

29a. Debois V, Herz R, Berghmans D, et al: Soft cervical disk herniation. Influence of cervical spinal canal measurements on development of neurologic symptoms. Spine 24:1996–2002, 1999.

30. DePalma AF, Subin DK: Study of the cervical syndrome. Clin Orthop 38:135–142, 1965.

31. Dillin W, Booth R, Cuckler J, et al: Cervical radiculopathy: A review. Spine 11:988–991, 1986.

32. Dillin W, Uppal GS: Analysis of medications used in the treatment of cervical disk degeneration. Orthop Clin North Am 23:421–433, 1992.

33. Dwyer A, Aprill C, Bogduk N: Cervical zygapophyseal joint pain patterns I: A study in normal volunteers. Spine 15:453–457, 1990.

34. Emery SE, Bolesta MJ, Banks MA, Jones PK: Robinson anterior cervical fusion: Comparison of the standard and modified techniques. Spine 19:660–663, 1994.

35. Fager CA: Management of cervical disc lesions and spondylosis by posterior approaches. Clin Neurosurg 24:488–507, 1977.

36. Flynn TB: Neurologic complications of anterior cervical interbody fusion. Spine 7:536–539, 1982.

37. Friedenberg ZB, Miller WT: Degenerative disc disease of the cervical spine. J Bone Joint Surg 45:1171–1178, 1963.

38. Garvey TA, Eismont FJ: Diagnosis and treatment of cervical radiculopathy and myelopathy. Orthop Rev 20:595–603, 1991.

39. George B, Laurian C: Impairment of vertebral artery flow caused by extrinsic lesions. Neurosurg 24:206–214, 1989.

40. Gore DR, Sepic SB: Anterior cervical fusion for degenerated or protruded disks. A review of one hundred forty-six patients. Spine 9:667–671, 1984.

41. Gore DR, Sepic SB, Gardner GM: Roentgenographic findings of the cervical spine in asymptomatic people. Spine 11:521–524, 1986.

42. Gore DR, Sepic SB, Gardner GM, Murray MP: Neck pain: A long-term follow-up of 205 patients. Spine 12:1–5, 1987.

42a. Grieve JP, Kitchen ND, Moore AJ, Marsh HT: Results of posterior cervical foraminotomy for treatment of cervical spondylitic radiculopathy. Br J Neurosurg 14:40–43, 2000.

43. Groen GJ, Baljet B, Drukker J: Nerves and nerve plexuses of the human vertebral column. Am J Anat 188:282–296, 1990.

44. Hanus SH, Homer TD, Harter DH: Vertebral artery occlusion complicating yoga exercise. Arch Neurol 34:574–575, 1977.

45. Hardin CA, Williamson WP, Streegman AT: Vertebral artery insufficiency produced by cervical osteoarthritic spurs. Neurology 10:855–858, 1960.

46. Heller JG: The syndromes of degenerative cervical disease. Orthop Clin North Am 23:381–394, 1992.

47. Henderson CM, Hennessy RG, Shuey HM, Shackelford EG: Posterior-lateral foraminotomy as an exclusive operative technique for cervical radiculopathy: A review of 846 consecutively operated cases. Neurosurgery 13:504–512, 1983.

48. Hilding DA, Tachdjian MO: Dysphagia and hypertrophic spurring of the cervical spine. N Engl J Med 263:11–14, 1960.

49. Hollinshead WH: General survey of the upper limb. In Hollinshead WH (ed): Anatomy for Surgeons, vol 3, 3rd ed. Philadelphia, Harper and Row, 1982, pp 203–257.

50. Hong CZ, Lee S, Lum P: Cervical radiculopathy. Clinical, radiographic and EMG findings. Orthop Rev 15:433–439, 1986.

51. Hult L: The Munkfors investigation. Acta Orthop Scand 16:1–76, 1954.

52. Jackson R: Headaches associated with disorders of the cervical spine. Headache 1:175–179, 1967.

53. Kadoya S, Nakamura T, Kwak R: A microsurgical anterior osteophytectomy for cervical spondylotic myelopathy. Spine 9:437–441, 1984.

54. Keyes DC, Compere EL: The normal and pathological

physiology of the nucleus pulposus of the intervertebral disk. J Bone Joint Surg Am 14A:897–938, 1932.

55. Krueger BR, Okazaki H: Vertebral-basilar distribution infarction following chiropractic cervical manipulation. Mayo Clin Proc 55:322–332, 1980.

56. Krupp W, Schattke H, Muke R: Clinical results of the foraminotomy as described by Frykholm for the treatment of lateral cervical disc herniation. Acta Neurochir 107:22–29, 1990.

57. Lees AF, Turner JWA: Natural history and prognosis of cervical spondylosis. Br Med J 2:1607–1610, 1963.

58. Lestini WF, Wiesel SW: The pathogenesis of cervical spondylosis. Clin Orthop 239:69–93, 1989.

59. Macnab I, McCulloch J: Cervical disk disease: Clinical assessment. In Passano WM (ed): Neck Ache and Shoulder Pain. Baltimore, Williams & Wilkins, 1994, pp 54–78.

60. Macnab I, McCulloch J: Cervical disc degeneration—Pathogenesis of symptoms. In Passano WM (ed): Neck Ache and Shoulder Pain. Baltimore, Williams & Wilkins, 1994, pp 42–53.

61. Maran A, Jacobson I: Cervical osteophytes presenting with pharyngeal symptoms. Laryngoscope 81:412–417, 1971.

62. Marzo JM, Simmons EH, Kallen F: Intradural connections between adjacent cervical spinal roots. Spine 12:964–968, 1987.

63. McCormick PC: Clinical manifestations of myelopathy and radiculopathy. In Cooper PC (ed): Degenerative Disease of the Cervical Spine. Rolling Meadows, IL, American Association of Neurological Surgeons, 1992, pp 1–8.

64. McCrae DL: The significance of abnormalities of the cervical spine. Am J Roentgenol 84:3–25, 1960.

65. Mehalic TM, Farhat SM: Vertebral artery injury from chiropractic manipulation of the neck. Surg Neurol 2:125–129, 1974.

66. Mixter WJ, Barr JS: Rupture of the intervertebral disc with involvement of the spinal canal. N Engl J Med 211:210–215, 1934.

67. Montgomery DM, Brower RS: Cervical spondylotic myelopathy: Clinical syndrome and natural history. Orthop Clin North Am 23:487–493, 1992.

68. Murphy F, Simmons JCH, Brunson B: Surgical treatment of laterally ruptured cervical disk: Review of 648 cases, 1939 to 1972. J Neurosurg 38:679–683, 1973.

69. Nagashima C: Surgical treatment of vertebral artery insufficiency caused by cervical spondylosis. J Neurosurg 32:512–521, 1970.

70. Okawara BS, Nibblink D: Vertebral artery occlusion following hyperextension and rotation of the head. Stroke 5:640–642, 1974.

71. Parkin PJ, Wall WE, Wilson JL: Vertebral artery occlusion following manipulation of the neck. N Z Med J 88:441–443, 1978.

72. Payne EE, Spillane JD: The cervical spine: An anatomico-pathological study of 70 specimens (using a special technique) with particular reference to the problem of cervical spondylosis. Brain 80:571–596, 1957.

73. Rahim KA, Stambough JL: Radiographic evaluation of the degenerative cervical spine. Orthop Clin North Am 23:395–403, 1992.

74. Raynor RB: Pathophysiology of bony and ligamentous changes in cervical spondylosis. In Cooper PR (ed): Degenerative Disease of the Cervical Spine. Rolling Meadows, IL, American Association of Neurological Surgeons, 1992, pp 9–15.

75. Raynor RB, Carter FW: Cervical spine strength after facet injury and spine plate application. Spine 16S:558–560, 1991.

76. Riley LH, Robinson RA, Johnson KA, Walker AE: The results of anterior interbody fusion of the cervical spine. J Neurosurg 30:127–133, 1969.

77. Robinson RA, Smith GW: Anterolateral disk removal and interbody fusion for cervical disk syndrome. Bull Johns Hopkins Hosp 96:223–224, 1955.

78. Robinson RA, Walker AE, Ferlic DC, et al: The results of anterior interbody fusion of the cervical spine. J Bone Joint Surg 44:1569–1587, 1962.

79. Schellhas KP, Latchaw RE, Wendling LR, Gold LHA: Vertebrobasilar injuries following cervical manipulation. JAMA 244:1450–1453, 1980.

80. Schmorl G: Uber verlagerung von bandscheibengewebe und ihre folgen. Arch Klin Chir 172:240–276, 1997.

81. Scoville WB, Dohrmann GJ, Corkill G: Late results of cervical disk surgery. J Neurosurg 45:203–210, 1976.

82. Sheehan S, Bauer RB, Meyer JS: Vertebral artery compression in cervical spondylosis. Neurology 70:968–986, 1960.

83. Shelokov AP: Evaluation, diagnosis, and initial treatment of cervical disk disease. Spine 5S:167–176, 1991.

84. Sherman MR, Smialek JE, Zane WE: Pathogenesis of vertebral artery occlusion following cervical spine manipulation. Arch Pathol Lab Med 111:851–853, 1987.

85. Simmons EH, Bhalla SK: Anterior cervical diskectomy and fusion: A clinical and biomechanical study with eight-year follow-up. J Bone Joint Surg Br 51B:225–237, 1969.

86. Smith GW, Robinson RA: The treatment of certain cervical-spine disorders by anterior removal of the intervertebral disk and interbody fusion. J Bone Joint Surg Am 40A:607–623, 1958.

87. Smith MD, Emery SE, Dudley A, et al: Vertebral artery injury during anterior decompression of the cervical spine: A retrospective review of ten patients. J Bone Joint Surg Br 75B:410–415, 1993.

88. Southwick WO, Robinson RA: Surgical approaches to the vertebral bodies in the cervical and lumbar regions. J Bone Joint Surg 39:631–644, 1957.

89. Spurling RG, Scoville WB: Lateral rupture of the cervical intervertebral disks: A common cause of shoulder and arm pain. Surg Gynecol Obstet 78:350–358, 1944.

90. Stookey B: Compression of the spinal cord due to ventral extradural cervical chondromas. Arch Neurol Psychiat 20:275–291, 1928.

91. Sugar O: Spinal cord malfunction after anterior cervical discectomy. Surg Neurol 15:4–8, 1981.

92. Sullivan HG, Hardison JW, Vines FS, Becker D: Embolic posterior cerebral artery occlusion secondary to spondylotic vertebral artery compression. J Neurosurg 43:818–822, 1975.

93. Tan JC, Nordin M: Role of physical therapy in the treatment of cervical disk disease. Orthop Clin North Am 23:435–449, 1992.

94. Tew JC, Mayfield FH: Complications of surgery of the anterior cervical spine. Clin Neurosurg 23:424–434, 1975.

94a. Thorell W, Cooper J, Hellbusch L, Leibrock L: The long-term clinical outcome of patients undergoing anterior cervical discectomy with and without intervertebral bone graft placement. Neurosurgery 43:268–273, 1998.

95. Tsai CP, Huang CI, Wang V, et al: Evaluation of cervical radiculopathy by cervical root stimulation. Electromyogr Clin Neurophysiol 34:363–366, 1994.

96. Veidlinger OF, Colwill JC, Smyth HS, Turner D: Cervical myelopathy and its relationship to cervical stenosis. Spine 6:550–552, 1981.

97. White AA, Hirsch C: An experimental study of the immediate load bearing capacity of some commonly used iliac bone grafts. Acta Orthop Scand 42:482–490, 1971.

98. Whitecloud TS III, Seago RA: Cervical discogenic syndrome. Results of operative intervention in patients with positive discography. Spine 12:313–316, 1987.

99. Wilkinson HA, LeMay ML, Ferris EJ: Clinical-radiographic correlations in cervical spondylosis. J Neurosurg 30:213–218, 1969.

100. Williams RW: Microcervical foraminotomy: A surgical alternative for intractable radicular pain. Spine 8:708–716, 1983.

100a. Wirth FP, Dowd GC, Sanders HF, Wirth C: Cervical discectomy. A prospective analysis of three operative techniques. Surg Neurol 53:340–346, 2000.

100b. Woertgen C, Rothoerl RD, Henkel J, Brawanski A: Long term outcome after cervical foraminotomy. J Clin Neurosci 7:312–315, 2000.

101. Wolf BS, Khilnani M, Malis L: The sagittal diameter of the bony cervical canal and significance in cervical spondylosis. J Mount Sinai Hosp 23:283–292, 1956.

102. Young P: Degenerative cervical disk disorders: Pathophysiology and clinical syndromes. In Young P (ed): Microsurgery of the Cervical Spine. New York, Raven, 1991, pp 49–63.

103. Zdeblick TA, Abitbol J, Kunz DN, et al: Cervical stability after sequential capsule resection. Spine 18:2005–2008, 1993.

104. Zdeblick TA, Zou D, Warden KE, et al: Cervical stability after foraminotomy: A biomechanical in vitro analysis. J Bone Joint Surg 74:22–27, 1992.

105. Zeidman SM, Ducker TB: Posterior cervical laminoforaminotomy for radiculopathy: Review of 172 cases. Neurosurgery 33:356–362, 1993.

8

CERVICAL SPONDYLOTIC MYELOPATHY AND CERVICAL KYPHOSIS

Sanford E. Emery, M.D.

By trying, we can easily learn to endure adversity.
Another man's, I mean.
— Mark Twain

HISTORICAL PERSPECTIVE

Although Bailey and Casamajor had described degenerative changes in the thoracic and lumbar spine causing spinal cord compression in 1911,[5] Stookey was the first to discuss cervical spondylosis and cord impingement in 1928.[65] It was not until 1934 that Peet and Echols showed "chondromas" of the spine to be disk protrusions.[53] The best understanding of the pathophysiology of cervical spondylosis causing cord compression and myelopathy came in the 1950s with classic papers by Brain et al.,[10] Payne and Spillane,[52] Clarke and Robinson,[15] and Wilkinson.[73] Interestingly, this expansion in knowledge of cervical spondylosis and myelopathy paralleled the development of surgical approaches to the spine for treatment of this disorder.

In 1892, Horsley performed probably the first successful operation, a C6 laminectomy, for cervical cord compression.[68] In 1912, Bailey and Elsberg[6] used the term "spinal decompression" to describe seven cases of laminectomy in the thoracic and lumbar region. Reports of cervical laminectomy for treatment of disk herniations with radiculopathy began to appear in the 1940s.[64, 66] The following two decades demonstrated larger series of patients with spondylosis and myelopathy treated by posterior laminectomy techniques.[17, 20, 59, 62, 67]

During this same period, the anterior approach to the cervical spine had been developed and used initially in the treatment of patients with neck pain and later radiculopathy.[16, 57, 58, 71] In 1966, Crandall and Batsdorf included 28 patients with myelopathy treated by anterior interbody fusion and compared the results to a laminectomy group.[17] In 1970, Nurick published his thesis on a large group of patients using the Cloward technique of anterior fusion.[45] In 1977, Bohlman published a series of patients with moderate to severe myelopathy using the Smith-Robinson fusion technique with excellent results.[8]

The evolution of neuroradiologic imaging techniques fostered a better appreciation of the pathoanatomy present in patients with cervical myelopathy. More aggressive anterior procedures were described in the Japanese[35, 41] and then the English literature in the late 1970s and early 1980s. Whitecloud and LaRocca published the first article using a fibula strut graft following partial corpectomy at multiple levels.[72] Abe et al.[1] and Hanai et al.[29] described the technique of anterior cervical corpectomy followed by bone strut fusion for patients with ossification of the posterior longitudinal ligament (OPLL). Boni et al. used this technique for patients with spondylotic myelopathy.[9] Many more publications in the 1980s and 1990s followed that described the concept of subtotal anterior vertebrectomy and strut fusion to treat spondylotic myelopathy.[7, 19, 28, 48, 61, 76] Although initially described for OPLL, laminoplasty has evolved through these same decades as an alternative method to treat certain patients with cervical spondylotic myelopathy. We have come a long way since Horsley's surgical success more than 100 years ago, but there is undoubtedly more to be learned about this disorder and its management.

PATHOPHYSIOLOGY

Cervical spondylosis is a result of degenerative processes in the soft tissue and bony structures of the cervical spine. These changes are largely related to aging and are present in approximately 50% of the population at 50 years of age.[37] Biochemical alterations in the disk with proteoglycan changes and loss of water result in decreased disk elasticity and settling. These changes in nature's "shock absorbers" for each vertebral motion segment alter the biomechanics of the disk as well as the surrounding ligamentous structures and facet joints. Osteophytes form in response to the altered mechanical environment. Typically spurs form at the insertion of annular fibers, the facet joints, and particularly the uncovertebral joints (joints of Luschka). This uncovertebral joint hypertrophy is very important in the pathophysiology of root compression. Large spurs compromise the neural foramen and also can contribute to spinal cord compression along with transverse osseous ridges, disk herniations, and OPLL. Disk settling and loss of height at the motion segment can lead to inward buckling of the ligamentum flavum posteriorly, contributing to canal stenosis or, rarely, resulting in focal dorsal spinal cord compression. Patients with cervical spondylosis can also develop *compensatory subluxation*, defined as excessive motion at a level one or two disk spaces above stiffened spondylotic segments. This finding needs to be identified (usually by flexion–extension x-rays) to help guide the surgical plan. The presence of cervical kyphosis also can significantly

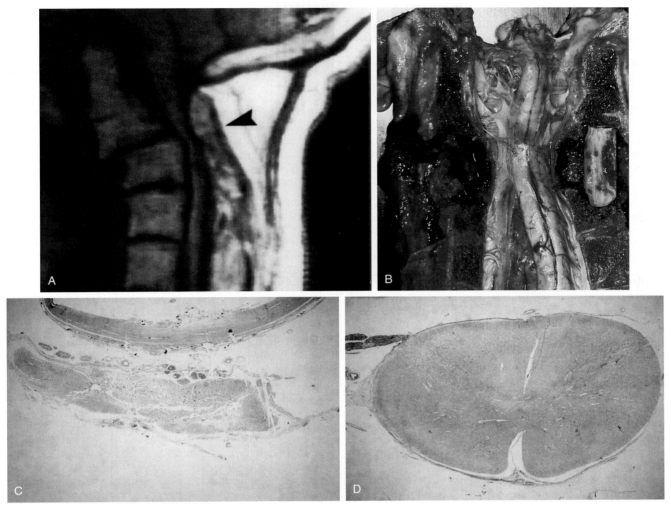

Figure 8–1. *A 40-year-old Caucasian male complained of gait difficulty with upper and lower extremity weakness of 1 year's duration. He was ambulatory but required a walker. Examination showed obvious long tract signs with bilateral upper and lower extremity weakness. A, A sagittal MRI shows severe spinal cord compression at the level of the subluxation. The patient underwent anterior cervical vertebrectomy of C4 and fibular strut fusion followed by halo vest placement. The immediate postoperative period was uneventful, but 1 week postoperatively the patient died of a myocardial infarction. B, Gross pathologic examination of the spinal cord illustrates the area of indentation where the chronic anterior compression has been. C, Histology shows severe flattening of the cord with distorted architecture. D, Section from the C1 level shows normal cord histology for comparison. (From Emery SE: Cervical spondylotic radiculopathy and myelopathy: Anterior approach and pathology. In White AH, Schofferman JA (eds): Spine Care. St. Louis, Mosby Inc., 1995, p. 178.)*

contribute to cord compression. With a kyphotic deformity, the neural elements will be draped over any protruded disks, osteophytes, or OPLL areas and aggravate the already compromised physiology of the spinal cord.

Cervical spondylosis can result in spinal cord compression at one level or multiple levels. There can be focal cord impingement with deformation or more generalized canal stenosis with circumferential narrowing around the cord. The inherent size of the spinal canal plays an important role, and patients with a narrow canal and spondylosis are at increased risk for cord compression with resultant myelopathy.[4, 24] A spinal canal of 12 mm or less on plain films is likely to produce neural compression, because the midcervical cord is usually 9 to 10 mm in diameter. A Pavlov's ratio of canal:vertebral body width < 0.8 indicates a congenitally narrow spinal canal. Fujiwara et al.[25] used

computed tomography (CT)/myelography to correlate the transverse area of the cord with the severity of pathologic changes in cadaver spinal cords. Koyanagi et al.[39] and Fujiwara et al.[24] demonstrated that patients with a transverse area of the cord < 30 mm^2 preoperatively had poorer neurologic recovery postoperatively.

Chronic compression of the spinal cord first results in demyelination in the white matter. Continued compression can lead to cell necrosis in the gray matter which can at times be seen on cross-sectional imaging studies such as CT/myelography and magnetic resonance imaging (MRI).[47] This cell death can be attributed to direct neural compression as well as to ischemia. Breig et al.[11] showed that the transverse arterioles are subject to mechanical distortion with flattening of the cord in the anteroposterior direction, leading to relative ischemia of the central gray matter and

Table 8–1. *Long Tract Signs for Cervical Myelopathy*

Babinski's sign	Extension of the great toe instead of the normal flexion reflex to plantar stimulation
Hoffmann's reflex	Elicited by positioning the hand and wrist at rest and flicking the terminal phalanx of the middle finger by snapping it between the examiner's thumb and index finger. A positive response is when the patient's thumb and index terminal phalanx flex simultaneously.
Inverted radial reflex	Tapping of the distal brachioradialis tendon produces hyperactive finger flexion. This pathologic reflex is believed to result from compression at the C5 level.
Finger escape sign	Deficient adduction and/or extension of the ulnar two or three digits. With the arms out and palms down, the small finger tends to lie in slight abduction and cannot be held in adduction for more than 30 seconds.[49]
Myelopathy hand	Localized wasting and weakness of the intrinsic muscles of the hand with an inability to grip and release rapidly with the fingers.[49]

the medial white matter. With cell destruction and loss of axons, the spinal cord may appear small or atrophic. Neuroradiologic imaging studies and histologic changes can be remarkable (Fig. 8–1). Many of these patients can still recover substantially after surgical decompression, although some evidence suggests that patients with a small atrophic cord, particularly at multiple levels, have a worse prognosis.[24, 30, 39]

The actual biochemical and cellular events occurring with spinal cord compression and myelopathy are complex and an area of active research. More attention has been directed to acute spinal cord injury and associated cellular events.[13, 14] Glutamate toxicity, free radicals, cationic-mediated injury, programmed cell death (apoptosis), and other unknown mechanisms probably all play a role in compromised neural physiology.[23]

CLINICAL PRESENTATION

The earliest symptoms of cervical myelopathy usually involve an alteration in balance and gait. Patients may have a wide-based, spastic-type gait or, in more subtle cases, the inability to perform toe-to-heel tandem gait maneuvers. Patients may have numbness of the hands, usually in a global distribution.[26] Tasks requiring fine motor control, such as working buttons or handwriting, may become difficult. Although most patients with myelopathy report neck or arm pain, approximately 20% report no pain at all,[19] and the absence of pain should not keep the examiner from considering the diagnosis. Complaints of weakness in the upper or lower extremities also may be present. Any of the muscle groups in the upper extremities may be affected, unilaterally or bilaterally, including the hand intrinsics. In the lower extremities, the proximal musculature is typically affected before distal strength. Reflex examination reveals hyperreflexia, and gross long-tract signs (Table 8–1) including Babinski's, clonus, Hoffmann's (Fig. 8–2), and the inverted radial reflex (Fig. 8–3), are commonly present. The finger escape sign (Fig. 8–4), positive grip and release test or, in more advanced cases, "myelopathy hand" may be observed (Fig. 8–5).[49] In some cases, because of severe segmental compression, hyporeflexia may be present consistent with root or even anterior horn cell compromise at that specific level.

DIAGNOSTIC EVALUATION

Although cross-sectional neuroradiologic imaging has greatly enhanced our understanding of cervical spondylosis and spinal cord compression, plain x-rays still provide a substantial amount of information for any given patient. Disk space narrowing and posterior osteophytes are best appreciated on the lateral view. Oblique views can show foraminal encroachment by uncovertebral osteophytes, although these need not be routinely obtained. The sagittal diameter of the spinal canal can be measured from the lateral view and Pavlov's ratio[51] calculated. A ratio ≤ 0.8

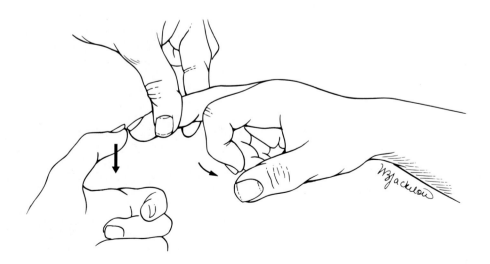

Figure 8–2. Hoffmann's reflex.

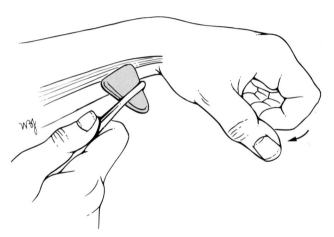

Figure 8–3. Inverted radial reflex.

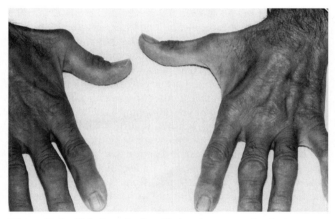

Figure 8–5. "Myelopathy hand" showing severe intrinsic muscle wasting in a patient with long-standing cervical spondylotic myelopathy.

indicates a congenitally narrow spinal canal. Although disk material will not be evident on plain films, the narrowest sagittal diameter of the spinal canal behind the largest osteophyte can be measured. A diameter ≤ 12 mm usually indicates some degree of cord compression. Flexion and extension lateral views should always be considered, as compensatory subluxation may occur above spondylotic segments; this can influence the type of surgical approach and the number of levels that need to be stabilized.

MRI has become the next step in evaluating patients with suspected cervical myelopathy. Improvements in resolution enable visualization of disks, osteophytes, OPLL, and the spinal cord. Areas of high signal intensity within the cord can be visualized, although these findings have not been correlated with outcomes.[42] MRI may be the only diagnostic and preoperative study needed to provide the spinal surgeon with sufficient information to make surgical decisions. We often still rely on cervical myelography and CT/myelography (Fig. 8–6) to determine where to stop— that is, to determine which levels do not have cord flattening or root cutoff and may not need to be included as an operative level. I depend on physical examination for our overall evaluation of the patient, but give the pathoanatomic

information provided by studies such as CT/myelography the most weight by far when choosing surgical levels.

I have not found electromyography (EMG) and nerve conduction velocity studies to be useful in the diagnosis and management of this patient population. This is not to say, however, that consultation with neurology colleagues is not useful. Other conditions that may clinically mimic cervical myelopathy include amyotrophic lateral sclerosis, benign familial spasticity, and cerebral vascular disease.

INDICATIONS FOR SURGERY

The natural history of cervical myelopathy has been documented by Clarke and Robinson to be progressive in nature.[15] This often occurs in a step-like fashion, in which the patient may function at a given level for some time and then deteriorate with or without any known minor trauma. For this reason, if the patient has spinal cord compression

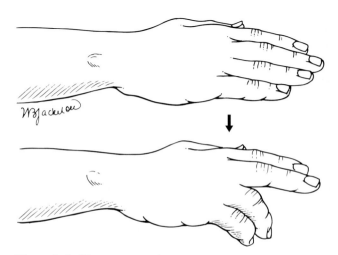

Figure 8–4. Finger escape sign.

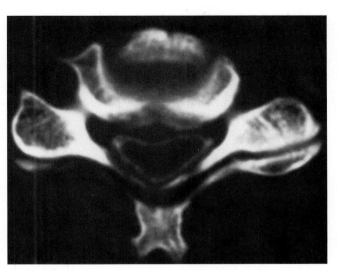

Figure 8–6. This CT myelogram shows some osteophytic ridging and disk herniation causing moderately severe compression of the spinal cord.

with clinical evidence of myelopathy and can tolerate the stress of general anesthesia and surgery, then surgical intervention is recommended. This usually can be done on an elective basis, although I recommend protecting the patient with a soft cervical collar while awaiting surgery. Occasionally more rapid neurologic deterioration is evident and more urgent surgical treatment is indicated.

Some patients may have significant spinal cord compression from spondylosis yet not manifest clinical signs of myelopathy. Severe neck pain with or without concomitant radiculopathy may be an indication for surgery in these patients. A patient without pain or neurologic abnormalities but with spinal cord compression revealed on cross-sectional imaging studies needs to be counseled about the relative risk of any spinal cord injury with a traumatic episode. This is a judgment call on the part of the physician, and my recommendation depends on the degree of cord compression present. Only in the rare case of severe compression in an asymptomatic patient will I recommend surgical intervention to prevent spinal cord injury from minor trauma.

SURGICAL TREATMENT ALTERNATIVES

Once the decision has been made to perform operative decompression in a patient with cervical myelopathy, the next choice is whether to take an anterior or a posterior approach. Certain authors favor anterior decompression and fusion, whereas others favor posterior decompression with or without fusion. Many choose an approach based on the pathoanatomy present in a given patient. Traditionally, posterior multilevel laminectomy was performed for operative decompression of myelopathy.[21, 22, 46] Some reports showed satisfactory results, but late deterioration has been a problem,[27] at times related to postlaminectomy instability. Laminoplasty has emerged as an alternative to laminectomy by enlarging the spinal canal without removing the posterior bony elements, allowing the posterior cervical musculature to reattach and minimize the chance of late kyphosis. The results of laminoplasty were initially reported for patients with severe OPLL, but subsequently were also reported for patients with cervical spondylosis and myelopathy.[18, 32, 38, 62a] Potential advantages of posterior laminoplasty include a straightforward approach, dissection that can span many levels, and no requirement that bony fusion occur. Decreased motion following laminoplasty is seen in most patients[18, 38]; however, relative preservation of motion might be an advantage compared to arthrodesis. There is some evidence that laminoplasty might be less satisfactory in relieving axial neck pain.[33] Laminectomy or laminoplasty is not recommended in patients with cervical kyphosis, because the spinal cord will not migrate posteriorly away from anterior compression and the deformity is at risk to worsen after a posterior procedure.[2] If a posterior approach is desired for patients with evidence of instability (such as compensatory subluxation), then a concomitant posterior arthrodesis with a facet fusion is indicated.

If the surgeon chooses an anterior approach to treat cervical myelopathy, then the next step is to choose either diskectomy and fusion or corpectomy and fusion. This decision depends largely on the pathoanatomy seen on cross-sectional imaging studies. Pathology such as disk herniations and spondylosis at the level of the endplates can be addressed by performing a diskectomy and, if necessary, burring off limited endplate osteophytes to adequately decompress the spinal canal. If there are large osteophytes, disk material tracking up or down behind vertebral bodies, or concomitant ossification of the posterior longitudinal ligament behind the vertebral bodies, then vertebral corpectomy is indicated. This allows the surgeon to burr down directly to the posterior longitudinal ligament and avoid reaching behind any vertebral body with instruments that may cause neural injury. Hemicorpectomy (or partial corpectomy) may also be done at a level where some but not all of the vertebral body needs to be removed to adequately decompress the canal. If the posterior longitudinal ligament is ossified (i.e., OPLL), then typically it is removed to adequately decompress the cord. An alternative is the floating method of decompression, where an island of OPLL is left centrally on the dura and allowed to expand or "float" anteriorly as the dura expands.[42a, 74] A slightly different approach was recently reported by Onari et al. using interbody fusion without decompression for patients with OPLL and myelopathy; 24 of 30 patients improved neurologically and 6 were unchanged or worse.[48a]

Anterior plate instrumentation for the cervical spine is a more recent option for the spinal surgeon. I recommend plate fixation for patients treated with multilevel diskectomy and fusions, single-level corpectomy, and many two-level corpectomy procedures, as discussed in the next section. Anterior plating generally allows for less restrictive brace wear postoperatively, but has some inherent risks of loosening, breakage, and added expense.

CERVICAL KYPHOSIS

Many patients with myelopathy have concomitant cervical kyphosis, with the spinal cord draped over the back of the vertebral bodies. The severity of the kyphosis is an important factor in making decisions about treatment. Many patients with cervical spondylosis have slight kyphosis (10 degrees or less) and generally can be treated surgically with anterior corpectomy and strut grafting alone[77] (Fig. 8–7). If the deformity is flexible (i.e., the patient's head and neck can be brought into near-normal alignment), then posterior laminectomy and posterior instrumentation and fusion may be a satisfactory option. This is often the case in patients in whom musculature insufficiency (e.g., postradiation myelopathy) is the cause of kyphosis.

Most patients with kyphosis due to cervical spondylosis are relatively stiff, though not necessarily ankylosed. In my experience, higher-magnitude, stiff kyphotic deformities usually necessitate anterior strut grafting and posterior stabilization to ensure graft stability and maintenance of correction. If true ankylosis is present, then posterior osteotomy may be necessary as a first step in correction, followed by anterior decompression (usually corpectomy).

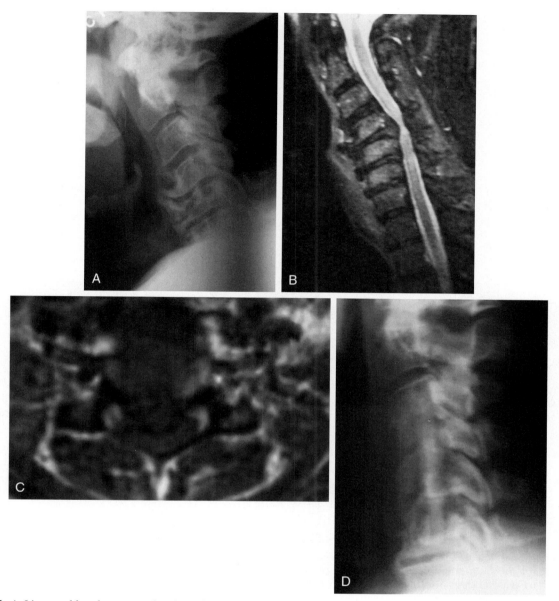

Figure 8–7. *A 64-year-old male presented with neck pain, increasing weakness and numbness in both upper extremities, and long tract signs consistent with cervical myelopathy. A, A lateral x-ray shows hypertrophic osteophytic changes at multiple levels with mild kyphosis (13 degrees by measurement). B, A sagittal MRI demonstrates the kyphosis and the disk material producing severe cord compression. C, A transverse MRI image showing a deformed kidney bean–shaped spinal cord at the C4–C5 level. D, A two-level corpectomy and fibular strut procedure was performed with uneventful healing and recovery of his myelopathy. This lateral plain film shows mild residual kyphosis (5 degrees by measurement), which in this author's experience is of no clinical significance.*

During the posterior ostectomy, the head is brought into extension to lengthen the anterior column and shorten the posterior column, hinging the osteotomy level on the posterior longitudinal ligament, followed by rigid posterior instrumentation (e.g., lateral mass plating).[3] Anterior decompression and strut grafting is then performed. These complex patients are obviously at high risk for neurologic complications; high-quality spinal cord monitoring, thoughtful preoperative planning, adequate internal fixation, plus a halo vest postoperatively are usually needed.

Postlaminectomy kyphosis is an especially difficult clinical problem.[3, 12, 31, 36, 43, 44, 55, 60, 63, 75] Removal of the lamina and posterior ligamentous structures eliminates the posterior tether that helps maintain lordosis. Removal of part or all of the facet joints potentiates the problem.[54, 78] These patients usually need multilevel corpectomy and strut grafting to decompress the canal and correct the deformity in the face of limited inherent posterior stability. This problem is best treated with circumferential arthrodesis using anterior strut grafts and lateral mass plates to achieve

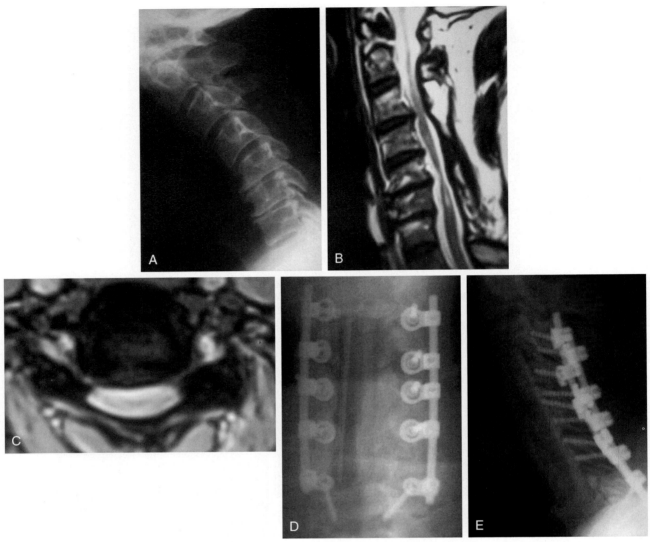

Figure 8–8. *A 75-year-old male presented with neck pain, balance trouble, and progressive weakness in both upper extremities. Approximately 15 years earlier he had a multilevel cervical laminectomy. A, A lateral x-ray in the neutral position shows the patient's postlaminectomy kyphosis. B, A sagittal MRI demonstrates spondylotic changes, increased signal changes in the cord consistent with myelomalacia, and spinal cord atrophy. C, A transverse MRI image shows the flattened, atrophic cord due to long-standing compression over the kyphotic deformity and spondylotic bars. D and E, The patient underwent a three-level anterior corpectomy and fibular strut grafting, followed by a posterior instrumentation and fusion. Lateral mass screws were used from C3 to C6; some mild subluxation prompted inclusion of the C7–T1 level, so T1 pedicle screws were utilized for the lowest point of fixation. Excellent stability and correction has been achieved with this circumferential approach. A rigid two-poster type brace was used postoperatively.*

maximum stability (Fig. 8–8).[55] Poor bone stock may warrant a "belt-and-suspenders" approach by using a halo vest postoperatively.

AUTHOR'S PREFERRED METHOD

Choice of Approach

For most patients with cervical spondylosis and myelopathy, I favor the anterior approach with decompression and arthrodesis. This is the most direct way to remove all bone and disk pathology compressing the anterior aspect of the dura and spinal cord. The operative approach is straightforward with clear fascial planes. Potential complications involving the esophagus, recurrent laryngeal nerve, and vertebral artery should be minor with good surgical technique. Many patients with spondylosis have a loss of lordosis or kyphosis, which can best be corrected and maintained with strut graft arthrodesis. There is some evidence that fusion provides superior pain relief, presumably by eliminating motion at spondylotic segments, than that afforded by posterior laminoplasty.[33] With experience and meticulous surgical technique, the incidence of graft complications should be very low.[19]

For patients with myelopathy and diffuse multilevel canal stenosis, normal lordosis, and little to no neck pain, I perform posterior laminoplasty; for most patients with cervical spondylosis and myelopathy, however, anterior decompression and fusion is my procedure of choice. The relative advantages and disadvantages of the anterior and posterior approaches for the treatment of cervical myelopathy are summarized in Table 8–2.

Operative Positioning and Surgical Approach

Because of the spinal cord compression in this patient population, patient positioning is a crucial step that demands attention to detail. Neck extension narrows the spinal canal and can result in cord injury if hyperextension is produced by positioning. Spinal cord monitoring is used for these procedures, including during patient preparation. A short, rolled-up sheet is placed transversely under the patient's upper thoracic area to help the shoulders drop posteriorly. Intraoperative traction is applied, but care is taken to use no more than 5 to 10 lb until decompression is completed. The shoulders are pulled distally with tape without excessive vigor, to avoid stretching the brachial plexus. I use a left-sided approach with the patient's head turned slightly to the right. The left-sided incision minimizes the chance of recurrent laryngeal nerve injury, because the nerve is more constant in its course on this side. A transverse incision is made at the appropriate level from just to the right of the midline over to the left sternocleidomastoid muscle. After the superficial cervical fascial layer is incised, the deep cervical fascia is incised superiorly and inferiorly along the border of the sternocleidomastoid to facilitate retraction superiorly and inferiorly. This allows for multilevel corpectomy and strut fusion through a transverse incision without struggling, provided that two assistants are present to provide retraction in multilevel procedures. The intervening fascia between the carotid sheath and the trachea and esophagus is dissected, and the spine is then palpable. Cautery is used along the

Table 8–2. *Anterior Versus Posterior Approaches to Treating Cervical Myelopathy*

Advantages	Disadvantages
Anterior Approach	
1. Direct removal compressive pathology	1. Technically demanding
2. Stabilization with arthrodesis	2. Graft complications
3. Correction of deformity	3. Postoperative bracing
4. Good axial pain relief	4. Loss of motion
	5. Adjacent segment degeneration
Posterior Approach	
1. Less loss of motion	1. Indirect decompression
2. Not as technically demanding	2. Preoperative kyphosis and/ or instability limitations
3. Less bracing	3. Inconsistent axial pain results
4. Avoids graft complications	

edges of the longus colli bilaterally to prevent venous bleeding. At this point, an x-ray should be obtained to ensure the appropriate operative level.

Technique of Anterior Cervical Corpectomy

The discussion here is limited to cervical corpectomy. The anterior diskectomy and fusion procedure is described in Chapter 7, and strut graft reconstruction of the spine for arthrodesis is described in Chapter 4.

After exposure of the anterior cervical spine and identification of the appropriate levels, the first step in a corpectomy procedure is removing the disks above and below the appropriate vertebrae. Incision of the anterior longitudinal ligament is followed by curettage of the bulk of the disk using small curettes. Fragments can be retrieved from the disk space using small pituitary rongeurs. The operative microscope can be used or $3\frac{1}{2}\times$ loupe magnification with a headlight. The key is the use of magnification in conjunction with adequate lighting to ensure excellent visualization. The disk and endplate cartilage is removed back to the posterior longitudinal ligament. In most cases, the disk space can be gently distracted using a Cloward-type lamina spreader or Caspar screw post distractors. If severe cord compression is present, however, then this step must be done with great care or even omitted, because any distraction may further impinge a compromised cord and result in injury. If the disk is narrow from spondylosis and quite stiff, then the burr can be used to remove the endplates and disk down toward the posterior longitudinal ligament to obtain adequate visualization. I prefer to expose the posterior longitudinal ligament to establish the depth for the ensuing vertebra resection. It is also important to identify the uncovertebral joints bilaterally. These anatomic landmarks provide orientation to the midline, minimizing the risk of vertebral artery injury with the burr.

After the disks are removed above and below the vertebra, a rongeur may be used to remove the anterior aspect of the vertebral body, staying within the boundaries of the uncovertebral joints as mentioned earlier. A power burr with a carbide tip is then used to remove the bulk of the vertebral body, heading posteriorly toward the back wall of the vertebra (Fig. 8–9A). When the posterior wall is reached, a 5-mm diamond burr is used, which minimizes the risk of soft tissue injury (Fig. 8–9B). The posterior wall is thinned in the left and right gutters. The remnants of the posterior shell of bone can then be carefully picked away from the posterior longitudinal ligament or from the dura in case of an ossified ligament (Fig. 8–9C). Any remnant disk material is also elevated off of the dura, allowing the dura and its contents to expand anteriorly (Fig. 8–9D). The foramina are cleaned out by removing osteophytes and disk material, using small curettes and a small 3-mm diamond burr as needed. In cervical spondylosis, it is often necessary to remove the superior endplate and a few millimeters of vertebral body above and below the corpectomy level, because osteophytic compression is usually present on each side of the disk at those motion segments. I prefer a 16- to 18-mm wide vertebrectomy channel, depending on the

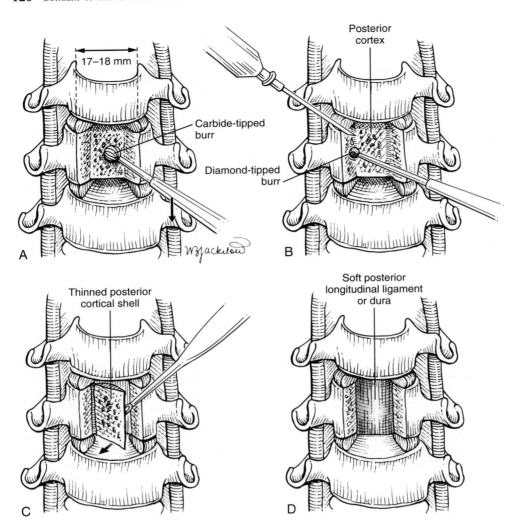

Figure 8–9. Technique of subtotal vertebral corpectomy. A, A carbide-tipped burr is used to remove most of the central portion of the body, back to a thin bony shell. B, A diamond-tipped burr is then used to remove bone in the gutters back to the posterior longitudinal ligament. C, The thinned posterior cortical shell is then carefully lifted off the posterior longitudinal ligament. D, The posterior longitudinal ligament (or dura if the posterior longitudinal ligament is removed) should reexpand into the decompressed area.

patient's size. If centered, this distance will adequately decompress the spinal canal (Fig. 8–10). Some authors remove part of the pedicles for a wider decompression,[48] but I have not found this to be necessary for neural recovery or graft placement.

Choice of Strut Graft

There are three main choices for strut graft materials following cervical corpectomy. A tricortical iliac crest is a satisfactory graft for one-level or two-level corpectomy, provided that the patient does not have severe osteoporosis. For anything more than a one-level corpectomy, I prefer autogenous fibula strut grafting. I have found the donor site morbidity to be low and the healing rate extremely high for this particular type of graft.[19] Some settling commonly occurs, particularly in older patients with osteoporotic vertebral bodies, but in my experience this has not resulted in clinical morbidity.[34] Allograft fibula is an alternative that some have found satisfactory,[40] but I have found to have a slower and less successful fusion rate.

Use of Instrumentation

The evolution of internal fixation for the spine has greatly enhanced the surgeon's ability to provide additional stability, maintain correction of deformity, and promote arthrodesis. Anterior plating is increasingly used in degenerative conditions, particularly for multilevel diskectomy and fusion procedures. For patients with myelopathy, corpectomy is usually necessary, as discussed earlier. For one-level corpectomy and iliac strut grafting procedures, anterior plating is an excellent adjunct that can minimize postoperative bracing requirements with a soft collar or Philadelphia-type brace. The use of anterior plates for multilevel corpectomy and strut graft procedures is more controversial, with mixed results reported in the literature.[31, 40, 50] Because of the long lever arm with only two screws above and two screws below, a higher rate of loosening and displacement has been reported. Vaccaro et al.[69] found an early failure rate of approximately 10% for two-level corpectomy constructs and 50% for three-level constructs, when several surgeons were involved. Some surgeons now choose to perform concomitant posterior instrumentation (e.g., lateral mass plating) for multilevel corpectomy procedures to avoid graft complications. Others use a buttress-type plate at the superior pole and/or inferior pole to help prevent graft dislodgment, with mixed results.[56, 70]

If there is good bone stock and minimal kyphosis, anterior plating is useful for, but not essential to, two-level corpectomy procedures. Meticulous sculpting of the docking sites and centralization of the graft are extremely important to minimize graft complications. I do not recommend anterior plating for three-level corpectomy–strut graft constructs, because of the biomechanical limitations. Most of the patients can be treated with autogenous fibula strut grafting alone and a two poster–type of brace. Poor bone stock or kyphosis warrants adjunct posterior stabilization, usually with wiring plus lateral mass plates and bone grafting. This is a lot of surgery for some patients but does provide maximum stability postoperatively.

Postoperative Care

With good reconstruction technique, a stable strut graft construct should result. Most of my corpectomy and strut graft patients are treated postoperatively in a rigid head-cervical-thoracic orthosis with underarm straps. Indications for halo vest immobilization include severely osteoporotic vertebral bone, lack of posterior elements from remote surgical procedures if a concomitant facet fusion is not performed, and questionable stability of the graft at the time of the surgery. In these situations, a concomitant posterior fusion would be an advisable alternative.

Immobilization with a rigid brace or halo vest is generally maintained for 8 weeks postoperatively. A soft collar is then used for several days or a few weeks as a step down, depending on the patient's comfort level.

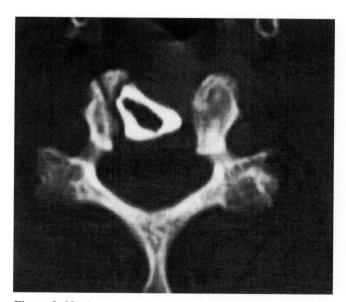

Figure 8–10. *A postoperative CT scan following a multilevel corpectomy and fibula strut procedure. The canal has been decompressed, and the fibula is seen in cross-section.*

Results

Many authors have reported high levels of neurologic recovery and successful arthrodesis after anterior decompression and fusion.[19, 48, 61, 76] The patient usually will begin to notice a difference in walking ability or hand function within several weeks after surgery. Spinal cord recovery will continue to occur in most patients over 1 to 2 years. Motor strength can be expected to improve by one or two grades and becomes normal in many patients. Numbness of the hands usually takes longer to resolve and may resolve incompletely. In our review, pain relief and functional outcome were found to be quite satisfactory in this patient population.[19] Long-term follow-up is recommended, not only to monitor improvement, but also to identify any significant adjacent level degeneration or compensatory subluxation.

REFERENCES

1. Abe H, Tsuru M, Ito T, et al: Anterior decompression for ossification of the posterior longitudinal ligament of the cervical spine. J Neurosurg 55:108–116, 1981.
2. Aita I, Hayashi K, Wadano Y, Yabuki T: Posterior movement and enlargement of the spinal cord after cervical laminoplasty. J Bone Joint Surg Br 80B:33–37, 1998.
3. Albert TJ, Vacarro A: Postlaminectomy kyphosis. Spine 23:2738–2745, 1998.
4. Arnold JG Jr: The clinical manifestations of spondylochondrosis of the cervical spine. Ann Surg 141:872–889, 1955.
5. Bailey P, Casamajor L: Osteo-arthritis of the spine as a cause of compression of the spinal cord and its roots: With reports of five cases. J Nerv Ment Dis 38:588–609, 1911.
6. Bailey P, Elsberg CA: Spinal decompression: Reports of seven cases and remarks on the dangers of and justification for exploratory operations. JAMA 58:675–679, 1912.
7. Bernard TN Jr, Whitecloud TS III: Cervical spondylotic myelopathy and myeloradiculopathy: Anterior decompression and stabilization with autogenous fibula strut graft. Clin Orthop 221:149–160, 1987.
8. Bohlman HH: Cervical spondylosis with moderate to severe myelopathy: A report of 17 cases treated by Robinson anterior cervical discectomy and fusion. Spine 2:151–162, 1977.
9. Boni M, Cherubino P, Denaro V, Benazzo F: Multiple subtotal somatectomy: Technique and evaluation of a series of 39 cases. Spine 9:358–362, 1984.
10. Brain WR, Northfield D, Wilkinson M: The neurological manifestations of cervical spondylosis. Brain 75:187–225, 1952.
11. Breig A, Turnbull I, Hassler O: Effects of mechanical stresses on the spinal cord in cervical spondylosis: A study on fresh cadaver material. J Neurosurg 25:45–56, 1966.
12. Callahan RA, Johnson RM, Margolis RN, et al: Cervical facet fusion for control of instability following laminectomy. J Bone Joint Surg Am 59A:991–1002, 1977.
13. Carlson GD, Gorden CD, Nakazowa S, et al: Perfusion-limited recovery of evoked potential function after spinal cord injury. Spine 25:1218–1226, 2000.
14. Carlson GD, Warden KE, Barbeau JM, et al: Viscoelastic relaxation and regional blood flow response to spinal cord compression and decompression. Spine 22:1285–1291, 1997.
15. Clarke E, Robinson PK: Cervical myelopathy: A complication of cervical spondylosis. Brain 79:483–510, 1956.

16. Cloward RB: The anterior approach for removal of ruptured cervical disks. J Neurosurg 15:602–617, 1958.

17. Crandall PH, Batzdorf U: Cervical spondylotic myelopathy. J Neurosurg 25:57–66, 1966.

18. Edwards CC II, Heller JG, Silcox DH III: T-saw laminoplasty for the management of cervical spondylotic myelopathy: Clinical and radiographic outcome. Spine 25:1788–1794, 2000.

19. Emery SE, Bohlman HH, Bolesta MJ, Jones PK: Anterior cervical decompression and arthrodesis for the treatment of cervical spondylotic myelopathy: Two- to seventeen-year follow-up. J Bone Joint Surg Am 80A:941–951, 1998.

20. Epstein JA, Davidoff LM: Chronic hypertrophic spondylosis of the cervical spine with compression of the spinal cord and nerve roots. Surg Gynecol Obstet 93:27–38, 1951.

21. Epstein JA, Janin Y, Carras R, Lavine LS: A comparative study of the treatment of cervical spondylotic myeloradiculopathy. Experience with 50 cases treated by means of extensive laminectomy, foraminotomy, and excision of osteophytes during the past 10 years. Acta Neurochir 61:89–104, 1982.

22. Fager CA: Results of anterior posterior decompression in the relief of spondylotic cervical myelopathy. J Neurosurg 38:684–692, 1973.

23. Fehlings MG, Skaf G: A review of the pathophysiology of cervical spondylotic myelopathy with insights for potential novel mechanisms drawn from traumatic spinal cord injury. Spine 23:2730–2736, 1998.

24. Fujiwara K, Yonenobu K, Ebara S, et al: The prognosis of surgery for cervical compression myelopathy. An analysis of the factors involved. J Bone Joint Surg Br 71B:393–398, 1989.

25. Fujiwara K, Yonenobu K, Hiroshima K, et al: Morphometry of the cervical spinal cord and its relation to pathology in cases with compression myelopathy. Spine 13:1212–1216, 1988.

26. Good DC, Couch JR, Wacaser L: "Numb, clumsy hands" and high cervical spondylosis. Surg Neurol 22:285–291, 1984.

27. Gregorius FK, Estrin R, Crandall PH: Cervical spondylotic radiculopathy and myelopathy. A long-term follow-up study. Arch Neurol 33:618–625, 1976.

28. Hanai K, Fujiyoshi F, Kamei K: Subtotal vertebrectomy and spinal fusion for cervical spondylotic myelopathy. Spine 11:310–315, 1986.

29. Hanai K, Inouye Y, Kawai K, et al: Anterior decompression for myelopathy resulting from ossification of the posterior longitudinal ligament. J Bone Joint Surg Br 64B:561–564, 1982.

30. Hayashi H, Okada K, Hashimoto J, et al: Cervical spondylotic myelopathy in the aged patient. A radiographic evaluation of the aging changes in the cervical spine and etiologic factors of myelopathy. Spine 13:618–625, 1988.

31. Herman JM, Sonntag VK: Cervical corpectomy and plate fixation for postlaminectomy kyphosis. J Neurosurg 80:963–970, 1994.

32. Hirabayashi K, Satomi K: Operative procedure and results of expansive open-door laminoplasty. Spine 13:870–876, 1988.

33. Hosono N, Yonenobu K, Ono K: Neck and shoulder pain after laminoplasty. Spine 21:1969–1973, 1996.

34. Hughes S, Pringle T, Phillips F, Emery SE: Multilevel cervical corpectomy and fibular start grafting: Intermediate clinical and radiographic follow-up. Submitted to Spine, 2002.

35. Kamikozuru M, Yamaura I, Fujii K, et al: Anterior decompression for ossification of the posterior longitudinal ligament of the multiple cervical spine. Clin Orthop Surg 12:416–424, 1977.

36. Katsumi Y, Honma T, Nakamura T: Analysis of cervical instability resulting from laminectomies for removal of spinal cord tumor. Spine 14:1171–1176, 1989.

37. Kellgren JH, Lawrence JS: Osteoarthritis and disk degeneration in an urban population. Ann Rheum Dis 17:388–397, 1958.

38. Kimura I, Shingu H, Nasu Y, et al: Long-term follow-up of cervical spondylotic myelopathy treated by canal-expansive laminoplasty. J Bone Joint Surg Br 77B:956–961, 1995.

39. Koyanagi T, Hirabayashi K, Satomi K, et al: Predictability of operative results of cervical compression myelopathy based on preoperative computed tomographic myelography. Spine 18:1958–1963, 1993.

40. Macdonald RL, Fehlings MG, Tator CH, et al: Multilevel anterior cervical corpectomy and fibular allograft fusion for cervical myelopathy. J Neurosurg 86:990–997, 1997.

41. Manabe S, Nomura S: Anterior decompression for ossification of the posterior longitudinal ligament of the cervical spine. Neurol Surg 5:1253–1259, 1977.

42. Matsumoto M, Toyama Y, Ishikawa M, et al: Increased signal intensity of the spinal cord on magnetic resonance images in cervical compressive myelopathy. Does it predict the outcome of conservative treatment? Spine 25:677–682, 2000.

42a. Matsuoka T, Yamaura I, Kurosa Y, et al: Long-term results of the anterior floating method for cervical myelopathy caused by ossification of the posterior longitudinal ligament. Spine 26:241–248, 2001.

43. Mikawa Y, Shikata J, Yamamuro T: Spinal deformity and instability after multilevel cervical laminectomy. Spine 12:6–11, 1987.

44. Miyazaki K, Tada K, Matsuda Y, et al: Posterior extensive simultaneous multisegment decompression with posterolateral fusion for cervical myelopathy with cervical instability and kyphotic and/or S-shaped deformities. Spine 14:1160–1170, 1989.

45. Nurick S: The Natural History of the Neurological Complications of Cervical Spondylosis [thesis]. Oxford, UK, Oxford University, 1970.

46. Nurick S: The pathogenesis of the spinal cord disorder associated with cervical spondylosis. Brain 95:87–100, 1972.

47. Ohshio I, Hatayama A, Kaneda K, et al: Correlation between histopathologic features and magnetic resonance images of spinal cord lesions. Spine 18:1140–1149, 1993.

48. Okada K, Shirasaki N, Hayashi H, et al: Treatment of cervical spondylotic myelopathy by enlargement of the spinal canal anteriorly, followed by arthrodesis. J Bone Joint Surg Am 73A:352–364, 1991.

48a. Onari K, Akiyama N, Kondo S, et al: Long-term follow-up results of anterior interbody fusion applied for cervical myelopathy due to ossification of the posterior longitudinal ligament. Spine 26:488–493, 2001.

49. Ono K, Ebara S, Fuji T, et al: Myelopathy hand: New clinical signs of cervical cord damage. J Bone Joint Surg Br 69B:215–219, 1987.

50. Paramore CG, Dickman CA, Sonntag VK: Radiographic and clinical follow-up review of Caspar plates in 49 patients. J Neurosurg 84:957–961, 1996.

51. Pavlov H, Torg JS, Robie B, Jahre C: Cervical spinal stenosis: Determination with vertebral body ratio method. Radiology 164:771–775, 1987.

52. Payne EE, Spillane JD: The cervical spine: An anatomico-pathological study of 70 specimens (using a special technique) with particular reference to the problem of cervical spondylosis. Brain 80:571–596, 1957.

53. Peet MM, Echols DH: Herniation of the nucleus pulposus: A cause of compression of the spinal cord. Arch Neurol Psychiatry 32:924–932, 1934.

54. Raynor RB, Moskovich R, Zidel P, Pugh J: Alterations in primary and coupled neck motions after facetectomy. Neurosurgery 21:681–687, 1987.

55. Riew KD, Hilibrand AS, Palumbo MA, Bohlman HH: Anterior cervical corpectomy in patients previously managed with a laminectomy: Short-term complications. J Bone Joint Surg Am 81A:950–957, 1999.

56. Riew KD, Sethi NS, Devney J, Goette K, Choi K: Complications of buttress plate stabilization of cervical corpectomy. Spine 24:2404–2410, 1999.

57. Robinson RA, Smith GW: Anterolateral cervical disc removal and interbody fusion for cervical disc syndrome [abstract]. Bull Johns Hopkins Hosp 96:223–224, 1955.

58. Robinson RA, Walker AE, Ferlic DC, Wiecking DK: The results of anterior interbody fusion of the cervical spine. J Bone Joint Surg Am 44A:1569–1587, 1962.

59. Rogers L: The surgical treatment of cervical spondylotic myelopathy: Mobilisation of the complete cervical cord into an enlarged canal. J Bone Joint Surg Br 43B:3–6, 1961.

60. Saito T, Yamamuro T, Shikata J, et al: Analysis and prevention of spinal column deformity following cervical laminectomy. I. Pathogenetic analysis of postlaminectomy deformities. Spine 16:494–502, 1991.

61. Saunders RL, Bernini PM, Shirreffs TG Jr, Reeves AG: Central corpectomy for cervical spondylotic myelopathy: A consecutive series with long-term follow-up evaluation. J Neurosurg 74:163–170, 1991.

62. Scoville WB: Cervical spondylosis treated by bilateral facetectomy and laminectomy. J Neurosurg 18:423–428, 1961.

62a. Seichi A, Takeshita K, Ohishi I, et al: Long-term results of double-door laminoplasty for cervical stenotic myelopathy. Spine 26:479–487, 2001.

63. Sim FH, Svien HJ, Bickel WH, Janes JM: Swan-neck deformity following extensive cervical laminectomy. A review of twenty-one cases. J Bone Joint Surg Am 56A:564–580, 1974.

64. Spurling RG, Scoville WB: Lateral rupture of the cervical intervertebral discs: a common cause of shoulder and arm pain. Surg Gynecol Obstet 78:350–358, 1944.

65. Stookey B: Compression of the spinal cord due to ventral extradural cervical chondromas. Arch Neurol Psychiatry 20:275–291, 1928.

66. Stookey B: Compression of spinal cord and nerve roots by herniation of the nucleus pulposus in the cervical region. Arch Surg 40:417–432, 1940.

67. Stoops WL, King RB: Chronic myelopathy associated with cervical spondylosis: its response to laminectomy and foramenotomy. JAMA 192:281–284, 1965.

68. Taylor J, Collier J: The occurrence of optic neuritis in lesions of the spinal cord. Injury, tumor, myelitis. (An account of twelve cases and one autopsy.) Brain 24:532–550, 1901.

69. Vaccaro AR, Falatyn SP, Scuderi GJ, et al: Early failure of long segment anterior cervical plate fixation. J Spinal Disord 11:410–415, 1998.

70. Vanichkachorn JS, Vaccaro AR, Silveri CP, Albert TJ: Anterior junctional plate in the cervical spine. Spine 23:2462–2467, 1998.

71. White AA III, Southwick WO, Deponte RJ, et al: Relief of pain by anterior cervical-spine fusion for spondylosis. A report of sixty-five patients. J Bone Joint Surg Am 55A:525–534, 1973.

72. Whitecloud TS III, LaRocca H: Fibular strut graft in reconstructive surgery of the cervical spine. Spine 1:33–43, 1976.

73. Wilkinson M: The morbid anatomy of cervical spondylosis and myelopathy. Brain 83:589–617, 1960.

74. Yamaura I, Kurosa Y, Matuoka T, Shindo S: Anterior floating method for cervical myelopathy caused by ossification of the posterior longitudinal ligament. Clin Orthop 359:27–34, 1999.

75. Yasuoka S, Peterson HA, MacCarty CS: Incidence of spinal column deformity after multilevel laminectomy in children and adults. J Neurosurg 57:441–445, 1982.

76. Yonenobu K, Fuji T, Ono K, et al: Choice of surgical treatment for multisegmental cervical spondylotic myelopathy. Spine 10:710–716, 1985.

77. Zdeblick TA, Bohlman HH: Cervical kyphosis and myelopathy. Treatment by anterior corpectomy and strut grafting. J Bone Joint Surg Am 71A:170–182, 1989.

78. Zdeblick TA, Zou D, Warden KE, et al: Cervical stability after foraminotomy. A biomechanical in vitro analysis. J Bone Joint Surg Am 74A:22–27, 1992.

9

Cervical Myelopathy with Ossification of the Posterior Longitudinal Ligament

Rick B. Delamarter, M.D.
J. Scott Smith, M.D.

*You can lead a horse to water but you can't grow
moss on a rolling stone.*
—Anonymous

Ossification of the posterior longitudinal ligament (OPLL) is a progressive disorder of the spine that may result in spinal cord compression, leading to myelopathy or radiculomyelopathy. The posterior longitudinal ligament is intimately attached to the annulus fibrosis at each intervertebral space. When affected by OPLL, this ligament not only ossifies, but also thickens significantly. This process leads to narrowing of the spinal canal, reducing the space available for the passing neurologic structures, including the spinal cord.

Although OPLL was first described in 1838 by Key,[32] the entity received little attention until 1960, when Tsukimoto[72] first described autopsy findings associated with the disease. Since that time, a great deal has been discovered and written on the subject, primarily in the Japanese literature, where OPLL is now recognized as a common cause of myelopathy.

OPLL is most common in individuals of Asian descent, but also occurs in other populations.[13, 34, 44] In an attempt to determine the prevalence of OPLL, the Japanese Ministry of Public Health and Welfare instituted a special commission for the investigation of this disease. Lateral x-rays of more than 2000 patients were evaluated for signs of OPLL, namely, abnormal ossification posterior to the vertebral bodies. Tsuyama and colleagues reported the commission's findings in 1981.[74] The prevalence of OPLL from radiographic criteria was determined to be 2.4% among the Japanese and similar among other eastern Asiatic countries. Other published reports have also estimated that between 2% and 3% of Asian individuals have OPLL.[54, 55, 64, 77] After looking at the Japanese population, the Japanese Ministry of Public Health dispatched agents across the world to study the rate of OPLL among other racial groups. Only 3 of 1834 white individuals (0.16%) were found to be affected by the condition.[74] Because OPLL is often difficult to see and frequently overlooked on cervical spine x-rays, the true prevalence may well be higher than any of these studies report. Indeed, some authors have reported OPLL to be the primary contributing factor in 20% to 25% of North Americans who are frankly myelopathic.[12, 13]

Regardless of race, the number of individuals with OPLL increases with the age of the study population.[69, 70] Various studies have reported up to an 11% incidence of OPLL in asymptomatic Asian persons over age 50.[8, 48, 68, 70] It is in this age group that OPLL is likely to present as a clinical problem.

In an attempt to determine if OPLL represents the same clinical condition in all racial groups, Trojan et al. looked at the demographic features, clinical presentation, types and location of OPLL, associated diseases, and treatment outcomes in Japanese and non-Japanese patients.[70] Multiple similarities were found in the two populations, leading the authors to conclude that although the prevalences differ, OPLL represents the same condition in both groups.

PATHOPHYSIOLOGY

Although the exact etiology of OPLL remains unknown, the importance of genetic factors has been demonstrated by Terayama, who studied the cervical spine x-rays of family members of 347 individuals with documented OPLL.[68] The x-rays were critically evaluated to determine the prevalence of OPLL among related individuals. Overall, 26% of parents and 29% of siblings were found to be affected.[68] These prevalences are significantly higher than those found within the general population, indicating a genetic component. Because of the relatively high percentages, the authors suggested that OPLL might be transmitted via an autosomal dominant inheritance pattern.

An association exists between OPLL and hyperostotic disorders such as diffuse idiopathic skeletal hyperostosis and ankylosing spondylitis.[11, 18, 37, 44, 54, 60] Other associated conditions include obesity and various endocrinopathies including diabetes mellitus, acromegaly, and hyperparathyroidism.[12, 13, 27] Although vitamin A has been suggested as a possible etiologic factor in the development of OPLL, further studies are needed to determine the relative importance of retinol in the disease process.[59]

A clinicopathologic study of OPLL reported in 1977 by Ono et al. used cross-sectional microscopy to study the postmortem spines of two patients with OPLL.[57] Findings included marked flattening of the spinal cord secondary to

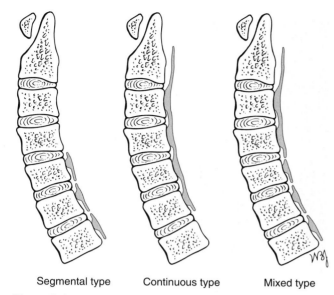

Segmental type   Continuous type   Mixed type

Figure 9–1. *Types of ossification of the posterior longitudinal ligament.*

the protruding ossified mass, infarction of the gray matter, and demyelination of the long tracts. Ossification was found to advance particularly in the superficial layer of the posterior longitudinal ligament.

McAfee et al. analyzed surgical specimens containing the ossified portion of the posterior longitudinal ligament taken from six different patients with myelopathy secondary to OPLL, during treatment by anterior cervical spinal decompression and fusion.[44] Histologic evaluation revealed ossified segments of osteoid arising from hypervascular fibrous tissue (Fig. 9–1). The authors described the ossified section of the posterior longitudinal ligament as follows:

> The ossified mass was mainly lamellar bone in the periphery farthest from the vertebral body with occasional islands of calcified and woven bone closer to the ligamentous attachment to the vertebral body. Protruded segments of nucleus pulposus, as described by Tsuyama, were occasionally observed within the ossified mass posterior to the vertebral body.

The authors then compared their histologic findings with those known to exist in Asian patients. Comparative slides were provided by Dr. Terayama, Chairman of the Investigation Committee on OPLL of the Japanese Ministry of Public Health and Welfare. No significant identifiable difference was found between the material retrieved from non-Asian patients and that from patients of Asian ancestry.

CLINICAL PRESENTATION

Because of the slowly progressive nature of OPLL, affected patients may present with varying symptoms and physical findings ranging from mild neck pain to quadriplegia. Symptoms and neurologic dysfunction result from various mechanisms including direct compression, vascular insufficiency, and dynamic mechanical factors. Direct compression of the anterior spinal cord and exiting nerve roots, with eventual flattening of the spinal cord, occurs as

the ossified mass enlarges and fills the spinal canal. This process of ossification proceeds slowly over time, with the spinal canal gradually becoming increasingly stenotic. Usually, the patient remains asymptomatic until the stenosis ratio reaches the critical point of 40%,[63, 69] or in one study, 30 mm² in transverse area.[13a] At approximately this degree of central stenosis, the patient will begin to develop signs and symptoms of cervical myelopathy.

As is the case with cervical spondylitic myelopathy, interruption of the vascular supply to the neurologic tissue may also be responsible for at least a portion of the patient's physical limitations.[22] Ischemia is believed to occur through stretching of the terminal branches of the anterior spinal artery as the cord is deflected posteriorly by the growing area of ossification.[58] Instability may be induced either above or below an area of ossification that becomes relatively immobile. This instability can lead to a dynamic compressive myelopathy. In any of these situations, the condition of the spinal cord may be extremely tenuous such that even minor trauma, such as a fall, can lead to a major neurologic deficit.[8, 14, 41, 44, 67]

In 1984, Tsuyama published information obtained from a study organized by the Investigation Committee on OPLL of the Japanese Ministry of Public Health and Welfare.[73] Subjects included 1448 men and 677 women with OPLL. The age distribution showed that the highest incidence was in patients age 50 to 60, with no particular sex difference. The reported frequency of presenting symptoms is listed in Table 9–1.[44, 69]

In this study, 85% of the patients noted a gradual onset of symptoms. At the time of the diagnosis, nearly 20% of the patients had become so affected in their upper extremities that they were dependent on others for routine activities of daily living. About 10% had lost the ability to walk, and an additional 13% were only able to walk with assistive support. The authors found that the OPLL was progressive in nearly 20% of the subjects followed radiographically for more than 1 month.

NATURAL COURSE

Until recently, information regarding the natural course of myelopathy caused by OPLL in the cervical spine was not known. Matsunaga et al. studied the natural course of the disease, particularly the relationship between the onset of myelopathy and the factors associated with its aggravation.[41] They followed 207 patients for an average period of

Table 9–1. *Prevalence of Presenting Symptoms in OPLL*

Presenting Symptom	Percentage (%)
Neck pain	42
Upper extremity dysesthesia	48
Upper extremity motor dysfunction	19
Lower extremity weakness	15
Bladder disturbance	1

From Tsuyama N: Ossification of the posterior longitudinal ligament of the spine. Clin Orthop 184:71–84, 1984.

more than 10 years. Myelopathic signs were present in 37 (18%) patients at the time of initial examination. Of these 37, 14 deteriorated during the observation period. Myelopathy developed in 33 (16%) of the remaining 170 individuals. The remaining 137 patients, or 66% of the initial study group, were found to be free of myelopathic signs after the observation period.

Some of these asymptomatic patients were found to have severe cervical stenosis secondary to their OPLL. The range of motion in this subgroup of patients was severely restricted, suggesting that dynamic factors may play an important role in the development of myelopathy. They concluded that both static and dynamic factors play a role in the deterioration of patients with stenosis secondary to OPLL.

Even with the use of computed tomography (CT) scanning, no direct correlation has been found to exist between the remaining space available for the spinal cord and the degree of neurologic deficit.[76] This may be because of the spinal cord's ability to adapt to gradual compression, combined with the decrease in cervical mobility from the ossification.[45, 73] One cadaveric study did find that the transverse area of the cord correlated best with the severity of the pathologic change.[13b] The transverse area of a normal spinal cord in the mid cervical spine is 80 to 100 mm^2.[9a, 9b] A cord of 5 mm^2 had grade 1 (mild) pathologic changes, and another cord of 10 mm^2 had grade 3 (severe) histologic changes in Fujiwara's study.[13b]

Even minor trauma in patients with OPLL can produce disastrous outcomes. McAfee et al. reported on four patients

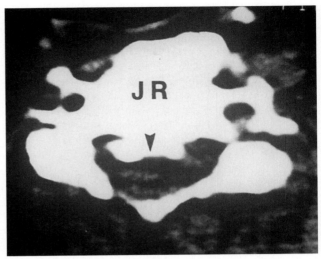

Figure 9–3. A CT scan clearly identifying ossification of the posterior longitudinal ligament in the anterior spinal canal (arrow). Note the significant decrease in space available for the cord because of the mass of the ossification.

who developed tetraparesis following a minor fall.[44] Others have also reported on rapid and severe neurologic deterioration under similar circumstances.[8, 70]

DIAGNOSTIC EVALUATION

Hirabayashi et al. have classified OPLL into four subtypes, depending on the configuration and extent of the ossification.[23] These subtypes are segmental, continuous, mixed, and circumscribed (Fig. 9–2).

The posterior longitudinal ligament comprises superficial and deep layers. The pattern of ligamentous ossification may depend on the relative involvement of these layers. The deep layer connects adjacent annulus fibrosi that fan out at each level. The more superficial layer is made up of longer collagen fibers, which extend over two to four vertebral bodies.[18, 70]

Segmental OPLL likely involves the fibers of the deep layer, whereas the continuous type requires extensive involvement of the superficial fibers over multiple segments. The mixed and circumscribed subtypes may represent combinations of the segmental and continuous subtypes as well as points along a spectrum of disease.[18]

On a lateral view of the cervical spine, OPLL is seen as a radiodense strip occupying the anterior spinal canal (Fig. 9–3). Despite its distinct radiographic appearance, OPLL is frequently overlooked on plain cervical x-rays.[44, 70] This may be because of overlying structures that may make visualization difficult. Whereas cervical spondylotic myelopathy is characterized radiographically by horizontal osteophytes extending into the spinal canal from the vertebral endplates, OPLL is more often found directly posterior to the vertebral bodies. True lateral views are essential, because obliquity causes the posterior aspects of the vertebral bodies to simulate OPLL. Nose et al. summarized the distribution of OPLL in 1987.[51] In

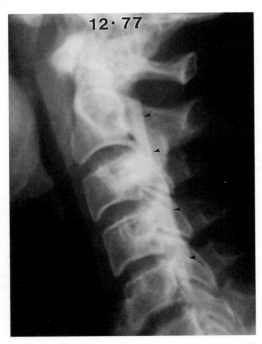

Figure 9–2. A lateral cervical spine x-ray showing ossification of the posterior longitudinal ligament (arrows). Seen as a radial dense strip occupying the anterior spinal canal, ossification of the posterior longitudinal ligament is frequently overlooked on plain cervical x-rays.

decreasing order of frequency, the C5, C6, and C4 levels are most commonly involved.

Today, CT scanning after injection of intrathecal contrast material provides the best available imaging for OPLL.[15, 70, 76] CT scanning provides superior visualization of the ossified mass and the space available for the cord (Fig. 9–4). The addition of intrathecal contrast material aids evaluation of the anatomic effects of OPLL on neurologic tissue. With the help of sagittal reconstructions, the full extent of the ossification can be appreciated in all dimensions. Reconstructions are also useful in differentiating between endplate osteophytes and OPLL located posterior to the vertebral bodies. This information is invaluable during preoperative planning to ensure that complete decompression can be performed to avoid postoperative deterioration. Accurate measurement of the space available for the spinal cord can prevent intraoperative damage to the spinal cord.

Magnetic resonance imaging (MRI) has also been used as a diagnostic study for OPLL. The region of ligamentous ossification appears as an area of very low signal between the vertebral body and the thecal sac on both T1- and T2-weighted imaging.[39, 75] Although CT scanning provides superior detail in evaluating the extent of the ligamentous ossification, MRI is invaluable in assessing the condition of the spinal cord.[43] Close review of T2-weighted images may show evidence of localized edema or myelomalacia. MRI

also offers the advantage of imaging the cervical spine in both flexion and extension, which may provide additional information regarding any dynamic factors that may be contributing to the clinical situation.

Although CT myelography and MRI are capable of accurately describing the degree of spinal cord compression and the anatomic extent of the ossification process as well as dynamic factors contributing to the patient's symptoms, neither can evaluate the functional capacity of the neurologic tissues. As a result, it is very difficult to determine with certainty the level of the responsible lesion in a multilevel continuous or mixed-type OPLL. In an excellent clinical study using evoked spinal cord potentials (ESCPs), Shinomiya et al. monitored 26 patients during decompressive surgery for symptomatic OPLL.[65] ESCPs were recorded from the cervical epidural space to make a precise level diagnosis in OPLL myelopathy. In cases in which the ESCP disappeared across the narrowed cervical canal, another stimulating electrode was placed cephalad in the cysterna magna, and descending potentials were performed. In this manner, the authors were able to accurately identify the level of physiologic cord dysfunction. In their series, 11 patients were found to have changes in potentials at the level of greatest cord compression, whereas another 11 demonstrated these same changes at the site of OPLL termination. Four other cases showed both findings. White column lesions were localized, but gray

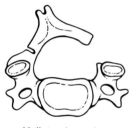

Unilateral opening
(Hirabayashi)

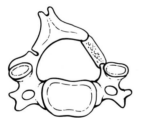

Unilateral opening
with bone graft
(Itoh, Matsuzaki)

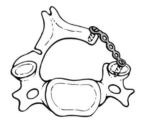

Unilateral opening
with titanium plate

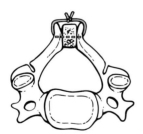

Midline open door
with bone graft
(Kurokawa)

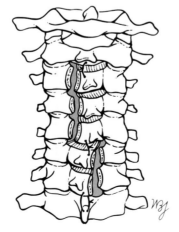

Unilateral alternate trap door opening
(C3–5 one way, C6–7 the opposite way)
(Chiba University)

Figure 9–4. Examples of the five main laminoplasty techniques used by various authors.

matter lesions were unexpectedly extensive. The authors concluded that both static and dynamic factors are significant in the genesis of OPLL myelopathy.

INDICATIONS FOR SURGERY

Because there currently is no way to recover the function of irreversibly damaged neurologic tissue within the spinal canal, and because of the progressive nature of the ossification in OPLL, operative intervention is indicated in patients who present with or develop signs of cord compression. Because it has been demonstrated that many patients with OPLL remain asymptomatic despite cord compression, positive radiologic findings alone are insufficient to warrant surgical intervention. Intractable nerve root pain or radiculopathy that fails to respond to conservative treatment is also an indication for surgery.

A trial of conservative therapy for patients with OPLL is appropriate, provided that there are no signs of myelopathy. Conservative measures include bed rest, continuous skull traction, observation with application of a neck brace, short courses of oral steroids, and rehabilitation.[70] These measures should minimize repetitive trauma to the cervical cord and decrease edema. Of course, the patient should avoid contact sports and other activities that could result in cervical trauma or hyperextension.

Surgical intervention not only must allow for decompression of the spinal cord over the entire area of ossification, but also must prevent the development of postoperative instability and resultant deformity by stabilizing the cervical spine. With these goals in mind, various surgical treatments have been used to treat myeloradiculopathy secondary to OPLL. Traditional laminectomy or laminoplasty provides for decompression via a posterior approach, whereas anterior decompression with or without fusion may also be appropriate, depending on the clinical situation.

Posterior procedures, including laminectomy and laminoplasty, are appropriate when the alignment of the cervical spine is either straight or lordotic, because the spinal cord will drift posteriorly after decompression, relieving the pressure on the neural tissue. Posterior approaches have the advantage of providing relatively safe and easy access to the neural elements and avoiding the need for fusion in many cases. Posterior decompression, on the other hand, will universally fail in the kyphotic spine. In the presence of kyphosis, the spinal cord will remain draped over the kyphotic deformity, unable to move away from the compressive lesion, and the patient will fail to improve.

To assess the results of operative treatment, the Japanese Orthopedic Association (JOA) developed a clinical scoring system based on the ability to perform activities of daily living (Table 9–2).[28] A normal person is given the maximum score of 17. This system is used extensively throughout the OPLL literature.

Laminectomy

Posterior decompression via laminectomy was used extensively before the 1970s, but has been avoided because of concerns over the development of postoperative instabil-

Table 9–2. *The Japanese Orthopedic Association's Evaluation Criteria*

Upper limb ADL
  0: Unable to feed oneself with either chopsticks or a spoon
  1: Able to feed oneself with a spoon but not with chopsticks
  2: Able to feed oneself with chopsticks, though awkwardly
  3: Feeds oneself regularly with chopsticks, but a bit awkwardly
  4: Normal
Lower limb ADL
  0: Unable to walk
  1: In need of a cane or support even in walking on a level
  2: In no need of a cane or support in walking on a level, but needs either of them in climbing up stairs
  3: In no need of a cane or support in either walking on a level or climbing up stairs, but awkward
  4: Normal
Sensory disturbances of upper limbs
  0: Definite sensory disturbance on physical examination
  1: Slight sensory disturbance or only numbness
  2: None
Sensory disturbances of trunk
  0, 1, and 2 are same as for upper limbs
Urinary disturbance
  0: Urinary incontinence
  1: Severe dysuria and/or residual urine
  2: Mild dysuria, i.e., pollakisuria or delayed start
  3: Normal

From the Japanese Orthopedic Association: Criteria on the evaluation of the treatment of cervical myelopathy. J Jpn Orthop Assoc 50:Addendum 5, 1976.

ity and resultant kyphosis, swan neck deformity, or multiple-level subluxation.[6, 20, 30, 38, 46, 47, 66] There is no question that postlaminectomy deformity occurs at a high incidence in children and should be avoided or combined with prophylactic fusion.[3, 5, 7] In the adult population, however, postoperative instability and the development of kyphosis are less common and likely depend on a number of factors, including the preoperative alignment and preservation of the facet joints.[2, 10, 29, 30, 46, 47, 50, 61]

In clinical reviews, Jenkins and Rogers reported that in most adult patients with cervical myelopathy, extensive laminectomy was not followed by instability. However, in patients with misalignment of the cervical spine, a tendency to develop deformity was noted.[29, 61]

Katsumi et al. reviewed 34 patients after laminectomy for the removal of spinal cord tumors and identified risk factors associated with the development of postoperative deformity or instability.[30] Younger patients, patients with preoperative kyphosis, and patients undergoing extensive laminectomy (four or more laminae removed) were more susceptible to developing deformity. In addition, it was found that interruption or destruction of the facet joints led to deformity or instability in 50% of patients.

The importance of the facet joint and associated capsular tissue in the maintenance of stability following laminectomy has been studied in the laboratory. Zdeblick et al. studied the effects of progressive facetectomy and capsular resection on cervical stability.[79] They tested human specimens after sequential bilateral facetectomy or capsular resection in 25% increments. They found that removing more than 50% of either the facet joint or associated capsular tissue caused a significant loss of stability in both flexion and torsion.

In another biomechanical experiment, Nowinski et al. found that kyphosis could be induced after as little as 25% facetectomy, and recommended combining multilevel cervical laminectomy with prophylactic fusion if the integrity of the facet joints was violated during the decompression.[52] Laminoplasty appeared to negate the need for fusion.

In addition to biomechanical studies showing the fundamental importance of the facet joints, clinical experience has also confirmed the importance of preoperative alignment and sparing of the facet joint to avoid postoperative instability and deformity. Mikawa et al. reported on 64 patients who underwent multilevel cervical laminectomy.[46] Within the treatment group were 24 patients with cervical spondylotic myelopathy (CSM) and 25 with OPLL. Laminectomy was performed with an air drill, removing between one-third and one-half of the medial facets. No patients demonstrated kyphosis before surgery. Interestingly, none of the cervical spondylosis (CS) patients developed deformity, but 6 of the 25 patients with OPLL developed either kyphotic or meandering-type curves, as did 3 children. None of these adult patients needed further surgery to correct deformity or instability.

Miyazaki and Kirita reviewed 155 cases of multisegment laminectomy for myelopathy from OPLL.[47] A review of their technique, however, revealed that no specific attempts were made to preserve the facet complex. In their series, 25 cases (17%) demonstrated either postoperative cervical kyphosis or enhancement of preoperative kyphosis, and another 4 cases developed an S-shaped alignment. Although the follow-up was short, no corrective surgery was performed for alignment correction. Unfortunately, the authors made no statement regarding postoperative alignment and clinical improvement.

One might assume that the incidence of deformity after laminectomy of the cervical spine is low in cases of OPLL, because the ossification foci create a condition similar to anterior spinal fusion. Based on a review of the relevant studies, however, it appears premature to conclude that even continuous OPLL will provide adequate stability of the cervical spine after laminectomy, particularly when the facet joints are disrupted.

Nakano et al. compared results of posterior decompression laminectomy with open-door laminoplasty for myeloradiculopathy in patients with OPLL.[50] Based on the preoperative and postoperative JOA scores, no significant difference in the level of recovery was noted, with both groups demonstrating an average improvement of 81%. No evidence of instability was found in any patient, and no patient undergoing laminectomy developed a clinically significant postoperative kyphosis. The authors emphasized that the laminectomies were performed with careful attention given to preserving the facet joints and capsular tissues.

A review of these clinical studies and the biomechanical work of Zdeblick et al.[79] clearly shows that the facet complex provides essential stability to the cervical spine after laminectomy and must not be compromised to prevent instability and subsequent kyphosis. Indeed, Epstein has

recommended that not more than 25% of the facet joint be removed during the decompression.[10] The presence of kyphosis preoperatively is a risk factor for postoperative deformity and should be considered in surgical planning.

Laminectomy Plus Fusion

Some authors favor the straightforward decompression offered by multilevel laminectomy coupled with instrumented arthrodesis. This avoids the instability and late deformity complications associated with laminectomy alone, although it limits motion and invites complications of graft harvest related to laminoplasty. Typically, lateral mass plating plus facet joint bone grafting is used for this operative option. As of this writing, only a few series have been published in the literature, but one study showed good results.[36a]

Laminoplasty

Because of the fear of developing postlaminectomy kyphosis, laminoplasty was developed as a surgical treatment alternative. Advantages of laminoplasty over laminectomy include retention of the lamina with decreased likelihood of surgically induced instability and decreased perineural scarring.

The surgical technique of laminoplasty was developed in the late 1960s and 1970s. Different authors have proposed various methods for expanding the available space for the spinal cord (Fig. 9–5). Hattori advocated the Z-shaped laminoplasty, in which two sections of lamina are pried open in opposite directions to increase the canal size. Kawai et al. reported on 118 patients with CSM or OPLL undergoing canal expansion laminoplasty by this method, with 84% demonstrating good to excellent short- and long-term results.[31]

Other techniques include spinous process splitting and open-door laminoplasty (Fig. 9–6). The spinous process splitting technique involves making laminar grooves both in the midline and at the laminar/facet junction.[26, 49, 62a, 78] The laminae are then opened and sutured in place. Tomita et al. described cutting through the midline from ventral to dorsal using a thin wire passed under the lamina and pulled upward in a reciprocating motion (T-saw laminoplasty).[69a] Autogenous bone and hydroxyapatite spacers have been used to maintain the opened position of the lamina. Yoshida et al. found a 53% to 63% improvement in the JOA score after spinous process splitting laminoplasty with a bone graft spacer.[78] Although the number of study subjects was small, Hukuda et al. found no difference in long-term functional improvement with midline open-door laminoplasty versus laminectomy.[26]

Hirabayashi developed the expansive open-door laminoplasty technique after noting the development of symptomatic osteoarthritic changes and postoperative malalignment in 43% of patients undergoing laminectomy.[24, 25] Modifications of this technique include placing bone grafts (e.g., allograft rib or autogenous spinous processes) on the open hinged side to maintain the lamina position (see Fig. 9–4). O'Brien et al. published a series of unilateral

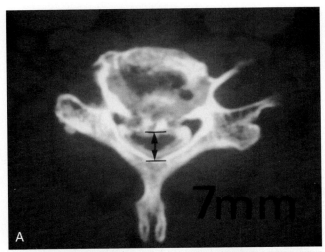

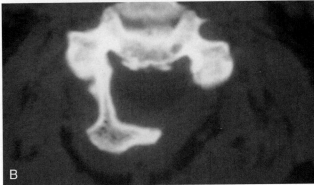

Figure 9–5. Open-door laminoplasty. A, CT scan with ossification of the posterior longitudinal ligament narrowing the spinal canal down to 7 mm. This patient had a 3-year progressive history of myelopathy. B, CT scan showing the opening of the spinal canal with lamina fused on the right side in this open position. Note the complete spinal decompression even though the anterior ossification remains.

open-door laminoplasties using a small titanium plate and screws to hold the "trap door" open.[52a]

We have used the technique as described by Hirabayashi for treating myelopathy secondary to CSM or OPLL when appropriate. In our experience, the procedure is both safe and reliable.

Surgical Technique

The posterior elements are exposed through a midline approach, with care taken to avoid damaging the facet joint capsules and interspinous ligaments. The entire area of stenosis is exposed, including one level above and below the pathology, generally C3 to C7 (Fig. 9–7). Extending the dissection lateral to the facet joints will denervate the local musculature and should be avoided. Decompression foraminotomy may be performed as needed for radiculopathy.

The laminoplasty grooves are then prepared. We prefer to perform this portion of the procedure with a high-speed air drill, such as a Midas Rex with an AM 8 attachment. A trough extending the length of the stenosis is made

through both laminar cortices at the junction of the lamina and facet joint. A 2-mm Kerrison rongeur is helpful in removing any bony connections, and a small forward-angled curette is used to free the ligamentum and any dural adhesions.

A unicortical trough is then created on the opposite side to act as an opening hinge on canal expansion. This trough should be started slightly more laterally than the opening groove on the opposite side and needs to be wide enough to allow space for the opening hinge maneuver so that the dorsal laminar cortices do not abut until an adequate opening of the spinal canal has been achieved.

Before the laminoplasty is opened, the ligamentum flavum and interspinous ligaments should be released above and below the end lamina and stay sutures placed through the facet capsular tissue at each level on the hinge side. Placement of these sutures is much more difficult after the laminoplasty has been opened. The laminoplasty is then opened 45 to 60 degrees by creating a greenstick fracture at the unicortical trough. This procedure should be performed slowly and carefully to avoid complete fracture of the cortical hinge. If the hinge fails, the lamina may fall into the spinal canal, producing nerve root compression and radiculopathy.

The stay sutures are then passed around the spinous processes or through the ligamentum flavum and tied to the facet capsule to keep the laminoplasty open between 45 and 60 degrees. All bleeding should be controlled throughout the procedure and before closure with bipolar cautery, bone wax, and Gelfoam. After closure, the patient is immobilized in a cervical orthosis for 8 to 10 weeks.

Results

In 1988, Hirabayashi reported his short-term results on 90 patients treated with this technique. The average recovery rate for patients with OPLL, based on an improved JOA score, was 58%. Postoperatively, seven patients noted transient C5–C6 motor paresis secondary to cervical root damage.[24] Longer-term follow-up on this same group of patients was later reported by Satomi et al.[62] This study reviewed 51 patients who underwent expansive open-door laminoplasty at an average follow-up of 7.8 years; 33 of these had OPLL as the cause of myelopathy. The average recovery rate in this subgroup was also 58%. Patients noted to have more than 5 mm of canal widening postoperatively had statistically higher recovery rates than those with widening less than 2 mm. Functional improvements continued for up to 3 years after the procedure.

Although the avoidance of fusion is a potential benefit of laminoplasty, Satomi reported a pronounced loss of cervical range of motion (measured on flexion and extension x-rays) after open-door laminoplasty. On average, less than 10 degrees of motion was found after 1 year, decreasing to less than 7 degrees after 5 years. This decrease did not correlate with worsened clinical symptoms, however. No patient developed a clinically significant kyphotic deformity, although 4 of the 33 patients with OPLL worsened during the follow-up period secondary to either progression or new formation of OPLL.

Other authors have reported similar success with this procedure,[8a, 21, 33, 53, 62a, 71] and with good patient selection, the results of neurologic recovery are consistent. One potential problem with laminoplasty, however, is persistent axial neck pain, as noted by Hosono et al.[25a] Thus, patients with significant preoperative neck pain may not be ideal candidates for this type of operative approach.

ANTERIOR APPROACHES

Although laminoplasty is technically easier to perform in patients with multilevel involvement, it does not permit removal of the pathologic ossification and is contraindicated in patients with cervical kyphosis. Laminectomy does not stop motion at pathologic segments.[22] Anterior decompres-

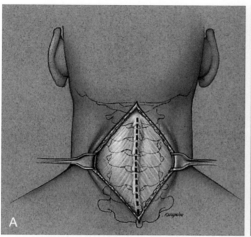
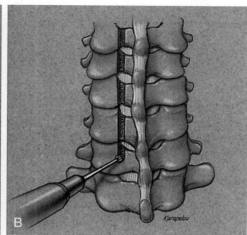
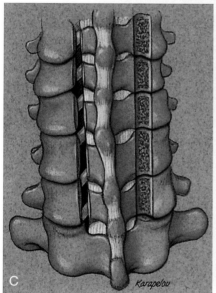
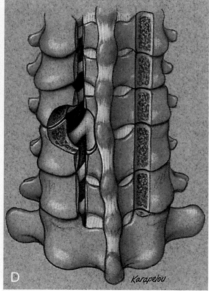
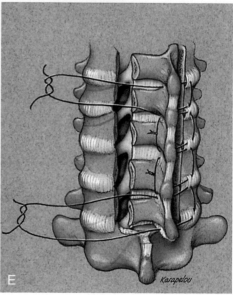

Figure 9–6. *Illustrations of open-door laminoplasty. A, Approach to the cervical spine. The cervical spine is exposed through a posterior midline approach. Supraspinous and intraspinous ligaments and facet capsules are generally preserved, and care is taken not to extend beyond the edge of the lateral masses to avoid denervating the posterior cervical musculature. B, The laminoplasty grooves are first created at the junction of the lamina and facet joints on the most affected side with the aid of a high-speed drill and Kerrison rongeur. Once the groove is completed, the ligamentum flavum is freed with forward-angle curettes and a Kerrison rongeur. C, The hinge lamina resection. The hinge groove is performed slightly more lateral than the open-door lamina resection. Using a high-speed air drill, a unicortical groove is made in the lamina. The groove is made slightly wider than the open-door side to allow a maximum opening. D, Foraminotomy for myeloradiculopathy. The foraminotomy may be performed at the affected levels in patients with myeloradiculopathy. Foraminotomy is generally performed on the open side before creation of the laminoplasty. In general, the open side of the laminoplasty should always be on the side of most significant cord compression and most radicular complaints. E, Opening and anchoring of the lamina. The securing, nonabsorbable sutures are passed into each facet capsule and through each corresponding interspinous ligament or spinous process. The sutures are tied down securely, holding the lamina door open.*

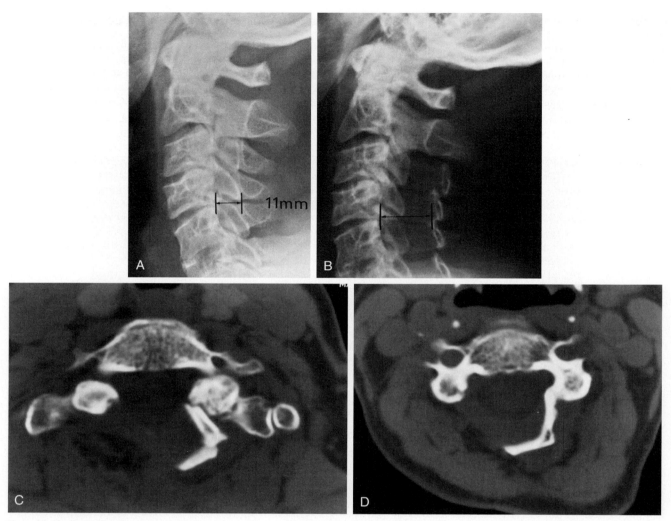

Figure 9–7. *This 67-year-old male had a 3-year history of progressive gait disturbance and poor hand coordination, consistent with progressive myelopathy. A, A lateral cervical spine x-ray revealed cervical spondylosis, ossification of the posterior longitudinal ligament, and narrowing of the spinal canal down to 11 mm. An open-door laminoplasty was performed, allowing resolution of the cervical myelopathy. B, A cervical spine lateral x-ray taken 6 months after open-door laminoplasty. Note the substantial opening of the cervical spinal canal, measuring 23 mm, compared with the preoperative opening of 11 mm. C, A CT scan taken 3 days after open-door laminoplasty. Note the completely decompressed spinal canal and the nonunited hinge side of the laminoplasty. D, A CT scan taken 1 year after open-door laminoplasty. Note the continued wide-open spinal canal and the fused hinge on the laminoplasty. The hinge side of the open-door laminoplasty generally fuses solid within 2 to 3 months of the surgery.*

sion procedures allow for removal of the pathologic tissue and elimination of motion throughout the decompressed region by way of fusion. Anterior procedures also avoid damaging the radicular blood supply, which may already be compromised by the disease process.[18] But these procedures are technically more difficult to perform and require extensive experience with anterior cervical approaches. Anterior dissection of the neck risks injury to the carotid artery, esophagus, trachea, and recurrent laryngeal nerve. Halo immobilization may be required postoperatively for stability until fusion is achieved.

Abe et al. first recommended the anterior approach for resection of OPLL after noting symptomatic recurrences in their patients treated with laminectomy.[1] Since then, other

authors also have reported successful treatment of symptomatic OPLL through an anterior approach.[8, 17, 35, 40]

Goto and Kita published a summary of their surgical experience in the treatment of OPLL.[14] They reported on 50 patients who underwent anterior surgery and 65 patients who underwent posterior surgery between 1968 and 1993. As the authors gained experience and confidence in the anterior technique, the surgical indications for anterior decompression expanded from single-level disease treated with subtotal spondylectomy to multilevel disease treated with sequential vertebrectomy and fibular strut grafting. The selection criteria for anterior versus posterior surgery varied during the study period, making precise comparisons of the surgical results difficult. Nonetheless, the authors were able to identify a subgroup of patients undergoing surgery for treatment of multilevel ossification involving four vertebral bodies. Those treated with posterior laminoplasty improved on average by 58.7%, whereas those treated with anterior débridement and strut grafting improved by 88.2% ($p <$ 0.05). Factors associated with a poor outcome or subsequent deterioration after anterior decompression surgery included insufficient removal of lateral, superior, or inferior OPLL; kyphotic malalignment; and reossification. Careful review revealed that only 38% of patients undergoing anterior decompression had complete surgical extirpation of ossification; however, of these, 89% followed a stable clinical course. This number is impressive when compared with a deterioration rate of 36.4% only 7 years after laminoplasty in the same study.

A number of serious complications were seen in the anterior group. Four patients developed spinal fluid fistulas. Two of these were controlled in the operating room, and the other two were treated with a pressure dressing for 3 weeks after surgery. More importantly, three of five patients with a cord space of less than 3 mm became quadriplegic after anterior decompression. In this group of patients, posterior decompression should be seriously considered to avoid this disastrous complication. If the patient has a kyphotic deformity requiring an anterior procedure and a spinal canal of less than 5 mm, posterior decompression will provide space for the cord to move posteriorly while the anterior procedure is being performed. Placing even a 1-mm Kerrison rongeur into a canal with only 3 mm of space available for the cord causes a 33% compression of the neurologic elements.

Smith and Bohlman reported a series of 22 patients who underwent anterior decompression of the spinal canal for OPLL.[67] Seven of the 22 were found to have a dural defect on removal of the ossified segment, despite meticulous surgical technique. In all cases, the dural defect was located in the area corresponding to the region of greatest cord compression. Even though the arachnoid membrane appeared competent in most patients, five patients developed a postoperative cerebrospinal fluid fistula; three of these patients required a second operation to repair the defect in the dura. The authors determined that the dural defects were secondary to chronic pressure in the region of ossification, and now recommend taking the following precautions and interventions if a dural defect is anticipated or encountered:

1. Appropriate preparation and operative draping of a potential donor site for a dural patch, if needed

2. Patching of any dural defect with an onlay graft of muscle and fascia before insertion of the bone graft

3. Prophylactic placement of a subarachnoid lumbar shunt as described by Eismont et al. before awakening the patient from anesthesia.[9] The drain is continued for at least 4 days. The patient is placed on bed rest with the head elevated between 10 and 30 degrees while the drain is in place and for an additional day after its removal.

4. Efforts to prevent dramatic increases in the intrathecal pressure, including administration of both antiemetic and antitussive medications, as well as extubation from mechanical ventilation as quickly as safety permits.

PREDICTING POSTOPERATIVE IMPROVEMENT

Several authors have evaluated the association between morphologic changes in the spinal cord and clinical recovery.[4, 16, 36, 56] No clear, consistent relationship has been established between the compression ratio or cross-sectional area of the spinal cord at the region of maximum stenosis and clinical recovery. Although patients with high-grade stenosis generally do poorly following decompression, some do well despite their severe compression.

Ono et al. noted that cord signs were generally not produced until the ossified mass occupied more than 60% of the sagittal diameter of the spinal canal.[57] In a postmortem examination of cervical spines from myelopathic patients secondary to OPLL, these authors found a close relationship between the severity of compression and histologic degeneration of the cord. Severe compression was associated with infarction of the gray matter, ascending demyelination in the posterior white column, and descending demyelination in the lateral columns.

Shinomiya et al. noted that patients with intraoperative conduction velocities across the OPLL stenosis of less than 40 m/sec tended to have unsatisfactory clinical results.[65] They concluded that the electrical abnormalities and poor outcomes were because of central demyelination, indicative of irreversible neurologic damage.

Matsuyama et al. analyzed 44 patients with cervical myelopathy, 18 from OPLL.[42] Although there was no relationship between clinical recovery and compression ratio, the authors noted a correlation between good recovery and gradual expansion of the cord postoperatively. Immediate expansion, assessed by intraoperative sonography, was not a predictor of good outcome and was felt to be due to edematous changes of the parenchyma.[19] In comparison, gradual expansion measured 1 month postoperatively was an indicator of good recovery and was thought to indicate the return of axonal transport in the lateral funiculi, which is more important for clinical recovery.

Based on these findings, recovery appears to be inversely proportional to the degree of demyelination or wallerian degeneration present at the time of surgical decompression. Intervention before this degenerative process becomes irreversible is certainly desirable.

AUTHORS' PREFERRED METHOD

Once the need for operative treatment has been determined, the type of surgical approach is selected. Anterior, posterior, or combined approaches may be appropriate, depending on the patient's specific circumstances. The extent of the ossified mass and the sagittal alignment of the cervical spine are the primary determining factors in selecting a surgical approach. Other factors to consider include the patient's general medical condition and the surgeon's experience.

Isolated anterior approaches should be used in kyphotic deformities and in one- or two-level disease. Posterior approaches are effective in neutral or lordotic spines with ossification extending over multiple levels. Combined approaches are reserved for cases in which kyphosis coexists with severe neurologic compression (< 5 mm space available for the cord). In these cases, posterior decompression will not effectively treat the pathology, but anterior decompression carries a high risk of paralysis. Removal of the posterior elements will provide space for the cord to move back during subsequent anterior decompression and fusion.

We prefer laminoplasty to laminectomy for posterior decompression. Although multiple laminoplasty techniques have been described, we have used the open-door technique as described by Hirabayashi[25] with good results. We have found the procedure to be technically simple, safe, and reliable for treating myelopathy. We include foraminotomy as needed for radiculopathy.

In a prospective study performed at our institution from 1990 to 1993, 22 patients with cervical spondylotic myeloradiculopathy were treated with expansion open-door laminoplasty. Overall, the average JOA score of these patients improved by 67%. Only one patient showed no clinical improvement after the procedure. We have found laminoplasty to be an excellent procedure for multilevel cervical stenosis when the spine is aligned in either a neutral or lordotic position.

Although we have not critically reviewed our experience with anterior decompression and fusion, we agree with Goto,[14] Kojima,[35] and others who believe that anterior procedures are superior for treating OPLL in the presence of kyphosis. We have also experienced the problem of dural erosion posterior to an area of severe compression, and recommend that the surgeon prepare preoperatively for this possibility. Because of the potential for complications and the difficult nature of decompression, we feel that anterior decompression and fusion are best performed by those surgeons with extensive experience in this area.

REFERENCES

1. Abe H, Tsuru M, Ito T, et al: Anterior decompression for ossification of the posterior longitudinal ligament of the cervical spine. J Neurosurg 55:108–116, 1981.
2. Aronson N, Filtzer DL, Bagan M: Anterior cervical fusion by the Smith-Robinson approach. J Neurosurg 29:397–404, 1968.
3. Aronson D, Kahn R, Canady A: Cervical spine instability following suboccipital decompression and cervical laminectomy for Arnold-Chiari syndrome (abstract). Presented at the 56th Annual Meeting of the American Academy of Orthopaedic Surgeons, Las Vegas, 1989.
4. Batzdorf U, Flanningan BD: Surgical decompressive procedures for cervical spondylotic myelopathy: A study using magnetic resonance imaging. Spine 16:123–127, 1991.
5. Bell DF, Walker JL, O'Connor G, Tibshirani R: Spinal deformity after multiple-level cervical laminectomy in children. Spine 19:406–411, 1994.
6. Callahan RA, Johnson RM, Margolis RN, et al: Cervical facet fusion for control of instability following laminectomy. J Bone Joint Surg Am 59A:991–1002, 1977.
7. Cattell HS, Clark GL Jr: Cervical kyphosis and instability following multiple laminectomies in children. J Bone Joint Surg Am 49A:713–720, 1967.
8. Cheng WC, Chang CN, Lui TN, et al: Surgical treatment for ossification of the posterior longitudinal ligament of the cervical spine. Surg Neurol 41:90–97, 1994.
8a. Edwards CC Jr, Heller JG, Silcox DH Jr: T-saw laminoplasty for the management of cervical spondylotic myelopathy: Clinical and radiographic outcome. Spine 25:1788–1794, 2000.
9. Eismont FJ, Wiesel SW, Rothman RH: Treatment of dural tears associated with spinal surgery. J Bone Joint Surg Am 63A:1132–1136, 1981.
9a. Eliot HC: Cross-sectional diameters and areas of the human spinal cord. Anat Rec 287–293, 1945.
9b. Tanaka Y: Morphological changes of the cervical spinal canal and cord due to aging. J Jpn Orthop Assoc 58:873–886, 1984.
10. Epstein JA: The surgical management of cervical spinal stenosis, spondylosis, and myeloradiculopathy by means of the posterior approach. Spine 13:864–869, 1988.
11. Epstein N: The surgical management of ossification of the posterior longitudinal ligament in 51 patients. J Spinal Disord 6:432–455, 1993.
12. Epstein NE: Ossification of the posterior longitudinal ligament in evolution in 12 patients. Spine 19:673–681, 1994.
13. Epstein NE: The surgical management of ossification of the posterior longitudinal ligament in 43 North Americans. Spine 19:664–672, 1994.
13a. Fujiwara K, Yonenobu K, Ebara S, et al: The prognosis of surgery for cervical compression myelopathy: An analysis of the factors involved. J Bone Joint Surg Br 71B:393–398, 1989.
13b. Fujiwara K, Yonenobu K, Hiroshima K, et al: Morphometry of the cervical spinal cord and its relation to pathology in cases with compression myelopathy. Spine 13:1212–1216, 1988.
14. Goto S, Kita T: Long-term follow-up evaluation of surgery for ossification of the posterior longitudinal ligament. Spine 20:2247–2256, 1995.
15. Hanai K, Adachi H, Ogasawara H: Axial transverse tomography of the cervical spine narrowed by ossification of the posterior longitudinal ligament. J Bone Joint Surg Br 59B:481–484, 1977.
16. Harada A, Mimatsu K: Postoperative changes in the spinal cord in cervical myelopathy demonstrated by magnetic resonance imaging. Spine 17:1275–1280, 1992.
17. Harsh GR IV, Sypert GW, Weinstein PR, et al: Cervical spine stenosis secondary to ossification of the posterior longitudinal ligament. J Neurosurg 67:349–357, 1987.
18. Heller JG, Johnston RB III, Goodrich A: Ossification of the posterior longitudinal ligament: A report of nine cases in non-Asian patients. Skeletal Radiol 23:601–606, 1994.
19. Henderson FC, Crockard HA, Stevens JM: Spinal cord oedema due to venous stasis. Neuroradiology 35:312–315, 1993.
20. Herkowitz HN: A comparison of anterior cervical fusion, cervical laminectomy, and cervical laminoplasty for the surgical management of multiple level spondylotic radiculopathy. Spine 13:774–780, 1988.
21. Herkowitz HN: The surgical management of cervical spondylotic radiculopathy and myelopathy. Clin Orthop 239:94–108, 1989.
22. Hirabayashi K, Bohlman HH: Multilevel cervical spondylosis:

Laminoplasty versus anterior decompression. Spine 20:1732–1734, 1995.

23. Hirabayashi K, Miyakawa J, Satomi K, et al: Operative results and postoperative progression of ossification among patients with ossification of the cervical posterior longitudinal ligament. Spine 6:354–364, 1981.

24. Hirabayashi K, Satomi K: Operative procedure and results of expansive open-door laminoplasty. Spine 13:870–876, 1988.

25. Hirabayashi K, Watanabe K, Wakano K, et al: Expansive open-door laminoplasty for cervical spinal stenotic myelopathy. Spine 8:693–699, 1983.

25a. Hosono N, Yonenobu K, Ono K: Neck and shoulder pain after laminoplasty: A noticeable complication. Spine 21:1969–1973, 1996.

26. Hukuda S, Ogata M, Mochizuki T, Shichikawa K: Laminectomy versus laminoplasty for cervical myelopathy: Brief report. J Bone Joint Surg Br 70B:325–326, 1988.

27. Ikegawa S, Kurokawa T, Hizuka N, et al: Increase of serum growth hormone-binding protein in patients with ossification of the posterior longitudinal ligament of the spine. Spine 18:1757–1760, 1993.

28. Japanese Orthopedic Association: Criteria on the evaluation of the treatment of cervical myelopathy. J Jpn Orthop Assoc 50:Addendum 5, 1976 (in Japanese).

29. Jenkins DH: Extensive cervical laminectomy: Long-term results. Br J Surg 60:852–854, 1973.

30. Katsumi Y, Honma T, Nakamura T: Analysis of cervical instability resulting from laminectomies for removal of spinal cord tumor. Spine 14:1171–1176, 1989.

31. Kawai S, Sunago K, Doi K, et al: Cervical laminoplasty (Hattori's method): Procedure and follow-up results. Spine 13:1245–1250, 1988.

32. Key C: On paraplegia depending on disease of the ligaments of the spine. Guy's Hospital Report 3:17–34, 1838.

33. Kimura I, Oh-Hama M, Shingu H: Cervical myelopathy treated by canal-expansive laminoplasty: Computed tomographic and myelographic findings. J Bone Joint Surg Am 66A:914–920, 1984.

34. Klara P, McDonnell DE: Ossification of the posterior longitudinal ligament in Caucasians: Diagnosis and surgical intervention. Neurosurgery 19:212–217, 1986.

35. Kojima T, Waga S, Kubo Y, et al: Anterior cervical vertebrectomy and interbody fusion for multi-level spondylosis and ossification of the posterior longitudinal ligament. Neurosurgery 24:864–872, 1989.

36. Koyanagi T, Hirabayashi K, Satomi K, et al: Predictability of operative results of cervical compression myelopathy based on preoperative computed tomographic myelography. Spine 18:1958–1963, 1993.

36a. Kumar VG, Rea GL, Mervis LJ, McGregor JM: Cervical spondylotic myelopathy: Functional and radiographic long-term outcome after laminectomy and posterior fusion. Neurosurgery 44:771–777, 1999.

37. Kurihara A, Tanaka Y, Tsumura N, Iwasaki Y: Hyperostotic lumbar spinal stenosis: A review of 12 surgically treated cases with roentgenographic survey of ossification of the yellow ligament at the lumbar spine. Spine 13:1308–1316, 1988.

38. Lonstein J: Post-Laminectomy Kyphosis Spinal Deformities and Neurologic Dysfunction. New York, Raven Press, 1978, pp 53–63.

39. Luetkehans TJ, Coughlin BF, Weinstein MA: Ossification of the posterior longitudinal ligament diagnosed by MR. Am J Neuroradiol 8:924–925, 1987.

40. Manabe S, Nomura S: Anterior decompression for ossification of the posterior longitudinal ligament of the cervical spine. Neurol Surg 5:1253–1259, 1977 (in Japanese).

41. Matsunaga S, Sakou T, Taketomi E, et al: The natural course of myelopathy caused by ossification of the posterior longitudinal ligament in the cervical spine. Clin Orthop 305:168–177, 1994.

42. Matsuyama Y, Kawakami N, Mimatsu K: Spinal cord expansion after decompression in cervical myelopathy: Investigation by computed tomography myelography and ultrasonography. Spine 20:1657–1663, 1995.

43. McAfee PC, Bohlman HH, Han JS, Salvagno RT: Comparison of nuclear magnetic resonance imaging and computed tomography in the diagnosis of upper cervical spinal cord compression. Spine 11:295–304, 1986.

44. McAfee PC, Regan JJ, Bohlman HH: Cervical cord compression from ossification of the posterior longitudinal ligament in non-Asians. J Bone Joint Surg Br 69B:569–575, 1987.

45. Merlini L, Granata C, Albisinni U, et al: Severe cervical stenosis due to ossification of the posterior longitudinal ligament without neurological manifestations ("silent OPLL"). Ital J Neurol Sci 10:93–96, 1989.

46. Mikawa Y, Shikata J, Yamamuro T: Spinal deformity and instability after multilevel cervical laminectomy. Spine 12:6–11, 1987.

47. Miyazaki K, Kirita Y: Extensive simultaneous multisegment laminectomy for myelopathy due to the ossification of the posterior longitudinal ligament in the cervical region. Spine 11:531–542, 1986.

48. Nakanishi T, Mannen T, Toyokura Y: Asymptomatic ossification of the posterior longitudinal ligament of the cervical spine: Incidence and roentgenographic findings. J Neurol Sci 19:375–381, 1973.

49. Nakano K, Harata S, Suetsuna F, et al: Spinous process-splitting laminoplasty using hydroxyapatite spinous process spacer. Spine 17S:41–43, 1992.

50. Nakano N, Nakano T, Nakano K: Comparison of the results of laminectomy and open-door laminoplasty for cervical spondylotic myeloradiculopathy and ossification of the posterior longitudinal ligament. Spine 13:792–794, 1988.

51. Nose T, Egashira T, Enomoto T, Maki Y: Ossification of the posterior longitudinal ligament: a clinico-radiological study of 74 cases. J Neurol Neurosurg Psychiatry 50:321–326, 1987.

52. Nowinski GP, Visarius H, Nolte LP, Herkowitz HN: A biomechanical comparison of cervical laminoplasty and cervical laminectomy with progressive facetectomy. Spine 18:1995–2004, 1993.

52a. O'Brien MF, Peterson D, Casey AT, Crockard HA: A novel technique for laminoplasty augmentation of spinal canal area using titanium miniplate stabilization: A computerized morphometric analysis. Spine 21:474–484, 1996.

53. Ogino H, Tada K, Okada K, et al: Canal diameter, anteroposterior compression ratio, and spondylotic myelopathy of the cervical spine. Spine 8:1–15, 1983.

54. Ohtsuka K, Terayama K, Yanagihara M, et al: An epidemiological survey on ossification of ligaments in the cervical and thoracic spine in individuals over 50 years of age. J Jpn Orthop Assoc 60:1087–1098, 1986.

55. Ohtsuka K, Terayama K, Yanagihara M, et al: A radiological population study on the ossification of the posterior longitudinal ligament in the spine. Arch Orthop Trauma Surg 106:89–93, 1987.

56. Okada Y, Ikata T, Yamada H, et al: Magnetic resonance imaging study on the results of surgery for cervical compression myelopathy. Spine 18:2024–2029, 1993.

57. Ono K, Ota H, Tada K, et al: Ossified posterior longitudinal ligament: A clinicopathologic study. Spine 2:126–138, 1977.

58. Parke WW: Correlative anatomy of cervical spondylotic myelopathy. Spine 13:831–846, 1988.

59. Pennes DR, Martel W, Ellis CN: Retinoid-induced ossification of the posterior longitudinal ligament. Skeletal Radiol 14:191–193, 1985.

60. Resnick D, Guerra J Jr, Robinson CA, Vint VC: Association of diffuse idiopathic skeletal hyperostosis (DISH) and calcification and ossification of the posterior longitudinal ligament. AJR Am J Roentgenol 131:1049–1053, 1978.

61. Rogers L: The surgical treatment of cervical spondylotic myelopathy: Mobilisation of the complete cervical cord into an enlarged canal. J Bone Joint Surg Br 43B:3–6, 1961.

62. Satomi K, Nishu Y, Kohno T, Hirabayashi K: Long-term follow-up studies of open-door laminoplasty for cervical stenotic myelopathy. Spine 19:507–510, 1994.

62a. Seichi A, Takeshita K, Ohishi I, et al: Long-term results of double-door laminoplasty for cervical stenotic myelopathy. Spine 26:479–487, 2001.

63. Shibasaki H, Nagamatsu K: Calcification of the posterior longitudinal ligament: Its relation with cervical spondylosis. Clin Neurol 7:22–29, 1968 (in Japanese).

64. Shinoda Y, Hanzawa S, Nonaka K, Owada O: Ossification of the longitudinal ligament of the posterior cervical vertebrae. Orthop Surg 22:383–391, 1971.

65. Shinomiya K, Furuya K, Sato R, et al: Electrophysiologic diagnosis of cervical OPLL myelopathy using evoked spinal cord potentials. Spine 13:1225–1233, 1988.

66. Sim FH, Svien HJ, Bickel WH, Janes JM: Swan neck deformity following extensive cervical laminectomy: A review of twenty-one cases. J Bone Joint Surg Am 56A:564–580, 1974.

67. Smith MD, Bolesta MJ, Leventhal M, Bohlman HH: Postoperative cerebrospinal-fluid fistula associated with erosion of the dura: Findings after anterior resection of ossification of the posterior longitudinal ligament in the cervical spine. J Bone Joint Surg Am 74A:270–277, 1992.

68. Terayama K: Genetic studies on ossification of the posterior longitudinal ligament of the spine. Spine 14:1184–1191, 1989.

69. Terayama K, Mamiya N, Suzuki A: Ossification of the posterior longitudinal ligament of the cervical spine: Clinical symptoms, roentgenographic changes and treatment. Clin J Orthop 23:478–487, 1972 (in Japanese).

69a. Tomita K, Kawahara N, Toribatake Y, Heller JG: Expansive midline T-saw laminoplasty (modified spinous process-splitting) for the management of cervical myelopathy. Spine 23:32–37, 1998.

70. Trojan DA, Pouchot J, Pokrupa R, et al: Diagnosis and treatment of ossification of the posterior longitudinal ligament of the spine: Report of eight cases and literature review. Am J Med 92:296–306, 1992.

71. Tsuji H: Laminoplasty for patients with compressive myelopathy due to so-called spinal canal stenosis in cervical and thoracic regions. Spine 7:28–34, 1982.

72. Tsukimoto H: A case report-autopsy of syndrome of compression of spinal cord owing to ossification within spinal canal of cervical spines. Arch Japanische Chir 29:1003–1007, 1960.

73. Tsuyama N: Ossification of the posterior longitudinal ligament of the spine. Clin Orthop 184:71–84, 1984.

74. Tsuyama N, Terayama K, Ohtani K, et al: The Investigation Committee on OPLL of the Japanese Ministry of Public Health and Welfare. The ossification of the posterior longitudinal ligament of the spine (OPLL). J Jpn Orthop Assoc 55:425–440, 1981.

75. Widder DJ: MR imaging of ossification of the posterior longitudinal ligament. AJR Am J Roentgenol 153:194–195, 1989.

76. Yamamoto I, Kageyama N, Nakamura K, Takahashi T: Computed tomography in ossification of the posterior longitudinal ligament in the cervical spine. Surg Neurol 12:414–418, 1979.

77. Yanagi T, Yamamura Y, Ando K, Sobve I: Ossification of the posterior longitudinal ligament of the cervical spine: Analysis of 37 cases. Clin Neurol 7:727, 1967.

78. Yoshida M, Otani K, Shibasaki K, Ueda S: Expansive laminoplasty with reattachment of spinous process and extensor musculature for cervical myelopathy. Spine 17:491–497, 1992.

79. Zdeblick TA, Abitbol JJ, Kunz DN, et al: Cervical stability after sequential capsule resection. Spine 18:2005–2008, 1993.

Traumatic Injuries of the Surgical Spine

10

SPINAL CORD TRAUMA: PATHOPHYSIOLOGY AND MEDICAL MANAGEMENT

Gregory D. Carlson, M.D.
Jeffery C. Wang, M.D.

Hope is the feeling you have that the feeling you have isn't permanent.

— Jean Kerr

Spinal cord trauma has devastating and long-lasting consequences for those injured. Approximately 10,000 new cases of acute paralysis are documented per year in the United States alone. Societal costs are estimated at $10 billion dollars per year; the personal costs are incalculable.[185] The combination of younger patients being injured and increased patient longevity conspire to create an increasing financial and social burden on society. Highly specialized regional spinal cord injury (SCI) centers have evolved to better handle the complex problems of patients with SCI. Advances in neuroimaging have opened the door for more accurate assessment of spinal column disruption and intramedullary cord injury. Early medical management of SCI has improved the outcomes for some patients. Modern neuroscience techniques have led to a better understanding of the neuropathophysiology of permanent neural injuries. Investigators have recognized

the importance of both primary (passive) and secondary (active) events surrounding the progressive loss of neural function.[187] Clinical and experimental evidence supports the role of intra-medullary microvascular injury, ischemia, neurochemical and electrolyte imbalances, free radical damage, and programmed cell death as major factors affecting cellular function and ultimate morbidity.[2, 5, 7, 14, 16, 17, 34, 52, 58, 62, 75, 106, 109, 187] These advances point to possible breakthrough strategies to improve the medical[98, 99] and surgical treatments[11, 25, 26, 98, 99] for SCI patients. Laminectomies previously performed for spinal cord decompression have been replaced by more sophisticated anterior spinal column procedures for improved neural decompression and stabilization.[24] Still controversial, issues of timing for spinal cord decompression and stabilization are currently being debated.[53] Recent outcome studies strongly support early spinal column stabilization within the first 24 hours after injury for shortened hospitalization and a more rapid rehabilitation.[45, 132] Despite 50% declines in mortality rate and average length of hospital stay since 1974, rates of permanent paralysis are still unacceptably high.[104, 114]

EPIDEMIOLOGY

The true incidence of acute SCI ranges from 22 to 32 per 1 million persons at risk in the United States.[59, 83, 119, 126, 154, 156, 180] The prevalence has been estimated at approximately 906 per million.[129, 180] This rate represents a nearly 50% increase over estimates made in 1975. The rate is significantly lower than that in developing countries, where accident prevention and health care are less accessible.

The rate of SCI is two to four times greater in males than in females, and is two times higher in nonwhite ethnic groups than in whites.[119, 180] This racial variation is attributed to the increased accident rate in minorities.[119, 126, 127] Fatalities associated with SCIs are more common in females than in males, and more common in African Americans than in whites.[127]

SCI occurs most often in persons age 15 to 20, with 19 the most common age.[59, 180] This young age of persons at most risk is particularly devastating when the life expectancy of these individuals is examined.

The etiology of SCIs is similar in all industrialized countries. Motor vehicle accidents (47.7%) is the most common cause of SCI in the United States. Falls (20.8%), acts of violence (14.6%), and sports-related accidents (14.2%) are some of the other more common reasons for SCIs.[119, 126, 127, 180] Factors such as sex, race, and age also correlate within the different etiologic factors.[83] Not surprisingly, injuries tend to occur more frequently around the summer months of the year and many are alcohol related.[83]

There is a trend toward more incomplete neurologic injuries. This may be due in part to the efficacy of regional trauma centers that are expertly trained in the management of spinal cord injured patients.[186] When broken into sub-categories incomplete quadriparesis is most common, followed by complete paraplegia and then complete quadriplegia. Incomplete paraparesis is the least common pattern.[119, 127, 180] The most common neurologic level of injury is the C6 level. This correlates with the most common spinal column injury levels which are the C4, C5, and then the C6 level. The least common levels of injury are at C1, C2, and C3.[83]

Mortality rates of spinal cord injured patients have also declined. Patients who survive the first post-injury year have a much better prognosis, with younger patients living longer. The leading causes of death include pneumonia, accidents, and suicide.[119, 126, 180]

In addition to the enormous toll of human suffering endured by the individual and family, the economic costs largely borne by society over the lifetime of the patient are high. The average annual costs of caring for spinal cord injured patients depend primarily on the degree of impairment and range from $58,000 to $170,000 according to the level of spinal injury.[112, 119, 180, 198]

EARLY MANAGEMENT

Care of the SCI patient involves early immobilization, medical stabilization, restoration of spinal alignment, spinal cord decompression, and finally spinal stabilization. The first step is to recognize the patient with potential spinal column instability or SCI and immobilize the spine appropriately. Movement of the patient from the accident scene should be performed with a rigid cervical collar and backboard.

The physical examination begins with an analysis of the historical account of injury. Factors to investigate include: circumstances of trauma, the position of the patient, seat belt history, type of treatment at the scene, and important questions regarding transient sensory or motor loss. Evidence of head trauma and history of high velocity trauma or mechanisms such as falls in the elderly or child should be carefully evaluated for spinal column instability.[24] Patients who are unconscious or have an altered sensorium (drug or alcohol intoxication) should be treated as though they have spinal column instability. Failure to initially recognize an unstable cervical spine injury has been reported in as many as 33% of patients hospitalized with cervical trauma.[24] Factors that contribute to a missed or delayed diagnosis include an altered state of consciousness, incomplete radiographic evaluation, and severe concomitant injuries.[174]

Medical stabilization follows the basic principles of the advanced trauma life support (ATLS) protocol.[81] Airway and breathing take first priority followed by hemodynamic stabilization. Aspiration of gastric contents and shock are the two most common causes of death before hospital admission for spinal cord–injured patients.[97] SCI may be associated with hypotension and bradycardia as a result of traumatic sympathectomy. Peripheral resistance and cardiac output are decreased with loss of autonomic tone. The systemic effects of neurogenic shock may precipitate progressive microcirculatory cord injury. Levi and colleagues at Maryland Shock Trauma Center have postulated that the pulmonary vascular resistance is a more sensitive measure of sympathectomized effect of acute cervical SCI than traditional measures of systemic vascular resistance. They recommend early aggressive hemodynamic monitoring with arterial line and Swan-Ganz catheter and support with fluids and dopamine and/or dobutamine, titrated to maintain a hemodynamic profile with adequate cardiac output (to be determined by oxygen consumption and delivery) and a mean blood pressure of greater than 90 mm Hg.[131] Volume replacement should proceed with caution due to fluid redistribution that may precipitate congestive heart failure and pulmonary edema. The treatment of neurogenic shock involves redistributing the blood volume back into the central venous system from the dilated peripheral circulation. By maintaining adequate circulatory perfusion, the effects of secondary SCI and damage to other organ systems may be minimized.[131, 187]

Important steps of the physical examination include inspection, palpation, and neurologic testing of motor and sensory function. Head and facial abrasions may coincide with cervical injury. Observation of chest wall abrasions or paradoxical motion may lead to findings of mediastinal injury and possible thoracic column trauma. Palpation of soft tissue crepitus is indicative of pulmonary injury and pneumothorax. Ecchymosis in the abdominal region may be associated with seat belt trauma and thoracolumbar fractures. Flexion-distraction lumbar fractures caused by seat belts are commonly associated with intra-abdominal injury to liver, spleen, bowel, and urologic structures.[95]

The initial neurologic status of the spinal cord–injured patient should be thoroughly documented using the American Spinal Cord Injury Association/International Medical Society of Paraplegia (ASIA/IMSOP) standards (Fig. 10–1).[143] The neurologic examination comprises sensory, motor, and reflex function. Each of the 28 dermatomes on the right and left sides of the body are examined for sensitivity to light touch and pin prick (Fig. 10–2). Upper cervical roots, C-2 and C-3, innervate the skin of the posterior occiput and upper neck to the angle of the jaw. C-4 supplies fibers to the nape of the neck and clavicular region. C-5 classically extends to the deltoid and anterolateral upper arm. C-6 provides sensation to the radial forearm, thumb and index finger. C-7 innervates the skin over the long finger and C-8 provides sensation to the ring and small fingers as well as ulnar hand and forearm. In addition, position sense and awareness of deep pressure or pain is suggested for each limb.

Motor examination of a key muscle in the 10 paired myotomes should be examined from rostral to caudal. Muscle strength is graded by a scale of function: grade 0 for no function; grade 1 for palpable contraction without joint motion; grade 2 for complete joint active range of motion with gravity eliminated; grade 3 for full joint active range of motion against gravity; grade 4 for full active range of joint motion with some resistance; and grade 5 for normal strength and full range of motion against gravity and resistance. The external anal sphincter is graded for muscle contraction around the finger and sensation. Motor level determination is by convention assigned to the caudal level with at least a grade of three. This assumes that the proximal adjacent level must test to a grade of 5. Sparing of function below the level of the injury, no matter how trivial may significantly alter the long-term prognosis. A recent study demonstrated that 86% of patients with only a flicker of motor sparing below the level of the injury recovered useful motor function.[86] The best long-term prognostic factor is early motor recovery.[188] Besides the conventional deep tendon reflexes, superficial and pathologic reflexes may provide valuable insight into the extent of neurologic damage. The abdominal (upper T7–T10 and lower T11–T12) and cremasteric reflexes (T12–L2) are mediated through the central nervous system (CNS) and elicited by stroking the skin of the abdomen and inner thigh. Umbilical deviation toward the stimulated side indicates an intact

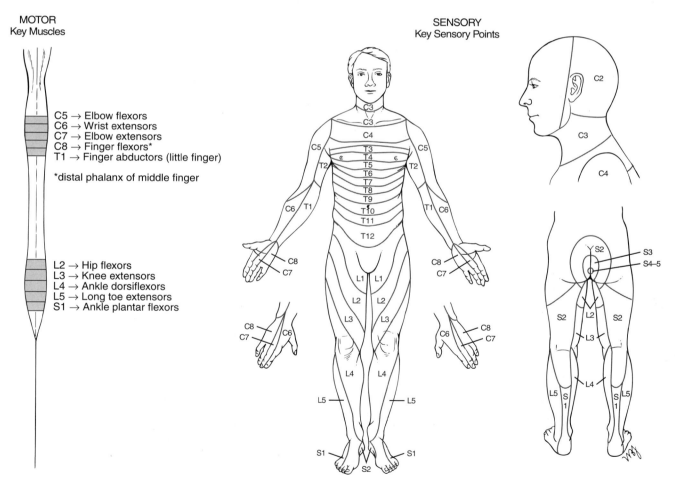

MOTOR
Key Muscles

C5 → Elbow flexors
C6 → Wrist extensors
C7 → Elbow extensors
C8 → Finger flexors*
T1 → Finger abductors (little finger)

*distal phalanx of middle finger

L2 → Hip flexors
L3 → Knee extensors
L4 → Ankle dorsiflexors
L5 → Long toe extensors
S1 → Ankle plantar flexors

SENSORY
Key Sensory Points

Figure 10–1. Standard neurologic classification of spinal cord injuries. (Modified from American Spinal Injury Association: International Standards for Neurologic and Functional Classification of Spinal Cord Injury. Atlanta, American Spinal Injury Association, 1996.)

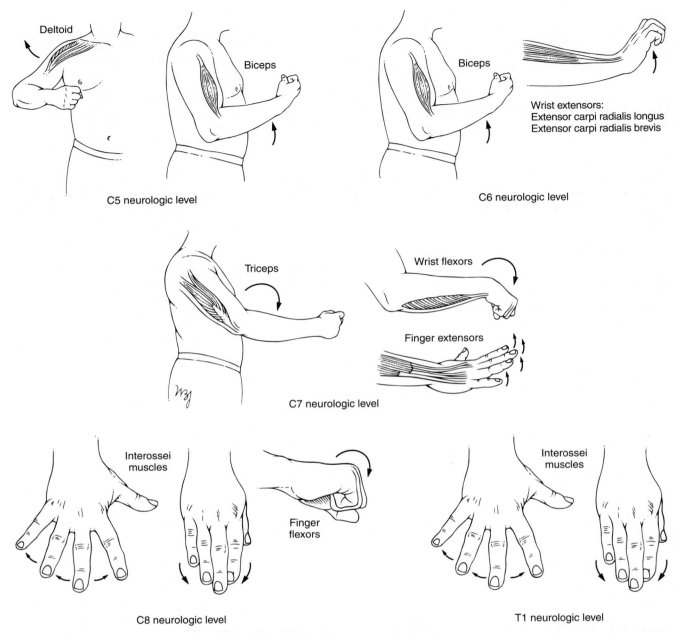

Figure 10–2. *Cross-section of the lower cervical spinal cord with common spinal pathways.*

response. Contraction of the scrotum on the side stimulated is also normal. Upper motor neuron loss is indicated by a positive pathologic reflex. The Babinski reflex, elicited by stimulation of the plantar surface, is positive if the great toe extends with simultaneous plantar flexion of the remaining toes. A similar test, the Oppenheim reflex, is elicited by running an object along the tibial spine with results similar to the Babinski.

The ASIA impairment scale, a modification of the Frankel scale, is the most widely accepted tool for comparison of neurologic injury (Table 10–1).[194] Patients in grade A have complete neurologic injury without sensory or motor function preserved in the sacral segments.[188, 196] Grade B (incomplete) suggests a patient has sensory preservation below the level of injury including sacral segments but no motor function. Grade C classifies patients with more than half of key muscle groups below the neurologic level with muscle grade of less than 3. In grade D, motor function is preserved below the neurologic level with a motor grade of 3 or greater in at least half of the key muscle groups. Grade E is a normal neurologic exam.[143]

Functional independence measurement (FIM) is one of several disability scales that estimate the cost of disability in terms of self-care and provide an approach for assessing the impact of SCI on the individual's daily life and activities. The FIM focuses on six areas of function: self-care, sphinter control, mobility, locomotion, communication, and social cognition. The best means of patient care assessment is probably a combination of both impairment and disability scale.[196]

Conclusive evidence of a complete injury cannot be made until the resolution of spinal shock, the physiologic blockade of all or most spinal reflex activity below the level of the injury.[194] The return of the bulbocavernosus reflex or by definition a window of 48 hours surrounding the injury, signals the resolution of spinal shock. By this time, if no sensory or motor recovery has occurred below the neurologic injury, functional recovery is not expected. Spinal shock may mask deleterious secondary changes that occur in the hours immediately following contusion injury. The inability to monitor neurologic functional recovery during this time may place certain patients at risk of being treated as complete injuries when in fact early aggressive treatments may be efficacious in an unknown percentage of patients.

Damage to specific regions of the spinal cord typically produce neurologic findings grouped into classic partial injury syndromes. Functional neurologic injury can be correlated with anatomic regions of damage (see Fig. 10–2). Function of the dorsal column is assessed using a tuning fork to detect vibration or distal position sense of a limb in space. Pain and temperature sensation are relayed to the brain in the ascending anterolateral spinothalamic tract. Regional damage to these structures will present as loss of distal contralateral pain and temperature. Ipsilateral pain and temperature may be affected at the injury level. Distal motor function is innervated through the lateral corticospinal tracts.

The central cord syndrome is the most common (Fig. 10–3). These patients typically suffer a hyperextension injury and usually have some preexisting cervical spondylosis. The cord injury occurs through a pincer affect caused by the posterior hypertrophied ligamentum flavum and the anterior osteophytes/disk complex. A central cord lesion occurs with relatively greater loss of gray matter. The neurologic deficit is one of upper extremity weakness greater than lower with sacral sensory sparing. The prognosis is fair, with a large percentage of patients recovering the ability to walk.

Anterior cord syndromes commonly result from burst fracture, flexion injury, or fracture dislocation. The anatomic injury occurs in the anterior two-thirds of the cord (Fig. 10–4). The dorsal columns conveying proprioception and vibratory sense are usually spared. Variable motor loss can occur usually greatest in the lower limbs. The prognosis for recovery is poor.

Injury to one anatomic half of the cord results in Brown-Séquard syndrome (Fig. 10–5). Clinical presentation shows ipsilateral loss of motor, position, and proprioception, with contralateral sparing of pain and temperature. This syndrome has the best prognosis, most patients can be expected to recover long tract function. Bowel and bladder function should recover based on the unilateral nature of the injury.

Mixed cord syndromes are not uncommon. They may occur in combination with nerve root lesions. The most common roots involved are the fifth and sixth roots with corresponding deltoid or biceps weakness. Prognosis for nerve root recovery is good after either complete or incomplete injury.[11, 20, 25]

NEUROIMAGING
Radiography

High-quality cervical x-rays are the first imaging study needed for accurate and timely diagnosis. The cervical vertebra must be visualized caudal to the C7 and T1 junction. In addition to the lateral cervical spine x-ray, which should be instrumental in picking up 85% of significant injuries, an anteroposterior view and an open mouth odontoid view should be obtained to fully assess the spine. In patients with a large upper body mass, the cervicothoracic junction may not be easily visualized. A lateral swimmer's view or computed tomography (CT) scan should be obtained to adequately view the caudal region to the T1 junction. Dynamic radiography is of limited value in the acute trauma setting. Early postinjury flexion-extension views may be inadequate to rule out serious injury because of muscle spasms or guarding.

A normal cervical spine will demonstrate a lordotic curvature; however, up to 20% of the population without neck problems will have a neutral or kyphotic spine.[92] Expansion of the retropharyngeal space may suggest spinal column injury. Measurements greater than 7 mm below C2 have a statistical probability of underlying injury.[189] Radiologic imaging may be helpful in determining spinal instability. White and Panjabi have popularized the understanding of spinal instability determined by abnormal displacement or translation of greater than 3.5 mm and/or segmental angulation exceeding 11 degrees measured from standard lateral x-rays.[197] Instability may be assumed by finding asymmetric interspinous widening suggestive of posterior ligamentous injury. Subtle asymmetry on lateral

Table 10–1. *ASIA Impairment Scale*

A = Complete	No motor or sensory function is preserved in the sacral segments S4–S5.
B = Incomplete	Sensory but not motor function is preserved below the neurologic level and includes the sacral segments S4–S5.
C = Incomplete	Motor function is preserved below the neurologic level, and more than half of the key muscles below the neurologic level have a muscle grade less than 3.
D = Incomplete	Motor function is preserved below the neurologic level, and at least half of the key muscles below the neurologic level have a muscle grade of 3 or more.
E = Normal	Motor and sensory function are normal.

From the International Standards for Neurological and Functional Classification of Spinal Cord Injury, 2001.

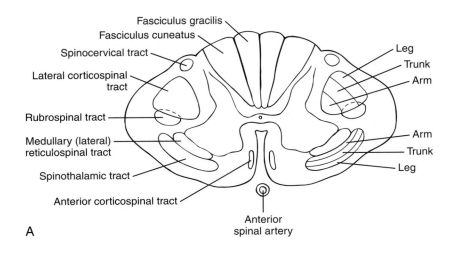

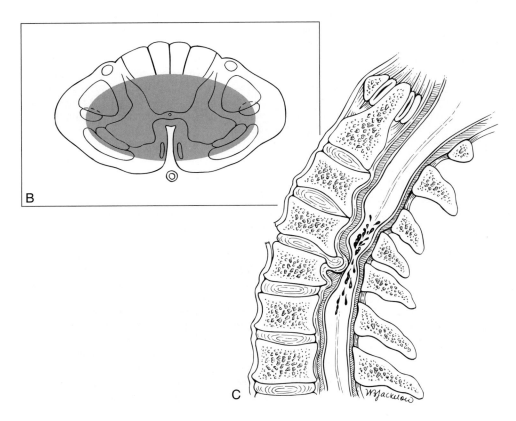

Figure 10–3. *Central cord injury illustrated in a cross-section of the spinal cord.*

x-rays of the lateral mass or facet may be the only finding associated with unilateral facet fracture or dislocation. Subluxation of up to 8 mm at the C2–C3 joint may be physiologic "pseudosubluxation" in the pediatric population. In contradistinction to the pathologic condition, the posterior spinolaminar line should be undisrupted in the nonpathologic conditions. Hyperextension injuries may present with mild anterior widening of the intervertebral space with an occasional small avulsion fracture of the adjoining endplate. Extensive soft tissue disruption through the intervertebral disk and concomitant posterior longitudi-

nal ligamentous injury may be associated with the severe injury pattern. The highly unstable "teardrop" fracture of the anterior vertebrae associated with hyperflexion injury mechanisms should not be confused with the unrelated endplate avulsion type of injury. Asymmetry and narrowing of the intervertebral space in combination with subluxation/ dislocation may signify disk disruption and possible concomitant intracanal herniation. Patients with these findings should undergo magnetic resonance imaging (MRI) before closed reduction maneuvers to prevent further neurologic injury.[68]

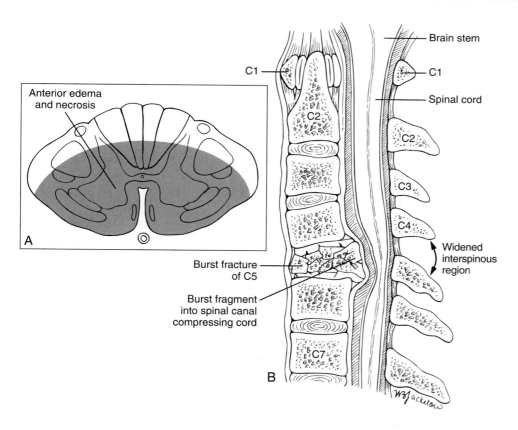

Figure 10–4. Anterior spinal cord injury with a burst fracture displaced bone fragment.

Computed Tomography

New high-resolution "spiral" CT scans have improved the speed and accuracy of three-dimensional spinal column imaging. The osseous detail provided by CT is unsurpassed by MRI and may be the study of choice for fracture assessment. Thin section cuts combined with sagittal and coronal reconstruction techiques provide excellent detail of the bony architecture and are particularly useful for odontoid and pedicle fractures, as well as facet fracture-subluxations. The modern CT scanner may collect data from the entire cervical spine within minutes and is of particular importance in ruling out concomitant spinal injuries. The incidence of concomitant noncontiguous spine fractures ranges from 3.2% to 16.7%.[19, 44] The most common pattern is a fracture of C1 or C2 with a noncontiguous subaxial cervical fracture.[48] Although thin section scanning provides high definition for fracture recognition, nondisplaced fractures or ligamentous injuries oriented in the axial plane can remain unrecognized, suggesting an additional role for MRI in the traumatized patient.

CT-myelography remains a useful study in some cases of acute cervical trauma. Particular uses include delineation of extent and location of residual cord compression after injury. Although noninvasive studies like MRI may provide complementary information, there are situations when myelography-enhanced CT provides unsurpassed detail for treatment planning.

Magnetic Resonance Imaging

MRI provides the greatest tool for detecting intramedullary cord damage, traumatic disk herniation, soft tissue injury, or epidural hematoma. The role of MRI in the management of cervical spine trauma is expanding. Reports of neurologic deterioration associated with disk prolapse into the canal with reduction techniques highlight the need for MRI scanning in patients at risk.[68] These cases usually involve facet joint injuries with some amount of dislocation Closed reduction without MRI has been the standard of care in awake patients without intervertebral disk space narrowing.[175] If the patient is not awake and alert, then MRI imaging is indicated before open or closed manipulation.

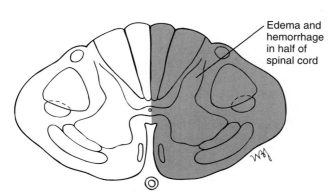

Figure 10–5. Brown-Séquard injury.

MRI can be a useful prognostic tool. Cord damage has been correlated with neurologic deficit and recovery.[82, 85, 105, 142, 152, 168, 169] The presence of cord edema is predictive of neurologic impairment.[85] Regions of hypointense signal within the cord substance (T2 image) represent hemorrhage. Small focal regions have better prognosis for neural recovery than larger diffuse multisegmental regions.

Disadvantages of MRI include longer study time, higher cost, relative difficulty managing unstable patients in the scanner tube, poor image quality in noncompliant patients, and sometimes inconvenient location related to the trauma facility. Growth and development of MRI technology will certainly enhance image quality and patient accessibility in the future.

CLASSIFICATION OF CERVICAL SPINAL COLUMN INJURY

Cervical spinal column injuries are classified by location, mechanism of injury, relative stability, fracture type, and presence of neurologic involvement. The craniocervical region encompassing the occiput to the atlas (C2) is anatomically distinct from the lower subaxial region. Ligamentous supports provide the main stabilizers to the craniocervical region. The unique anatomic configuration of this region allows for significant freedom of motion, particularly in the rotation planes. Because of the relatively large size of the head in relation to the body, 75% of cervical injuries involve the craniocervical junction in children under age 7.[48] The spinal canal and space available for the spinal cord are largest in the craniocervical region; however, injury to the region by high-speed trauma is commonly fatal because of involvement of the breathing centers, which are in proximity to the brainstem. Relatively rare atlanto-occipital dislocations have been classified by direction of displacement and presence or absence of distraction on lateral x-ray.[190] Powers ratio, a difficult measurement on some studies, has been classically used to describe injury to this region.[159] Traction is contraindicated because of the significant ligamentous instability. Early surgical stabilization is important, because halo vest immobilization is inadequate.

Atlas fractures are associated with concomitant cervical injury in many cases, most commonly C2 fractures. The atlas fractures can be classified by fracture type, mechanism of injury, and potential instability.[134] Posterior arch fractures with an intact transverse ligament can be treated with hard collar immobilization. Burst fractures of the ring involve multiple fragments and by definition are unstable. The classic Jefferson fracture is defined by measuring the spreading of the lateral masses on the open-mouth anteroposterior x-ray. Excursion of the lateral masses greater than 8 mm signifies transverse ligament rupture and instability of the C1–C2 articulation. In many cases, treatment of the concomitant bony fracture dictates the approach of treatment for the C1 ring. In isolated fractures, unstable ring injuries are treated with halo vest for at least 2 months, followed by hard-collar immobilization. Isolated atlantoaxial instability without fracture is uncommon, but when identified should be treated with posterior C1–C2 arthrodesis.

Odontoid fractures may result from high-velocity injury or seemingly insignificant falls in elderly persons. The Anderson and D'Alonzo classification system is still widely regarded as an important prognostic tool.[10] Type II fractures through the waist of the odontoid have a high rate of pseudarthrosis, which can lead to late instability. Early surgical stabilization has been advocated for displaced fractures, elderly patients, smokers, and patients who present more than 7 days after injury.[48] The Levine and Edwards classification system has been widely accepted for treatment of traumatic spondylolisthesis through the pedicle of C2.[133]

Subaxial injuries can be classified as anterior wedge fractures without canal compromise, vertebral burst fractures with retropulsion into the canal, facet-lateral mass injuries with and without dislocation, and hyperextension injuries. These injuries are discussed in greater detail in other chapters of this text.

PATHOPHYSIOLOGY

Primary Mechanisms of Injury

Increasing evidence indicates that the pathophysiology of acute SCI involves primary and secondary mechanisms of injury.[204] The primary injury usually involves blunt cord compression from dislocation of spinal vertebral motion segments or displaced bone fragments. The nature of the primary insult varies from initial dynamic cord contusion to sustained cord compression after displacement. The vast majority of cord injuries do not involve complete cord transection.[43] Morphologic characteristics and clinical outcomes vary with the force of compression, duration of compression, displacement, acceleration, and kinetic energy.[178, 179]

Various experimental models have been developed to determine the mechanical effects of cord compression on physiologic outcome parameters. Models in current use reflect either a dynamic contusion impact injury or a sustained compression such as small vascular clip or static application of weights to the surface of the cord.[12] Modifications of Allen's original weight drop technique are still the most widely used today.[4, 117] The severity of injury is quantified by the g-cm product of drop weight mass and thus gives a measure of the energy sustained at contact. Variability in testing may be dependent on the impactor contact area, stabilization of the spinal column in relation to the loading device, and the possibility of multiple impacts. More recent models with controlled contusion techniques have allowed precise control over injury severity and biomechanics, resulting in consistent populations of animals for comparison.[12, 41, 120] The probability of neurologic recovery after cord contusion can now be reliably computed based on the displacement, force, and acceleration.[12] Spinal cord tissue responds to load application in a predictable manner that can be mathematically modeled under precise loading conditions.[12, 50, 178]

Spinal cord trauma usually involves an initial impact, followed by residual spinal cord displacement or compression. To more precisely model the interaction between dynamic compression and residual spinal cord compression, Carlson and colleagues developed a consistent dynamic, sustained compression canine SCI model.[49, 50] They demonstrated that although interface pressures between the loading piston and displaced spinal cord decreased to 13% of maximum within 30 minutes after dynamic loading, no measurable recovery of electrophysiologic recovery occurred without early spinal cord decompression. This suggests that even though pressure gradients relax to baseline levels, residual spinal cord displacement is a significant factor in the propagation of secondary mechanisms of injury.[49]

Pathologic Changes

The pathophysiology of SCI can be divided into acute and chronic phases of injury. After the acute contusion, the spinal cord undergoes a series of pathologic changes including hemorrhage, edema, neuronal necrosis, axonal fragmentation, demyelination, and eventually cyst formation.[14, 15, 62, 187] Electron microscopy studies have demonstrated erythrocyte distension of the venules in the gray matter within the first 5 minutes after injury, followed by small hemorrhages within the perivascular spaces and some axonal changes 15 to 30 minutes after injury.[62] Within 1 hour after injury, damage characteristic of chromatolysis and ischemia begins to appear in the anterior ventral horn cells.[192] By 4 hours after injury, a central region of hemorrhagic necrosis forms and extends centifugally and proximally in the shape of a spindle.[65, 67]

White matter changes begin at the gray matter junction with progressive edema noted as spongiform changes on light microscopy.[63] Axonal swelling, attributed to axoplasmic stasis,[14, 15, 40, 42] affects multiple organelles, mitochondria, neurofilaments, and smooth endoplasmic reticulum, which undergo granular dissolution. Damage to the myelin sheath occurs through vesicular disruption.[14] Initially, polymorphonuclear cells infiltrate the injured region. These are replaced by macrophages within days after injury.[22, 148] Within 1 week, the central necrotic region begins to show cystic changes. Within 4 weeks, chronic changes have occurred, and a cystic cavity remains with astrocytic gliosis and demyelination of the remaining axons.[192]

Secondary Mechanisms of Injury

The original concept of secondary neurologic injury is attributed to Allen, who in 1911 postulated that a noxious biochemical factor is present in the hemorrhagic material within the midsubstance of the traumatized spinal cord, which if removed resulted in improvement of function after experimental injury.[4] Modern neuroscience techniques and research have implicated a number of mechanisms associated with progressive neurologic damage after trauma. These include vascular ischemia, electrolyte abnormalites, edema,[185] and biochemical events such as the release of excitatory amino acids that disrupt normal cellular homeostasis.[75, 78] Spinal cord ischemia and reperfusion are accompanied by early lipid peroxidation.[32, 138] Abrupt increases in extracellular lactate concentrations combined with biochemical alterations in intracellular pH and energy metabolites suggest factors of energy failure.[162, 191] Intracellular calcium homeostasis disruption results in proteolytic enzyme activation.[16, 207] Early postinjury events may trigger other irreversible delayed mechanisms of apoptosis.[136] Ongoing investigations into secondary mechanisms of injury suggest a "window of opportunity" shortly after injury during which pharmacotherapy and other treatment strategies provide future neuroprotective benefits for patients with SCI.[28, 29]

Systemic Vascular Changes

The early systemic effects of SCI manifest as neurogenic shock, with bradycardia, hypotension, and decreased cardiac output. These systemic changes were found to be due to a combination of decreased sympathetic tone and myocardial effects.[101] In combination with the systemic effects of hypotension, local microvascular changes occur that further reduce the traumatized regional spinal cord blood flow.[66, 161, 187] Vasospasm, mediated through increased neurotransmitter accumulation, noradrenaline, dopamine, and seratonin, may only further restrict blood flow and the delivery of oxygen to an already ischemic environment.[72, 77]

Regional Blood Flow Changes

Experimental evidence supports an ischemic mechanism of secondary injury. Various studies demonstrate posttraumatic ischemia during and after spinal cord compression.[49, 50, 100, 122, 123, 161, 166, 167, 205] Investigators have demonstrated that the severity of cord injury correlates significantly with the degree of posttraumatic ischemia and axonal dysfunction.[80] Not all studies of posttraumatic spinal cord blood flow agree, however. A consistent finding is hypoperfusion in the gray matter. Examination of the blood flow within the white matter has not always been consistent.[123] The variablity in reported series may result from numerous factors, including technique of blood flow measurement, method of cord injury, use of an animal model, and systemic factors of blood pressure and temperature.

Carlson and coworkers postulated that return of blood flow to baseline levels or above during and after sustained cord compression would improve neurologic recovery.[46, 47] They demonstrated that animals that recovered neurologic function after time-dependent spinal cord decompression had greater return of blood flow during sustained cord displacement and immediately after decompression. Earlier spinal cord decompression led to proportionally greater blood flow above baseline levels and coincidentally improved neural functional recovery.[46, 47]

The exact cause of posttraumatic ischemia remains unknown. Numerous theories postulate various etiologies, including vasospasm secondary to mechanical trauma or release of vasoactive amines. Trauma may cause endothelial swelling or disruption leading to hemorrhage, platelet aggregation, and excitatory neurotransmitter release.[187]

Autoregulation and Spinal Cord Injury

Considerable evidence shows that the normal autoregulatory mechanisms of spinal cord blood flow are damaged in acute SCI.[171] Under normal circumstances, the spinal cord autoregulates blood flow within the range of 50 to 130 mm Hg, similar to the brain.[121, 139] With SCI and loss of autoregulation, the systemic blood pressure range becomes more important. Spinal cord blood flow becomes passively dependent on systemic arterial pressure.

Experimentally, posttraumatic spinal cord blood flow has been improved with various methods, alone or in combination, including dextran and hemodilution,[193] whole blood transfusion, adrenaline, calcium channel blockers,[80, 102] and steroids.[54, 205] Recent clinical data from the Maryland Shock Trauma Center suggests that early hemodynamic stabilization of acute spinal cord shock may improve neurologic function. Levi and colleagues recommend aggressive titration of the hemodynamic profile with fluids, dopamine, and/or dobutamine to maintain adequate cardiac output and mean blood pressure above 90 mm Hg.[131]

Biochemical Alterations

Electrolyte Changes

Traumatic injury causes ionic cellular fluxes. Intracellular Na^+ and Ca^{2+} levels increase, whereas extracellular K^+ rises, resulting in neuron depolarization and activation of ligand-gated ion channels primarily associated with excitatory amino acids.[149] There is evidence that intracellular Na^+ entry potentiates hypoxic-ischemic cell death by causing cytotoxic edema, intracellular acidosis, and gating of Ca^{2+} entry by reverse activation of the Na^+–Ca^{2+} exchanger.[2]

Calcium ions are widely acknowledged as universal regulators of intracellular function.[13, 15] SCI initiates a cascade of Ca^{2+}-mediated events that are deleterious to cell survival.[203] SCI is known to markedly increase the local excitatory amino acids glutamate and aspartate, which can result in increased intracellular calcium and formation of free radicals.[78, 155] Evidence supporting the detrimental role of calcium in SCI includes a rapid decrease in extracellular calcium concentration after injury[176] in combination with an increase in total calcium in the injured spinal cord segment.[203]

Calcium ions bind to mitochondrial membranes halting adenosine triphosphate (ATP) production and diverting mitochondrial electron transport to form oxygen free radicals.[34] The increased intracellular calcium activates calcium-dependent phospholipase A2, which incites the release of arachidonic acid from membrane phospholipids.[203] These free fatty acids may then form free radicals, which cause further cellular damage.[182] In addition, free fatty acids may be metabolized to form leukotrienes, thromboxanes, or prostaglandins. These substances in turn may directly destroy or destabilize cell membranes, mediate platelet aggregation, vasospasm, vasoconstriction, or lead to lysosomal enzyme release.[7, 34–36, 107, 109, 110]

Excitotoxicity

Cell injury mediated by the excitatory neurotransmitters glutamate and aspartate has been termed *excitotoxicity.*[7] The excitatory pathway is one of the most important mediators of neuronal cell death.[52] The importance of excitotoxicity as a significant mechanism of secondary injury after spinal cord trauma is suggested by various observations including increased excitatory amino acid concentrations in the extracellular tissues,[78, 155] spinal cord ischemia associated with excitotoxic phenomena in experimental models,[118] and the beneficial effects of receptor antagonist.[146, 147] Glutamate exerts its harmful effects through several receptors, the most important being the N-methyl-D-aspartate (NMDA) receptor. Activated receptors trigger an inward Ca^{2+} influx, which ultimately leads to neuronal death. Research aimed at blocking the secondary effects of glutamate toxicity has been directed toward pharmacologic blockade of the NMDA receptor. In 1988, Faden and Simon demonstrated the therapeutic effect of MK-801, an NMDA receptor blocker, on experimental SCI.[75] There appears to be strong evidence supporting the efficacy of excitotoxic blockade through both NMDA and non-NMDA receptors.[7, 52, 71, 75, 78, 155, 208]

Neurotransmitter Accumulation

Naloxone and thyrotropin-releasing hormone (TRH) are opiate receptor antagonists that have proven beneficial in the treatment of experimental SCI.[72, 73, 77] Naloxone has been shown to reverse the hypotension produced by cervical spinal cord transection,[115] suggesting a role of endogenous opioids in the secondary injury cascade. To support the role of opioid-mediated injury, large elevations in endogenous endorphins have been found in the plasma after experimental SCI.[77] Naloxone and TRH antagonists have been shown to improve posttraumatic spinal cord blood flow independent of the systemic vascular effects.[206] The results from studies conducted by Faden have implicated the endogenous opioid dynorphin A (1 to 17), the ligand for the kappa opioid receptor, as the opioid most likely to be involved in SCI.[70] This is supported by the findings of selectively increased dynorphin immunoreactivity immediately after injury in direct proportion to the severity of injury.[74] Kappa opioid receptors have been shown to increase in a time-dependent manner with spinal trauma, and antagonists selective for the kappa receptors have shown the most promise in treating experimental SCI.[18, 128] Although considerable evidence points to an opioid-mediated component to SCI, clinical trials comparing naloxone, methylprednisolone, and placebo demonstrated no significant improvements in neurologic function in the naloxone-treated group.[31]

Lipid Peroxidation and Free Radical Formation

A growing body of evidence suggests that oxygen free radical formation and lipid peroxidation likely enhance adverse mechanisms of neuronal injury, such as spinal cord hypoperfusion, formation of edema, axonal conduction failure, and breakdown of energy metabolism.[106] Free radicals are molecules that have unpaired electrons in their outer orbits that predispose to increased reactivity and may propagate via chain reactions. Experimental studies suggest that oxygen free radicals and lipid peroxidation play key roles in posttraumatic damage of brain and spinal cord tissue.[32, 58, 109, 153] Early investigators postulated that CNS tissue is particularly susceptible to free radical damage because of its high concentration of polyunsaturated fatty acids and cholesterol.[58, 153] Oxygen free radicals are generated by many sources, including mitochondria, auto-oxidation of catecholamines, conversion of xanthine oxidase, production by activated neutrophils, activation of the arachidonic acid cascade, and the iron-catalyzed Haber–Weiss reaction.[144] Free radical–mediated injury occurs through disruption of cell and mitochondrial membranes, denaturation of proteins, and breakdown of DNA.[172] A significant mechanism of injury appears to be related to cellular swelling, with resulting edema characterized by increased water and sodium and reduced potassium in the affected CNS tissue. Separately, oxygen radicals appear to produce lesions of the vascular endothelium and a breakdown of the blood-brain barrier, resulting in vasogenic edema and impaired electrolyte and water homeostasis in CNS tissue.[195] The importance of free radicals and lipid peroxidation in SCI is supported by numerous studies demonstrating the potential neuroprotective efficacy of pharmacologic agents with antioxidant properties.[8, 9, 30, 31, 36, 51, 54, 87, 88, 106, 107, 109, 110, 182, 205]

Immune Response

Trauma-induced CNS inflammation occurs rapidly at the site of injury and involves the activation of resident and recruited immune cells.[22] Popovich and colleagues described the morphologic inflammatory cellular response to SCI in a rat model. Peak microglial activation was observed within the lesion epicenter between 3 and 7 days postinjury, preceding the bulk of monocyte influx and macrophage activation occurring 7 days postinjury. Rostral and caudal to the injury site, microglial activation plateaued between 2 and 4 weeks postinjury in the dorsal and lateral funiculi. T lymphocytes maximally infiltrated the lesion epicenter between 3 and 7 days postinjury. Reactive astrocytes, although present in the acute lesion, were more prominent later (7 to 28 days). These cells were interspersed with activated microglia but appeared to surround and enclose tissue sites occupied by reactive microglia and phagocytic macrophages.[158] Trauma-induced local expression of TGF-beta 1 within the CNS parenchyma can enhance immune cell infiltration and intensify the CNS impairment resulting from peripherally triggered autoimmune responses.[200]

Energy Metabolism

Injury to CNS tissue creates a significant energy demand on cells attempting to regulate normal ionic balance.[116] Coupled with decreased regional blood flow and disruption of normal oxidative metabolism, acute injury demands are met with hyperglycolysis, which leads to the accumulation of lactic acid and acidosis.[5, 6] SCI is followed by a decrease in tissue oxygen tension that may last for hours.[66, 177] Increased glucose use in the early period after SCI have been attributed to enhanced glycolysis and continued delivery of blood and glucose to an ischemic environment.[160] ATP stores are depleted in the hypoxic environment, leading to inactivation of calcium-dependent ATPase and the sodium/potassium ATPase. This may precipitate cellular membrane depolarization and uncontrolled influx of calcium ions.[207]

Apoptosis

Apoptosis is a mechanism of cell death characterized by nuclear fragmentation and histologic appearance of apoptotic bodies, seen as small balls of basophilic material within the nucleus or as similar balls extruded from the cell within blebs of cytoplasm.[199] Apoptosis is activated by a genetic program. In contrast to necrotic cell death, apoptosis results in cellular shrinkage and eventual phagocytosis by macrophages. Classically, necrosis is characterized by cell swelling and nuclear shrinkage without apoptotic bodies. Cells undergoing necrosis release chemicals that injure surrounding tissue and produce an inflammatory response typified by polymorphonuclear cells.[163] Experimental evidence supports both a necrotic pathway and an apoptotic pathway of final cell death in brain and SCI.[55, 137]

THERAPIES FOR ACUTE SPINAL CORD INJURY

Current progress in SCI research can be traced back to the original experiments described by Allen in 1911.[4] His model of a cord contusion injury has given rise to an array of different experimental techniques that have not always led to similar findings.[12] Early therapies were surgical in nature. Allen first described myelotomy for intramedullary hematoma expression and described the histopathology of cord injury.[3]

Hypothermia, a technique to decrease cerebral metabolic demand and reduce swelling, gained favor in the 1960s for SCI but was eventually abandoned for reasons of technical implementation.[164] Recent experimental studies have sparked a resurgent interest in cooling to treat traumatic brain injury. In animal models of brain injury, moderate hypothermia has been reported to attenuate neurologic motor dysfunction, decrease histopathologic damage and neuronal cell loss, attenuate cerebral edema and blood-brain barrier disruption, and reduce mortality.[145] Preliminary results from clinical trials suggest that this treatment improves outcome and decreases mortality in head-injured patients.[140] Although therapeutic hypothermia for traumatic brain injury is enjoying a comeback, whether it is effective and feasible for SCI remains unclear.

Surgical Decompression and Stabilization

The goal of treatment for any spinal injury must be to arrive at an anatomically reconstructed spine that will allow patient mobilization and support neurologic recovery. There is little controversy over the benefits of spinal cord decompression. Recovery in functional long-tract motor capacity has been described after anterior decompression surgery performed more than 1 year after injury.[25] Modern surgical techniques using both anterior and posterior approaches have been described for various spinal injury patterns, making comparative analysis of one particular approach difficult.[79, 91, 111, 165] The surgical approach to the spine should be dictated by the specific injury pattern. In many circumstances, realignment of the spinal canal is the most efficacious means of spinal cord decompression. Laminectomies without instrumented fusion have no place in modern treatment schemes of SCI.[26] Although many spinal injuries present with complex injury patterns, timely attention to spinal column realignment and decompression through either manual closed methods or open surgical decompression plays a role in the recovery of neurologic deficits.[1]

Timing of Spinal Cord Decompression

Experimental studies support a time-dependent course of events starting with the initial spinal cord impact.[64, 103, 124, 183, 184] Besides the duration of cord compression, impact velocity and displacement also determine the extent of injury.[12] Tarlov, in the 1950s, showed that duration of compression was an important factor in determining final neurologic outcome. Using a balloon compression model with increasing inflation and duration, he observed recovery after 1 hour in the medium balloons but only after 5 minutes in the large balloons.[183, 184] Kobrine observed that acute balloon compression in the thoracic spine of monkeys resulted in somatosensory evoked potential recovery only in those animals decompressed within 1 minute.[124] Guha and coauthors evaluated the interaction between graded clip compression strengths of 2.3, 16.9, and 53.0 g and increasing sustained compression times of 15, 60, 120, and 240 minutes in rats. They observed that duration of compression was a significant determinant of neurologic recovery, but only with clips of lower force. Based on this finding, they suggested that enhanced neurologic recovery may be realized by early decompression in patients with incomplete injuries, whereas little may be gained from early decompression in patients with complete injuries (more severe primary trauma).[103] Nystrom and Berglund also found that recovery varied directly with duration of compression in a static weight compression model, although the maximum compression times (19 minutes) were too short to be clinically applicable.[151]

Carlson and coworkers demonstrated a time-dependent window of opportunity for evoked potential recovery with early spinal cord decompression using a consistent SCI model that characterized both the dynamic and sustained compression phases of injury.[49] Increasing duration of spinal cord compression resulted in greater histopathologic lesion volume and diminished motor recovery 4 weeks after injury (Fig. 10–6).[47] Although mechanical factors differ between models, these studies suggest that final neurologic function is not only a result of the initial impaction forces of injury, but also a combination of these forces with secondary time-dependent events that follow shortly after initial impact.

The surgical treatment of SCI continues to evolve as a result of better pathophysiologic understanding of cord injury, improved surgical techniques, and advancements in neuroradiographic imaging such as MRI.[190a] Techniques including laminectomy with or without myelotomy and cord cooling have been tried with limited success. Clinical experience has demonstrated that laminectomy without

stabilization for acute cord injury did not improve neural function and in many circumstances led to increased spinal instability and late diminished neural function.[23, 24]

The clinical efficacy of early spinal surgery has been hotly debated. The results of early postinjury surgery in 1975 were such that Heiden wrote, "surgery during the first seven days following cervical cord injury is associated with a significant increase in morbidity and should be avoided."[113] In the 1970s, he felt that the only indication for early surgery was progressive neurologic deterioration, which occurred in less that 5% of patients after arrival to the hospital.[89, 113]

In a prospective randomized study of 283 patients with SCI, Marshall and coauthors identified 14 patients who deteriorated neurologically after hospitalization. A specific management event was associated with neurologic decline in 12 of the 14 patients. Cervical spine surgery performed within 5 days after injury was associated with neurologic deterioration in three patients with cervical injuries. In comparison, no deterioration in neurologic function was noted in patients who underwent surgery 6 or more days after injury. This led the authors to recommend avoidance of early surgery in patients with cervical cord injury, except in the incomplete patient with progressive neurologic deterioration.[141]

Levi and coworkers reviewed 103 consecutive patients with cervical spinal cord trauma who underwent anterior decompression and stabilization during a 5-year period at the Maryland Shock Trauma Center. Comparisons were made between early surgery (less than 24 hours after injury) and delayed surgery (more than 24 hours after injury). Although no statistical differences in the level of functional motor recovery between early and delayed surgery were seen in the patients who presented complete, early surgery resulted in faster mobilization and less intensive respiratory physiotherapy, which translated into shorter hospitalizations and rehabilitation time.[132] Although not statistically significant, one 19-year-old patient in the series who presented as a C5 complete tetraplegic recovered ambulatory function after early decompression.

In an effort to determine the effect of timing of stabilization on length of stay and medical complications, Campagnolo and coauthors reviewed 38 cervical spine–injured patients split equally between complete and incomplete injury. They noted significantly lower hospitalization times without increased complications in the early stabilized groups (<24 hours), leading them to conclude that active rehabilitation within the first 2 weeks after SCI is critical in reducing complications of long-term immobilization.[45] Similar findings were observed by Mirza et al. for patients stabilized within 72 hours of injury.[148a]

In a review of 38 patients with acute cervical SCIs treated with surgical stabilization, Krengel and coauthors reported greater improvement in Frankel grade (one level per patient vs. one-half level per patient) in patients treated within 72 hours of injury. Although the study was limited in patient numbers, they noted fewer pulmonary complications and a trend toward shorter hospitalizations and mechanical ventilation in those patients treated early. Similar findings were noted by Schlegel and colleagues, after review of 138 patients surgically treated for cervical spine injury. In those

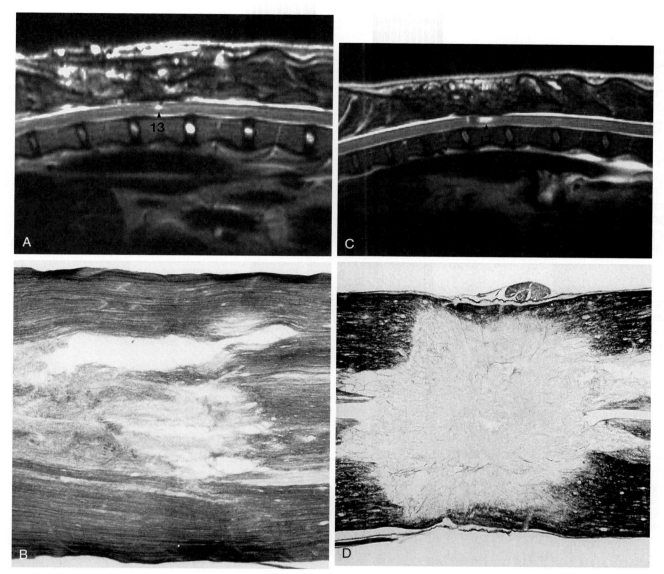

Figure 10–6. *Progressive neurologic damage caused by sustained spinal cord displacement. A, Sagittal MRI of T2 through T13 injury section taken 4 weeks after experimental cord injury (30 minutes of sustained displacement). B, Longitudinal histologic sections with luxol fast blue stain for myelin in same specimen (30 minutes of sustained compression). Note the cavitary changes in the gray matter. Early decompression was associated with recovery to almost completely normal gait pattern within 4 weeks after injury. C, Sagittal MRI of T2 through T13 injury segment taken after 3-hour sustained compression. Note the high signal lesion extending from the gray matter into the white matter. D, Histology section through the same region after 3 hours of sustained compression. There is significantly greater lesional volume and damage to surrounding myelinated tracts. This animal never regained significant ambulatory function 4 weeks after experimental injury.*

patients with neurologic injury, operative treatment within 72 hours of injury greatly reduced medical complications and morbidity. However, timing of surgery did not affect the functional neurologic recovery.[170]

The clinical question of whether earlier spinal decompression and stabilization can improve long-tract function still remains to be definitively answered. Clinical and laboratory studies suggest a window of opportunity for treatment in the hours immediately following spinal trauma.[31, 47, 49, 57] Early reduction is supported by Aebi and colleagues, who reported on 100 cervical spinal injuries. Overall, only 31% of patients showed neurologic improve-

ment after manual or surgical reduction in long-term follow-up of more than 1 year. Of those who improved, 75% were reduced within the first 6 hours after the accident, whereas 85% of the remaining 69 patients without neurologic recovery were reduced later than 6 hours after injury.[1]

The neuroprotective effects of early pharmacotherapy have been well documented. The second National Acute Spinal Cord Injury Study (NASCIS-2) demonstrated that the highest proportion of all neurologic recovery is associated with pharmacotherapy administered within the first 8 hours after injury.[28] Further study of the initial 8-hour window after injury demonstrated that steroid pharmaco-therapy administered within the first 3 hours after injury was more efficacious than that initiated 3 to 8 hours after injury.[29] These studies strongly support the earliest possible initiation of both pharmacotherapy and spinal realignment and/or decompression for maximal neurologic recovery.

Pharmacotherapy

The goals of SCI treatment include preservation of intact neurons, restoration of injured but surviving cells to optimal function, and regeneration of new neural connecting tissue. Improved understanding of the complex pathophysiology initiated by SCI has led to the testing of numerous pharmacotherapies aimed at modifying the secondary injury cycle. Clinical trials with methylprednisolone suggest that future treatments aimed at neuroprotection will involve combinations of drugs that target certain damaging processes in the cycle.[29]

Pharmacotherapy may have a therapeutic role in three stages of SCI.[98, 99] In the acute stage, methylprednisolone or other drugs aimed at decreasing the immune or inflammatory response administered early after injury will limit secondary mechanisms of injury.[31] In the subacute stage, neuroregenerative or neurotrophic therapies may help reconstitute the damaged tissue.[93, 94] Interventions in the

chronic stage of SCI will more than likely involve neurotrophic substances in combination with some neural tissue or mesenchymal stem cell transplantation.[37–39, 60, 61]

A better understanding of the bioreactive mechanisms of injury after CNS trauma have led to numerous potential treatments including corticosteroids, antioxidants or free radical scavengers, drugs that modify arachidonic acid metabolism, platelet-activating factor antagonists, gangliosides, modulators of monoamine actions, opioid receptor antagonists, thyrotropin-releasing hormone and thyrotropin-releasing hormone analogues, glutamase receptor antagonists, calcium channel blockers, agents that modify the inflammatory/immune response and trophic factors (Fig. 10–7).[76]

Methylprednisolone, a glucocorticoid, is the first pharmacologic agent proven to alter the neurologic outcome in randomized clinical trials comparing methylprednisolone, naloxone, and placebo. In the NASCIS-2 trial, the methyl-prednisolone group (30 mg/kg IV bolus and 5.4 mg/kg/hr for 23 hours) showed improved neurologic outcome only if administered within 8 hours of injury. Unfortunately, significant functional motor improvement was minimal. Corticosteroids have been shown to improve neural recovery through a combination of mechanisms.[7, 17, 21, 28–33, 35, 36, 51, 54, 58, 76, 87, 88, 106–110, 125, 150, 172, 195, 202, 205] Serum cortisol decreases in the first 24 hours after SCI.[56] Corticosteroids

STRATEGIES FOR NEURONAL PROTECTION

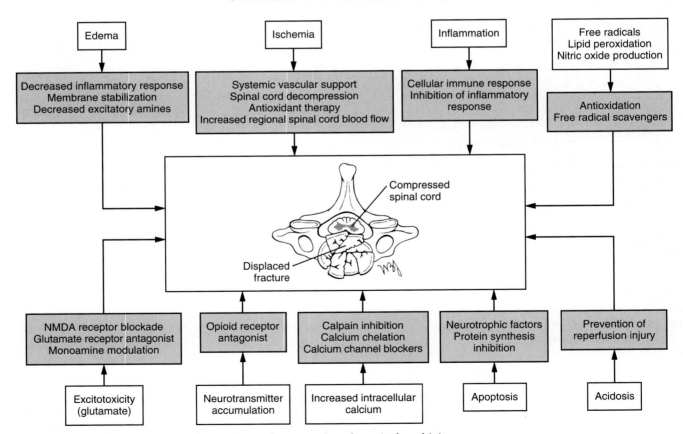

Figure 10–7. Strategies for neuronal protection and regeneration after spinal cord injury.

aid in normal homeostasis of plasma glucose and electrolytes.[135] Membrane stabilization and prevention of lipid peroxidation may be one of the most important mechanisms of corticosteroid neuroprotection.[106, 109] Steroids have strong anti-inflammatory properties and may decrease spinal cord edema.[135] Methylprednisolone administered in animals has been associated with a reduction in the zone of injury and improved axonal conduction.[150] Neuroprotective effects include preservation of vascular and cellular membranes through potentiation of free oxygen radical scavengers and stabilization of white matter in hemorrhagic lesions.[7]

The NASCIS-1 trial demonstrated significant side effects with the administration of high-dose (1000 mg/day) steroids for 10-day courses.[27] These effects include wound infections and gastic ulcers. Other reports cite increased hospital stays and increased risk of pneumonia for patients receiving high-dose steroids.[90] Tirilazad, a synthetic 21-aminosteroid developed as a powerful lipid peroxidation inhibitor, has been advocated as an alternative to glucocorticoid treatment. Experimental studies using tirilazad have demonstrated cell membrane stabilization and improved posttraumatic spinal cord blood flow by inhibiting oxygen radical microvascular lipid peroxidation and attenuating the injury-stimulated decline in tissue concentrations of vitamin E, a natural antioxidant.[33, 36, 88, 107, 108, 110] Animals treated with tirilazad have demonstrated neurologic recovery after injury.[8, 9, 87] The NASCIS-3 clinical trials compared the efficacy of methylprednisolone administered for 24 hours with methylprednisolone administered for 48 hours or tirilazad mesylate administered for 48 hours in patients with acute SCI. The trials showed that patients treated with methylprednisolone for 48 hours had improved motor recovery at 6 weeks ($p = 0.09$) and 6 months ($p = 0.07$) after injury. Although the tirilazad group tended to have fewer complications, these differences were small, and the neurologic motor recovery of these patients did not match that of patients who received 48 hours of methylprednisolone.[29] The NASCIS-3 study underscores the benefits of early treatment after acute injury. Improved neurologic recovery was demonstrated when methylprednisolone maintenance dosing was extended to 48 hours in patients treated 3 to 8 hours after injury.[29]

Gangliosides are complex acidic glycolipids that form a major component of the cell membrane. They are present in high concentrations in the cells of the CNS, located primarily in the outer leaflet of bilayer cell membranes.[130] They are thought to induce neuronal regeneration of neurons and restore function after injury.[201] In vitro studies have demonstrated that GM-1 ganglioside protects against excitatory amino acid–related neurotoxicity. In animal models, GM-1 ganglioside appears to reduce acute nerve cell damage and aid functional recovery following trauma.[173]

A small (34 patients), prospective, randomized, double-blind trial of GM-1 ganglioside demonstrated neurologic improvement in patients up to 1 year after the initial injury. Thirty-four patients were given either 100 mg of GM-1 ganglioside intravenously per day for 18 to 32 days or placebo. Treatment was initiated within 72 hours of initial injury.[93] A larger randomized multicenter trial is currently being concluded in the United States.[96] The concurrent use of methylprednisolone with GM-1 ganglioside is controversial. GM-1 ganglioside may counteract some of the desirable anti-inflammatory properties of methylprednisolone.[29] GM-1 modulates protein kinase activity, which inhibits lipocortins, substances responsible for the anti-inflammatory effects of glucocorticoids.[208]

Faden and colleagues demonstrated that spinal cord ischemia was associated with increased levels of plasma endorphins, which can be blocked with naloxone, an opiate receptor antagonist.[73] Various investigators have demonstrated potential benefits of naloxone in SCI.[72, 74, 77, 84] However, in human trials (i.e., NASCIS-2), naloxone did not show significant benefits.[31] Thyrotropin-releasing hormone, initially hypothesized to act as a physiologic opiate antagonist, has demonstrated neuroprotective benefits in models of SCI.[73, 181] A small clinical trial with TRH did not appear to have significant neuroprotective effects in patients with complete neurologic injuries; however, the study group was too small to make conclusive determinations of efficacy, suggesting the need for more study.[157] Because the effective half-life of TRH is short, later studies have focused on synthetic analogs with longer effective durations of action.[18, 69]

FUTURE DIRECTIONS

Experimental studies continue to provide a better understanding of the complex interaction of pathophysiologic events immediately following traumatic SCI. Clinical and experimental studies have determined that earlier intervention in the form of spinal cord decompression/stabilization and neuroprotective pharmacotherapy is efficacious in decreasing neurologic damage. Future pharmacologic approaches will be aimed at modifying the delayed injury response by blocking one or more components of the reactive biochemical and metabolic cascade. As the mechanisms of action of the neurotrophic compounds become better understood, treatment strategies can be developed to encourage regeneration of the injured CNS.

REFERENCES

1. Aebi M, Mohler J, Zach GA, Morscher E: Indication, surgical technique, and results of 100 surgically treated fractures and fracture-dislocations of the cervical spine. Clin Orthop 203:244–257, 1986.
2. Agrawal SK, Fehlings MG: Mechanisms of secondary injury to spinal cord axons in vitro: Role of Na, Na-K-ATPase, the Na-H exchanger, and the Na-Ca exchanger. J Neurosci 16:545–552, 1996.
3. Allen A: Remarks on the histopathological changes in the spinal cord due to impact: An experimental study. J Nerv Ment Dis 41:141–147, 1914.
4. Allen AR: Surgery of experimental lesion of spinal cord equivalent to crush injury of fracture dislocation of spinal column: a preliminary report. JAMA 57:878–880, 1911.
5. Anderson D, Means E, Waters T, Spears C: Spinal cord

energy metabolism following compression trauma to the feline spinal cord. J Neurosurg 53:375–380, 1980.

6. Anderson D, Prockop L, Means E, Hartley L: Cerebrospinal fluid lactate and electrolyte levels following experimental spinal cord injury. J Neurosurg 44:715–722, 1976.

7. Anderson DK: Chemical and cellular mediators in spinal cord injury. J Neurotrauma 9:143–145, 1992.

8. Anderson DK, Braughler JM, Hall ED, et al: Effects of treatment with U-74006F on neurological outcome following experimental spinal cord injury. J Neurosurg 69:562–567, 1988.

9. Anderson DK, Hall ED, Braughler JM, et al: Effect of delayed administration of U74006F on recovery of locomotor function after experimental spinal cord injury. J Neurotrauma 8:187–192, 1991.

10. Anderson L, D'Alonzo R: Fractures of the odontoid process of the axis. J Bone Joint Surg Am 56A:1663–1674, 1974.

11. Anderson PA, Bohlman HH: Anterior decompression and arthrodesis of the cervical spine: Long-term motor improvement. Part II: Improvement in complete traumatic quadriplegia. J Bone Joint Surg Am 74A:683–692, 1992.

12. Anderson TE, Stokes BT: Experimental models for spinal cord injury research: Physical and physiological considerations. J Neurotrauma 9:S135–142, 1992.

13. Balentine J, Spector M: Calcifications of axons in experimental spinal cord trauma. Ann Neurol 2:520–523, 1977.

14. Balentine JD: Pathology of experimental spinal cord trauma: ultrastructure of axons and myelin. Lab Invest 39:254–266, 1978.

15. Balentine JD, Hilton CW: Ultrastructural pathology of axons and myelin in calcium-induced myelopathy. J Neuropathol Exp Neurol 39:339, 1980.

16. Banik N: Pathogenesis of myelin breakdown in demyelinating diseases: Role of proteolytic enzymes. J Crit Rev Neurobiol 6:257–271, 1992.

17. Barut S, Canbolat A, Bilge T, et al: Lipid peroxidation in experimental spinal cord injury: Time–level relationship. Neurosurg Rev 16:53–59, 1993.

18. Behrmann D, Bresnahan J, Beattie M: A comparison of YM-146743, U-50488H, and nalmefene after spinal cord injury in the rat. Exp Neurol 119:258–267, 1993.

19. Bentley G, McSweeney T: Multiple spinal injuries. Br J Surg 55:565–570, 1968.

20. Benzel EC, Larson SJ: Recovery of nerve root function after complete quadriplegia from cervical spine fractures. Neurosurgery 19:809–812, 1986.

21. Black P, Markowitz RS: Experimental spinal cord injury in monkeys: Comparison of steroids and local hypothermia. Surg Forum 22:409, 1971.

22. Blight A: Delayed demyelination and macrophage invasion: A candidate for secondary cell damage in spinal cord injury. CNS Trauma 2:299–315, 1985.

23. Bohlman H, Ducker T: Spine and spinal cord injury. In Herkowitz H, Garfin S, Balderston R, et al (eds): The Spine, 3rd ed. Philadelphia, WB Saunders, 1992, pp 973–1103.

24. Bohlman HH: Acute fractures and dislocations of the cervical spine: An analysis of three hundred hospitalized patients and a review of the literature. J Bone Joint Surg Am 61A:1119–1142, 1979.

25. Bohlman HH, Anderson PA: Anterior decompression and arthrodesis of the cervical spine: Long-term motor improvement. Part I—Improvement in incomplete traumatic quadriparesis. J Bone Joint Surg Am 74A:671–682, 1992.

26. Bohlman HH, Ducker T: Spine and spinal cord injuries. In Rothman RH, Simeone FA (eds): The Spine. Philadelphia, WB Saunders, 1992, pp 973–1104.

27. Bracken M, Collins W, Freeman D, et al: Efficacy of methylprednisolone in acute spinal cord injury. JAMA 251:45–52, 1984.

28. Bracken M, Holford T: Effects of timing of methylprednisolone or naloxone administration on recovery of segmental and long-tract neurologic function in NASCIS 2. J Neurosurg 79:500–507, 1993.

29. Bracken M, Shepard M, Holford T, et al: Administration of methylprednisolone for 24 or 48 hours or tirilazad mesylate for 48 hours in the treatment of acute spinal cord injury. JAMA 277:1597–1604, 1997.

30. Bracken MB: Treatment of acute spinal cord injury with methylprednisolone: Results of a multicenter, randomized clinical trial. J Neurotrauma 8:S47–51, 1991.

31. Bracken MB, Shepard MJ, Collins WF, et al: A randomized, controlled trial of methylprednisolone or naloxone in the treatment of acute spinal cord injury. N Engl J Med 322:1405–1411, 1990.

32. Braughler J, Hall E: Involvement of lipid peroxidation in CNS injury. J Neurotrauma 9(suppl):S1–S7, 1992.

33. Braughler JM, Chase RL, Neff GL, et al: A new 21-aminosteroid antioxidant lacking glucocorticoid activity stimulates adrenocorticotropin secretion and blocks arachidonic acid release from mouse pituitary tumor (AtT-20) cells. J Pharmacol Exp Ther 244:423–427, 1988.

34. Braughler JM, Duncan LA, Goodman T: Calcium enhances in vitro free radical-induced damage to brain synaptosomes, mitochondria, and cultured spinal cord neurons. J Neurochem 45:1288–1293, 1985.

35. Braughler JM, Hall ED, Means ED, et al: Evaluation of an intensive methylprednisolone sodium succinate dosing regimen in experimental spinal cord injury. J Neurosurg 67:102–105, 1987.

36. Braughler JM, Pregenzer JF, Chase RL, et al: Novel 21-amino steroids as potent inhibitors of iron-dependent lipid peroxidation. J Biol Chem 262:10438–10440, 1987.

37. Bregman BS, Broude E, McAtee M, Kelley MS: Transplants and neurotrophic factors prevent atrophy of mature CNS neurons after spinal cord injury. Exp Neurol 149:13–27, 1998.

38. Bregman BS, Diener PS, McAtee M, et al: Intervention strategies to enhance anatomical plasticity and recovery of function after spinal cord injury. Adv Neurol 72:257–275, 1997.

39. Bregman BS, McAtee M, Dai HN, Kuhn PL: Neurotrophic factors increase axonal growth after spinal cord injury and transplantation in the adult rat. Exp Neurol 148:475–494, 1997.

40. Bresnahan J: An electron-microsopic analysis of axonal alterations following blunt contusion of the spinal cord of the rhesus monkey (Macaca mulatta). J Neurol Sci 37:59–82, 1978.

41. Bresnahan J, Beattie M, Todd F, Noyes D: A behavioral and anatomical analysis of spinal cord injury produced by a feedback-controlled impaction device. Exp Neurol 95:548–570, 1987.

42. Bresnahan J, King J, Martin G, et al: A neuroanatomical analysis of spinal cord injury in the rhesus monkey. J Neurol Sci 28:521–542, 1976.

43. Bunge RP, Puckett WR, Becerra JL, et al: Observations on the pathology of human spinal cord injury. A review and classification of 22 new cases with details from a case of chronic cord compression with extensive focal demyelination. Adv Neurol 59:75–89, 1993.

44. Calenoff L, Chessare JW, Rodgers LF, et al: Multiple level

spinal injuries: Importance of early recognition. AJR 130:665–669, 1978.

45. Campagnolo D, Esquieres R, Kopacz K: Effect of timing of stabilization on length of stay and medical complications following spinal cord injury. J Spinal Cord Med 20:331–334, 1997.

46. Carlson GD, Gorden CD, Nakazowa S, et al: Perfusion-limited recovery of evoked potential function after spinal cord injury. Spine 25:1218–1226, 2000.

47. Carlson G, Gorden C, Wada E, et al: Vascular re-perfusion and neural preservation after spinal cord injury. J Neurotrauma 15:860, 1998.

48. Carlson G, Heller J, Abitbol J, Garfin S: Odontoid fractures. In Levine A, Eismont F, Garfin S, Zigler J (eds): Spine Trauma. Philadelphia, WB Saunders, 1998.

49. Carlson GD, Minato Y, Okada A, et al: Early time-dependent decompression for spinal cord injury: Vascular mechanisms of recovery. J Neurotrauma 14:951–962, 1997.

50. Carlson GD, Warden KE, Barbeau JB, et al: Viscoelastic relaxation and regional blood flow response to spinal cord compression and decompression. Spine 22:1285–1291, 1997.

51. Chen A, Xu XM, Kleitman N, Bunge MB: Methylprednisolone administration improves exonal regeneration into Schwann cell grafts in transected adult rat thoracic spinal cord. Exp Neurol 138:261–276, 1996.

52. Choi D, Rothman S: The role of glutamate neurotoxicity in hypoxic-ischemic neuronal death. Annu Rev Neurosci 13:171–182, 1990.

53. Collins WF: Surgery in the acute treatment of spinal cord injury: A review of the past forty years. J Spinal Cord Med 18:3–8, 1995.

54. Constantini S, Young W: The effects of methylprednisolone and the ganglioside GM-1 on acute spinal cord injury in rats. J Neurosurg 80:97–111, 1994.

55. Crowe MJ, Bresnahan JC, Shuman S, et al: Apoptosis and delayed degeneration after spinal cord injury in rats and monkeys. Nat Med 3:73–76, 1997.

56. De La Torre JC: Spinal cord injury: Review of basic and applied research. Spine 6:315–335, 1981.

57. Delamarter RB, Sherman J, Carr JB: Pathophysiology of spinal cord injury. J Bone Joint Surg Am 77A:1042–1049, 1995.

58. Demopoulous H, Flamm E, Seligman M, Pietronigro D: Oxygen free radicals in central nervous system ischemia and trauma. In Autor AP (ed): Pathology of Oxygen. New York, Academic Press, 1982, pp 127–155.

59. DeVivo MJ, Rutt RD, Black KJ, et al: Trends in spinal cord injury demographics and treatment outcomes between 1973 and 1986. Arch Phys Med Rehabil 73:424–430, 1992.

60. Diener PS, Bregman BS: Fetal spinal cord transplants support growth of supraspinal and segmental projections after cervical spinal cord hemisection in the neonatal rat. J Neurosci 18:779–793, 1998.

61. Diener PS, Bregman BS: Fetal spinal cord transplants support the development of target reaching and coordinated postural adjustments after neonatal cervical spinal cord injury. J Neurosci 18:763–778, 1998.

62. Dohrman G, Wagner FJ, Bucy P: The microvasculature in transitory traumatic paraplegia. An electron microscopic study of the monkey. J Neurosurg 35:263–271, 1971.

63. Dohrman G, Wagner FJ, Bucy P: Transitory traumatic paraplegia: Electron microscopy of early alterations in myelinated nerve fibers. J Neurosurg 36:407–415, 1972.

64. Dolan EJ, Tator CH, Endrenyi L: The value of decompression for acute experimental spinal cord compression injury. J Neurosurg 53:749–755, 1980.

65. Ducker T: Experimental injury of the spinal cord. In Vinken P, Bruyn GW (eds): Handbook of Clinical Neurology. New York, Elsevier, 1976, pp 9–26.

66. Ducker T, Saleman M, Perot P, et al: Experimental spinal cord trauma: I. Correlation of blood flow, tissue oxygen and neurologic status in the dog. Surg Neurol 10:60–63, 1978.

67. Ducker TB, Kindt GW, Kempe LG: Pathological findings in acute experimental spinal cord trauma. J Neurosurg 35:700–708, 1971.

68. Eismont FJ, Arena MJ, Green BA: Extrusion of an intervertebral disc associated with traumatic subluxation or dislocation of cervical facets. Case report. J Bone Joint Surg Am 73A:1555–1560, 1991.

69. Faden A: TRH analog YM-14673 improves outcome following traumatic brain and spinal cord injury in rats: Dose-response studies. Brain Res 486:228–235, 1989.

70. Faden A: Opioid and nonopioid actions mechanisms may contribute to dynorphin's pathophysiological actions in spinal cord injury. Ann Neurol 27:67–74, 1990.

71. Faden A, Demediuk P, Panter S, et al: The role of excitatory amino acids and NMDA receptors in traumatic brain injury. Science 244:798–800, 1989.

72. Faden A, Jacobs P, Holaday J: Opiate antagonist improves neurologic recovery after spinal injury. Science 211:493–494, 1981.

73. Faden A, Jacobs T, Holaday J: Thyrotropin-releasing hormone improves neurologic recovery after spinal trauma in cats. N Engl J Med 305:1063–1067, 1981.

74. Faden A, Molineaux C, Rosenberger J, et al: Endogenous opioid immunoreactivity in rat spinal cord following traumatic injury. Ann Neurol 17:386–390, 1985.

75. Faden A, Simon R: A potential role for excitotoxins in the pathophysiology of spinal cord injury. Ann Neurol 23:623–626, 1988.

76. Faden AI: Pharmacological treatment of central nervous system trauma. Pharmacol Toxicol 78:12–17, 1996.

77. Faden AI, Jacobs TP, Mougey E, Holaday JW: Endorphins in experimental spinal injury: Therapeutic effect of naloxone. Ann Neurol 10:326–332, 1981.

78. Farooque M, Hillered L, Holtz A, Olsson Y: Changes of extracellular levels of amino acids after graded compression trauma to the spinal cord: An experimental study in the rat using microdialysis. J Neurotrauma 13:537–548, 1996.

79. Fehlings M, Cooper P, Errico T: Posterior plates in the managment of posterior instability: Long-term results in 44 patients. J Neurosurg 81:341–349, 1994.

80. Fehlings M, Tator C, Linden R: The relationships among the severity of spinal cord injury, motor and somatosensory evoked potentials and spinal cord blood flow. Electroencephalogr Clin Neurophysiol 74:241–259, 1989.

81. Fehlings MG, Louw D: Initial stabilization and medical management of acute spinal cord injury. Am Fam Physician 54:155–162, 1996.

82. Felsberg GJ, Tien RD, Osumi AK, Cardenas CA: Utility of MR imaging in pediatric spinal cord injury. Pediatr Radiol 25:131–135, 1995.

83. Fine PR, Kuhlemeier KV, DeVivo MJ, Stover SL: Spinal cord injury: an epidemiologic perspective. Paraplegia 17:237–250, 1980.

84. Flamm E, Young W, Demopulus H, et al: Experimental spinal cord injury: Treatment with naloxone. Neurosurgery 10:227–231, 1982.

85. Flanders AE, Schaefer DM, Doan HT, et al: Acute cervical spine trauma: Correlation of MR imaging findings with degree of neurologic deficit. Radiology 177:25–33, 1990.

86. Folman Y, el Masri W: Spinal cord injury: Prognostic indicators. Injury 20:92–93, 1989.

87. Fowl RJ, Patterson RB, Gewirtz RJ, Anderson DK: Protection against postischemic spinal cord injury using a new 21-aminosteroid. J Surg Res 48:597–600, 1990.

88. Francel PC, Long BA, Malik JM, et al: Limiting ischemic spinal cord injury using a free radical scavenger 21-aminosteroid and/or cerebral spinal fluid drainage. J Neurosurg 79:742–751, 1993.

89. Frankel HL, Hancock DO, Hyslop G, et al: The value of postural reduction in the initial management of closed injuries of the spine with paraplegia and tetraplegia. Paraplegia 7:179–192, 1969.

90. Galandiuk S, Raque G, Appel S, Polk HJ: The two-edged sword of large-dose steroids for spinal cord trauma. Ann Surg 218:419–425, 1993.

91. Garvey T, Eismont F, Roberti L: Anterior decompression, structural bone grafting, and Caspar plate stabilization for unstable cervical spine fractures and/or dislocations. Spine 17(suppl):S431–S435, 1997.

92. Gehweiler J, Osborne R, Becker, R: The Radiology of Vertebral Trauma. Philadelphia, WB Saunders, 1980.

93. Geisler FH, Dorsey FC, Coleman WP: Recovery of motor function after spinal cord injury—A randomized placebo-controlled trial with GM-1 ganglioside. New Engl J Med 324:1829–1838, 1991.

94. Geisler FH, Dorsey FC, Coleman WP: GM-1 ganglioside in human spinal cord injury. J Neurotrauma 9:S517–S530, 1992.

95. Gertzbein S, Count-Brown C: Flexion-distraction injuries of the lumbar spine. Clin Orthop 1988;227:50–52.

96. Giesler F: National Neurotrauma Sixteenth Annual Meeting, Los Angeles, CA, 1998.

97. Green BA, Callahan RA, Kose KJ, De La Torre J: Acute spinal cord injury: Current concepts. Clin Orthop 154:125–135, 1981.

98. Greene KA, Marciano FF, Sonntag VKH: Pharmacological strategies in the treatment of spinal cord injuries: A critical review. Crit Rev Neurosurg 4:254–264, 1994.

99. Greene KA, Marciano FF, Sonntag VKH: Pharmacological management of spinal cord injury: Current status of drugs designed to augment functional recovery of the injured human spinal cord. J Spinal Disord 9:355–366, 1996.

100. Griffiths I, Trench J, Crawford R: Spinal cord blood flow and conduction during experimental cord compression in normotensive and hypotensive dogs. J Neurosurg 1979;50:353–360.

101. Guha A, Tator C: Acute cardiovascular effects of experimental spinal cord injury. J Trauma 28:481–490, 1988.

102. Guha A, Tator C, Smith C, Piper I: Improvement in posttraumatic spinal cord blood flow with a combination of a calcium channel blocker and a vasopressor. J Trauma 29:1440–1447, 1989.

103. Guha A, Tator CH, Endrenyi L, Piper I: Decompression of the spinal cord improves recovery after acute experimental spinal cord compression injury. Paraplegia 25:324–339, 1987.

104. Guin P: Standardized nursing care plans for acute care SCI: improved documentation. SCI Nurs 7:4–7, 1990.

105. Hackney DB, Finkelstein SD, Hand CM, et al: Postmortem magnetic resonance imaging of experimental spinal cord injury: Magnetic resonance finding versus in vivo functional deficit. Neurosurgery 35:1104–1111, 1994.

106. Hall E, Braughler J: Free radicals in CNS injury. Res Publ Assoc Res Nerv Ment Dis 71:81–105, 1993.

107. Hall ED: Effects of the 21-aminosteroid U74006F on post-traumatic spinal cord ischemia in cats. J Neurosurg 68:462–465, 1988.

108. Hall ED, McCall JM, Chase RL, et al: A nonglucocorticoid steroid analog of methylprednisolone duplicates its high-dose pharmacology in models of central nervous system trauma and neuronal membrane damage. J Pharmacol Exp Ther 242:137–142, 1987.

109. Hall ED, Yonkers PA, Andrus PK, et al: Biochemistry and pharmacology of lipid antioxidants in acute brain and spinal cord injury. J Neurotrauma 9:S425–S442, 1992.

110. Hall ED, Yonkers PA, Horan KL, Braughler JM: Correlation between attenuation of posttraumatic spinal cord ischemia and preservation of tissue vitamin E by the 21-aminosteroid U74006F: Evidence for an in vivo antioxidant mechanism. J Neurotrauma 6:169–176, 1989.

111. Hamilton A, Webb J: The role of anterior surgery for vertebral fractures with and without cord compression. Clin Orthop 300:79–89, 1994.

112. Harvey C, Wilson SE, Greene CG, et al: New estimates of the direct costs of traumatic spinal cord injuries: Results of a nationwide survey. Paraplegia 30:834–850, 1992.

113. Heiden JS, Weiss MH, Rosenberg AW, et al: Management of cervical spine cord trauma in Southern California. J Neurosurg 43:732–736, 1975.

114. Hixon AK: Implementation of standards of practice: A spinal cord injury program. ACI Nurs 7:8–11, 1990.

115. Holaday J, Faden A: Naloxone acts at central opiate receptors to reverse hypotension, hypothermia and hypoventilation in spinal shock. Brain Res 189:295–299, 1980.

116. Hovda DA, Becker DP, Katayama Y: Secondary injury and acidosis. J Neurotrama 9:S47–S60, 1992.

117. Huang PA, Young W: The effects of arterial blood gas values on lesion volumes in a graded rat spinal cord contusion model. J Neurotrauma 11:547–562, 1994.

118. Jorgensen M, Diemer N: Selective neuron loss after cerebral ischemia in the rat: Possible role of transmitter glutamate. Acta Neurol Scand 79:536–546, 1982.

119. Kalnbeek WD, McLaurin RL, Harris BSH, Miller JD: The national head and spinal cord injury survey: Major findings. J Neurosurg 53:S19–S31, 1980.

120. Kearney P, Ridella S, Viano D, Anderson T: Interaction of contact velocity and cord compression in determining severity of spinal cord injury. J Neurotrauma 5:187–208, 1988.

121. Kobrine A, Doyle T, Martins A: Autoregulation of spinal cord blood flow. Clin Neurosurg 22:573–581, 1975.

122. Kobrine A, Evans D, Rizzoli H: Correlation of spinal cord blood flow and function in experimental compression. Surg Neurol 9:54–59, 1978.

123. Kobrine AI, Doyle TF, Martins AN: Local spinal cord blood flow in experimental traumatic myelopathy. J Neurosurg 42:144–149, 1975.

124. Kobrine AI, Evans DE, Rizzoli HV: Experimental acute balloon compression of the spinal cord. Factors affecting disappearance and return of the spinal evoked response. J Neurosurg 51:841–845, 1979.

125. Koc RK, Akdemir H, Kurtsoy A, et al: Lipid peroxidation in experimental spinal cord injury. Comparison of treatment with Ginkgo biloba, TRH and methylprednisolone. Res Exp Med 195:117–123, 1995.

126. Kraus JF: A comparison of recent studies on the extent of the head and spinal cord injury problem in the United States. J Neurosurg 53:S35–S43, 1980.

127. Kraus JF, Franti CE, Riggins RS, et al: Incidence of traumatic spinal cord lesions. J Chron Dis 28:471–492, 1975.

128. Krumins S, Faden A: Traumatic injury alters opiate receptor binding in rat spinal cord. Ann Neurol 19:498–501, 1986.

129. Kurtzke JF: Epidemiology of spinal cord injury. Exp Neurol 48:163–236, 1975.

130. Ledeen RW: Ganglioside structures and distribution: Are they localized at the nerve ending? J Supramol Struct 8:1–17, 1978.

131. Levi L, Aizik W, Belzberg H: Hemodynamic parameters in patients with acute cervical cord trauma: Description, intervention, and prediction of outcome. Neurosurgery 33:1007–1016, 1993.

132. Levi L, Wolf A, Ragamonti D, et al: Anterior decompression in cervical spine trauma: Does the timing of surgery affect the outcome. J Neurosurg 29:216–222, 1991.

133. Levine A, Edwards C: The management of traumatic spondylolisthesis of the axis. J Bone Joint Surg Am 67A:217–226, 1985.

134. Levine A, Edwards C: Fractures of the atlas. J Bone Joint Surg Am 73A:680–691, 1991.

135. Lewin MG, Hansebout RR, Pappius HM: Chemical characteristics of spinal cord edema in cats: Effects of steroids on potassium depletion. J Neurosurg 40:65, 1974.

136. Liu X, Xu X, Hu R, et al: Neuronal and glial apoptosis after traumatic spinal cord injury. J Neurosci 17:5395–5406, 1997.

137. Ibid.

138. Lukacova N, Halat G, Chavko M, Marsala J: Ischemia-reperfusion injury in the spinal cord of rabbits strongly enhances lipid peroxidation and modifies phospholipid profiles. Neurochem Res 21:869–873, 1996.

139. Marcus M, Heistad D, Ehrhardt J, et al: Regulation of total and regional spinal cord blood flow. Circ Res 41:128–134, 1977.

140. Marion D, White M: Treatment of traumatic brain injury with moderate hypothermia. N Engl J Med 336:540–546, 1997.

141. Marshall L, Knowlton S, Garfin S, et al: Deterioration following spinal cord injury: A multicenter study. J Neurosurg 66:400–404, 1987.

142. Mascalchi M, Dal Pozzo G, Dini C, et al: Acute spinal trauma: prognostic value of MRI appearances at 0.5T. Clin Radiol 48:100–108, 1993.

143. Maynard FR: International Standards for Neurological and Functional Classification of Spinal Cord Injury, rev ed. Chicago, American Spinal Injury Association, 1996.

144. Maza S, Frishman W: Therapeutic options to minimize free radical damage and thrombogenicity in ischemic/reperfused myocardium. Am Heart J 114:1206–1215, 1987.

145. McIntosh T, Juhler M, Wieloch T: Novel pharmacologic strategies in the treatment of experimental traumatic brain injury: 1998. J Neurotrauma 15:731–769, 1998.

146. McIntosh TK, Vink R, Soares H, et al: Effects of the N-methyl-D-aspartate receptor blocker MK-801 on neurologic function after experimental brain injury. J Neurotrauma 6:247–259, 1989.

147. McIntosh TK, Vink R, Soares H, et al: Effect of noncompetitive blockade of N-methyl-D-aspartate receptors on the neurochemical sequelae of experimental brain injury. J Neurochem 55:1170–1179, 1990.

148. Means E, Anderson D: Neuronophagia by leukocytes in experimental spinal cord injury. J Neuropathol Exp Neurol 42:707–719, 1983.

149. Moriya T, Hassan AZ, Young W, Chesler M: Dynamics of extracellular calcium activity following contusion of the rat spinal cord. J Neurotrauma 11:255–263, 1994.

150. Nacimiento AC, Bartels M, Herrmann HD: Dexamethasone prevents loss of axonal conduction and reflex activity, and reduces spread of structural damage in acute spinal cord trauma. Soc Neurosci Abstr 5:727, 1979.

151. Nystrom B, Berglund J: Spinal cord restitution following compression injuries in rats. Acta Neurol Scand 78:467–472, 1988.

152. Ohshio I, Hatayama A, Kaneda K, et al: Correlation between histopathologic features and magnetic resonance images of spinal cord lesions. Spine 18:1140–1149, 1993.

153. Ortega B, Demopoulos H, Ransohoff J: Effect of antioxidants on experimental cold-induced cerebral edema. In Reulen HJ, Schurmann K (eds): Steroids and Brain Edema. New York, Springer, 1972, pp 167–175.

154. Palma V, Ambrosio G, Scarano E, et al: Spinal cord injury: Some epidemiological data. A review of 233 cases. Acta Neurol 14:29–38, 1992.

155. Panter S, Yum S, Faden A: Alteration in extracellular amino acids after traumatic spinal cord injury. Ann Neurol 28:594–595, 1990.

156. Pedersen V, Muller PG, Biering-Sorensen F: Traumatic spinal cord injuries in Greenland 1965–1986. Paraplegia 27:345–349, 1989.

157. Pitts LH, Ross A, Chase GA, Faden AI: Treatment with thyrotropin-releasing hormone (TRH) in patients with traumatic spinal cord injuries. J Neurotrauma 12:235–243, 1995.

158. Popovich PG, Wei P, Stokes BT: Cellular inflammatory response after spinal cord injury in Sprague–Dawley and Lewis rats. J Comp Neurol 377:443–464, 1997.

159. Powers B, Miller M, Kramer R, et al: Traumatic atlanto-occipital dislocation. J Neurosurg 4:12–17, 1979.

160. Rawe S, Lee W, Perot P: Spinal cord glucose utilization after experimental spinal cord injury. Neurosurgery 9:40–47, 1981.

161. Rivilin A, Tator C: Regional spinal cord blood flow in rats after severe cord trauma. J Neurosurg 49:844–853, 1978.

162. Robertson C, Goodman J, Grossman R, Priessman A: Reduction in spinal cord postischemic lactic acidosis and functional improvement with dichloroacetate. J Neurotrauma 7:1–12, 1990.

163. Rosenblum W: Histopathologic clues to the pathways of neuronal death following ischemia/hypoxia. J Neurotrauma 14:313–326, 1997.

164. Rosomoff H, Gilbert R: Brain volume and cerebrospinal fluid pressure during hypothermia. Am J Physiol 183:19–22, 1955.

165. Roy-Camille R, Saillant G, Laville C, et al: Treatment of lower cervical spine injuries—C3 to C7. Spine 17 (suppl): S442–S446, 1991.

166. Sandler A, Tator C: Regional spinal cord blood flow in primates. J Neurosurg 45:647–659, 1976.

167. Sandler AN, Tator CH: Effect of acute spinal cord compression injury on regional spinal cord blood flow in primates. J Neurosurg 45:660–676, 1976.

168. Schaefer DM, Flanders A, Northrup BE, et al: Magnetic resonance imaging of acute cervical spine trauma. Correlation with severity of neurologic injury. Spine 14:1090–1095, 1989.

169. Schaefer DM, Flanders AE, Osterholm JL, Northrup BE: Prognostic significance of magnetic resonance imaging in the acute phase of cervical spine injury. J Neurosurg 76:218–223, 1992.

170. Schlegel J, Bayley J, Yuan H, et al: Timing of surgical decompression and fixation of acute spinal fractures. J Orthop Trauma 10:323–330, 1996.

171. Senter HJ, Venes JL: Loss of autoregulation and posttraumatic ischemia following experimental spinal cord trauma. J Neurosurg 50:198–206, 1979.

172. Siesjo B, Agardh C, Bengtsson F: Free radicals and brain damage. Cerebrovasc Brain Metabol Rev 1:165–211, 1989.

173. Skaper SD, Leon A: Monosialogangliosides, neuroprotection, and neuronal repair processes. J Neurotrauma 9:S507–S516, 1992.

174. Slucky AV, Eismont FJ: Treatment of acute injury of the cervical spine. J Bone Joint Surg Am 76A:1882–1896, 1994.

175. Star AM, Jones AA, Cotler JM, et al: Immediate closed reduction of cervical spine dislocations using traction. Spine 15:1068–1072, 1990.

176. Stokes B, Fox P, Hallinden G: Extracellular calcium activity in the injured spinal cord. Exp Neurol 80:561–572, 1983.

177. Stokes B, Garwood M: Traumatically induced alterations in the oxygen fields in the canine spinal cord. Exp Neurol 75:665–677, 1982.

178. Stokes BT: Experimental spinal cord injury: A dynamic and verifiable injury device. J Neurotrauma 9:129–131, 1992.

179. Stokes BT, Noyes DH, Behrmann DL: An electromechanical spinal injury technique with dynamic sensitivity. J Neurotrauma 9:187–195, 1992.

180. Stover SL, Fine PR: The epidemiology and economics of spinal cord injury. Paraplegia 25:225–228, 1987.

181. Takami K, Hashinoto T, Shino A, Fukuda N: Effect of thyrotropin-releasing hormone (TRH) in experimental spinal cord injury: a quantitative histopathologic study. Jpn J Pharmacol 57:405–417, 1991.

182. Taoka Y, Naruo M, Koyanagi E, et al: Superoxide radicals play important roles in the pathogenesis of spinal cord injury. Paraplegia 33:450–453, 1995.

183. Tarlov I: Spinal cord compression studies. III. Time limits for recovery after gradual compression in dogs. Arch Neurol Psych 71:588–597, 1954.

184. Tarlov I, Klinger H: Spinal cord compression studies II. Time limits for recovery after acute compression in dogs. Arch Neurol Psych 71:271–290, 1954.

185. Tator CH: Experimental and clinical studies of the pathophysiology and management of acute spinal cord injury. J Spinal Cord Med 19:206–214, 1996.

186. Tator CH, Duncan EG, Edmonds VE, et al: Neurological recovery, mortality and length of stay after acute spinal cord injury associated with changes in management. Paraplegia 33:254–262, 1995.

187. Tator CH, Fehlings MG: Review of the secondary injury theory of acute spinal cord trauma with emphasis on vascular mechanisms. J Neurosurg 75:15–26, 1991.

188. Tator CH, Rowed DW, Schwartz ML: Sunnybrook Cord Injury Scales for Assessing Neurological Injury and Neurological Recovery in Early Management of Acute Spinal Cord Injury. New York, Raven Press, 1982.

189. Templeton P, Young J, Mirvis S, et al: The value of retropharyngeal soft tissue measurement in trauma of the adult cervical spine. Skeletal Radiol 16:98–104, 1987.

190. Traynelis V, Marano G, Dunker T, et al: Traumatic atlanto-occipital dislocation: Case report. J Neurosurg 65:863–870, 1988.

191. Vink R, Noble L, Knoblack S, et al: Metabolic changes in rabbit spinal cord after trauma: Magnetic resonance spectroscopy studies. Ann Neurol 25:26–31, 1989.

192. Wagner F, Dhormann G, Bucy P: Histopathology of transitory traumatic paraplegia in the monkey. J Neurosurg 35:272–276, 1971.

193. Wallace M, Tator C: Successful improvement of blood pressure, cardiac output, and spinal cord blood flow after experimental spinal cord injury. Neurosurgery 18:433–439, 1987.

194. Waters RL, Adkins RH, Yakura, JS: Definition of complete spinal cord injury. Paraplegia 9:573–581, 1991.

195. Wei E, Christman C, Kontos H, Povlishock J: Effects of oxygen radicals on cerebral arterioles. Am J Physiol 248:H157–H162, 1985.

196. Wells JD, Nicosia S: Scoring acute spinal cord injury: A study of the utility and limitations of five different grading systems. J Spinal Cord Med 18:33–41, 1995.

197. White A, Panjabi M.: Clinical Biomechanics of the Spine. Philiadelphia, JB Lippincott, 1978.

198. Whiteneck GG, Menter RR, Charlifue SW, et al: Initial and long-term costs of spinal cord injury. Paraplegia 26:135, 1988.

199. Wyllie A, Kerr J, Currie A: Cell death: The significance of apoptosis. In Bourne G, Danielli J (eds): International Review of Cytology. New York, Academic Press, 1980, pp 251–306.

200. Wyss-Coray T, Borrow P, Brooker MJ, Mucke L: Astroglial overproduction of TGF-beta 1 enhances inflammatory central nervous system disease in transgenic mice. J Neuroimmunol 77:45–50, 1997.

201. Young W: Recovery mechanisms in spinal cord injury: Implications for regenerative therapy. In Seil F (ed): Neural Regeneration and Transplantation. New York, Liss, 1989, pp 157–169.

202. Young W: Methylprednisolone treatment of acute spinal cord injury: An introduction. J Neurotrauma 8:S43–S46, 1991.

203. Young W: Role of calcium in central nervous system injuries. J Neurotrauma 9:S9–S25, 1992.

204. Young W: Secondary injury mechanisms in acute spinal cord injury. J Emerg Med 1:13–22, 1993.

205. Young W, Flamm ES: Effect of high-dose corticosteroid therapy on blood flow, evoked potentials, and extracellular calcium in experimental spinal injury. J Neurosurg 57:667–673, 1982.

206. Young W, Flamm ES, Demopoulos HB, et al: Effect of naloxone on posttraumatic ischemia in experimental spinal contusion. J Neurosurg 55:209–219, 1981.

207. Young W, Koreh I: Potassium and calcium changes in injured spinal cords. Brain Res 365:42–53, 1986.

208. Zeidman SM, Ling GSF, Ducker TB, Ellenbogen RG: Clinical applications of pharmacologic therapies for spinal cord injury. J Spinal Disord 9:367–380, 1996.

11

FRACTURES AND DISLOCATIONS OF THE UPPER CERVICAL SPINE

Steven C. Scherping, Jr., M.D.
James D. Kang, M.D.

Great spirits have always found violent opposition from mediocrities.
— Albert Einstein

Traumatic injuries of the upper cervical spine, or the occipitoatlantoaxial complex, require separate consideration from other spinal trauma. Injuries to this area include occipital condyle fractures, occipitoatlantal dislocations, subluxations and dislocations of the atlantoaxial articulation, atlas fractures, odontoid fractures, and fractures of the arch of the axis. It is difficult to establish the true incidence of these injuries, because their consequences are often fatal.[2, 3, 21, 30] A review of 312 victims of fatal traffic accidents revealed that nearly 20% had evidence of an injury to the craniocervical junction.[2] Nevertheless, many of the traumatic injuries of the upper cervical spine are uncommon in clinical practice. The potentially grave consequences of misdiagnosis or improper treatment mandates that considerable attention be given to each entity.

HISTORICAL PERSPECTIVE

In his classic review of 300 patients with acute cervical spine injuries, Bohlman found a delay in diagnosis ranging from 1 day to 1 year for 100 of these patients.[15] A more recent review of traumatic spinal injuries demonstrated little improvement in this unsettling finding, with a delay in diagnosis in more than 20% of patients with acute cervical spine trauma.[88] The most common factors cited for the delay in diagnosis were similar in both studies and included altered level of consciousness due to a head injury or intoxication, multiple trauma, or multiple noncontiguous spine injuries. Because 50% to 60% of patients with acute spinal cord injuries have other significant skeletal or visceral trauma, and as many as 20% are hypotensive on arrival to the emergency room, the initial clinical evaluation of these patients necessitates an organized, meticulous approach to ensure that important clinical and radiographic findings are not overlooked.[52]

ANATOMY AND KINEMATICS

The craniocervical junction is an anatomically and biomechanically distinct area with several key features that must be appreciated before consideration is given to the management of upper cervical spine trauma. First, injuries to this region are greatly influenced by the mass and position of the cranium relative to the cervical spine at the time of impact. Second, in the upper cervical spine, the ratio between the diameter of the neural canal and the enclosed neural structures is large. Third, a high degree of mobility exists between the cranium and upper cervical spine, with the ligamentous structures providing a disproportionate amount of the stability to this region. And finally, despite a similar mechanism of injury for many of these traumatic conditions, the incidence of neurologic injury and the optimal form of treatment vary greatly from one entity to another. Consequently, in this chapter we discuss each injury and its treatment options independently, beginning with a brief review of the clinically relevant anatomic and kinematic features of the cervicocranium.

A thorough understanding of the anatomy of the cervicocranium is critical in the diagnosis and treatment of patients with upper cervical spine trauma. The cervicocranium, or occipitoatlantoaxial complex, begins superiorly with the occipital condyles and the paired atlanto-occipital joints. The occiput sends two convex condyles to join with the reciprocally concave superior articular facets of the atlas to form the atlanto-occipital joints. This bony configuration allows for approximately 10 to 15 degrees of flexion and extension and 8 degrees of lateral flexion while precluding essentially all axial rotation at the atlanto-occipital articulation.[58, 98, 114] The articular capsules of the atlanto-occipital joint are thin and provide only marginal stability to this articulation. Stability at the craniocervical junction is provided mainly by the ascending ligamentous structures. Anteriorly, the anterior longitudinal ligament gives origin to the anterior atlanto-occipital membrane, which extends from the anterior arch of the atlas to the anterior rim of the foramen magnum. The posterior longitudinal ligament also extends to the cranium in the form of the tectorial membrane. This important stabilizer travels from the posterior surface of the dens to the anterior surface of the foramen magnum. Between the atlas and the skull, the paired ligametum flavum, typical of other interspaces, are represented by the posterior atlanto-occipital membrane. These relatively thin membranes are pierced by the vertebral arteries as they run from the posterior arch of the atlas to the posterior segment of the foramen magnum (Fig. 11–1).[112a]

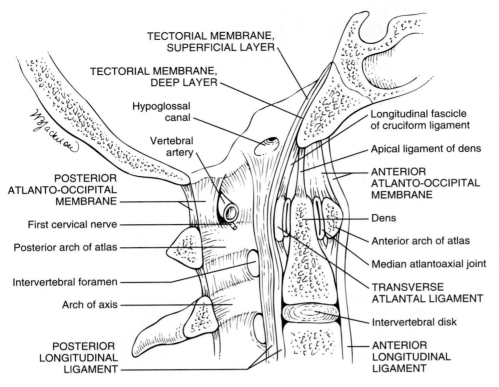

TECTORIAL MEMBRANE, SUPERFICIAL LAYER

TECTORIAL MEMBRANE, DEEP LAYER

Hypoglossal canal

Vertebral artery

POSTERIOR ATLANTO-OCCIPITAL MEMBRANE

First cervical nerve

Posterior arch of atlas

Intervertebral foramen

Arch of axis

POSTERIOR LONGITUDINAL LIGAMENT

Longitudinal fascicle of cruciform ligament

Apical ligament of dens

ANTERIOR ATLANTO-OCCIPITAL MEMBRANE

Dens

Anterior arch of atlas

Median atlantoaxial joint

TRANSVERSE ATLANTAL LIGAMENT

Intervertebral disk

ANTERIOR LONGITUDINAL LIGAMENT

Figure 11–1. *Lateral cross-sectional view of the upper cervical spine demonstrating the osseous and ligamentous anatomy responsible for the stability in this region. Notice the continuation of the anterior and posterior longitudinal ligaments to the cranium as the anterior atlanto-occipital and tectorial membranes, respectively. The ligamentum flavum forms the posterior atlanto-occipital membrane as it projects into the cranium.*

The atlas is an atypical cervical vertebra that consists of an anterior and posterior arch bridged by two lateral masses. The anterior arch has anteriorly a small tubercle, to which the longus colli muscles insert, and posteriorly a facet for articulation with the odontoid process. The posterior arch is a thin, bony ring that is more round than flat and has a tubercle for the origin of the suboccipital muscles. Immediately posterior to the lateral masses, the posterior arch is grooved as a sulcus for the vertebral arteries. This feature makes this portion of the ring extremely susceptible to failure under supraphysiologic loading. The superior articular surfaces of the lateral masses face cephalad and slightly medially. The inferior articular surfaces face caudad and slightly medially to join with the opposing, saddle-shaped biconvex surfaces of the superior articular facets of the axis.

The axis is also atypical with the largest body of all of the cervical vertebrae and a vertical projection termed the dens or odontoid process. With its odontoid process, the axis forms a unique articulation between the axis and the anterior arch of the atlas, the central or median atlantoaxial joint. This joint, through its bony configuration and ligamentous restraints, provides a central pivot for the atlantoaxial junction and allows for tremendous axial rotation while resisting anteroposterior translation. The paired lateral atlantoaxial joints are almost flat and more nearly in the transverse plane than the other cervical facet joints. There is, however, a slight sloping to this articulation such that with rotation between the atlas and the axis, a slight downward and backward sliding of the atlas occurs on the side toward which rotation is occurring and a slight upward and forward movement on the contralateral side. The capsules of the lateral atlantoaxial joints are relatively loose

to accommodate the great amount of motion at this level. Approximately 50 degrees of axial rotation, or about half of all of the axial rotation of the cervical spine, occurs through the atlantoaxial junction.[98, 114] An estimated 10 degrees of flexion and extension but little or no lateral flexion also occurs at the atlantoaxial junction.

The principal restraint to anterior translation at the atlantoaxial junction is the transverse atlantal ligament. This ligament is the strongest portion of the cruciform ligament and runs just posterior to the dens as it traverses the ring of the atlas. The transverse ligament inserts on tubercles

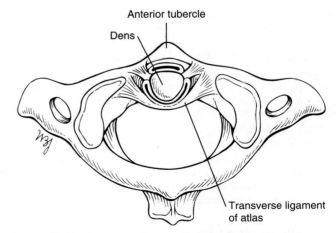

Anterior tubercle

Dens

Transverse ligament of atlas

Figure 11–2. *Transverse view at the level of the atlas ring demonstrating the relationship between the odontoid process and the atlas. The transverse atlantal ligament prevents anterior translation of the atlas on the axis.*

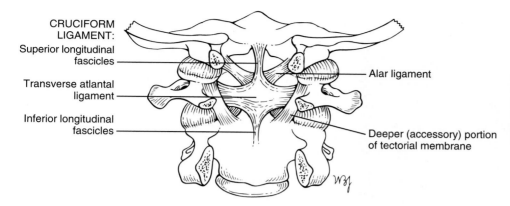

Figure 11–3. A posterior view of the upper cervical spine (with the posterior arch and spinal cord removed) demonstrating the important ligamentous stabilizers.

CRUCIFORM LIGAMENT:
Superior longitudinal fascicles
Transverse atlantal ligament
Inferior longitudinal fascicles

Alar ligament

Deeper (accessory) portion of tectorial membrane

projecting from the medial side of the lateral masses on either side of the C1 ring (Fig. 11–2). Paired alar ligaments that run from both sides of the dens to attach to tubercles on the lateral rim of the foramen magnum near the occipital condyles also provide important stability. The alar ligaments act as secondary restraints to anterior translation of the atlas and play a crucial role in providing stability with axial rotation.[38, 42, 98] The apical dental ligament runs from the tip of the dens to the ventral ridge of the foramen magnum. This ligament provides only a minor contribution to the stability of the cervicocranium (Fig. 11–3).

ASSESSMENT OF PATIENTS WITH UPPER CERVICAL SPINE TRAUMA

As alluded to in the introductory remarks, suspicion of a cervical spine injury must be entertained in every patient involved in a traumatic event, particularly those complaining of neck pain or presenting with altered level of consciousness. The examining physician must seek a thorough history regarding the nature of the accident and carefully probe for the presence of any neurologic symptoms either immediately after the incident or on presentation to the emergency room. An accurate reconstruction of the accident and the possible mechanisms of injury will often give valuable clues to the injury pattern sustained by the patient. Obviously, the comatose or intoxicated patient can provide little assistance in determining an injury pattern, and thus continued spinal immobilization along with a vigilant physical and radiographic examination must be performed. It cannot be overemphasized that the most critical factor in the initial evaluation of the patient with a spinal injury is the examining physician's suspicion that such an injury might exist.

The physical examination should initially focus on the hemodynamic stability of the patient. Up to 70% of patients with a cervical spine injury who present with systolic blood pressure below 100 mm Hg have some component of neurogenic shock contributing to their hemodynamic instability.[101] Treatment of the neurogenic shock with fluid and vasopressors as needed should be initiated as the systematic evaluation continues. Inspection and palpation of the entire spine, as well as a complete neurologic

examination, including evaluation of cranial nerve function, should be performed by an experienced physician. It is also crucial to make note of any lacerations, contusions, or fractures of the skull, face, or upper thorax, because these injuries provide valuable clues as to both the mechanism of injury and the energy involved. The presence of significant head trauma should arouse great suspicion of a cervical or cervicocranial injury in every patient.

The initial radiographic evaluation of the patient should include an anteroposterior (open-mouth) view of the atlantoaxial articulation, an anteroposterior view of the lower cervical spine, and a lateral view of the cervical spine from the occiput to T1. Oblique lateral views may at times provide useful information. The need for computed tomography (CT) scans and magnetic resonance imaging (MRI) depends on the specific injury and clinical scenario, as discussed later in this chapter. When interpreting radiographic studies, the examiner must be alert to the possibility of noncontiguous spinal column injuries. The incidence of noncontiguous spine fractures is reported to be between 4% and 16% and most commonly occurs with at least one of the fractures involving the upper cervical spine.[63, 64, 89, 111] Continued awareness of this and attention to detail so as not to miss subtle radiographic clues, such as prevertebral soft tissue swelling, will help avoid missed diagnoses.

OCCIPITAL CONDYLE FRACTURES

Although recognized since 1817, fracture of the occipital condyle is a rarely reported traumatic lesion.[10, 18, 55, 68, 121] In Alker's series of 312 patients with fatal craniovertebral trauma, fracture of the occipital condyle was found in only 2 patients.[2] Virtually all of the reported cases have involved patients in motor vehicle accidents, and the occipital condyle fractures have occurred in conjunction with other significant cranial or spinal trauma. Fractures of the atlas are the most commonly associated spine injury. The often nonspecific symptoms and physical examination findings, in light of the difficulty identifying these fractures on routine x-rays, make diagnosis of this injury a clinical challenge. The examiner must be wary though, as patients with an occipital condyle fracture may present with lower cranial nerve findings if the fracture extends to involve the jugular

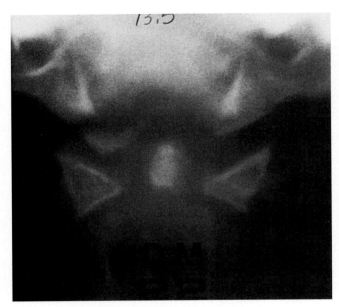

Figure 11–4. This anteroposterior CT scan demonstrates an avulsion fracture of the occipital condyle (type 3) in a 22-year-old man involved in a motor vehicle accident. (From Anderson PA, Montesano PX: Morphology and treatment of occipital condyle fractures. Spine 13:731–736, 1988.)

foramen and hypoglossal canal.[16] Less commonly, vertebrobasilar symptoms may arise from either compression of a vertebral artery or the brainstem by a displaced bony fragment.[7, 18]

Occipital condyle fractures occur in two patterns.[7] The first pattern is an avulsion fracture of the alar ligament. The second, and by far the more common pattern is a compression fracture. This injury is due to a combination of lateral bending and axial loading in which the condyle fails under direct compression. Generally, only one condyle is involved. A classification scheme proposed by Anderson and Montesano categorizes these fractures into one of three types.[7] Type 1 is an impaction fracture of the condyle, a type 2 fracture has an associated basilar skull fracture, and type 3 is a condylar avulsion fracture (Fig. 11–4).

Treatment of these injuries begins with fracture recognition. A CT scan through the craniovertebral junction is nearly always necessary for diagnosis and should be used in evaluating any patient with suspected occipital condyle fracture.[7, 16, 18, 121] The treatment approach is then dictated by the degree of associated atlanto-occipital instability. Patients without any evidence of atlanto-occipital instability may be treated in a hard collar for 6 to 8 weeks, or until symptoms abate. In patients with evidence of atlanto-occipital instability due to disruption of the alar ligament complex, definitive treatment involves halo immobilization or occiput to C1 arthrodesis.

OCCIPITOATLANTAL DISLOCATIONS

Traumatic occipitoatlantal dislocations are rare injuries. Their rarity is surpassed only by survivorship of

these generally fatal insults.[2, 3, 21] First described in 1908 by Blackwood, occipitoatlantal dislocations are believed to represent less than 1% of all acute cervical spine injuries.[12] However, the exact incidence of this dislocation remains unknown and is likely underestimated, because a great percentage are quickly fatal and escape diagnosis. Bucholz and Burkhead found that 8% of patients involved in fatal motor vehicle accidents had sustained an occipitoatlantal dislocation, whereas Alker et al. found that 19% of fatal motor vehicle–related cervical spine injuries were from craniovertebral junction dislocations.[2, 21] Although survivorship of this injury is unusual, it is being increasingly reported over the past 1 to 2 decades.[17, 25, 32, 40, 41, 73, 77, 84, 110, 117, 119] Proper spinal immobilization and aggressive cardiorespiratory management of trauma victims in the field is likely responsible for this notable improvement.

Occipitoatlantal dislocations are high-energy injuries nearly always reported after motor vehicle accidents or after pedestrian and motor vehicle accidents.[2, 3, 17, 21, 25, 32, 40, 41, 73, 77, 84, 110, 117, 119] They are usually accompanied by other significant trauma, especially head injuries. This injury is more common in children, perhaps even twice that in adults (Fig. 11–5).[51, 62] The rationale for this is based on the proportionately larger head to body mass found in children and the developing anatomy of the craniovertebral junction. In children, the inclination of the occipitoatlantal joints is more horizontal and the occipital condyles and C1

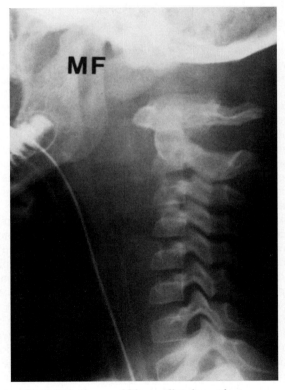

Figure 11–5. This 7-year-old boy suffered an atlanto-occipital dislocation after a pedestrian motor vehicle accident. Despite responsive care, this injury proved fatal for this unfortunate child.

facets are more shallow. Both of these anatomical variations from a mature skeleton predispose children to dislocation rather than another injury under the same loading conditions. Although definitive distinction between the types probably does not exist in the clinical setting, these dislocations have been classified as anterior, posterior, and longitudinal distractions.[108] Anterior dislocations whereby the occiput is displaced anteriorly relative to the atlas, is the most commonly reported type.[32, 86] The forces responsible for this injury involve a combination of hyperextension, distraction, and possibly rotation. The evidence to support this is founded in both clinical experience and Werne's anatomic dissections of the craniovertebral junction.[113] Clinical observation frequently uncovers submental and mandibular trauma in patients with anterior dislocation, indicative of an extension loading vector.[21, 25, 32, 51, 86] In Werne's anatomic dissections of the craniovertebral junction, he was able to identify the tectorial membrane and the alar ligaments as the primary ligamentous stabilizers of the craniovertebral junction. The tectorial membrane limits hyperextension and longitudinal distraction, with the alar ligaments also contributing to limit hyperextension as well as lateral bending. He found flexion to be limited by bony contact between the odontoid apex and the anterior margin of the foramen magnum. Moreover, he demonstrated that when the tectorial membrane and alar ligaments were transected, as they would be with hyperextension, anterior dislocation of the craniovertebral junction was possible.[113]

The diagnosis of occipitoatlantal dislocation or instability is at times quite obvious, and at other times quite subtle. Particularly among survivors of this injury, difficulty in making a diagnosis based on plain films alone has been consistently reported.[32, 66, 77, 86] This, in part, is related to the widely variable clinical manifestations with which survivors can present. As mentioned, most victims die immediately or prior to presentation at the hospital. Victims suffering transection of the medulla oblongata or the spinomedullary junction develop immediate respiratory arrest and die at the scene unless prompt respiratory resuscitation is initiated. Others may present with no or mild neurologic deficits, a Brown-Sequard–like picture, or a high cervical quadriplegia. It is important to suspect this diagnosis in patients with cardiorespiratory arrest and a high or mixed quadriplegia. Moreover, as patients may present with no neurologic deficit, severe upper occipital neck pain mandates expeditious evaluation of the craniovertebral junction to rule out this grossly unstable injury.[32] Among survivors it is also important to fully evaluate the function of cranial nerves, which are commonly involved. The abducens is the cranial nerve most often damaged with this injury.[32, 41] Lastly, injury to the vertebral arteries is a possibility and the status of these vessels may need to be investigated.

The radiographic diagnosis of an occipitoatlantal dislocation is usually evident on the lateral cervical spine roentgenogram in the patient with a profound neurologic deficit. Marked diastasis or translation between the occiput and atlas proves diagnostic. In contrast, patients with incomplete or minimal neurologic deficits may have nondiagnostic or subtle evidence on plain film examination. Prevertebral soft tissue swelling is universally present and

should be identified.[50, 66] A number of other measurements based on plain x-rays may also be used to detect an aberrant craniovertebral relationship. The three most commonly used relationships are Wackenheim's clival line, the dens–basion relationship, and Power's ratio. Wackenheim's line, which extends caudally along the posterior surface of the clivus, should run tangential to the posterior tip of the dens.[112] In anterior dislocations this line will traverse a portion of the dens, and in distracted or posterior dislocations it will completely miss the dens. The dens is in vertical alignment with the basion with the head in a neutral position. The normal distance between the dens and basion is 4 to 5 mm in adults and roughly 10 mm in children.[36, 115, 116] Any increase in the dens–basion distance is considered significant and necessitates further investigation. Furthermore, flexion and extension x-rays should show less than 1 mm of translation between these two landmarks.[116] More than 1 mm of translation constitutes instability.

Whereas the aforementioned techniques depend on proper positioning of the cranium relative to the torso, Power's ratio assesses the relationship between two lines and is unaffected by positioning and magnification (Fig. 11–6).[86] A ratio of the distance between the basion (B) and the posterior arch of the atlas (C), and of the opisthion (O) and the anterior arch of the atlas (A) constitutes Power's ratio. This ratio, BC/OA, normally averages 0.77. A ratio greater than 1 establishes the radiographic diagnosis of an anterior occipitoatlantal dislocation. Ratios less than 0.77 may be found with posterior dislocations. Power's ratio is not applicable in children, in persons with congenital craniovertebral anomalies, or in instances where the odontoid or C1 ring is fractured.[86] Using these techniques, plain film interpretation will detect approximately 50% to 75% of occipitoatlantal dislocations.[66] Difficulties in accurately identifying anatomic landmarks or clinical suspicion not substantiated by plain film findings are indications for tomography or computed tomography through the craniovertebral junction.[32, 73, 77] Power's ratio may be determined on a lateral tomogram or sagittal reconstruction of a CT scan, and importantly, the occipitoatlantal joints may be clearly visualized to identify any occult pathology. An MRI of the region is indicated in most situations, but its use and timing will be dictated by the clinical scenario.

Treatment of patients with an occipitoatlantal dislocation should allow for the simultaneous, coordinated management of the spine injury and any cardiorespiratory compromise. For patients who arrive at the hospital with no or an incomplete neurologic deficit it must be recognized that this represents an extremely unstable injury with a high risk of progressive neurologic deterioration. There is some disagreement as to the preferred method of emergent spinal immobilization. Although it has been suggested that skeletal traction with 1 to 2 kg is a safe and effective measure for acute immobilization and realignment, others caution about the use of traction.[32, 68, 86, 108] Most prefer the immediate application of a halo vest, ideally under fluoroscopic guidance. Once the patient's cardiorespiratory status has been stabilized and other life-threatening injuries addressed, acute surgical stabilization of the cervicocranium is the preferred treatment algorithm.[11, 32, 41, 51, 73, 77, 86] The re-

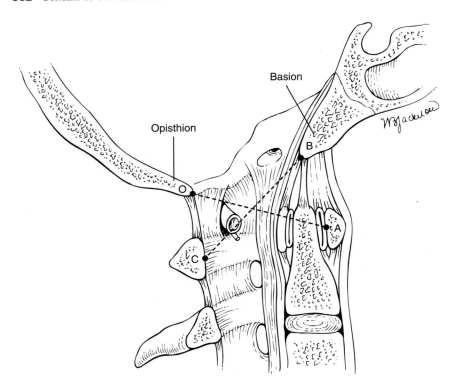

Basion

Figure 11–6. *Power's ratio is calculated as BC:OA. If this ratio is greater than 1, then an anterior atlanto-occipital dislocation exists. Ratios below 1 are normal except in posterior dislocations, associated fractures of the odontoid process or ring of the atlas, and congenital anomalies of the craniocervical junction.*

sults of treatment with immobilization alone have not been favorable. Posterior spinal fusion from the occiput to C1 or C2 with continued postoperative immobilization in a halo vest is the procedure of choice in patients with a salvageable neurologic status. Operative intervention should proceed as soon after the injury as the patient's overall cardiopulmonary and neurologic status allow.

RUPTURE OF THE TRANSVERSE LIGAMENT

Ligamentous attenuation and resultant subluxation of the atlantoaxial articulation is a common sequela of long-standing inflammatory arthritidies.[13] Conversely, traumatic injuries to the ligamentous structures of the atlantoaxial articulation, and specifically the transverse atlantal ligament, are relatively rare clinical entities.[31, 33, 42] Transverse atlantal ligament ruptures may be isolated or seen in conjunction with C1 ring fractures or atlantoaxial rotatory fixation. Noteworthy is that these injuries typically occur in older adults. Patients are often in their fifth decade or older as opposed to the third decade and younger when most other traumatic spinal injuries occur.[68, 69] The mechanisms of injury, however, are similar, with falls and motor vehicle accidents being responsible for the vast majority of transverse ligament ruptures.[31, 33, 42, 68] Forced flexion of the neck is responsible for creating this purely ligamentous injury.

Rupture of the transverse ligament is a major destabilizing injury to the atlantoaxial articulation. As previously discussed in the anatomy section, the transverse ligament is the primary anterior stabilizer of the atlantoaxial joint with

the alar ligaments playing a secondary role.[38, 42, 114] Posterior stability is provided by abutment of the anterior part of the ring of the atlas against the odontoid process. According to Fielding, after rupture of the transverse ligament, the secondary and tertiary stabilizers are inadequate to prevent further anterior translation of the atlas on the axis when a force of similar magnitude to that which ruptured the ligament is applied.[42] Fielding's work also created parameters for assessing the integrity of the transverse ligament. An atlanto-dens interval (ADI) of less than or equal to three millimeters indicates that the transverse ligament is intact. An ADI between three to five millimeters implies rupture of the transverse ligament, and an ADI greater than five millimeters suggests incompetence of the transverse ligament and secondary restraints (Fig. 11–7). In Fielding's studies and other more recent work, the transverse ligament was discovered to fail with either a midsubstance rupture or with an osteoperiosteal avulsion at the tubercle.[33, 34, 42]

The clinical presentation of patients with a traumatic transverse ligament rupture is quite variable.[31, 33, 42, 68, 69] In Fielding's series, all 11 patients had an associated severe head injury, whereas in the series of DeBeer et al., only two of seven patients had a significant head injury.[31, 42] The presence of a neurologic deficit is also quite variable and the spectrum broad. Patients may die immediately at the scene, may develop long-tract signs and a Brown-Séquard–type picture, or present with no neurologic deficit and only severe upper neck pain. Neurologic deficit is roughly predicted by the degree of anterior displacement of the atlas.

The radiographic diagnosis of this injury may be difficult.[68] If the lateral cervical spine film is taken with the patient in a supine position with the neck in slight extension, the ADI may be within normal limits as a result of a positional reduction. The detection of prevertebral soft tissue swelling may provide a clue, as will the finding of a bony fleck from a tubercle avulsion on the open-mouth odontoid view. This bony fleck from an avulsion of the transverse ligament may be more readily seen on a CT scan. In the alert patient who is neurologically intact, physician-supervised flexion-extension views may provide a radiographic diagnosis. Unfortunately, this may also fail to provide a definitive diagnosis as protective paraspinal muscle spasm may obscure the atlantoaxial instability.[68] Levine and Edwards suggest that in the patient with suspected instability and obvious paraspinal muscle spasm, the examiner immobilize the patient until the spasm resolves and then repeat the flexion-extension views. A second option, in their opinion, is to inject the paraspinous muscles with a local anesthetic, thereby relieving the pain and spasm, and then repeat the exam. More recently, some authors have espoused the use of MRI to evaluate the transverse ligament.[34] The clinical applicability of an MRI scan remains uncertain, but this is the study of choice in those patients with a neurologic deficit in which flexion-extension views are contraindicated.

Following the dictum that ligamentous injuries of the cervical spine fail to reliably heal, there is a general consensus that the treatment of a transverse ligament rupture is surgical stabilization.[31, 42, 43, 68, 69] A posterior atlantoaxial arthrodesis has achieved good success in this regard.[42, 43] Recently, though, one report in the literature has suggested that some traumatic transverse ligament disrup-

tions may be successfully treated with halo immobilization.[33] In this study an MRI of the transverse ligament was utilized to distinguish between a midsubstance rupture and a bony, insertional failure. Prior work had demonstrated that traumatically induced physiologic incompetence of the transverse ligament develops from one of these two failure modes.[34, 42] As expected, the midsubstance failures of the ligament failed to heal with external immobilization, and a delayed arthrodesis was necessary to restore atlantoaxial stability. Conversely, some of the failures associated with an insertional disruption of the ligament demonstrated a capability for spontaneous healing and restoration of atlantoaxial stability. If surgical stabilization is deemed necessary, a further area of controversy focuses on the type of arthrodesis. All agree that reduction followed by posterior atlantoaxial spinal fusion is the procedure of choice, but differing opinions arise on which particular type of fusion is best.[20, 49]

ATLANTOAXIAL ROTATORY SUBLUXATIONS AND DISLOCATIONS

Atlantoaxial rotatory subluxations and dislocations comprise a constellation of injuries ranging from the benign to the catastrophic. Although rotatory injuries of the atlantoaxial articulation have been recognized since the turn of the century, an organized appreciation for this continuum of pathology did not evolve until Fielding's work in the late 1970s.[27, 44] Fielding popularized the terminology of atlantoaxial rotatory fixation and helped to begin the differentiation between the self-limiting atlantoaxial subluxations in children, and the more severe, often traumatically induced injuries witnessed in adults. Overall, this spectrum of injuries is rarely encountered in clinical practice, and the exact etiology remains unclear.[27, 28, 37, 44, 61, 68, 69, 79, 109] A vast number of theories have been proposed, but none has gained widespread acceptance. Perhaps the most widely embraced theory is that of Fielding and Hawkins, who believe that reduction in the early stages after a subluxation of the atlantoaxial joints is prevented by swollen capsular and synovial tissues and by associated muscle spasm.[44] Over time, ligament and capsular contractures develop, holding the joint in a subluxated or dislocated position. Nevertheless, no single theory adequately describes all of the pathology evident with these rotatory disorders.

The foundation of concern with rotatory injuries dates back to Coutts' work in the 1930s.[28] Coutts, and more recently Massara and Fielding, demonstrated that with an intact transverse ligament, the atlantoaxial articulation pivots on the odontoid and complete bilateral dislocation of the articular processes occurs at approximately 65 degrees of rotation.[28, 74] Along with this rotation is a resultant narrowing of the neural canal to less than 1 cm, the approximate width of the spinal cord at this level. Coutts also noted that with rupture of the transverse ligament and 5 mm of anterior displacement of the atlas, complete unilateral dislocation and narrowing of the neural canal to

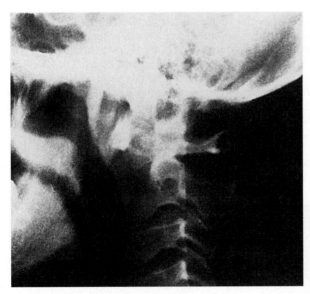

Figure 11–7. A lateral x-ray of a 26-year-old man with incompetence of the primary and secondary restraints to anterior atlantoaxial subluxation (rupture of the transverse and alar ligaments). Because the ADI is 11 mm, there is immediate risk to the spinal cord. (From Fielding JW, Cochran GV, Lawsing JF, Hohl M: Tears of the transverse ligament of the atlas. A clinical and biomechanical study. J Bone Joint Surg Am 56A:1683–1691, 1974.)

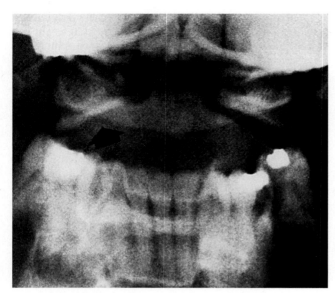

Figure 11–8. *This open-mouth x-ray demonstrates a wink sign, in which the lateral mass of C1 overlaps the lateral mass of C2 on the affected side. (From Levine AM, Edwards CC: Traumatic lesions of the occipitoatlanto-axial process. Clin Orthop 239:53–68, 1989.)*

12 mm occurs with 45 degrees of rotation. Although narrowing of the neural canal is of primary concern, injury to the vertebral arteries also becomes possible with severe rotatory deformity, especially those with anterior displacement.[79, 94] Brainstem and cerebellar infarction may follow as a consequence of the vertebrobasilar insufficiency.

The diagnosis of atlantoaxial rotatory fixation is difficult and often delayed.[44, 61, 68, 79, 109] Patients may present after either minor or major trauma complaining of neck pain but usually demonstrating no evidence of neurologic compromise. In patients with severe subluxation or frank dislocation, significant deformity in the form of torticollis or lateral bending of the neck may be present. Moreover, these are the patients that typically develop neurologic symptoms, ranging from the benign occipital neuralgia to complete compromise of the spinomedullary structures. However, with minimal amounts of subluxation there may be little or no demonstrable deformity and no evidence of neurologic

involvement.[44, 68, 79, 109] To make the diagnosis of atlanto-axial rotatory fixation, the physician must have a strong clinical suspicion and carefully scrutinize the radiographic studies.

Unfortunately, the radiographic diagnosis of these rotatory disorders is also fraught with potential pitfalls. The diagnosis begins with evaluation of the open-mouth odontoid view, looking for asymmetry of the clear space between the odontoid and lateral masses of the atlas. Normally on the anteroposterior view, with rotation to the right the left lateral mass of C1 appears wider and to approach the odontoid as the atlas rotates on the axis. Moreover, because of the configuration of the atlantoaxial facets, the facet joint appears to widen on the left and narrow on the right.[37, 45, 120] With rotation in excess of normal limits, this may produce a "wink sign," in which there is apparent overlap of the lateral masses and complete loss of the facet joint space (Fig. 11–8). If the open-mouth odontoid view demonstrates asymmetry in the clear space about the dens or in the facet joint space, then the physician should confirm the proper alignment of the patient's head and neck at the time of the x-ray. If there is a question about the position, then the open-mouth view with the head and neck in neutral alignment should be repeated. If the asymmetry persists, open-mouth views with the patient's head rotated 15 degrees to each side will confirm the diagnosis of atlantoaxial rotatory fixation (Figs. 11–9 and 11–10). A CT scan through the atlantoaxial articulation will give additional information as to the presence of any facet or ring fractures, the degree of subluxation, and the presence of any anteroposterior displacement.[37, 45] Proceeding with the CT scan before obtaining the rotated open-mouth odontoid views is commonly done because of technical difficulties in obtaining these views and the additional information available with the CT scan. It is crucial to determine the competence of the transverse ligament before rendering a diagnosis or treatment plan. The transverse ligament should be assessed by determining the ADI on the lateral cervical spine x-ray and CT scan. If the ADI is less than 3 mm and the patient is neurologically intact, then lateral flexion-extension views will help further delineate the physiologic integrity of the transverse ligament.

Fielding and Hawkins have divided atlantoaxial rotatory fixation into four types (Fig. 11–11).[44] In type I, there is

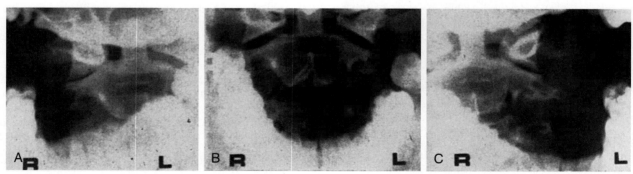

Figure 11–9. *Atlantoaxial joint with rotation to the right, in neutral position, and with rotation to the left, showing a normal range of movement. The slight asymmetry seen on the neutral film is due to minimal rotation to the left. (From Wortzman G, Dewar FP: Rotary fixation of the atlantoaxial joint: Rotational atlantoaxial subluxation. Radiology 90:479–487, 1968.)*

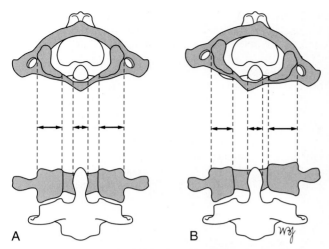

Figure 11–10. Atlantoaxial joint in neutral position (A) and on rotation to the right (B). With rotation, changes evident on the anteroposterior view include: (1) an apparent approximation of the left atlantal articular mass to the odontoid, (2) increase in the width of the left atlantal articular mass with a decrease in the width of the right atlantal articular mass, and (3) a widened left and a narrowed right atlantoaxial joint. (From Wortzman G, Dewar FP: Rotary fixation of the atlantoaxial joint: Rotational atlantoaxial subluxation. Radiology 90:479–487, 1968.)

that some form of traction with an attempted closed reduction should be the initial step.[44, 68, 79, 109] The success of traction in achieving an acceptable reduction is inversely proportional to duration of the deformity. Levine and Edwards advocate an attempted closed manipulation of the step-off of C1 on C2 through the oropharynx under local anesthesia in an awake patient.[68] If an acceptable reduction can be achieved, and the transverse ligament is intact, then halo immobilization for 3 months is suggested. At the conclusion of immobilization, if the patient is symptomatic or has any residual instability, C1–C2 posterior spinal fusion is the treatment of choice. All patients treated with halo immobilization should have flexion-extension views to assess the integrity of the transverse ligament once immobilization is discontinued. For patients with chronic or irreducible subluxations, recurrent subluxations, a neurologic deficit, or evidence of transverse ligament insufficiency, open reduction via a posterior approach and a posterior Brooks-type C1–C2 arthrodesis is the treatment of choice.[44, 68, 79, 109] This approach is unchanged from that initially recommended by Fielding and Hawkins in their 1977 paper, with the exception of the type of arthrodesis. Fielding and Hawkins favored a Gallie-type fusion. Because of the improved rotational control with a Brooks-type fusion, we believe this to be the procedure of choice. If adequate reduction is achieved, transarticular C1–C2 screw fixation is typically added for rigidity.

rotatory fixation without anterior displacement, with the ADI less than 3 mm. The fixed rotation is within the normal range of motion of the atlantoaxial articulation, and the transverse ligament is intact, allowing the dens to act as the pivot. This was the most common type seen in the Fielding and Hawkins series (Fig. 11–12). In type II, the second most prevalent type in the Fielding and Hawkins series, the rotatory fixation is associated with anterior displacement of the atlas with an ADI of 3 to 5 mm. In their scheme, the transverse ligament is deficient, and unilateral anterior displacement of one lateral mass occurs while the opposite facet joint remains intact and acts as a pivot. In this case the amount of fixed rotation is beyond the normal limits of atlantoaxial rotation. In type III, there is more than 5 mm of anterior displacement of the atlas on the axis. Both the transverse ligament and the secondary restraints, including the C1–C2 facet capsules, are deficient. Both lateral masses of the atlas are displaced anteriorly, but one more so than the other, creating the rotated position (Fig. 11–13). In type IV, the least common type, there is posterior displacement of the atlas on the axis in association with a deficient dens. Here too, one of the lateral masses is displaced more so than the other, creating the rotatory component.

The Fielding and Hawkins classification provides some guidance for the treatment of these deformities. Unfortunately, the management of atlantoaxial rotatory fixation usually follows a protracted period of misdiagnosis and inadequate treatment.[44, 68, 79, 109] In the Fielding and Hawkins series, the average delay in diagnosis was 11.6 months.[44] Levine and Edwards reported a delay in diagnosis ranging from 9 days to 6 months. Although the treatment remains somewhat controversial, most agree

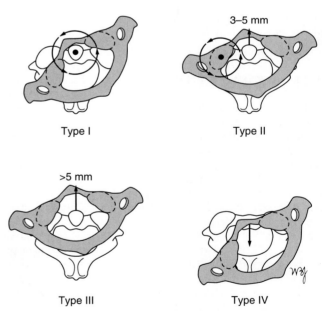

Figure 11–11. Diagram showing the four types of rotatory fixation in the Fielding classification scheme. A, Type I—rotatory fixation with no anterior displacement and the odontoid acting as the pivot. B, Type II—rotatory fixation with anterior displacement of 3 to 5 mm, one lateral articular process acting as the pivot. C, Type III—rotatory fixation with anterior displacement of more than 5 mm. D, Type IV—rotatory fixation with posterior displacement. (From Fielding WJ, Hawkins RJ: Atlanto-axial rotatory fixation [fixed rotatory subluxation of the atlanto-axial joint]. J Bone Joint Surg Am 59A:37–44, 1977.)

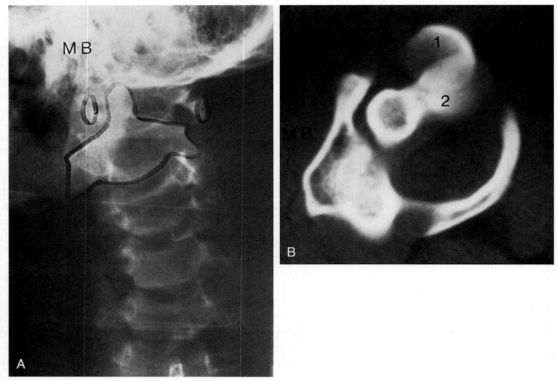

Figure 11–12. *A, Anteroposterior x-ray of an 18-year-old male presenting with acute painful torticollis after a minor fall. Note the malalignment and asymmetry of the atlas on the axis. B, A CT scan of the atlantoaxial complex demonstrates the obvious anterior subluxation of the C1 lateral mass on the C2 consistent with a type 1 C1–C2 rotatory subluxation. The patient underwent a successful closed reduction under mild intravenous sedation, and postreduction AP and lateral flexion and extension x-rays demonstrated an anatomic reduction without evidence of a transverse ligament injury.*

ATLAS FRACTURES

In describing 4 of his own cases and reviewing 42 others, Jefferson is generally acknowledged as the first to report on fractures of the atlas.[60] Although this may not be historically accurate, that the eponym for the bursting atlantal fracture bears his name is testimony to his important contribution to the early understanding of this fracture. Jefferson theorized a bursting mechanism of the C1 ring under axial loading of the occipital condyles. His conceptualization of atlas fractures has undergone some modification through the modern era, but the general principles remain without major changes.[65, 67, 68, 99] These injuries are related to impact of the skull on the arch of C1, with such factors as the force vector applied to the head and craniovertebral relationship at the time of impact determining the specific injury pattern. As a group, fractures of the atlas represent approximately 25% of all injuries to the atlantoaxial complex and 10% of all injuries to the cervical spine.[67, 69] The most common causes of these injuries are motor vehicle accidents, falls, and diving accidents. In the retrospective review of Levine and Edwards, all C1 ring fractures followed a major traumatic event.[67, 122] Rarely are atlas fractures the cause of a neurologic deficit. Patients with atlas fractures who present with a neurologic deficit generally do so as a result of an associated spinal column or head injury. The one exception to this rule involves crush injuries to the suboccipital and

greater occipital nerves. Dysesthetic symptoms in the suboccipital region may be present acutely, and their persistence has been reported in long-term studies.[67–69, 97]

Radiographic diagnosis of atlas fractures begins with routine anteroposterior, open-mouth anteroposterior, and lateral views of the cervical spine. The lateral cervical spine film may demonstrate a fracture in the posterior C1 ring; the anterior ring is not well visualized on plain films. This film must also be carefully evaluated for the presence of retropharyngeal soft tissue swelling, an abnormal ADI, or any evidence of other cervical spine fractures.[106] Patients with posterior arch fractures have a 50% incidence of associated cervical spine fractures.[67, 68] Other types of atlas fractures have a lower, but still significant, incidence of associated cervical spine trauma.[65, 67, 68, 72, 111] The open-mouth view should be used to reveal any lateral displacement of the C1 lateral masses on those of the axis.[103] If lateral displacement is present, it is important to note if both lateral masses are displaced symmetrically and to accurately quantify the amount of displacement. A CT scan is then obtained to precisely define the fracture pattern of the C1 ring. Evidence of a transverse ligament avulsion should also be sought on the CT scan. For patients with suspected type II or III odontoid fracture, three-dimensional sagittal reconstructions should be formatted to further evaluate the status of the dens. Linear tomography remains an excellent alternative for the radiographic evaluation of

C1 ring fractures and is a superior method for assessing fractures of the dens. However, in many centers, this technology is being increasingly supplanted by CT scans and CT reconstructions.

Atlas fractures have been classified as posterior arch, comminuted, bursting (or Jefferson), and anterior arch fractures.[67] These distinct types depend on the mechanism of injury and craniovertebral relationship at the time of injury. Their significance rests in understanding the mechanism, developing a treatment algorithm, and offering a reliable prognosis.

Bilateral fracture of the posterior arch is believed to result from hyperextension and axial loading as the posterior arch of C1 is caught between the occiput and posterior elements of C2.[67, 68, 99] This loading of the C1 ring leads to a tension failure of the posterior arch. Neurologic

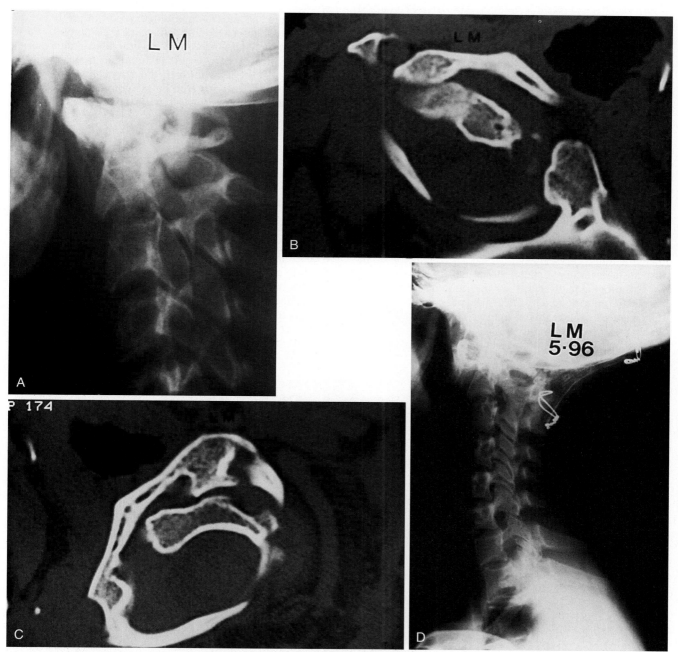

Figure 11–13. *A, Lateral x-ray of a 22-year-old female with a history of Marfan's syndrome presenting with acute neck pain and torticollis after a minor fall. Note the increased ADI measuring 7 mm. A dynamic CT scan with the head rotated to the right (B) shows the increased ADI. When the head is rotated to the left (C), the ADI decreases slightly, but the right lateral mass of C1 is completely dislocated anteriorly. These findings are consistent with a type 3 rotatory fixation. D, The patient underwent a successful occiput to C2 posterior fusion. The patient had a hypoplastic posterior C1 ring, which necessitated the fusion to the occiput.*

deficit is not associated with an isolated posterior arch fracture and should arouse suspicion of a second cervical spine fracture. In the series of Levine and Edwards, more than 50% of patients with a posterior arch fracture had an associated cervical spine fracture.[67] Most commonly, traumatic spondylolisthesis of the axis or odontoid fracture accompanies the posterior arch fracture. It is noteworthy that one patient in the Levine and Edwards series had a rupture of the transverse ligament in association with the posterior arch fracture; other authors have reported similarly rare associations.[67, 72, 82] Therefore, identification of a posterior arch fracture on plain films mandates that the examiner determine whether this is an isolated injury or one part of a combined injury. Retropharyngeal soft tissue swelling ordinarily is not present with an isolated posterior ring fracture; its presence indicates that either the anterior ring is fractured or there is an associated upper cervical spine injury. Similarly, with an isolated posterior ring fracture there should be no lateral displacement of the C1 articular masses on the open-mouth view. Retropharyngeal soft tissue swelling and lateral splaying of the articular masses are indications for obtaining a CT scan through the C1 ring.

Isolated posterior arch fractures are treated with a cervical orthosis for 6 to 8 weeks or until the patient is asymptomatic.[67] These fractures heal reliably with minimal long-term sequelae. For posterior arch fractures in association with other cervical spine fractures, treatment of the most unstable injury dictates the management. Generally, the posterior arch fracture is the more stable of the concurrent injuries and plays a secondary role. Specific injury patterns and treatment options are discussed later in this chapter.

A second type of atlas fracture is the comminuted fracture.[67, 97] Although this has previously been referred to as the lateral mass fracture, a distinction should be made between it and the isolated lateral mass fracture. The latter is a relatively rare injury that infers an intra-articular fracture through the C1 lateral mass without involvement of the anterior or posterior ring.[67, 68] It is a stable injury that may be treated with a cervical orthosis, although the long-term sequelae with regard to arthrosis and neck pain are not well defined. Alternatively, the comminuted fracture refers to an injury occurring on one side of the C1 ring with one fracture just anterior or within the anterior portion of the lateral mass and a second fracture line passing posterior to the ipsilateral lateral mass.[67, 97] Several other fractures may or may not also be present, including a more extensive intra-articular fracture through the lateral mass, a second fracture of the posterior arch on the contralateral side, and an ipsilateral osteoperiosteal avulsion of the transverse ligament.

This fracture pattern follows an axial loading to the cranium with some element of lateral flexion such that the C1 lateral masses are asymmetrically loaded. On the open-mouth view this is demonstrated by markedly disparate lateral displacement of the masses with the uninvolved side having no or minimal displacement and the involved side having essentially all of the total displacement (Fig. 11–14).[67, 97] The amount of displacement of the involved side is often comparable to the total displacement of both lateral masses in a bursting atlantal fracture. As in the case of posterior arch fractures, neurologic involvement is rare with this fracture pattern unless caused by an associated injury. Treatment for comminuted fractures follows the same algorithm as for bursting atlantal fractures. However, one retrospective review of atlas fractures has suggested that this fracture pattern is the most likely to

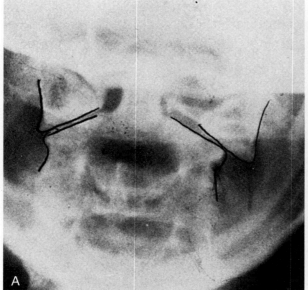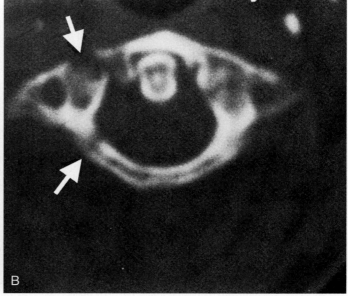

Figure 11–14. *Comminuted fracture of the atlas. A, The open-mouth view demonstrates no displacement of one lateral mass and marked displacement of the opposite side. B, The CT scan demonstrates similar findings with fracture lines anterior and posterior to the lateral mass on the affected side with no fractures in the arch on the opposite side. (From Levine AM, Edwards CC: Traumatic lesions of the occipitoatlanto-axial process. Clin Orthop 239:53–60, 1989.)*

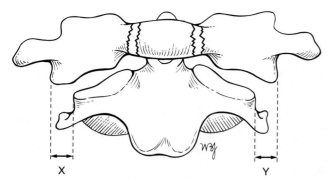

Figure 11–15. *Total atlantoaxial offset is calculated by adding X + Y. A total offset exceeding 6.9 mm implies transverse atlantal ligament rupture.*

result in nonunion and a poor functional outcome.[97] Therefore, accurate identification of the fracture pattern and strict adherence to the principles of immobilization must be the treatment goals.

The third type of atlas fracture is the bursting, or Jefferson fracture.[54, 60, 65, 67–69] This fracture is the result of axial loading through the cranium and occipital condyles flowing caudally through the lateral masses of the atlas. The bony geometry of the occipitoatlantal and atlantoaxial joints forces the lateral bursting of the C1 ring in tension and consequent lateral displacement of the masses. The C1 ring fails in one or two sites anteriorly and in two sites posteriorly with the development of the three- or four-part fracture, depending on the number of anterior ring fractures. Because this fracture effectively decompresses the thecal sac and neural elements, neurologic deficits are uncommon.[54, 60, 67–69, 122] A notable exception is that this fracture also is commonly associated with other upper and lower cervical spine fractures.

The radiographic evaluation of bursting atlantal fractures proceeds as for other atlas fractures with the inclusion of a CT scan through the upper spine. The central issue in the evaluation and treatment of bursting fractures is the status of the transverse atlantal ligament. Several methods are available to assess the competence of the transverse ligament. First, the ADI should be measured on lateral cervical spine x-ray. An ADI less than or equal to 3 mm provides little information, but an ADI greater than 4 mm indicates transverse ligament insufficiency.[42] Second, the open-mouth odontoid view and CT scan should be inspected for evidence of an osteoperiosteal avulsion of the transverse ligament insertion.[42, 67, 68] Third, the integrity of the transverse ligament can be predicted using the recommendations of Spence et al., who performed an in vitro experiment in which the transverse ligament was ruptured through distraction of the C1 lateral masses after the ring was sectioned to simulate a bursting fracture.[103] The cumulative lateral offset of the C1 lateral masses relative to the C2 lateral masses was recorded simultaneously during the distraction. These authors concluded that a cumulative offset of 5.7 mm or less was consistent with an intact ligament, whereas a cumulative offset greater than 6.9 mm indicated rupture of the transverse ligament (Figs. 11–15

and 11–16). More recently, the role of radiographic magnification has led some to question the strict interpretation of 6.9 mm as a measure of transverse ligament competence. Instead, these authors contend that a cumulative offset greater than 8 mm should define transverse ligament rupture.[56] Finally, should the status of the transverse ligament remain uncertain despite the aforementioned, MRI may be useful in determining its integrity.[34]

Some controversy surrounds the treatment of comminuted and bursting atlantal fractures. This controversy centers on three areas: the management of patients with radiographic evidence of transverse ligament rupture, the management of patients with associated odontoid fractures, and the role of fracture reduction in the prevention of posttraumatic symptoms and atlantoaxial arthrosis.[54, 65, 67–69, 97, 100] General guidelines for the treatment of these fractures have been outlined by Levine and Edwards.[67] Nondisplaced fractures (those with less than 2 mm of offset) can be treated with a cervical orthosis. Patients with fractures with 2 to 7 mm of offset are best managed with a halo vest until fracture union occurs. For patients with fractures with greater than 7 mm of offset, these authors recommend fracture reduction and maintenance through traction until stability to the C1 ring is restored. Traction is terminated when no loss of reduction occurs (as judged by an open-mouth view) after the traction has been removed for 1 hour with the patient in the supine position. This usually takes approximately 6 weeks. After removal from traction, the patient is placed into a halo vest until complete osseous healing occurs. After this regimen, reliable bony union is expected. Although of great concern, atlantoaxial instability is rarely a clinical problem after fracture treatment, even in situations in which transverse ligament rupture was implied or verified by radiographic criteria.[65a, 67–69, 97] In the Levine and Edwards series of atlas fractures, no patient had an ADI greater than 5 mm and no patient required an arthrodesis for atlantoaxial instability at the conclusion of treatment.[67] Transverse ligament ruptures in conjunction with comminuted and bursting atlantal fractures behave differently from those that follow a flexion injury and represent a purely ligamentous insult. With the former, the secondary restraints including the alar ligaments and facet capsules are not disrupted or attenuated, as they often are secondary to a hyperflexion injury. Moreover, in a series of atlas fractures in which the patients were evaluated with pretreatment and posttreatment CT scans, six of the seven transverse ligament failures were identified as avulsions, and 80% of these were shown to heal with osseous congruity in their posttreatment study.[97] Thus, although attention must be given to the competence of the transverse ligament, and all patients should have flexion-extension views of the cervical spine at the conclusion of treatment to assess its physiologic competence, clinically significant instability is rare.

The management of patients with comminuted or bursting atlantal fractures and concurrent type II or III odontoid fractures should generally follow a more conservative approach of initial halo vest immobilization or traction, followed by a delayed atlantoaxial arthrodesis, if necessary. Occiput to C2 arthrodesis is an option, but this involves significant morbidity in the form of lost cervical spine motion.[98, 114] Primary anterior screw fixation of a type

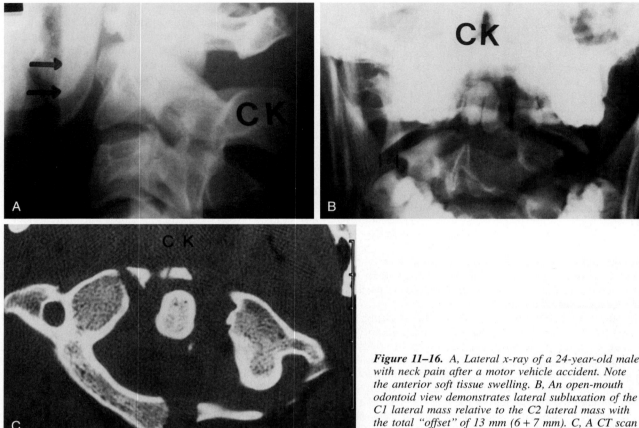

Figure 11–16. *A, Lateral x-ray of a 24-year-old male with neck pain after a motor vehicle accident. Note the anterior soft tissue swelling. B, An open-mouth odontoid view demonstrates lateral subluxation of the C1 lateral mass relative to the C2 lateral mass with the total "offset" of 13 mm (6 + 7 mm). C, A CT scan demonstrates the classic "Jefferson" bursting fracture.*

II odontoid fracture affords another option and, in the hands of a surgeon with adequate experience, a reasonable one in specific scenarios (Fig. 11–17).[1, 14, 23, 48, 78]

The role of fracture reduction in preventing delayed symptoms and atlantoaxial arthrosis is unclear. Although many authors report the relatively prevalent development of symptoms such as neck pain and occipital dysesthesias after these fractures, most believe them to be mild in nature.[67, 68, 97] To our knowledge, the development of posttraumatic arthrosis has not been characterized. What is clear, as Levine and Edwards have demonstrated, is that a permanent reduction is not possible without a protracted course of traction.[67] Ostensibly, this would be an overzealous approach to a problem heretofore considered to be relatively minor.

The fourth type of atlas fracture is the anterior arch fracture.[87, 105] This fracture is believed to follow a hyperextension mechanism and is usually directed horizontally across the anterior arch. Whether this fracture results from mechanical abutment of the dens and anterior arch, avulsion of the longus colli, or a combination of the two mechanisms is uncertain. It may be associated with other cervical spine trauma, particularly with odontoid fractures and traumatic spondylolisthesis of the axis. Isolated anterior arch fractures can be managed with a cervical orthosis with an expected good outcome.[69, 87, 105]

ODONTOID FRACTURES

The high degree of morbidity associated with the treatment of odontoid fractures has made this subject the focus of considerable controversy and ongoing study. No single method of management has gained universal acceptance, and clinical reports of odontoid fracture treatment continue to appear in the literature. Historically, odontoid fractures had a dismal prognosis with high incidences of neurologic involvement and death.[9, 29, 76, 81, 83] Early on it was recognized that union rarely occurred and that delayed myelopathy, thought to be secondary to a nonunion, threatened previously injured patients.[9, 29, 76, 81, 83] Consequently, primary surgical stabilization became a consideration in the management of these fractures, but the indications for it were unclear. Unfortunately, although our surgical expertise and experience with odontoid fractures has grown exponentially, a number of questions as to their optimal treatment remain unanswered.

Odontoid fractures represent 7% to 15% of all cervical spine fractures. Most patients present after a fall or motor vehicle accident, generally of high energy, except for elderly, osteoporotic patients and patients with long-standing rheumatoid arthritis.[6, 24, 91, 92] In patients with severe osteopenia or history of rheumatoid arthritis, spontaneous fractures of the odontoid process without a known history of antecedent trauma have been reported.[107] Despite extensive research efforts, the exact mechanism of odontoid fractures has eluded description.[4, 35, 69, 80] Research to date suggests that a pure extension moment through the cranium and upper cervical spine favors a fracture to the body of the axis (type III), whereas an oblique or lateral bending moment favors a fracture through the base of the odontoid (type II).[4, 35, 80] However, a definitive explanation of the mechanism of these fractures in vivo awaits further investigation. Most likely, a complex combination of several force vectors produces the various odontoid fractures seen in clinical practice.

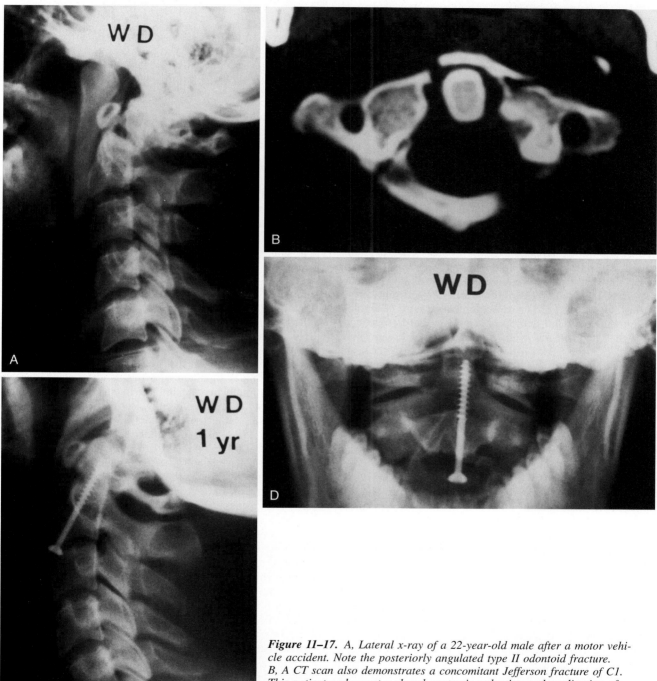

Figure 11–17. *A, Lateral x-ray of a 22-year-old male after a motor vehicle accident. Note the posteriorly angulated type II odontoid fracture. B, A CT scan also demonstrates a concomitant Jefferson fracture of C1. This patient underwent a closed anatomic reduction and application of a halo vest. The reduction of the odontoid fracture was lost, however, and the patient subsequently underwent an anterior odontoid screw fixation to stabilize the odontoid fracture. One-year follow-up AP (C) and lateral (D) x-rays show well-healed odontoid and atlas fractures.*

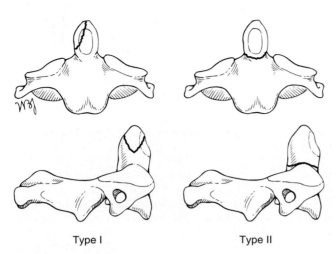

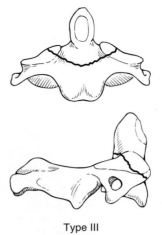

Type I   Type II   Type III

Figure 11–18. The three types of odontoid fractures as proposed by Anderson and D'Alonzo. (From Anderson LD, D'Alonzo RT: Fractures of the odontoid process of the axis. J Bone Joint Surg Am 56A:663–674, 1974.)

Patients with odontoid fractures often present with associated mental status changes from head trauma or intoxication, as well as other skeletal and visceral injuries.[6, 24, 90, 92] Consequently, localizing signs and symptoms may be subtle and these fractures may be missed on initial evaluation.[6, 15, 24, 90, 92] Patients who are alert generally complain of upper neck pain and tenderness on palpation of the posterior spine. Paravertebral muscle spasm is variably present. The incidence of neurologic involvement in patients with odontoid fractures ranges from 15% to 25% of cases.[6, 24, 90, 92] Neurologic deficits may be limited to a greater occipital neuropraxia or may be as extensive as high quadriplegia with respiratory center involvement.[6, 24, 90, 92, 102] Brown-Séquard syndrome and "cruciate paralysis" are other possible findings. At least one report in the literature associates an odontoid fracture with a lower cranial nerve palsy.[75]

The radiographic diagnosis of odontoid fractures sometimes may be difficult based on plain film studies alone.[6, 24] When suspicion is sufficiently aroused based on the plain films, linear tomography is the study of choice for evaluating the odontoid. Where tomography has been supplanted by CT, a CT scan with a three-dimensional reconstruction is the second-best option. The association of odontoid fractures with other cervical spine fractures, particularly those of the C1 ring, was noted earlier in this chapter.[67, 111] It is essential that any concomitant fractures of the atlas be detected before a treatment plan is determined.

Anderson and D'Alonzo created a classification system for odontoid fractures based on a retrospective review of their experience.[6] Because of its clinical applicability and anatomical significance, this classification system has gained universal acceptance (Fig. 11–18). A type I fracture is an oblique fracture through the upper part of the odontoid process. This pattern is believed to represent an avulsion fracture where the alar ligament attaches to the odontoid. It is the least common type, representing less than 5% of odontoid fractures.[6, 24] A type II fracture occurs at the junction of the odontoid process with the body of the axis. This is the most common type, accounting for approximately 60% of odontoid fractures, and is responsible for the

vast majority of the controversy surrounding the management of these injuries.[6, 24] A type III fracture extends downward into the cancellous portion of the body, representing a fracture through the body of the axis. This type accounts for 30% of odontoid fractures.[6, 24]

Before discussing the treatment options, a review of the relevant ligamentous, osseous, and vascular anatomy is warranted in gaining an appreciation for the reasons why difficulties healing these fractures, particularly those at the odontoid base, might be anticipated. As detailed in the anatomy section, the dens is connected to the occiput and atlas through several key ligaments.[38, 58] The apical dental ligament arises from the odontoid tip, and the paired alar ligaments originate from the superolateral sides of the odontoid. These ligaments travel in a cephalad direction until the apical ligament attaches to the basion and the paired alar ligaments attach to the lateral rim of the foramen magnum and occipital condyles. The tension in these ligaments in a static state is unknown, but probably is not negligible. Thus, in fractures of the odontoid tip or base, healing theoretically occurs in the absence of any compressive forces. Furthermore, with synovial tissue anterior and posterior to the odontoid base, fractures in this region adopt an intra-articular–like local environment with any bony displacement or distraction.

Histomorphometric studies of the osseous microanatomy of the axis and odontoid process have revealed markedly less trabecular bone at the base of the odontoid as compared to the odontoid process and the body of the axis.[5] The cortical thickness of the base of the odontoid is one-third that of the axis body. The relative paucity of trabecular and cortical bone at the base of the odontoid not only creates a predilection for fractures, but also suggests that in the fracture setting, osseous healing is unlikely to proceed with exuberance.

The vascular anatomy of the odontoid process was well described by Schiff and Parke in 1973.[93] Three main groups of arteries supply the odontoid process and its ligaments. Paired anterior ascending arteries originate from the vertebral arteries and follow a rostral course until most branching vessels penetrate at the anterior and lateral margins of the odontoid base. Similarly, paired posterior ascending arteries also originate from the vertebral arteries and send branches that pierce the odontoid at its base. Both pairs of vessels, which provide the majority of the blood supply to the odontoid, terminate in an anastomosis at the odontoid tip termed the apical arcade. This arcade is formed from branches of the ascending arteries that do not penetrate the base of the odontoid, but rather ascend along its lateral borders to the apex. The third arterial supply of the odontoid, of lesser magnitude, is the cleft perforators. These vessels originate from the most rostral extracranial portion of the internal carotid arteries and anastomose with the anterior ascending arteries at or near the odontoid base. Therefore, it is evident that fractures of the odontoid base are at great risk for significantly compromising the arterial supply to the odontoid and the surrounding structures. Taken together, the ligamentous, osseous, and vascular anatomy of the odontoid process create an environment that is most unfavorable for healing of any fracture, particularly one occurring at or near the odontoid's base.

Type I odontoid fractures are stable injuries, and treatment involves orthotic immobilization.[6, 24] However, it is worth noting that these injuries have been reported in association with atlanto-occipital instability.[96] Therefore, evaluation of the craniovertebral junction is part of the management of this uncommon fracture.

The treatment of type II odontoid fractures remains controversial; no single treatment algorithm has gained universal acceptance. There are strong advocates of primary surgical and nonsurgical management alike, as well as a foundation of literature to support either approach, and the surgeon is justified in selecting either form of treatment.[1, 6, 8, 14, 23, 24, 26, 43, 53, 59, 71, 78, 92, 102] The reported incidence of nonunion of type II fractures treated solely with some form of immobilization is 10% to 65%.[6, 8, 24, 53, 71, 92] A large, multicenter study sponsored by the Cervical Spine Research Society found that 66% of all type II fractures treated with halo vest immobilization united without secondary treatment.[24] In this study, all patients who had either no treatment or immobilization in a cervical orthosis alone failed to unite. Several factors have been identified as predisposing to nonunion or malunion of type II fractures. These include initial fracture displacement, either anterior

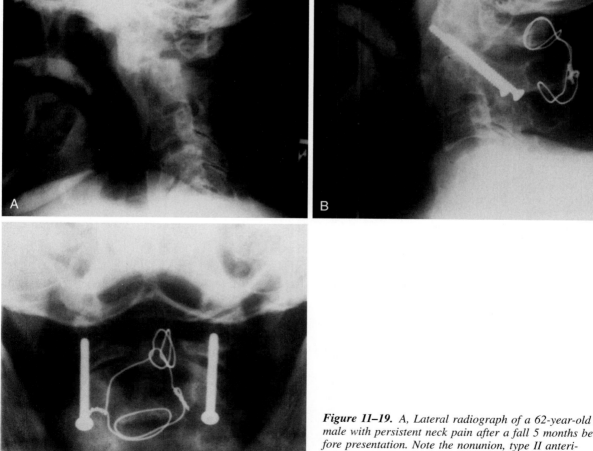

Figure 11–19. *A, Lateral radiograph of a 62-year-old male with persistent neck pain after a fall 5 months before presentation. Note the nonunion, type II anteriorly displaced odontoid fracture. B and C, The patient underwent a successful posterior C1–C2 fusion using the transarticular Magerl screw technique.*

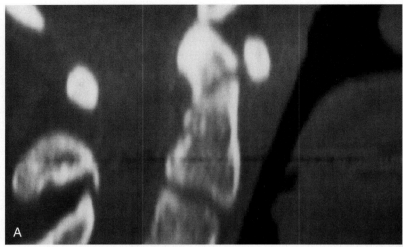

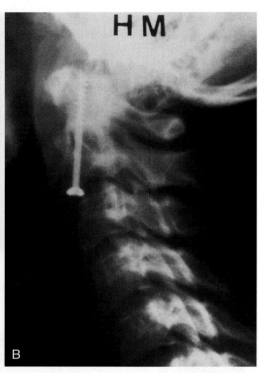

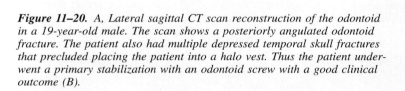

Figure 11–20. A, Lateral sagittal CT scan reconstruction of the odontoid in a 19-year-old male. The scan shows a posteriorly angulated odontoid fracture. The patient also had multiple depressed temporal skull fractures that precluded placing the patient into a halo vest. Thus the patient underwent a primary stabilization with an odontoid screw with a good clinical outcome (B).

or posterior, greater than 4 to 5 mm; angulation greater than 10 to 15 degrees; and patient age above 40 to 50 years (Fig. 11–19).[8, 24, 53, 71] Posterior displacement of the odontoid may also be a risk factor for nonunion.

The choice between primary surgical stabilization and halo vest immobilization is made based on these parameters and on other patient- and situation-specific variables. Primary posterior spinal fusion of C1 to C2 has proven highly successful.[24, 43, 59] Stabilization of the atlantoaxial articulation was achieved in 96% of the patients in the multicenter study treated with primary posterior fusion.[24] Nonetheless, primary posterior fusion carries the associated surgical risks and morbidity of lost atlantoaxial motion. Primary anterior stabilization of the odontoid with compressive screw fixation remains a third option.[1, 14, 23, 48, 57a, 78] The potential advantage of this method is the preservation of atlantoaxial motion. A high complication rate is associated with anterior screw fixation in elderly patients.[7a] The significant number of complications and persistent nonunions reported in the literature after anterior screw fixation, in addition to a recent report that raises doubt as to whether there is actual preservation of motion as compared to posterior procedures, relegates primary anterior stabilization to cases in which halo immobilization and posterior atlantoaxial fusion are unacceptable alternatives (Fig. 11–20). Most commonly, this situation arises in patients in whom surgical stabilization is deemed necessary, but who have a concomitant fracture of the C1 ring. Although posterior fusion to the occiput is an alternative in these patients, with sufficient surgical expertise and a relative or absolute contraindication to halo vest immobilization, anterior screw fixation provides another reasonable treatment option (see Fig. 11–17).

Although the treatment of type III fractures is less troublesome, these injuries are not benign and if treated inappropriately can result in significant morbidity.[24, 57] When initial fracture displacement exceeds 5 mm, a 40% nonunion rate, irrespective of method of immobilization, has been reported.[24] Angular deformity greater than 10 degrees has been shown to result in a nonunion rate of 22%.[24] Overall, reduction and halo vest immobilization can be expected to achieve union in more than 80% of patients and is the preferred treatment for this fracture (Fig. 11–21). A cervical orthosis is indicated only when the fracture is minimally displaced or impacted and the patient has a contraindication to halo vest immobilization.

TRAUMATIC SPONDYLOLISTHESIS OF THE AXIS

Since Schneider coined the term "hangman's fracture" in 1965, this term has gained widespread use in describing neural arch fractures of the axis.[95] The historical evolution of judicial hanging was reviewed in great detail by Fielding et al.[46] This form of punishment consistently produces a fatal, fracture-dislocation of the axis with a submental knot position.[118] The bilateral fracture lines extend through the pars interarticularis of the neural arch and are accompanied by complete disruption of the disk and the ligaments between the C2 and C3. This is in contrast to the clinically relevant fracture of the neural arch produced by motor vehicle accidents and falls in both the mechanism and the degree of soft tissue and disk disruption.[19, 22, 39, 46, 47, 70, 95]

In fact, the only similarity between an axis fracture from a hanging and the fracture commonly called a hangman's fracture is the radiographic appearance. Consequently, the more descriptive term of traumatic spondylolisthesis of the axis has gained popularity to refer to fracture of the posterior elements of the axis.

The exact incidence of these injuries is unknown, because only occipitoatlantal dislocations are more common in patients involved in fatal motor vehicle accidents.[21, 22] Similar to other upper cervical spine fractures, traumatic spondylolisthesis of the axis generally follows a fall or motor vehicle accident.[19, 39, 46, 47, 70, 95] Importantly, concomitant cervical spine fractures occur in roughly one-third of patients, with the vast majority of these in the upper

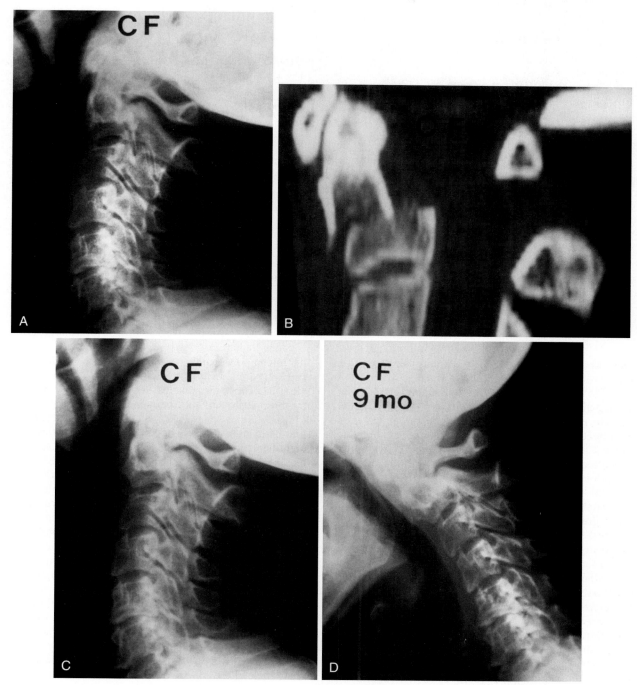

Figure 11–21. *A, Lateral x-ray of a 43-year-old female after a motor vehicle accident. Note the anteriorly angulated type III odontoid fracture through the base of the odontoid. B, A sagittal CT scan reconstruction clearly demonstrates the fracture line through the base of the odontoid. Lateral flexion (C) and extension (D) x-rays, taken after successful treatment in a halo vest, show a well-healed fracture and a stable C1–C2 complex.*

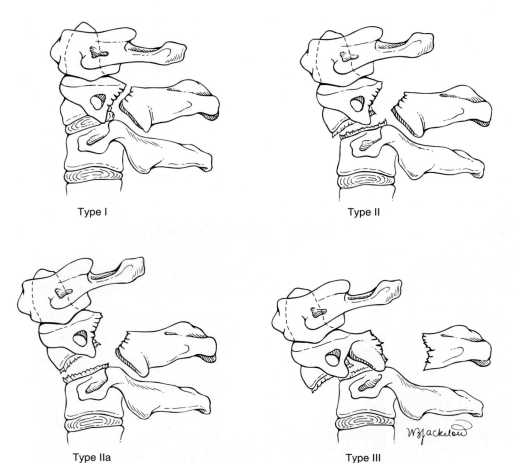

Type I

Type II

Type IIa

Type III

Figure 11–22. Classification scheme of Levine and Edwards for traumatic spondylolisthesis of the axis. (Adapted from Levine AM, Edwards CC: The management of traumatic spondylolisthesis of the axis. J Bone Joint Surg Am 67A:217–226, 1985.)

cervical spine.[19, 39, 46, 47, 70, 95, 111] Among survivors, the incidence of neurologic deficits is estimated to be 5% to 10%.[19, 39, 46, 47, 70, 95, 111] Most of the neurologic injuries occur in patients with a fracture-dislocation (type III) of C2 on C3. The overall low incidence of neurologic injury is due to the effective decompression of the neural canal created by this fracture pattern. Vertebral artery injury, though rare, has been reported.[15]

Effendi was the first to publish a systematic classification system of fractures of the arch of the axis.[39] This classification system was based on a retrospective review of the radiographic and clinical course of 131 patients and provided the framework to the currently accepted classification system of Levine and Edwards. This more recent classification scheme of Levine and Edwards attempts to correlate the mechanism of injury with the fracture type.[70] Conceptually related to this mechanistic understanding of neural arch fractures is the transitional role that the axis plays in cervical spine mechanics. The posterior elements of the axis join the relatively mobile upper cervical spine to the more constrained subaxial spine.[98, 114] In this junctional role, the inferior articular facets and spinous process, along with the robust nuchal muscles, anchor the posterior elements of the axis to the lower cervical spine, and the body and superior articular facets transmit loads from the cervicocranium. This places the uniquely elongated pars interarticularis of the axis under tremendous stress as it links

the disproportionately mobile segments. Understandably, supraphysiologic flexion and extension of the cervicocranium can stress this linkage, which is further compromised by the presence of the foramen transversarium, to failure.

The Levine and Edwards classification is based on pretreatment x-rays (Fig. 11–22).[70] After the fracture is identified, any displacement or angulation is measured. This displacement is measured as the distance, at the level of the C2–C3 disk space, between lines drawn along the posterior margins of C2 and C3. Angulation is calculated by measuring the angle subtended by lines drawn along the inferior endplates of C2 and C3. Type I fractures include all nondisplaced fractures and those with no angulation and less than 3 mm of displacement. Type I fractures (Fig. 11–23) are believed to result from a hyperextension vector along with concomitant axial loading. The energy involved in this injury is absorbed by the fracture of the neural arch, whereas the disk and anterior and posterior ligamentous structures are not significantly compromised. Because an intact soft tissue bridge remains with a type I fracture, bony displacement is minimal and a stable injury pattern is produced. However, because of the high association with other hyperextension cervical spine fractures, such as those of the atlas ring and odontoid, the physician must make sure that it is an isolated type I fracture before deciding on a treatment plan.

In the Levine and Edwards scheme, the type I fracture

represents the only stable injury pattern. The type II, IIA, and III fractures are all considered unstable injuries. Type II fractures are defined as having significant angulation and translation (Fig. 11–24).[70] Type II fractures are the most commonly reported type, nearly twice as prevalent as the second most commonly reported type I fracture. This fracture pattern is thought to have a dual mechanism in which an initial hyperextension-axial loading force is followed by an anterior flexion and compression force. The posterior bony elements of the axis are fractured similarly to their fracture pattern in a type I fracture, but the additional flexion-compression force causes the rupture of the posterior longitudinal ligament and the C2–C3 disk space in a posterior-to-anterior direction. Importantly, however, the anterior longitudinal ligament and a variable portion of the anterior disk space are not disrupted with this injury. Consequently, the body of C3 frequently incurs a compression-type fracture at its anterosuperior margin as a result of the cervicocranial mass hinging forward on the intact anterior longitudinal ligament. Proof that the anterior

longitudinal ligament remains intact is provided by the experience of Levine and Edwards, in which traction failed to produce widening of the C2–C3 disk space in any patient with a type II fracture. In fact, patients in whom the anterior longitudinal ligament is ruptured following this dual loading mechanism likely die acutely as the upper cervical segments translate anteriorly without restriction, thus compromising the integrity of the upper cervical cord.[70]

Type IIA fractures are differentiated from type II fractures in the proposed mechanism of injury and treatment approach.[70] Generally, the type IIA fracture is radiographically distinguished from the type II fracture by the presence of angulation with little or no displacement (Fig. 11–25). However, this radiographic distinction can often be difficult to see, and it is not until traction is applied that the two injury types become readily discernible. This is because the type IIA fracture, unlike the type II, is produced by a flexion-distraction mechanism with further soft tissue attenuation anteriorly. Therefore, the application of traction increases the deformity rather than decreasing it as normally

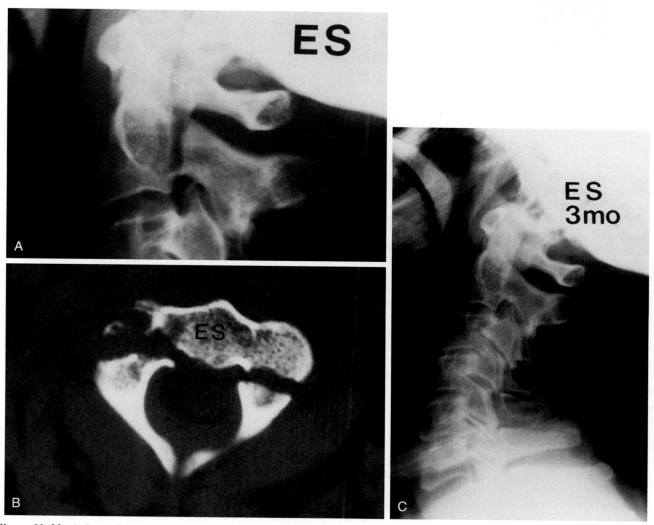

Figure 11–23. *A, Lateral x-ray of a 38-year-old female with acute neck pain after a motor vehicle accident. Note the type I non-displaced fracture line extending through the posterior element of C2 directly posterior to the C2 body. B, The CT scan confirms the diagnosis. C, The patient was successfully treated in a hard cervical collar.*

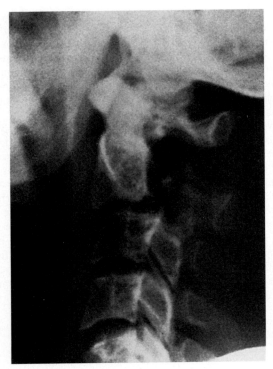

Figure 11–24. *Lateral x-ray of a type II hangman's fracture showing significant angulation and displacement. (From Levine AM, Edwards CC: The management of traumatic spondylolisthesis of the axis. J Bone Joint Surg Am 67A:217–226, 1985.)*

occurs with the mechanistically different type II fracture pattern. Moreover, the actual fracture pattern of the posterior bony structures is different in these two injuries. The fractures produced by hyperextension and axial loading, as in the case of type I and II fractures, tend to be in the anterior half of the neural arch and oriented longitudinally. In contrast, the fractures produced by a purely flexion vector tend to be in the posterior half of the arch with a more oblique orientation.

Type III fractures are defined as those showing severe angulation and translation as well as a unilateral or bilateral dislocation of the C2–C3 facet (Fig. 11–26).[70] The mechanism is postulated to be one of flexion and compression. Of all the fracture types, the type III injury carries the highest mortality rate and is by far the most likely to result in a permanent neurologic deficit.[70] Also differentiating the type III fracture from the others is the widely variable location of the fractures. The fractures may be either anterior, at the level of, or posterior to the facet joints. Establishing the exact fracture site is crucial, because this will determine whether there is any possibility of achieving a closed reduction of the facet dislocation. Nearly all of these fractures require operative intervention for treatment.

The last fracture type, known as the atypical hangman's fracture, is not part of any classification system.[104] Nonetheless, recogniton of this variant as a distinct fracture pattern is important in the management of patients with traumatic spondylolisthesis of the axis. In this variant, the

fracture configuration involves the posterior cortex of the axis rather than being isolated to the posterior elements. The significance of this fracture pattern is that instead of expanding the dimensions of the neural canal, as is normally seen when there is anterolisthesis and fractures restricted to the posterior elements, this fracture pattern may be canal compressive and place the spinal cord at risk with only moderate degrees of translation. In a review of 19 patients with traumatic spondylolisthesis of the axis, 6 were found to have an atypical variant.[104] All of these variants were found in patients with a type I or II fracture. More importantly, two out of the six had compression of the spinal cord resulting in a neurologic deficit at presentation. It is reasonable to conclude from this study that the atypical variant may be more prevalent and associated with a higher incidence of neurologic compromise than previously anticipated.

The treatment of traumatic spondylolisthesis of the axis was described by Levine and Edwards after they developed their classification system based on a rational explanation of fracture mechanism.[70] Type I fractures are considered stable injuries and may be treated with a cervical orthosis. Generally, only 6 weeks of immobilization is required. Type II, IIA, and III fractures are unstable injuries because of the significant disruption of the soft tissues at the C2–C3 interspace. Type II fractures are treated with cervical tong traction in extension until an adequate reduction (defined by Levine and Edwards as one with less than 4 to 5 mm of

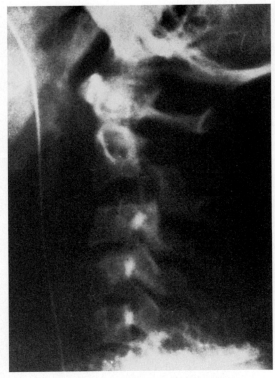

Figure 11–25. *Lateral x-ray of a type IIa hangman's fracture showing minimal displacement but severe angulation, apparently hinging from the anterior longitudinal ligament. (From Levine AM, Edwards CC: The management of traumatic spondylolisthesis of the axis. J Bone Joint Surg Am 67A:217–226, 1985.)*

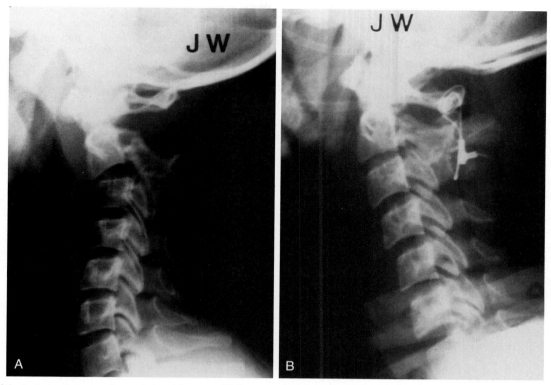

Figure 11–26. A, *Lateral x-ray of a patient with a type III hangman's fracture. Although this injury initially appears to be a type IIa, closer scrutiny shows that the C2–C3 facet joint is dislocated, making this a type III injury. Closed reduction was unsuccessful; therefore, an open reduction and posterior fusion was necessary (B). This patient was fused from C1 to C3, but a single-level C2–C3 fusion would be appropriate if adequate fixation could be achieved.*

displacement and less than 10 to 15 degrees of angulation) is maintained. Once a stable reduction is achieved, the patient is transferred to a halo vest until fracture union occurs. Whether or not a period of traction is necessary to achieve a stable reduction is debatable, however. Neither fracture union nor clinical outcome appears to be adversely affected by moderate amounts of residual fracture displacement or angulation.[70] Further study is needed to more precisely define what degree of residual deformity is acceptable before sequelae are seen in patient outcomes.

The most important aspect in the treatment of type IIA fractures is distinguishing these from the significantly more common type II fractures. Once a type IIA flexion-distraction injury is identified, it is treated by x-ray–guided reduction using compression and slight extension. A halo vest is then applied and maintained until fracture union is confirmed.

The type III fracture is the most unstable and the most difficult to treat of all the fracture types.[70] Although nearly all of these patients will eventually require operative treatment, the variability in injury pattern mandates a complete radiographic evaluation before definitive intervention is planned. Of paramount importance is determining whether the fractures are anterior, posterior, or at the level of the facets, and whether the dislocation is unilateral or bilateral. An MRI to evaluate the C2–C3 disk space and the space available for the cord is warranted when medically feasible. Acutely the patient is placed in a halo vest or tong traction to stabilize the spine and preliminarily reduce the deformity. In a patient with fractures of the neural arch anterior to the facets, the facet dislocation is free-floating and invariably irreducible by closed means. A posterior approach with an open reduction of the facet dislocation is completed before a single-level posterior fusion is performed. The patient is then placed in a halo vest for treatment of the neural arch fracture. In the patient with fractures at the level of or posterior to the facets, the dislocation may be amenable to a closed reduction. However, operative treatment is usually necessary to stabilize the spine and maintain the reduction in this unstable injury pattern. A single-level posterior fusion using a bilateral oblique wiring technique is usually sufficient, although this method requires healing of the neural arch fractures, if present, for ultimate stability. A posterior C1–C3 fusion provides surgical stability for the fracture dislocation pattern. Perhaps the best option, however, is an anterior C2–C3 interbody fusion, which provides stability and only a one level arthrodesis. A halo vest is worn until bony fusion is complete.

REFERENCES

1. Aebi M, Etter C, Coscia M: Fractures of the odontoid process. Treatment with anterior screw fixation. Spine 14:1065–1070, 1989.

2. Alker G, Oh YS, Leslie EV: High cervical spine and cranio-cervical junction injuries in fatal traffic accidents: A radiologic study. Orthop Clin North Am 9:1003–1010, 1978.

3. Alker GJ, Oh YS, Leslie EV, et al: Postmortem radiology of head and neck injuries in fatal traffic accidents. Radiology 114:611–617, 1975.

4. Althoff B: Fracture of the odontoid process. Acta Orthop Scand Suppl 177:3–94, 1979.

5. Amling M, Hahn M, Wening VJ, et al: The microarchitecture of the axis as the predisposing factor for fracture of the base of the odontoid process. A histomorphometric analysis of 22 autopsy specimens. J Bone Joint Surg Am 76A:1840–1846, 1994.

6. Anderson LD, D'Alonzo RT: Fractures of the odontoid process of the axis. J Bone Joint Surg Am 56A:663–674, 1974.

7. Anderson PA, Montesano PX: Morphology and treatment of occipital condyle fractures. Spine 13:731–736, 1988.

7a. Andersson S, Rodrigues M, Olerud C: Odontoid fractures: high complication rate associated with anterior screw fixation in the elderly. Euro Spine J 9:56–59, 2000.

8. Apuzzo ML, Heiden JS, Weiss MH, et al: Acute fractures of the odontoid process. An analysis of 45 cases. J Neurosurg 48:85–91, 1978.

9. Aymes EW, Anderson FM: Fracture of the odontoid process. Arch Surg 72:377–393, 1956.

10. Bell C: Surgical observations. Middlesex Hosp J 4:469, 1817.

11. Belzberg AJ, Tranmer BI: Stabilization of traumatic atlanto-occipital dislocation. Case report. J Neurosurg 75:478–482, 1991.

12. Blackwood NJ: Atlanto-occipital dislocations. Ann Surg 47:654–658, 1908.

13. Boden SA, Dodge LD, Bohlman HH, et al: Rheumatoid arthritis of the cervical spine. J Bone Joint Surg Am 75A:1282–1297, 1993.

14. Bohler J: Anterior stabilization for acute fractures and nonunions of the dens. J Bone Joint Surg Am 64A:18–27, 1982.

15. Bohlman HH: Acute fractures and dislocations of the cervical spine. J Bone Joint Surg Am 61A:1119–1142, 1979.

16. Bolander N, Cromwell LD, Wendling L: Fracture of the occipital condyle. Am J Roentgenol 131:729–731, 1978.

17. Bools JC, Rose BS: Traumatic atlanto-occipital dislocation: two cases with survival. Am J Neuroradiol 7:901–904, 1986.

18. Bozboga M, Unal F, Hepgul K, et al: Fracture of the occipital condyle. Spine 17:1119–1121, 1992.

19. Brashear HR, Venters GC, Preston ET: Fractures of the neural arch of the axis. A report of twenty-nine cases. J Bone Joint Surg Am 57A:879–887, 1975.

20. Brooks AL, Jenkins EB: Atlanto-axial arthrodesis by the wedge compression method. J Bone Joint Surg Am 60A:279–284, 1978.

21. Bucholz RW, Burkhead WZ: The pathologic anatomy of fatal atlanto-occipital dislocations. J Bone Joint Surg Am 61A:248–250, 1979.

22. Bucholz RW: Unstable Hangman's fractures. Clin Orthop 154:119–124, 1981.

23. Chiba K, Fujimura Y, Toyama Y, et al: Treatment protocol for fractures of the odontoid process. J Spinal Disord 9:267–276, 1996.

24. Clark CR, White AA: Fractures of the dens. A multicenter study. J Bone Joint Surg Am 67A:1340–1348, 1985.

25. Collato PM, De Muth WW, Schwentker EP, Boal DK: Traumatic atlanto-occipital dislocations. J Bone Joint Surg Am 67A:1106–1109, 1986.

26. Cooper PR, Maravilla KR, Sklar FH, et al: Halo immobilization of cervical spine fractures. Indications and results. J Neurosurg 50:603–610, 1979.

27. Corner ES: Rotary dislocations of the atlas. Ann Surg 45:9–26, 1907.

28. Coutts BM: Rotary dislocations of the atlas. Ann Surg 29:297–311, 1934.

29. Crooks F, Birkett AN: Fractures and dislocations of the cervical spine. Br J Surg 31:252–265, 1944.

30. Davis D, Bohlman HH, Walker AE, et al: The pathological findings in fatal craniospinal injuries. J Neurosurg 34:603–623, 1971.

31. De Beer JD, Thomas M, Walter J, Anderson P: Traumatic atlanto-axial subluxation. J Bone Joint Surg Br 70B:652–655, 1988.

32. Dickman CA, Papadopoulos SM, Sonntag VK, et al: Traumatic occipitoatlantal dislocations. J Spinal Disord 6:300–313, 1993.

33. Dickman CA, Greene KA, Sonntag VK: Injuries involving the transverse atlantal ligament: Classification and treatment guidelines based upon experience with 39 injuries. Neurosurgery 38:44–50, 1996.

34. Dickman CA, Mamourian A, Sonntag VKH, Drayer BP: Magnetic resonance imaging of the transverse atlantal ligament for the evaluation of atlantoaxial instability. J Neurosurg 75:221–227, 1991.

35. Doherty BJ, Heggeness MH, Esses SI: A biomechanical study of odontoid fractures and fracture fixation. Spine 18:178–184, 1993.

36. Dolan KD: Cervicobasilar relationships. Radiol Clin North Am 15:155–166, 1977.

37. Dvorak J, Hayek J, Zehnder R: CT-functional diagnostics of the rotatory instability of the upper cervical spine: II. An evaluation on healthy adults and patients with suspected instability. Spine 12:726–731, 1987.

38. Dvorak J, Schneider E, Saldinger P: Biomechanics of the craniocervical region: the alar and transverse ligaments. J Orthop Res 6:452–461, 1988.

39. Effendi B, Roy D, Cornish B, et al: Fractures of the ring of the axis. A classification based on the analysis of 131 cases. J Bone Joint Surg Br 63B:319–327, 1981.

40. Eismont FJ, Bohlman HH: Posterior atlanto-occipital dislocation with fracture of the atlas and odontoid process. Report of a case with survival. J Bone Joint Surg Am 60A:397–399, 1978.

41. Evarts CM: Traumatic occipito-atlantal dislocations. Report of a case with survival. J Bone Joint Surg Am 52A:1653–1660, 1970.

42. Fielding JW, Cochran GVB, Lawsing JF, Hohl M: Tears of the transverse ligament of the atlas. A clinical and biomechanical study. J Bone Joint Surg Am 56A:1683–1691, 1974.

43. Fielding JW, Hawkins RJ, Ratzan SA: Spine fusion for atlanto-axial instability. J Bone Joint Surg Am 58A:400–407, 1976.

44. Fielding WJ, Hawkins RJ: Atlanto-axial rotatory fixation (fixed rotatory subluxation of the atlanto-axial joint). J Bone Joint Surg Am 59A:37–44, 1977.

45. Fielding WJ, Stillwell WT, Chynn KY, Spyropoulos EC: Use of computed tomography for the diagnosis of atlanto-axial rotatory fixation. J Bone Joint Surg Am 60A:1102–1104, 1978.

46. Fielding JW, Francis WR, Hawkins RJ, et al: Traumatic spondylolisthesis of the axis. Clin Orthop 239:47–52, 1989.

47. Francis WR, Fielding JW, Hawkins RJ, et al: Traumatic

spondylolisthesis of the axis. J Bone Joint Surg Br 63B:313–318, 1981.

48. Fujii E, Kobayashi K, Hirabayashi K: Treatment of fractures of the odontoid process. Spine 13:604–609, 1988.

49. Gallie WE: Fractures and dislocation of the cervical spine. Am J Surg 46:495–499, 1939.

50. Gerlock AJ, Mirtakhraee M, Benzel EC: Computed tomography of traumatic atlanto-occipital dislocation. Neurosurgery 13:316–319, 1983.

51. Georgopoulos G, Pizzutillo PD, Lee M: Occipito-atlantal instability in children. A report of five cases and review of the literature. J Bone Joint Surg Am 69A:429–436, 1987.

52. Green BA, Eismont FJ, Oheir JT: Prehospital management of spinal cord injuries. Paraplegia 25:229–238, 1987.

53. Hadley MN, Dickman CA, Browner CM, et al: Acute axis fractures: A review of 229 cases. J Neurosurg 71:642–647, 1989.

54. Han SY, Witten DM, Musselman JP: Jefferson fracture of the atlas. Report of six cases. J Neurosurg 44:368–371, 1976.

55. Harding-Smith J, Macintosh PK, Sherbon KJ: Fracture of the occipital condyle. J Bone Joint Surg Am 63A:1170–1171, 1981.

56. Heller JG, Viroslav S, Hudson J: Jefferson fractures: The role of magnification artifact in assessing transverse ligament integrity. J Spinal Disord 6:392–396, 1993.

57. Heller JG, Levy MJ, Barrow DL: Odontoid fracture malunion with fixed atlantoaxial subluxation. Spine 18:311–314, 1993.

57a. Henry AD, Bohly J, Grosse A: Fixation of odontoid fractures by anterior screw. J Bone Joint Surg Br 81B:472–477, 1999.

58. Hollinshead WH, Rosse C: Textbook of Anatomy, 4th ed. Philadelphia, Harper and Row, 1985.

59. Jeanneret B, Magerl F: Primary posterior fusion C1/C2 in odontoid fractures: Indications, technique and results of transarticular screw fixation. J Spinal Disord 5:464–475, 1992.

60. Jefferson G: Fracture of the atlas vertebra. Report of four cases and a review of those previously recorded. Br J Surg 7:407–422, 1920.

61. Jones RN: Rotatory dislocation of both atlanto-axial joints. J Bone Joint Surg Br 66B:6–7, 1984.

62. Kauffman RA, Dunbar JS, Botsford JA, et al: Traumatic longitudinal atlanto-occipital distraction injuries in children. Am J Neuroradiol 3:415–419, 1982.

63. Keenen TL, Anthony J, Benson DR: Noncontiguous spinal fractures. J Trauma 30:489–501, 1990.

64. Kewalramani LS, Taylor RG: Multiple noncontiguous injuries of the spine. Acta Orthop Scand 47:52–58, 1976.

65. Landells CD, Petegher KV: Fractures of the atlas: Classification, treatment, and morbidity. Spine 13:450–452, 1988.

65a. Lee TT, Green BA, Petrin DR: Treatment of stable burst fracture of the atlas (Jefferson fracture) with rigid cervical collar. Spine 23:1963–1967, 1998.

66. Lee C, Woodring JH, Goldstein JS, et al: Evaluation of traumatic atlanto-occipital dislocations. Am J Neuroradiol 8:19–26, 1987.

67. Levine AM, Edwards CC: Fractures of the atlas. J Bone Joint Surg Am 73A:680–691, 1991.

68. Levine AM, Edwards CC: Traumatic lesions of the occipitoatlanto-axial complex. Clin Orthop 239:53–68, 1989.

69. Levine AM, Edwards CC: Treatment of injuries in the C1–C2 complex. Orthop Clin North Am 17:31–44, 1986.

70. Levine AM, Edwards CC: The management of traumatic spondylolisthesis of the axis. J Bone Joint Surg Am 67A:217–226, 1985.

71. Lind B, Nordwall A, Sihlbom H: Odontoid fractures treated with halo vest. Spine 12:173–177, 1987.

72. Lipson, SJ: Fractures of the atlas associated with fractures of the odontoid process and transverse ligament ruptures. J Bone Joint Surg Am 59A:940–942, 1977.

73. Matava MJ, Whitesides TE, Davis PC: Traumatic atlanto-occipital dislocation with survival. Serial computerized tomography as an aid to diagnosis and reduction: A report of three cases. Spine 18:1897–1903, 1993.

74. Massara JT, Fielding JW: Effect of C1–C2 rotation on canal size. Clin Orthop 237:115–119, 1989.

75. McCleary AJ: A fracture of the odontoid process complicated by tenth and twelfth cranial nerve palsies. A case report. Spine 18:932–935, 1993.

76. Mixter SJ, Osgood RB: Traumatic lesions of the atlas and axis. Ann Surg 51:193–207, 1910.

77. Montane I, Eismont FJ, Green BA: Traumatic occipitoatlantal dislocation. Spine 16:112–116, 1991.

78. Montesano P, Anderson PA, Schlehr F, et al: Odontoid fractures treated by anterior odontoid screw fixation. Spine 16(suppl):S33–S37, 1991.

79. Moore KR, Frank EH: Traumatic atlantoaxial rotatory subluxation and dislocation. Spine 20:1928–1930, 1995.

80. Mouradian WH, Fietti VG Jr, Cochran GVB, et al: Fractures of the odontoid: A laboratory and clinical study of mechanisms. Orthop Clin North Am 9:985–1001, 1978.

81. Nachemson A: Fracture of the odontoid process of the axis. A clinical study based on 26 cases. Acta Orthop Scand 29:185–217, 1960.

82. O'Brien JJ, Butterfield WL, Gossling JR: Jefferson fracture with disruption of the transverse ligament. A case report. Clin Orthop 126:135–138, 1977.

83. Osgood RB, Lund CC: Fractures of the odontoid process. N Engl J Med 198:61–72, 1928.

84. Papadopoulos SM, Dickman CA, Sonntag VK, et al: Traumatic atlantaloccipital dislocation with survival. Neurosurgery 28:574–579, 1991.

85. Pelker RR, Dorfman GS: Fracture of the axis associated with vertebral artery injury. A case report. Spine 11:621–623, 1986.

86. Powers B, Miller MD, Kramer RS, et al: Traumatic anterior atlanto-occipital dislocation. Neurosurgery 4:12–17, 1979.

87. Proubasta IR, Sancho RN, Alonzo JR, Palacio AH: Horizontal fracture of the anterior arch of the atlas. Spine 12:615–618, 1987.

88. Reid DC, Henderson R, Saboe L, et al: Etiology and clinical course of missed spine fractures. J Trauma 27:980–986, 1987.

89. Ryan MD, Henderson JJ: The epidemiology of fracture and fracture-dislocations of the cervical spine. Injury 23:38–40, 1992.

90. Ryan MD, Taylor TKF: Odontoid fractures. A rational approach to treatment. J Bone Joint Surg Br 64B:416–421, 1982.

91. Ryan MD, Taylor TK: Odontoid fractures in the elderly. J Spinal Disord 6:397–401, 1993.

92. Schatzker J, Rorabeck CH, Waddell JP: Fractures of the dens. An analysis of thirty-seven cases. J Bone Joint Surg Br 53B:392–405, 1971.

93. Schiff DCM, Parke WW: The arterial supply of the odontoid process. J Bone Joint Surg Am 55A:1450–1456, 1973.

94. Schneider KC, Schemm GW: Vertebral artery insufficiency in acute and chronic spinal trauma. With special reference to the syndrome of acute central cervical spinal cord injury. J Neurosurg 18:348–360, 1961.

95. Schneider KC, Livingston D, Cave A, et al: "Hangman's

fracture" of the cervical spine. J Neurosurg 22:141–154, 1965.

96. Scott EW, Haid RW, Peace D: Type I fractures of the odontoid process: implications for atlanto-occipital instability. J Neurosurg 72:488–492, 1990.

97. Segal LS, Grimm JV, Stauffer ES: Non-unions of fractures of the atlas. J Bone Joint Surg Am 69A:1423–1434, 1987.

98. Shapiro I, Frankel VH: Biomechanics of the cervical spine. In Frankel VH, Nordin M (eds): Basic Biomechanics of the Musculoskeletal System. Philadelphia, Lea and Febiger, 1988.

99. Sherk HH: Lesions of the atlas and axis. Clin Orthop 109:33–41, 1976.

100. Shilke LH, Calahan RA: A rational approach to burst fractures of the atlas. Clin Orthop 154:18–21, 1981.

101. Soderstrom CA, McArdle DQ, Ducker TB, et al: The diagnosis of intra-abdominal injury in patients with cervical cord trauma. J Trauma 23:1061–1065, 1983.

102. Southwick WO: Current concepts review. Management of fractures of the dens (odontoid process). J Bone Joint Surg Am 62A:482–486, 1980.

103. Spence KF, Decker S, Sell KW: Bursting atlantal fracture associated with rupture of the transverse ligament. J Bone Joint Surg Am 52A:543–549, 1970.

104. Starr JK, Eismont FJ: Atypical hangman's fractures. Spine 18:1954–1957, 1993.

105. Stewart GC, Gehweiler JA, Laib RH, et al: Horizontal fracture of the anterior arch of the atlas. Radiology 122:349–352, 1977.

106. Templeton PA, Young JW, Mirvis S, et al: The value of retropharyngeal soft tissue measurements in trauma of the adult cervical spine. Cervical spine soft tissue measurements. Skeletal Radiol 16:98–104, 1987.

107. Toyama Y, Hirabayashi K, Fujimura Y, et al: Spontaneous fracture of the odontoid process in rheumatoid arthritis. Spine 17(suppl):S436–S441, 1992.

108. Traynelis VC, Marano GD, Dunker RO, et al: Traumatic atlanto-occipital dislocation. Case report. J Neurosurg 65:863–870, 1986.

109. Van Hosbeeck EM, Mackay NN: Diagnosis of acute atlantoaxial rotatory fixation. J Bone Joint Surg Br 71B:90–91, 1989.

110. VanDenbout A, Dommisse GF: Traumatic atlanto-occipital dislocation. Spine 11:174–176, 1976.

111. Vaccaro AR, An HS, Lin S, et al: Noncontiguous injuries of the spine. J Spinal Disord 5:320–329, 1992.

112. Wackenheim A: Roentgen Diagnosis of the Craniovertebral Region. New York, Springer-Verlag, 1974, p 660.

112a. Weller SJ, Rossitch E Jr, Malek AM: Detection of vertebral artery injury after cervical spine trauma using magnetic resonance angiography. J Trauma Inj Inf Crit Care 46:660–666, 1999.

113. Werne S: Studies in spontaneous atlas dislocation. Acta Orthop Scand 23(suppl):122–126, 1977.

114. White AA III, Panjabi MM: The clinical biomechanics of the occipitoatlantoaxial complex. Orthop Clin North Am 9:867–878, 1978.

115. Wholey MH, Browner AJ, Baker HL: The lateral roentgenogram of the neck (with comments on the atlanto-odontoid-basion relationship). Radiology 71:250–256, 1958.

116. Wiesel SW, Rothman RH: Occipito-atlantal hypermobility. Spine 4:187–191, 1979.

117. Wigren A: Traumatic atlanto-axial dislocation without neurological disorder. A case report. J Bone Joint Surg Am 55A:642–644, 1973.

118. Wood Jones F: The ideal lesion produced by judicial hanging. Lancet 1:53–58, 1913.

119. Woodring JH, Selke AC, Duff DE: Traumatic atlanto-occipital dislocation with survival. Am J Radiol 137:21–44, 1981.

120. Wortzman G, Dewar FP: Rotatory fixation of the atlantoaxial joint: Rotational atlantoaxial subluxation. Radiology 90:479–487, 1968.

121. Young WF, Rosenwasser RH, Getch C, et al: Diagnosis and management of occipital condyle fractures. Neurosurgery 34:257–260, 1994.

122. Zielinski CJ, Gunther SF, Deeb Z: Cranial nerve palsies complicating Jefferson fracture. A case report. J Bone Joint Surg Am 64A:1382–1384, 1982.

12

FRACTIONS AND DISLOCATIONS OF THE LOWER CERVICAL SPINE AND CERVICOTHORACIC JUNCTION

A. Alexander M. Jones, M.D., F.A.C.S.
Paul A. Anderson, M.D.

Measure twice, cut once.
— Bob Vila
(Former host of "This Old House" on PBS)

Injuries to the lower cervical spine can be among the most devastating injuries to the musculoskeletal system because of the increased risk of injury to the spinal cord, and also because they so often occur in the younger members of the population. These injuries require prompt recognition and early treatment to try to minimize neurologic injury in the peri-injury period and to improve long-term outcome. Spinal cord injury is unfortunately not rare, with approximately 11,000 injuries, or an incidence of approximately 45 cases per million, occurring annually.[52]

Public health efforts (e.g., changes in driving laws and public education awareness programs regarding drunk driving and dangers of diving in pools) have led to a decrease in the etiologies of spinal cord injuries since the 1960s. However, several authors have noted increasing instances of spinal cord injuries secondary to gunshot wounds and violence. This has been reported both in predominantly urban settings and of late in more rural areas.

Historically, spinal cord injuries and cervical cord injuries were treated with a degree of nihilistic neglect. This attitude is probably not warranted now. With modern treatment techniques, including postaccident stabilization, pharmacologic intervention, and more advanced methods of internal stabilization, significant functional outcomes can be achieved. Mortality associated with these injuries is significant—approximately 3.6% the first year, decreasing to 1.6% to 2% thereafter. Spinal cord injury centers have documented a dramatic decrease of approximately 42% in mortality when comparing rates from 1992 to those of 1973.[39] The pattern of neurologic injury seems to have changed also, with a parallel decrease in the percentage of patients presenting with complete spinal cord injury (60% in 1973 vs. 48% in 1992).[40] This may be due to improvements in emergency medical management at the scene, and advances in initial and definitive treatment, including pharmacologic intervention and earlier stabilization.

Prognosis for neurologic recovery and functional rehabilitation has improved as well. In a study of 55 patients with incomplete quadriplegia, the American Spinal Injury Association (ASIA) score increased from 22 to 49 in the first year after injury. Both lower extremity and upper extremity recovery occurred simultaneously, implying that recovery was not based on upper motor neural regeneration alone. Of these patients, 47% regained the ability to ambulate with aids. Patients with complete motor paraplegia improved as well, albeit not as dramatically, with their average ASIA score increasing by only 9 points. No patient regained the ability to ambulate. Important determinants of the likelihood of recovery were the completeness of spinal cord preservation, perianal pinprick sensation, and the pattern of spinal cord syndrome, with patients with Brown-Sequard and central cord syndromes having a higher likelihood of recovery than those with anterior cord syndrome.[105]

In this chapter we review the anatomy and biomechanics of the normal and the injured cervical spine, both osseous and neural. Appreciation of the mechanism of injury and the resultant fracture pattern and injury pattern leads logically to an injury classification system (Table 12–1). This system then allows development of a logical treatment protocol based on the injury pattern and associated neurologic deficits. Emphasis is also placed on the anatomic considerations necessary for successful utilization of some of the more modern surgical techniques.

ANATOMY

The vertebral bodies and articulations of the subaxial spine (C3 to C7) and the first thoracic vertebra all have similar morphologic and kinematic characteristics. Therefore, injuries and disease processes usually can be thought to behave in similar fashion throughout the lower cervical spine. The major differences in anatomy involve variation in the lateral mass morphology and in identifying the varying course of the vertebral artery as it traverses from the lower and middle cervical spine.

Table 12–1. *Classification of Lower Cervical Spine Injuries*

I. Posterior column injuries
  A. Isolated fractures of the posterior elements
    1. Spinous processes
    2. Lamina
    3. Transverse processes
  B. Posterior ligamentous injury
    1. Mild ligamentous injury
    2. Severe ligamentous injury
  C. Hyperextension injury with spinal cord injury
II. Facet injuries
  A. Isolated facet or pedicle fractures
  B. Unilateral facet dislocation
    1. Pure unilateral facet dislocation
    2. Unilateral facet fracture dislocation
    3. Fracture separation of the lateral mass
  C. Bilateral facet dislocation
    1. Pure bilateral facet dislocation
    2. Bilateral facet fracture dislocation
    3. Bilateral facet fracture dislocation with traumatic disk herniation
    4. Distraction injury
III. Anterior column injuries
  A. Vertebral body compression fracture
  B. Vertebral body compression fracture with posterior ligamentous injury
  C. Discoligamentous extension injury

Osseous Anatomy

The basic structural arrangement of the subaxial cervical spine is similar to that of other vertebrae, consisting of an anterior vertebral body connected to a posterior neural arch complex by two intervening pedicles. The vertebral body is relatively small in comparison to thoracic and lumbar vertebrae and has a distinctive superior surface concavity. The edges of this concave superior surface project posterolaterally and are known as the uncinate processes. These help articulate with the inferior surface of the cephalad vertebral body, defining a matching concavity and convexity. The transverse processes are complex amalgamations of the rudimentary rib anteriorly and the true transverse process posteriorly. These form a contoured, gutter-like process that supports the exiting nerve root. The transverse process also contains the foramen transversarium through which the vertebral artery, C3 through C6, passes directly anterior to the nerve root (Fig. 12–1).[94] The pedicles are the short bony connections that connect the vertebral bodies to the lateral masses. The pedicles are angulated medially somewhere between 15 and 40 degrees and slightly cephalad.[76] The cervical lateral masses, or pillars, have a cuboid shape and are bounded by articulations on the superior and inferior surfaces. These are true synovial diarthral articulations and are angled upward approximately 30 to 45 degrees cephalad. The laminae are thin, bony connections that extend from the lateral masses to the base of the spinous process, covering the posterior aspect of the cervical cord. The valley that defines the junction of the laminae and the lateral mass is an important bony landmark in calculating screw placement for lateral mass plate fixation. The spinous processes arise from the posterior laminae, projecting posteriorly, and the tips are noted to be bifid C3 through C5 and often at C6. C7 and T1 (vertebrae prominens) are the most readily palpable spinous processes and can serve as surface landmarks.

Ligamentous Anatomy

Because of its enormous flexibility and range of motion requirements, the cervical spine has relatively little intrinsic bony stability. The surrounding ligamentous complex is necessary to maintain stability. The ligamentous anatomy can be divided from anterior to posterior, including the articulations between the vertebral bodies and the intervertebral discs and those ligaments spanning the posterior elements, including the facet joints and the posterior spinous processes.

The anterior and posterior longitudinal ligaments run the length of the bony spinal column, lying on the anterior and posterior vertebral surfaces, with relative widening at the level of the disks and narrowing in the midpoint of the vertebral bodies. The intervertebral disk consists of a cartilaginous endplate on each surface, a central nucleus, and the tough, dense ligamentous structure of the outer annulus fibrosis. The annulus is a powerful stabilizer and, if injured, can be the cause of pain or instability in patients who have sustained cervical trauma. Laterally, the disk is buttressed by the uncovertebral joints, which are pseudojoints (also known as the joints of Luschka) formed by the uncinate processes and their reciprocal articulation with the cephalad vertebral endplate.

The posterior neural arch bony structures are stabilized by the nuchal ligaments, the ligamentum flavum, and the joint capsules. The nuchal ligaments include the ligamentum nuchae, the supraspinous ligaments, and the interspinous ligaments. The ligamentum nuchae is a broad, strong structure that extends from the external occipital protuberance and attaches to the tips of the spinous processes. In comparative anatomy of quadrupeds, such as horses, this ligament serves as a suspensory element to allow energy-efficient head positioning. In bipeds, this

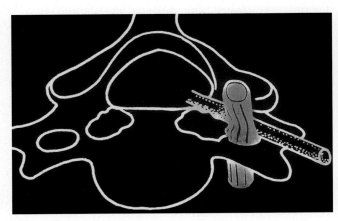

Figure 12–1. *Note the vertebral artery directly anterior to the nerve root.*

has more of a stabilization role. The supraspinous and interspinous ligaments connect the adjacent spinous processes, the ligamentum flavum is a more elastic structure that spans between adjacent laminae, and finally, the facet joint capsules have some redundancy in their dimensions to allow for physiologic motion between vertebrae.

Neurovascular Anatomy

Spinal cord dimensions show remarkably little variation between persons. However, the size and configuration of the bony spinal canal varies greatly and can be an important factor in the severity of spinal cord injuries.[47, 61] In the subaxial spine, the spinal cord has an average midsagittal diameter of approximately 9 mm. The midsagittal diameter of the bony spinal canal is measured from the base of the spinous process to the posterior margin of the vertebral body. When this diameter is less than 10 mm, it is believed to be stenotic and to predispose to the development of myelopathy. The Pavlov ratio (the midsagittal diameter of the canal, divided by the midsagittal diameter of the vertebral body) can also be used to estimate the size of the spinal canal on x-rays.[101] By definition, a Pavlov ratio below 0.8 is thought to define cervical stenosis.

The spinal nerves are formed from the ventral and dorsal roots and then pass through the neural foramina. The boundaries of the neural foramina consist of the pedicles above and below: posteriorly, the facet joint and capsules, and anteriorly, the disk annulus, the posterior vertebral body, and the posterolateral edge of the uncinate process. The dimensions of the neural foramina can be affected by displaced bone and disk fragments, vertebral malalignment, or loss of disk height. The neural foramina should be carefully evaluated in spinal-injured patients with an isolated root radiculopathy. After exiting the neural foramina, the spinal nerve lies on the transverse process before forming the brachial plexus. The nerve root in the cervical spine has a more horizontal course, exiting from the spinal cord and lying directly above the pedicle, in contrast to the lumbar spine, in which the nerve root has a more oblique course and is intimately applied to the inferior edge of the pedicle.

The vertebral arteries are the major source of blood supply to the vertebrae and spinal cord. They arise from the first branch of the subclavian artery bilaterally, enter the osseous spine, passing through the foramen transversarium at C6, and travel cephalad to enter the true spinal canal at the level of the atlas. Rarely, fractures of the transverse process, or fracture dislocations, can cause a significant occlusion of the vertebral artery that has clinical consequences.[110] A clinically significant vertebral artery injury is more likely in the upper cervical spine.

The cervical spine vasculature includes the anterior spinal artery, the paired posterior spinal arteries, and several (usually two to three) segmental arteries. The anterior and posterior spinal arteries originate intracranially from the vertebral artery and descend into the cord. The segmental vessels arise locally from the vertebral arteries and pass as tributaries through the neural foramina with the nerve root, and enter the spinal cord with the anterior root. These can be vulnerable to compromise by direct pressure of displaced bone or disk fragments and possibly contribute to cord ischemia.[20]

PATIENT ASSESSMENT

Each patient should be initially assessed according to Advanced Trauma Life Support (ATLS) protocols. Careful evaluation of the subaxial spine is mandatory because of the risk of catastrophic complications from missed injuries.[77] In every patient with deceleration injuries or other significant trauma, the cervical spine should be immobilized. Patients complaining of neck pain should be considered as having unstable fractures until proven otherwise. Clinical assessment includes posterior spinous process palpation. Focal reproducible spinous process tenderness is highly correlative of occult injury, even in the presence of negative x-rays. Anderson noted that in 50% of patients in his hospital experience, a fracture was discovered on computed tomography (CT) scan under these circumstances.[10] Palpable gaps in the spinous processes–although often difficult to identify–are evidence of severe injury and warrant further evaluation. Serial neurologic examinations should be performed, looking particularly for isolated motor weaknesses secondary to root injuries, long-tract signs indicative of cord-level injury, and, finally, changes consistent with deterioration and neurologic deficit progression.

To "clear" the cervical spine, a minimum of three radiographic views are required, including anteroposterior, lateral, and open-mouth odontoid views.[67, 68, 85] The entire cervical spine, from the occiput to T1, must be visualized. Approximately 5% of cervical trauma injuries occur at the cervicothoracic junction, and visualization to the superior endplate of T1 is required.[99a] Specialized techniques, including pull-down views (with the arms placed in gentle traction) or swimmer's views, can be used to facilitate visualization of this area (Fig. 12–2). Trauma oblique views, where the radiograph beam rather than the patient's neck is oriented 45 degrees off midline, can allow visualization of facet articulations and provide information on the cervicothoracic junction. CT scans with reconstructions can provide detailed information about the bony structure at the cervicothoracic junction. Noncontiguous spinal fractures are common (approximately 15%), and thus complete visualization of the entire spinal column by biplane x-rays is required once one spinal fracture has been identified.[62]

When a fracture has been identified on plain x-rays, subsequent evaluation with a CT scan or magnetic resonance imaging (MRI) is recommended. In patients with a neurologic deficit or facet fractures or dislocations, the MRI is preferable because it gives better visualization of any neural compression or intrinsic neural injury and thus allows the status of the intervertebral disk to be readily determined.[33, 87] Disk herniations are found in association with approximately 15% of bilateral facet dislocations (see Fig. 12–9).[46, 79] MRI may also reveal information about ligamentous injury, particularly posterior ligament injury, in the setting of a hyperflexion mechanism. Fat-suppression techniques, such as a T2-weighted or short time inversion

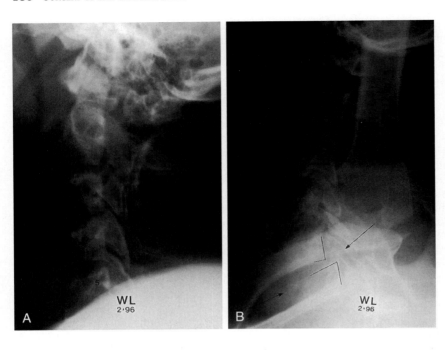

Figure 12–2. *A, A 300-lb male fell off a bar stool, hit his occiput, and presented with neck pain. No abnormality was seen on lateral x-ray; however, visualization was present only down to C5. B, Swimmer's view demonstrates C6–C7 subluxation (arrows).*

recovery (STIR) sequence, may be helpful. MRI recently has been shown to be substantially inferior to CT scans for identifying posterior element fractures.[62a] A CT scan is indicated in most patients with bony injuries, because it allows precise definition of fracture pattern, fragment location, and structure displacement. Moreover, CT scans, including reformatted images, allow precise preoperative surgical planning and are particularly useful if screw placement is anticipated.

MECHANISM OF INJURY

The mechanism of injury is defined by the direction and magnitude of forces that have been applied externally to the head and neck complex resulting in injury. The forces can be direct, from impaction on the cranium or neck, or indirect, from rapid deceleration of the thorax or head and neck. Knowledge of the mechanism of injury helps identify the major injury vector and aids in fracture classification.[108] Common injury vectors include flexion, compression, rotation, and extension. In reality, many injuries occur from a combination of these vectors. The pattern of injury is related not only to the external applied force, but also to the initial position or posture of the head and neck at the time of injury.

In reviewing postinjury x-rays in an attempt to determine mechanism of injury and major injury vectors, it is important that a physician recall that these x-rays are "snapshots" or a moment in time after the injury, and that the injury is, obviously, a dynamic event. Postinjury x-rays may not accurately record or reflect the maximum displacement or dislocation of osseous and neural elements and thus may underrepresent the magnitude of the injury. Chang et al. measured changes in the instantaneous cross-sectional spinal canal area in cadaver specimens during impact loading and found no correlation between the point of maximum transient displacement and the canal measurements as noted on postinjury CT scan.[28]

CLASSIFICATION

Classification systems are useful when they allow communication between physicians and researchers to determine prognosis and direct treatment. Although several systems have been developed for use in the cervical spine, none is uniformly accepted. The most important classification concept is that of stability. This is probably best defined using White's definition of "loss of ability of the spine under physiologic loads to maintain relationships in such a way that there is neither damage nor subsequent irritation of the spinal cord or nerve roots, and, in addition, there is no incapacitating deformity or pain."[108] Nicoll correlated fracture patterns with outcome and recognized that stable fracture patterns heal, allowing patients to return to work.[75] He further recognized that fractures with disruption of the ligamentous structures were generally unstable. Holdsworth confirmed Nicoll's observations and further refined understanding of fracture mechanics by dividing the spine into two theoretical columns.[57] The anterior column includes the vertebral body, the disk, and the longitudinal ligaments. The posterior column is defined by the neural arch and the associated posterior ligamentous structures. Stable injuries involve only one column, and unstable injuries involve both columns. The two-column framework continues to be very appropriate when considering the subaxial cervical spine, although it is probably not applicable to the thoracolumbar spine, for which a three-column model would appear to be more appropriate.

White and Panjabi performed cadaver testing of human cervical spines that confirms Holdsworth's two-column theory.[108] In addition, they defined parameters that can be used to help determine clinical instability. Experimentally, they sectioned ligamentous structures in a serial manner from a posterior-to-anterior direction and, subsequently, in an anterior-to-posterior direction. Flexion and extension moments were applied to specimens after each ligament division, and the subsequent kyphotic and angular displacements were measured. Significant increases in translation and/or vertebral angulation occurred when all posterior ligamentous structures and a single anterior structure, or all anterior structures and a single posterior structure, were divided. When the spine became unstable, 3.5 mm of anterior translation and 11 degrees of increased kyphotic angulation were observed (Fig. 12–3). On the basis of these experiments and other clinical observations, White and Panjabi developed a clinical checklist in an attempt to objectify cervical stability (Table 12–2). In this checklist, each factor is assessed and assigned a value of either 1 or 2 if present and 0 if absent. If the sum of all values is 5 or greater, then the spine is believed to be unstable. This does not directly indicate surgical treatment, but does suggest that in acute situations the patient should be treated with aggressive immobilization, including a halo vest. The checklist is not universally accepted and has not been clinically validated; however, it does provide useful clinical guidelines.

In this chapter, we present an adapted fracture classification as devised by Anderson. This is based on morphology, using terms that have been previously described and are widely accepted (see Table 12–1). Injuries are classified into three divisions, based on the location of the most obvious or significant point of injury. These divisions are the posterior column, the facets and their articulations, and the anterior column. In general terms, stable injuries are isolated to one division, whereas unstable injuries involve two or all three divisions.

Posterior Column Injuries
Isolated Fractures of Posterior Elements

Isolated fractures of the spinous processes, lamina, and transverse processes occur frequently and can be caused by all major injury vectors. These are stable as long as facet articulations are competent and there is no simultaneous vertebral body translation. Concomitant posterior ligament injury can occur and must be identified.[47a, 70a] Rarely, lamina fractures can be displaced into the spinal cord, necessitating removal to reconstitute the spinal canal dimension.

Posterior Ligamentous Injury

Rapid hyperflexion of the head and neck (usually from deceleration forces) creates large tensile forces in the posterior ligamentous structures, causing a variable amount of injury to the ligaments. Usually, large forces are required to create these injuries, except in elderly patients, whose ligaments may be more brittle from degeneration. Once the restraining ligamentous structures are injured, the vertebra is free to rotate in flexion over the lower caudal vertebral body, resulting in kyphotic angulation. Anterior translation also may occur if the tensile forces have injured the anterior structures, including the posterior longitudinal ligament or the disk annulus.

The severity of the posterior ligamentous injury is graded from mild to severe. In mild injuries, the forces can result in a grade I or grade II sprain, such that fibers are stretched but stability is maintained. Clinically, patients may have focal tenderness but no neurologic signs or symptoms.

Radiographic examination may show slight widening between the spinous processes, but no kyphosis or anterior translation. MRI reveals no evidence of hemorrhage with its increased signal intensity. These patients will score less than

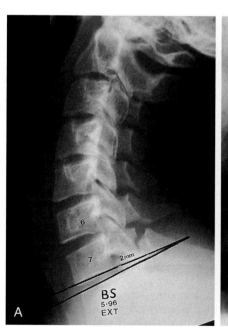
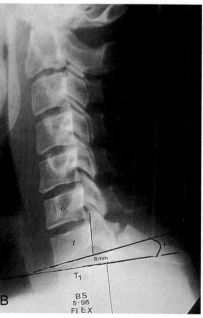

Figure 12–3. A 29-year-old skier sustained a flexion injury. Flexion (A) and extension (B) x-rays show translational and angular instability. (Note: White and Panjabi criteria are based on lines drawn parallel to the inferior endplates of two adjacent vertebral bodies. In this case, the inferior endplate of T1 cannot be visualized.)

Table 12–2. *Checklist for the Diagnosis of Clinical Instability*

Element	Point Value
Anterior elements destroyed or unable to function	2
Posterior elements destroyed or unable to function	2
Relative sagittal plane translation >3.5 mm	2
Relative sagittal plane rotation >11 degrees	2
Posterior stretch test	2
Cord injury	2
Root injury	1
Abnormal disk narrowing	1
Congenital spinal stenosis	1
Dangerous loading anticipated	1
	> 5 = clinical instability

5 points on the White and Panjabi checklist and, according to those parameters, are defined as clinically stable.

With increased hyperflexion, complete disruption of the posterior osteoligamentous complex can occur. These patients present with posterior tenderness, and often a gap is noted between the tips of the spinous processes, although this may be difficult to palpate because of posterior swelling. X-rays may show only subtle bony abnormalities. Local kyphosis, facet joint diastasis, malrotation of the facet joints, or interspinous widening may be seen. However, if patients are positioned in extension for lateral x-rays, the kyphotic angulation may be spontaneously reduced, making the diagnosis of ligamentous instability more difficult. Interspinous widening is a more consistent finding; however, this is often overlooked. This may be better visualized on the anteroposterior x-rays. The use of dynamic flexion-extension x-rays to assess stability and potential ligamentous injuries is controversial and probably not recommended, particularly in the acute setting. Currently, MRI with fat-suppression techniques is recommended to directly visualize the posterior ligaments (Fig. 12–4). Patients with the appropriate clinical scenario demonstrate areas of high signal intensity between the spinous processes on the MRI and are treated for a severe ligament injury.[47a] These patients are also evaluated using the White and Panjabi criteria, and any with a score exceeding 5 are similarly considered to have an unstable ligamentous injury.

Hyperextension Injury with Spinal Cord Injury

Taylor[100] and Schneider[90] have noted the association of central cord syndrome in older patients with stenotic or spondylotic spines. Additional observation has identified that many patients also have small amounts of posterior translation, on the order of 2 to 3 mm of retrolisthesis, and that this translation may be reducible with traction.[20, 69] MRI has also demonstrated disk and posterior ligamentous disruption at the site of spinal cord injury, indicating a more significant amount of injury and subsequent instability.

Although central cord syndromes are classically associated with this mechanism of injury, various spinal cord injury syndromes can occur.[69] Cervical traction is recommended as an initial treatment in an attempt to reduce retrolisthesis, which, although slight, can contribute to indirect decompression.

Facet Injuries

Isolated Facet and Pedicle Fractures

Isolated fractures to facets and pedicles are usually secondary to compression or lateral bending forces. These are often difficult to visualize on lateral x-rays because of overlying shadows. The anteroposterior view may show fracture of the lateral facet complex. Isolated fractures not associated with anterior or posterior subluxation are stable. Missed facet fractures can be the etiology of chronic neck pain after trauma. Bone scans may be helpful in identifying this injury.[34]

Unilateral Facet Dislocations

Unilateral facet dislocations, either with or without fractures, can have various mechanisms of injury and thus different prognoses. The typical unilateral facet fracture and dislocation results from exaggerated motion of the normal cervical spine.[108] Normal lateral bending and rotation involves coupled motion, so that as one facet moves upward, the contralateral facet moves downward. The spinous process moves laterally toward the convexity of the curve. With excessive loading, the inferior facet will move too far inferiorly and the superior facet will move too far cranially, with resultant facet dislocation. Fracturing of the facet articulation and occasionally disarticulation by fracture of the entire lateral mass will be present. These fractures result from the addition of shear or compressive forces, which cause excessive loading on the joint surfaces and commonly occur from falls, athletic trauma, or motor vehicle crashes.

Beatson carefully analyzed the structural injury necessary to cause a unilateral facet dislocation and found that a single facet can be dislocated only when the interspinous ligament, ligamentum flavum, and ipsilateral joint capsules are damaged.[12] If, in addition, the posterior longitudinal ligament adjacent to the side or the disk annulus is damaged, then the spine can be further displaced forward to just under 50% vertebral body displacement. Reduction by in-line traction is difficult because of the intact contralateral facet joints and ligamentous structures. A minimal amount of lateral bending to the side opposite of the dislocation can facilitate reduction, however.

Unilateral facet dislocations can be easily missed because the rotational nature of the injury is not well visualized on standard anteroposterior and lateral x-rays. Also, the small amounts of subluxation that may be present on initial x-rays may have reduced spontaneously. Unilateral facet dislocations occur most commonly at C5–C6 and C6–C7, at the junction between the most mobile portion of the cervical spine and the more rigid thoracic spine. Visualization at this level may be more difficult because of shadows of the overlying shoulders. In many cases, the injury is stable in the dislocated position, thereby minimizing pain and making the diagnosis more difficult.

Radiographic features include vertebral body displacement of about 25%. Rarely, a minimal compression fracture of the caudad vertebral body is present. Interspinous widening can be noted, although it is variable. The most consistent finding is asymmetry of the facets on the lateral view above and below the injury (Fig. 12–5). Normally, the

right and left facets superimpose and are viewed as a single unit on the lateral view. When a unilateral facet dislocation is present, the symmetry is lost because there is an element of rotation above the level of the dislocation. Most commonly, the two cranial facets are seen as separate shadows, whereas the caudal facets are still superimposed and viewed as a single unit. This creates the pathognomonic "bowtie" sign of unilateral facet dislocation. On the anteroposterior x-ray, rotation of the spinous processes

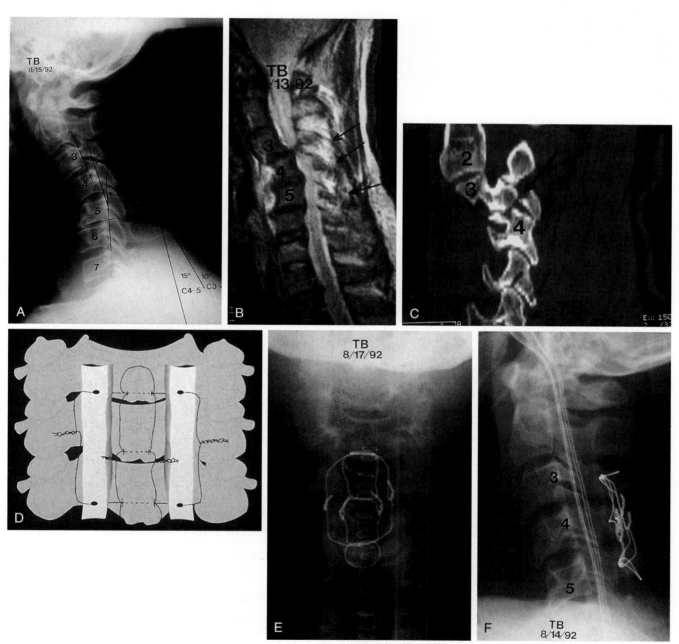

Figure 12–4. A, A 52-year-old male who suffered a deceleration injury after a vehicular crash presented with neck pain and no neurological deficit. Lateral x-ray shows translational and angular instability. B, A T2 MRI shows increased signal intensity in the interspinous ligaments (arrows), indicating significant posterior ligament disruption. C, A parasagittal reconstructed CT scan delineates fracture of the inferior articular process of C3 (arrow) and a fracture fragment anterior to C4. D, The Bohlman triple-wiring technique. E, An anteroposterior x-ray taken after the Bohlman triple-wiring technique. F, A lateral x-ray taken after the Bohlman triple-wiring technique.

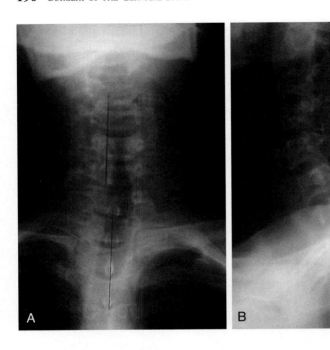

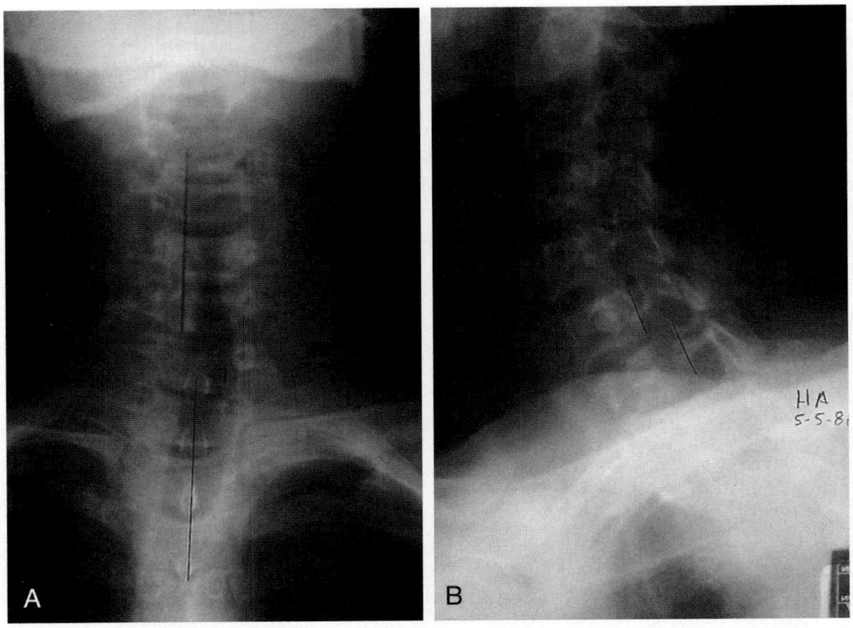

Figure 12–5. A, A 27-year-old bicyclist struck by a car sustained a unilateral facet dislocation of the left C6–C7. Note the rotation of the spinous process above the level of the dislocated facet on this anteroposterior view. B, Lateral view of this C6 unilateral facet dislocation. Note the 25% anterior subluxation of C6 on C7. Also note the change in appearance of the facets of C6 and above (oblique appearance) and C7 and below (lateral appearance).

(again above the level of the dislocation) may be noted. The cephalad spinous processes are rotated to the side of the dislocation. Oblique x-rays performed using the trauma technique (not turning the patient's head, but rotating the radiographic beam) may be helpful in demonstrating facet malalignment and possible foraminal encroachment. CT scans, particularly with sagittal and oblique reformatted images, provide clear visualization of the dislocated facets (Fig. 12–6). MRI may aid visualization of possible foraminal narrowing, but is of particular utility in visualizing the disk and ruling out a possible associated disk herniation, which occurs in approximately 15% of cases.

Clinically, patients with unilateral facet dislocations present with pain, usually radiculopathy, and/or a spinal cord injury. Detection of radiculopathies can be difficult and requires careful neurologic testing. Malrotation or gaps in the spinous processes can be difficult to determine by direct palpation. Unilateral facet dislocations can be classified as a "pure" unilateral facet dislocation, a unilateral facet dislocation with associated fracture, or, more severely, a fracture separation of the lateral mass. All three of these injuries are characterized by subluxation of approximately 25% (10% to 40%) displacement of the vertebral body and characteristic rotation of the spinous processes above the level of the injury to the side of the facet dislocation.

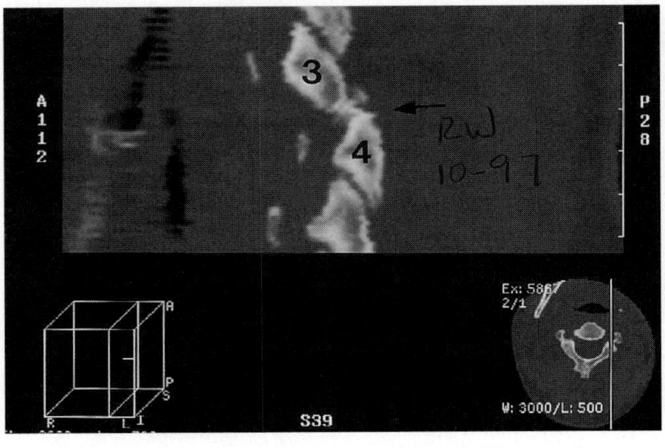

Pure Unilateral Facet Dislocation

This least common type of facet injury is characterized as having 25% vertebral body translation on lateral x-rays. Unfortunately, spinal cord injury can be present in up to 25% of cases. These dislocations may be difficult to reduce with cranial traction because of the intact ipsilateral bony structures and contralateral ligamentous structures; however, after reduction, they may also be stable and not require operative intervention.

Unilateral Facet Fracture Dislocations

This is the most common type of facet injury, occurring in up to 80% of cases.[64] The usual associated fracture is that of the superior articular facet and, less commonly, the inferior facet. Although these two fractures result from different mechanisms, both are unstable. This is because of the spine's inability to resist anterior shear or rotation due to the inadequate buttress provided by the fractured facet.

Fracture Separation of the Lateral Mass

Complete separation of the lateral mass can occur from fractures, usually caused by lateral extension and rotation forces (Fig. 12–7).[64, 66, 86] Compressive forces on the lateral masses fracture the pedicle and the lamina at its junction with the lateral mass. The lateral mass, or facet complex, is thus completely separated from the vertebral body and lamina and is free-floating. This side of the vertebral motion complex is rotationally unstable, allowing forward transla-

Figure 12–6. This parasagittal reconstructed CT scan shows C3–C4 facet dislocation.

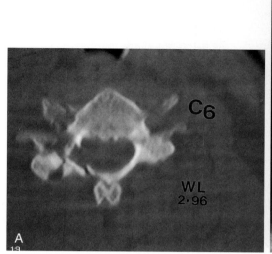

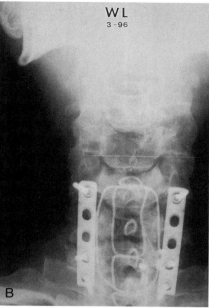

Figure 12–7. A, In this patient, whose lateral view is shown in Figure 2A–B, an axial CT scan shows fracture separation of a lateral mass with both lamina and pedicle fractures, creating a free-floating lateral mass. This is a two-motion segment injury. B, The patient was stabilized with lateral mass plates and screws and posterior cable tension wires of C5–T1.

tion of the vertebral bodies. Because the lateral mass with its superior and inferior facets participates in stabilization of two vertebral levels, fracture separation of the lateral mass may lead to instability at the two adjacent vertebral levels. Often, only minimal initial translation is noted, but despite bracing, progressive deformity will occur. Plain x-rays show malrotation of the entire facet joint on lateral views. On the anteroposterior view, facet joints may be rotated so that they can be seen end-on. The fracture of the lamina at the junction of the lateral mass is usually well visualized on the anteroposterior view.

Bilateral Facet Dislocations

Bilateral facet dislocations may result from several mechanisms, but occur most commonly from a combination of hyperflexion with some degree of rotation.[108] Allen has described these as either distraction-flexion stage III or stage IV lesions.[2] Roaf created spinal injuries in cadaver models and found that pure hyperflexion tended to result in compression fractures to the vertebral body.[80] However, the addition of small amounts of rotation loaded the ligaments and allowed bilateral facet dislocations to occur at much lower forces. Other researchers have created bilateral facet dislocations by putting compressive loading onto the skull with the neck in a slightly flexed posture, a common mechanism of injury in young athletes.[92] Regardless of the mechanism of injury, bilateral facet dislocations are highly unstable injuries that are associated with neurologic deficits in most cases. Cadaver dissections have demonstrated significant injury to all posterior ligamentous structures, in addition to the posterior longitudinal ligament and disk annulus. In patients with bilateral facet dislocations, the anterior longitudinal ligament often is the only remaining intact structure (Fig. 12–8).

The injury to the posterior disk annulus is of particular importance. The disk is avulsed from its vertebral attachments, allowing the nucleus pulposus, with portions of the annulus and endplate, to retropulse into the spinal canal, further compromising canal dimensions and compressing neural elements. MRI has documented associated disk herniations in 10% to 40% of patients with bilateral facet dislocations.[42, 46, 79] Clinically, patients with disk herniations may have increased or higher levels of neurologic deficit than skeletal injury or may deteriorate following closed reduction, a great concern. Bilateral facet dislocations classically have 50% vertebral body translation seen on lateral x-rays. Fracturing of the posterior elements is commonly seen in approximately 80% of cases. Disk space narrowing at the level of the facet dislocation is an ominous sign and can be associated with disk herniation.[108] The spine is usually kyphotic, with widening of the spinous processes. Bilateral laminar fractures, or fractures of the spinous processes, are common and complicate efforts at posterior fixation. Rarely, bilateral pedicle fractures are present, which create a spondylolisthetic slip and are difficult to reduce in a closed fashion.[72]

With more severe distractional forces, dislocation of the vertebral bodies can increase to 100% and result in true vertical separation between the vertebral bodies. This is a situation in which skull tong traction is absolutely contraindicated and can result in further neurovascular injury. In addition, these injuries appear to be associated with increased likelihood of later neurologic deterioration, progression of neurologic deficit (higher than the level of skeletal injury), and associated vertebral artery injury, along with an increased risk of death.

Anterior Column Injuries
Vertebral Body Compression Fractures

Vertebral body compression fractures can occur from hyperflexion injuries or axial loading. Lateral x-rays show

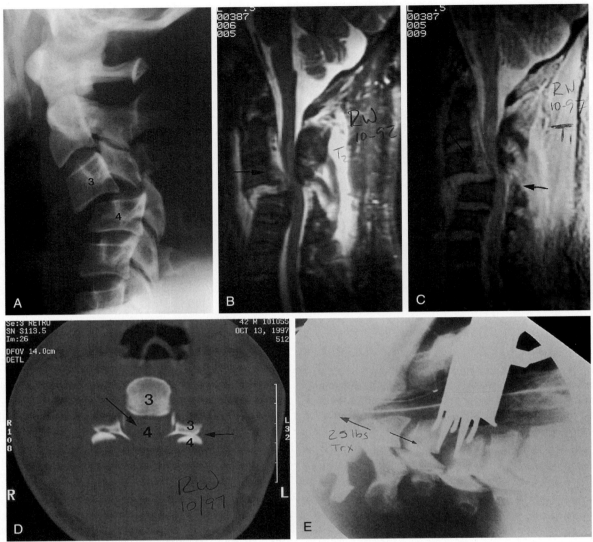

Figure 12–8. *A, A 42-year-old surgeon suffered a severe hyperflexion injury while mountain biking and was a temporary quadriplegic. The x-rays show a C3–C4 bilateral jumped facet fracture dislocation. Note that the arrows illustrate fracture fragments and greater than 50% anterior subluxation of C3 on C4. B, This preoperative MRI (T1 image) shows a very large posterior disk herniation (solid arrow) and marked soft tissue disruption posteriorly (open arrow). C, On this T2 image, again the large posteriorly displaced cervical disc herniation, posterior to the body of C3, is seen. Early cord changes can also be seen. The patient's neurologic status at this point was an incomplete combined central cord syndrome and Brown-Sequard syndrome, with greater motor deficit on the right side and greater involvement of the hands. D, An axial CT cut, showing (open arrow) the empty uncovertebral joint as the body of C3 is subluxed anteriorly. Note also the reversal of the normal arrangement of the facet joints, with the inferior articular process of C3 located anterior to the superior articular process of C4. The patient was stabilized and given the high-dose steroid protocol of the National Spinal Cord Injury Study No. II. Closed reduction of the jumped facets was unsuccessful, and he was transferred for definitive treatment. Because of the large posterior disk herniation, as noted on MRI, it was elected to proceed with an anterior decompression first. E, After completion of a formal diskectomy at C3–C4, an attempt was made at anterior reduction of the subluxation, increasing cervical traction to 25 lb and using an intervertebral body spreader (solid arrow). Spinal cord monitoring was used throughout the procedure. The reduction could not be performed from an anterior approach; accordingly, the anterior wound was closed. The patient was repositioned prone. (At the beginning of the case, the patient was placed on a Stryker turning frame, which facilitated the anterior-posterior-anterior approach used in this procedure.)*

the body to be wedge-shaped but the posterior vertebral wall to remain intact. In isolated compression fractures, the posterior osteoligamentous complex also remains intact, and fractures are stable. However, clinical suspicion is warranted, because compression fractures often occur in association with posterior ligament disruptions and, in this situation, are extremely unstable and usually do not respond well to nonoperative treatment.

Avulsion of the Anterior Longitudinal Ligament

Hyperextension forces applied to the neck create tensile forces in the anterior longitudinal ligament that can cause failure of this structure. This injury results in failure not only of the anterior longitudinal ligament, but also of the associated anterior disk annulus. More severe extension injuries can cause retrolisthesis of 50% or more. Radiographic examination shows increased widening of the anterior intervertebral disk or overall increased lordosis. MRI demonstrates increased signal intensity in the disk and retropharyngeal spaces on T2-weighted images consistent with edema or fluid accumulation secondary to the soft tissue injury.

Extension Teardrop Fractures

As noted previously, hyperextension can result in a benign avulsion fracture of the anteroinferior vertebral body. This indicates discoligamentous disruption, usually involving the anterior longitudinal ligament. This occurs most commonly at the C2–C3 interspace. This relatively benign fracture must be differentiated from the more severe flexion teardrop fracture described by Schneider.[51, 89]

Traumatic Retrolisthesis

Forced hyperextension of the neck, with resultant injury to the disk and longitudinal ligaments, can result in a traumatic retrolisthesis. This is usually a subtle finding, sometimes with only 2 to 3 mm of posterior translation present, and can be easily overlooked, or perhaps thought to be secondary to preexisting spondylosis. In patients with previously narrowed canals secondary to congenital narrowing or spondylosis, the addition of slight retrolisthesis can cause a significant reduction in the space available for the cord and lead to subsequent cord compression. Very rarely, greater degrees of retrolisthesis (up to 50%) can occur. Dramatic retrolisthesis is unstable and difficult to reduce and maintain in reduction.

Burst Fractures

Burst fractures occur secondary to increased hydraulic forces in the annulus and nucleus pulposus, causing a forced displacement of the disk down into the vertebral body with subsequent comminution of the vertebral body (Fig. 12–9). Displacement of the comminuted fragments occurs circumferentially and can lead to retropulsion of disk fragments into the canal. Plain x-rays show shortening of anterior and posterior vertebral body heights and, on the anteroposterior view, evidence of interpedicular widening (a classic finding). Burst fractures are associated with variable degrees of posterior ligamentous disruption, depending on the initial neck posture (e.g., flexion) or if an element of distraction was present also during injury. If interspinous widening is noted posteriorly or if facet disruptions are present—both consistent with severe posterior ligamentous injury—this injury should be considered unstable. Anderson has noted at his institution an increasing number of patients with

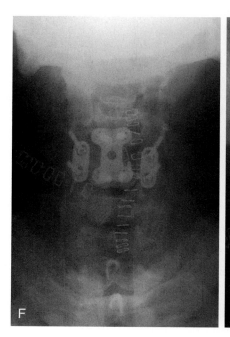
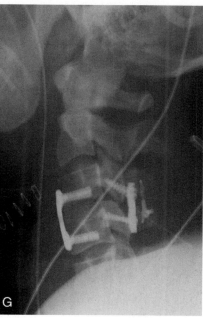

Figure 12–8 Continued. F and G, Postoperative plain x-rays show superior and lateral angulation of the lateral mass screws as described by Anderson, with good position of both the tricortical bone graft at C3–C4 and anterior plate and screws. After stabilization, patient's neurologic status continued to improve. He was able to regain independent ambulation and increasing use of his hands. He required postoperative immobilization in a cervical orthosis; use of a halo vest was not indicated.

bursting-type fractures and concomitant bilateral facet fracture dislocations.[4]

Flexion Teardrop Fractures

The flexion teardrop fracture of Schneider is a complex, severe injury, often associated unfortunately with spinal cord injury.[89, 102] The teardrop is the small bone fragment off the anteroinferior corner of the body rotated anteriorly (Fig. 12–10). (Some discussion has questioned whether the "teardrop" in its descriptive title refers to the shape of the bone fragment or to the unfortunate individuals who have sustained this severe injury.) Along with the anteroinferior bone fragment that is rotated anteriorly, the vertebral body is fractured in the coronal plane and retrolisthesed posteriorly into the canal, thus narrowing the space available for the cord. Posteriorly, there is interspinous widening and/or comminution of the lamina and spinous processes, consistent with posterior disruption of the osteoligamentous complex. Teardrop fractures are often seen after diving and football accidents and are usually

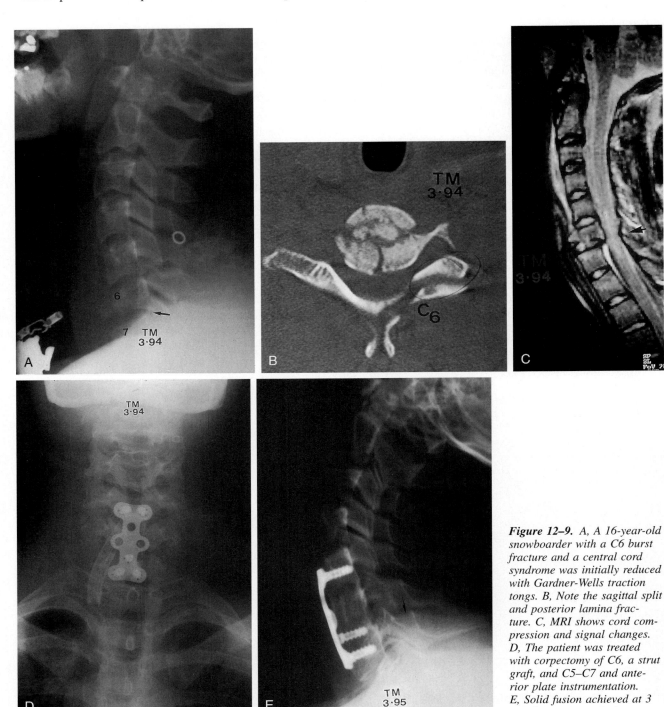

Figure 12–9. *A, A 16-year-old snowboarder with a C6 burst fracture and a central cord syndrome was initially reduced with Gardner-Wells traction tongs. B, Note the sagittal split and posterior lamina fracture. C, MRI shows cord compression and signal changes. D, The patient was treated with corpectomy of C6, a strut graft, and C5–C7 and anterior plate instrumentation. E, Solid fusion achieved at 3 months postoperatively.*

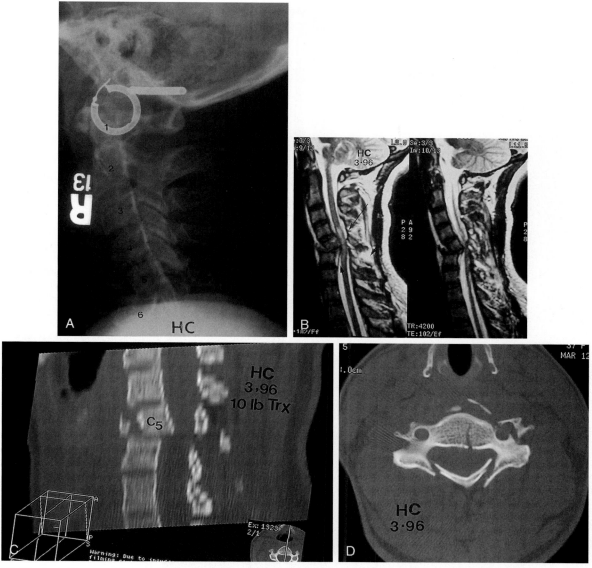

Figure 12–10. *A, A 35-year-old portrait artist sustained a flexion teardrop fracture of C5 and an incomplete central cord syndrome. Note the posterior displacement of C5 on C6. B, Note cord compression and avulsion of the anterior longitudinal ligament and posterior interspinous ligaments. The posterior longitudinal ligament appears to be intact. C, Sagittal CT shows displacement of C5 and canal narrowing. D, Displaced laminar fracture of C5.*

associated with significant spinal cord injury, with the classical injury being anterior spinal cord syndrome with loss of all motor and sensory functions distally, except proprioception.

GENERAL PRINCIPLES OF TREATMENT

The goals of treatment for all patients with cervical spine injuries are to protect the spinal cord from additional trauma, to reduce and stabilize dislocations and fractures, to decompress neurologic tissue, and to provide a long-term stable, painless spine.[29, 53, 83] The aim is to create an environment for maximal neurologic recovery, hopefully

within the first several hours after injury.[38, 43, 44, 78] The basic principles to follow include initial resuscitation; subsequent identification of the fracture pattern and classification; assessment of stability; early closed reduction, if possible, to effect indirect neurologic decompression; administration of appropriate pharmacologic agents in a timely fashion; and proceeding with definitive treatment. Definitive treatment, possibly including surgical intervention, is aimed at achieving complete decompression of the neural elements in patients with neurologic deficit, and at providing sufficient bony stabilization to allow early mobilization. These goals can be met by either operative or nonoperative methods. Most patients who exhibit radiographic evidence of neural compression but who remain neurologically intact do not require decompression. Surgical

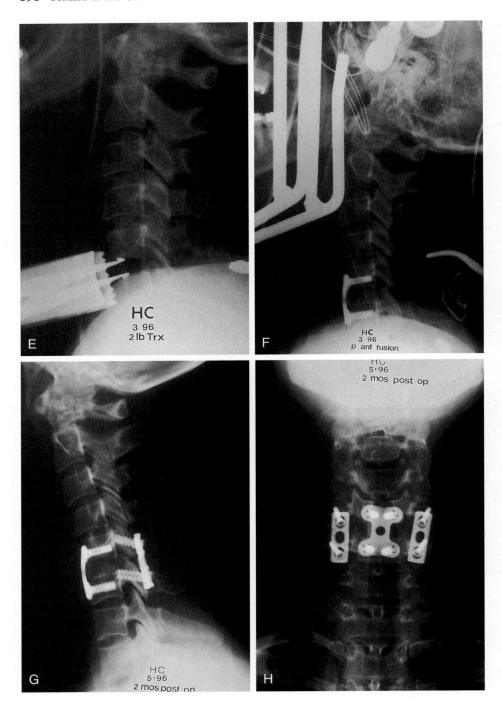

Figure 12–10 Continued. *E, Anterior approach and reduction; note the intervertebral spreaders. F, The patient after anterior decompression, stabilization, fusion with a Smith-Robinson graft, and anterior plate (the posterior approach to decompress the displaced laminae fracture). G and H, Anterior and posterior plates at C5–C6.*

stabilization, if necessary, should attempt to include as few motion segments as possible, and in neurologically impaired patients should be mechanically sound so as to allow early mobilization without the concomitant use of a halo brace.

The timing of closed reduction and surgical treatment is controversial. There are no definitive data in humans demonstrating that early treatment has any influence on ultimate neurologic recovery.[59] There are theoretical advantages to diminishing spinal cord compression trauma by operative and nonoperative treatment in the early hours after injury.[70] Several studies by institutions lend support to this intuitively logical relationship.[22, 46, 79] Marshall prospectively reviewed neurologic deterioration in 283 patients with spinal cord injuries.[70] He found that four patients deteriorated after surgery and that all had undergone surgery within 5 days of injury. No patient who underwent surgery after 5 days was noted to have deterioration; however, five patients deteriorated in the nonoperative period while awaiting surgery, including two from halo vest placement, two from rotation on a Stryker frame, and one from loss of reduction.

Animal studies have shown an inverse relationship between the timing of decompression and subsequent neurologic recovery, with the general rule being that a shorter time to decompression yields greater recovery.[11, 21, 38, 41, 43, 78] Delamarter created experimental stenosis in beagles by placing constricting bands on their spinal cords, which caused narrowing of approximately 50%.[38] The animals were decompressed by removing the constriction bands at various times. Those with early removal at time 0 (immediately) or at 1 hour postcompression made full clinical neurologic recovery, whereas those decompressed later—at 6 and 24 hours after placement of compression—did not. This correlates well with histopathologic studies demonstrating that axonal tracts in the white matter are intact immediately after experimental trauma.[11, 43] This is followed by progressive destruction over the next 24 to 48 hours from the secondary injury caused by adverse mechanical, biochemical, and vascular factors.[58, 60, 93, 111, 112]

Therefore, a short time period or "window of opportunity" may exist when prompt reduction of a deformity, with reestablishment of more normal canal dimensions and, hopefully, decreased neural compression and increased spinal cord perfusion may allow for complete reversal of spinal cord injury.[38, 63] Anderson has noted four cases of patients who underwent reduction of bilateral facet dislocation within 2 hours of injury and gratifyingly had complete reversal of their quadriplegia.[4] Based on these observations and review of animal studies, it seems reasonable that neurologically injured patients should have prompt reduction of dislocations or fractures, whenever feasible.[24, 37, 43, 44, 93]

A limitation of managing patients with cervical spine injuries with prolonged cervical traction is the deleterious effect on their general medical condition. Cranial tong traction requires continued recumbence, which can predispose a patient to pulmonary, urinary, gastrointestinal, and skin complications. Schlegel[88] and Anderson[10] reported decreased morbidity and length of hospitalization in patients with multiple injuries treated surgically within 72 hours as compared with those treated in a more delayed fashion.

MANAGEMENT OF SPECIFIC FRACTURE TYPES

Cervical Spinal Cord Injuries

It is recommended that after initial resuscitation and radiographic evaluation, if time allows, that patients with cord injuries be treated with high-dose methylprednisolone in accordance with National Acute Spinal Cord Injury Study (NASCIS) II guidelines.[22, 23] This study noted improved outcomes in patients treated with massive doses of methylprednisolone administered acutely after injury. A loading dose of 30 mg/kg is followed by a maintenance dose of 5.4 mg/kg/hr for the next 23 hours. This treatment must be initiated within 8 hours of injury; after this time, methylprednisolone may be deleterious. In patients with spinal malalignments and cord injuries or evidence of cord compression, immediate traction reduction should be

performed using cranial tongs. A later study has suggested that steroid treatment for 48 hours may be beneficial, if started 3 to 8 hours after injury.[23a]

Surgical Technique: Gardner-Wells Tongs Insertion and Reduction

Gardner-Wells tongs are inserted in line with the external auditory meatus 1 cm above the auricle. Between 5 and 10 lb of weight is applied, a repeat neurologic examination is performed, and a lateral x-ray is obtained (Fig. 12–11). The use of a flow sheet can facilitate information and record keeping. With each increase in traction weight, a serial neurologic examination is performed, findings are recorded, and repeat x-rays (lateral cervical) are obtained. The weight is increased in only 5- to 10-lb increments. The interval x-rays are carefully reviewed for signs of overdistraction, such as widening of the disk height or separation of the posterior facet joints. Traction up to 70% of body weight can be safely applied if meticulous attention is paid to both the neurologic examination findings and the x-rays.[35, 97] The use of C-arm fluoroscopy can facilitate radiographic surveillance. Once reduction of the facet joints has been achieved, the traction weight should be decreased, except in patients with bursting or teardrop-type fractures, where weight reduction allows redisplacement of fracture fragments into the canal. Cranial tong traction is obviously contraindicated in patients who have sustained skull fractures or extensive cranial injury. MRI-compatible tongs can allow for postreduction MRI; however, they cannot maintain as much traction weight as stainless steel tongs.[17] The final proviso should obviously be that traction must be used judiciously in patients with severe ligamentous injuries, to avoid the risk of overdisplacement or overdistraction. After reduction, MRI should be done in patients with cervical spinal cord injuries. Patients with persistent cord compression must be considered candidates for surgical decompression and stabilization. In most patients who have undergone successful reduction, the surgical approach and timing is based on the clinical course and fracture type. Indications for immediate surgery include patients with evidence of neurologic deterioration with persistent compressive lesions or malalignment. Patients in whom closed reduction has failed should also be considered to be candidates for early surgery, usually within the first 24 hours.[20, 93]

Stable Fractures

An approach to treating patients with stable fractures from any mechanism has already been discussed. To review briefly, these injuries are usually isolated to one side of the spinal column and are not associated with vertebral body translation or neurologic deficits. The injuries are assessed using the White and Panjabi criteria; stable injuries are those with scores of 4 or lower. Stable injuries commonly include vertebral body compression fractures, avulsion of the anterior longitudinal ligament, associated extension teardrop fractures, mild posterior longitudinal ligament injuries (e.g., sprains), and isolated fractures of the posterior elements (e.g., clay shoveler's fractures).

These patients are treated in a hard collar or cervicotho-

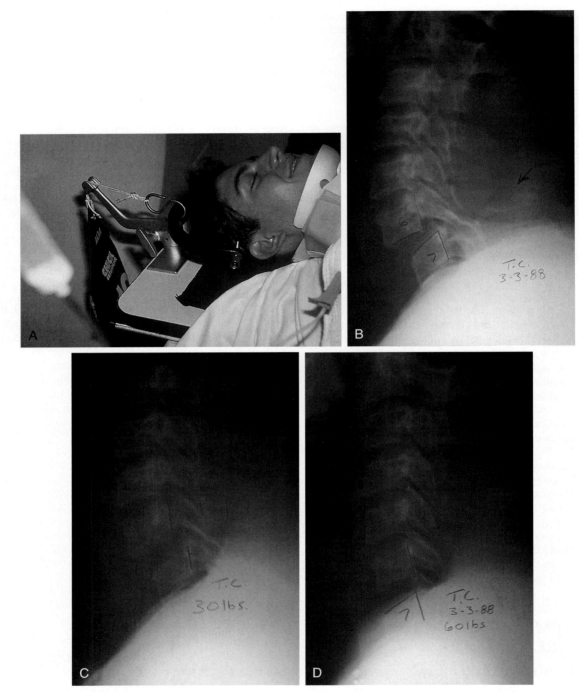

Figure 12–11. *A, Gardner-Wells MRI-compatible tongs and traction applied. The patient must be awake and alert to perform closed reduction. B, Unilateral jumped facet at C6–C7 and fracture of spinous process C6. C, Dislocation unreduced with 30 lb of traction. D, Dislocation reduced at 60 lb of traction. The traction weight was then discontinued and the patient immobilized.*

racic brace (Yale) for 6 to 8 weeks. After brace placement, an upright x-ray is performed to check alignment; this should be repeated biweekly until healing occurs (in about 6 to 8 weeks following injury). The physician needs to maintain a high degree of suspicion that his or her initial assessment of stability may be incorrect and may only be determined later by subsequent x-rays. Increased pain or development of new neurologic deficits may indicate fracture site motion or loss of position, and thus an unstable fracture. At approximately 6 to 8 weeks, supervised flexion-extension x-rays are obtained to assess healing. During the period of immobilization while in the collar, the patient performs isometric neck exercises and nonimpact aerobic exercises.

Posterior Column Injuries

Isolated Fractures of the Posterior Column

Stable hyperextension injuries are limited to one spinal column and are not associated with vertebral body displacement. Stable posterior injuries include isolated spinous process fractures, isolated laminar fractures, and facet fractures. Facet fractures should be carefully analyzed, because they may be the only clue of more significant instabilities that have spontaneously reduced. Isolated fractures of the transverse process are usually insignificant in terms of spinal stability, but can be associated with vertebral artery injury. Stable fractures of the posterior elements can be treated with a cervicothoracic brace or collar for 6 to 8 weeks; once again, after immobilization, supervised flexion-extension x-rays should be obtained to evaluate healing and to rule out unrecognized ligamentous instability. Displaced spinous process fractures may develop a nonunion, but are rarely symptomatic.

Posterior Ligamentous Injuries

Posterior ligamentous injuries are readily assessed using the White and Panjabi criteria. Patients who have ligamentous injuries and/or spinous process fractures from hyperflexion are stable and have a score below 4. Clinically, these patients have reproducible focal neck tenderness with palpation but have minimal kyphotic angulation, interspinous widening, or vertebral body translation. These injuries can be successfully treated with 6 to 8 weeks of immobilization in a hard collar or brace and isometric strengthening, as described in the previous section.

A more insidious fracture pattern is that of posterior ligamentous disruption associated with mild compression fractures. These injuries have a poor prognosis and are easily undertreated. Webb described six patients who had mild wedge compression fractures with unrecognized flexion injuries who became progressively unstable.[106] Mazur similarly reported five patients, all of whom had progressive kyphosis and failure of nonoperative treatment.[71] Patients with this injury pattern should be treated more aggressively, with either a halo brace or a posterior fusion. Patients treated nonsurgically should be carefully advised of the risks of poor outcome and of the possibility that they may need subsequent posterior fusion.

Common radiographic findings in patients suffering severe ligamentous injuries include interspinous widening, kyphotic angulation, but usually less than 3 mm of anterior translation. The facets can be in a perched position almost to the point of dislocation. Extension can reduce this deformity. The definitive treatment for severe hyperflexion injury is restoration of the deficient posterior tension band. This is done simply with an interspinous wiring technique and posterior cervical fusion, as described by Rogers[83] and Bohlman.[18] Alignment is readily restored by tightening the interspinous wire. If the need for postoperative MRI imaging is anticipated, then the use of titanium cable instead of stainless steel wire will decrease image distortion. The fixation is stable enough to allow early mobilization of the patient in an orthosis. Care must be taken to avoid overtightening the interspinous wire, which can lead to iatrogenic narrowing of the neural foramina. If the spinous processes or lamina are fractured and unavailable for a posterior wiring technique, then a posterior lateral mass plating and posterior fusion, or alternatively an anterior plate fixation and fusion, should be performed.

Posterior Cervical Fusion with Interspinous Wire

Posterior interspinous wiring fixation is utilitarian and has stood the test of time. This is one of the most common procedures performed to achieve posterior cervical stability. The two most commonly performed techniques are the simple Rogers interspinous wiring technique[83] and the slightly more complicated Bohlman triple-wire technique.[18] Posterior wire fixation is most effective in stabilizing one to two motion segments with intact posterior elements. If facet fractures are present, then the facets are unable to perform a buttressing role, and forward vertebral body translation may recur, leading to recurrent deformity after wire fixation. The Bohlman triple-wire technique increases rigidity, particularly resistance to rotation, but still may be insufficient to control subluxation.

Surgical Technique: Interspinous Wiring

The patient is positioned prone. The head may be held in a Mayfield three-point head holder or alternatively, in situations of instability, the patient may be turned prone on a Stryker turning frame while tong traction is maintained. Avoiding inadvertent ocular pressure is critical. Before skin incision, x-rays are taken to confirm adequate alignment.

A standard posterior midline exposure is performed. Dissection is carried out in a subperiosteal fashion, extending to the lateral masses. It is important to limit exposure only to those levels to be arthrodesed and to maintain a midline cuff of soft tissues to help prevent unintended extension of the fusion or iatrogenic instability by disruption of soft tissues at adjacent levels. The appropriate level is always confirmed with an intraoperative lateral x-ray.

If the closed reduction is unsuccessful and the facet remains dislocated, then an open reduction can be performed. Spinal cord monitoring should be maintained in all patients with preserved distal cord function. Several techniques are useful in performing open reduction of the dislocated facet joint. The spinous processes can be manipulated as levers, using Kocher clamps or towel clips. A small elevator can be inserted into the dislocated facet joint and levered to help unlock the joint. If necessary, the cephalad portion of the superior articular process can be partially removed with a bur to facilitate relocation. In a unilateral facet dislocation, gentle lateral bending to the opposite side can facilitate reduction. Rogers popularized the interspinous wiring technique and recommended its use for patients with unstable cervical spines.[83] A single stainless steel wire loop is passed through the cephalad spinous process and below the inferior edge of the caudad spinous process, restoring a mechanical tension band to the posterior column. Rogers reported that 35 of 37 patients experienced healed fusions, with 1 patient losing reduction. This technique is indicated in patients with hyperflexion injuries without posterior element fracture and without rotational instability.

Surgical Technique: Rogers Interspinous Wiring

After subperiosteal exposure, the bony structures are carefully inspected to identify any occult fractures that may prevent interspinous wiring fixation. Initially, a 3-mm hole is created with a bur at the base of the spinous process, at the junction of the spinous process in the lamina. This is gently enlarged with a Lewin clamp or a towel clip to allow passage of wires. Care must be taken not to place the hole too far anteriorly or laterally in the lamina, which might endanger the dura or spinal cord. At the lower level, a hole can be created in the spinous process or the wire simply passed beneath the caudal edge of the spinous process. Either 20-gauge stainless steel wires, braided 24-gauge stainless steel wires, or titanium cables can be used for this technique. The titanium cables offer the theoretical advantages of MRI compatibility and flexibility, allowing easier passage and more uniform tightening. The long-term use of these cables in cervical fusion has not been reported.[36, 96]

The facet joints are decorticated with a small curette, and a cancellous bone graft is gently packed into the facet joints. This is usually just the posterior third of the facet joint. The wire is subsequently passed through the hole at the base of the spinous process above and then below, creating a simple loop. The wire is gently tightened. If stainless steel wiring is used, kinking must be avoided, because this causes a marked stress riser and can lead to premature wire breakage. After tightening, lateral x-rays are obtained to ensure appropriate alignment. Overtightening, which can lead to retrolisthesis, must be avoided. The laminae are decorticated with a 3-mm bur, and additional bone graft (usually autologous iliac crest bone graft) is placed on the dorsal surfaces of the spinous processes and laminae. Rogers recommended placing a small amount of bone graft underneath the wire. The paraspinal muscles and nuchal ligaments are closed in two layers, and the neck is immobilized postoperatively in a hard collar or a cervicothoracic brace. The patient is rapidly mobilized, and an orthosis is worn for approximately 8 to 12 weeks. Fusion is assessed radiographically with flexion-extension x-rays at 3 months. After immobilization, the patient is placed on cervical isometric neck exercises and aerobic conditioning.

To increase rotational rigidity of the posterior wiring construct, Bohlman developed the triple-wire technique. This technique has been mechanically shown to increase flexion and rotational stiffness over the intact spine as compared with the Rogers single-wire technique.[30, 99]

Surgical Technique: Bohlman Triple-Wire

The first wire is placed similarly to the Rogers technique. A second wire is placed in the cephalad spinous process, using the same hole. A third wire is placed through the caudad spinous process hole. The loose ends of the wire are placed through two preformed corticocancellous autologous bone grafts approximately 1.5 cm wide, 3 to 4 mm thick, and approximately 3 to 4 cm long. The second and third wires are tightened onto each other, using needle drivers in a gentle twisting fashion, securing the outer bone grafts (see Fig. 12–4). Weiland has reported that 100 patients treated with the Bohlman triple-wire technique exhibited healed fusions.[107] Postoperatively, the course of immobilization with a brace is similar to that of the Rogers technique, as described earlier. Again, with the use of wire, notching or crimping of the wire must be avoided because of decreased fatigue strength. Modified techniques using titanium cables have been described, but again, long-term results are not available. The triple-wire technique is intended primarily to restore deficient posterior tension bands. Again, it must be noted that despite the increase in rotational rigidity, recurrent dislocations can occur if the facet articulation is incompetent.

Hyperextension Injury with Spinal Cord Injury

Taylor first reported this mechanism of spinal cord injury without obvious radiographic changes.[100] He postulated that the spinal cord was damaged by the pinching between the disk and bone spurs anteriorly and the infolded ligamentum flavum posteriorly. Schneider clarified the neuroanatomic basis for the development of the central cord syndrome so often seen in these extension injuries.[90] He postulated that the condition has a favorable prognosis and that surgery is rarely warranted. Marar reviewed 45 patients with spinal cord injuries from extension mechanisms and found that the neurologic injury was more variable than Schneider had reported and did not always conform to the typical central cord syndrome.[69] In that study, only 10 of the patients had normal x-rays; 11 were noted to have retrolisthesis, and 24 had extension teardrop fractures. Four of the patients died during treatment and underwent autopsy; all were noted to have transverse fractures through the vertebral body that were not apparent on preautopsy plain x-rays. The clinical outcome was correlated with initial hand strength. At long-term follow-up, 31 of the 32 patients could ambulate; however, only those patients with at least grade III hand strength at the time of admission had any significant recovery of hand function. Merriam also correlated clinical outcome with initial hand strength, as well as with the presence of perineal pinprick sensation.[73]

The initial treatment of extension injury and spinal cord injury is to apply longitudinal tong traction. This may reduce any malalignment and tends to lengthen the spinal column, hopefully reducing the redundant ligamentum flavum, thereby indirectly decompressing the spinal cord and stabilizing the spine to prevent further injury. Previous suggestions that these injuries do not require traction are probably incorrect, and we would advocate the use of traction, at least initially. Definitive treatment is based on imaging studies and the progression of neurologic recovery. Patients who are improving neurologically are mobilized within 5 to 7 days, in a collar. Upright x-rays are obtained with the collar on to verify alignment. Patients who are not improving or who have reached a neurologic recovery plateau can be considered candidates for surgical decompression. The approach depends on the site of cord compression and its extent. The approach is similar to that used for patients with cervical spondylotic myelopathy. Anterior decompression is indicated in patients with one to three levels of anterior or anteroposterior cord compression, and/or if the spine is in overall kyphotic alignment. Posterior decompression is indicated in rare cases where compression is focally localized posteriorly or, more commonly, when more than three levels of anteroposterior compression are present. To avoid later problems of kyphotic deformity, posterior decompression is performed only in patients in whom the spine is in neutral or lordotic alignment. After either anterior or posterior decompression, plate fixation can be added for additional stabilization.

Facet Injuries

Isolated Pedicle or Facet Fractures

Isolated pedicle or facet fractures without subluxation are usually stable and can be treated in a closed fashion with a cervical orthosis for 6 to 8 weeks. Careful follow-up x-rays are required because of the potential for late subluxation. Patients with chronic neck pain after trauma may have occult fractures of the facet that are not easily discernible on plain x-rays. These injuries can be identified with scintigrams or CT scans, and may be treated with late posterior fusion.

Unilateral Facet Dislocations

The treatment of this disorder is controversial. Important factors to consider when planning treatment include the stability, the ease of reduction, the presence or absence of facet fractures, the adequacy of the reduction, and associated neurologic deficits. Significant soft tissue injuries to the joint capsule, ligamentum flavum, nuchal ligaments, and posterior longitudinal ligament have occurred, and these disruptions then allow for the observed bony displacement.[12] Closed reductions can be achieved in a high percentage of cases. Difficulty in reduction may result from locking of the contralateral ligamentous structures that may have been spared or from an associated fracture or malrotation of the lateral mass. Closed reduction techniques have reported success rates of 70% to 90%.[35, 54, 97]

Several studies have documented that successful long-term outcome correlates with anatomic alignment, regardless of the method used to achieve it.[16, 84] Rorabeck analyzed 26 patients with unilateral facet dislocations and found that 7 of 10 who had healed in the displaced position unfortunately had chronic neck and arm pain, whereas none of the other 16 patients with anatomic positioning and healing had pain.[84] Beyer found that 75% of patients could achieve a closed reduction.[16] In patients with residual subluxation, he found a higher incidence of instability, neck pain, and stiffness. He recommended open reduction and fusion if attempts at closed reduction failed.

Controversies have arisen regarding whether patients should undergo surgery or be treated with a halo vest. In general, pure ligamentous injuries are not well treated by the halo vest, because torn ligaments have a poor healing capacity. In a unilateral facet dislocation without fractures, however, the contralateral ligaments may be spared, and with proper immobilization, recurrent dislocation may be prevented. If a facet fracture is present, the buttress to prevent rotation and anterolisthesis is lost, and in our experience, this frequently results in the loss of alignment. Based on these observations, we offer the following treatment recommendations:

- In all cases of unilateral facet dislocations, attempts at closed reduction should be performed initially.
- If this fails, then an open reduction and posterior fusion is recommended.
- Before any surgical procedure, the patient should be imaged fully to evaluate the intervertebral disk and the neural foramina. If a disk herniation is seen to be compressing the spinal cord, then the patient should be treated with an anterior cervical diskectomy, fusion, and anterior plating.
- Patients with foraminal encroachment and no significant anterior disk compression can be treated with posterior foraminotomy, performed in conjunction with the posterior fusion.
- In patients with significant neurologic deficits or spinal cord syndromes and a unilateral facet dislocation, the best treatment is emergent closed reduction followed by posterior fusion.
- In patients with spinal cord injury, the halo vest is best avoided, if at all possible. Their rehabilitation would be slowed by the halo, which interferes with nursing care and possibly pulmonary function and generally is poorly tolerated.

Pure Unilateral Facet Dislocations

These injuries may remain stable after reduction, and thus nonoperative treatment with a halo vest can be attempted. After successful reduction, keeping the head in slight extension and slight contralateral rotation may decrease the likelihood of redisplacement of the dislocation. The patient should be evaluated frequently to verify maintenance of the reduction. After 12 weeks, the halo vest is removed and flexion-extension x-rays are obtained. If instability is still present, then a late posterior fusion is indicated. Most patients with a pure unilateral facet dislocation without fracture can be treated with a posterior fusion augmented by the Rogers or Bohlman interspinous wire fixation technique.[18, 83]

Unilateral Facet Fracture Dislocations

Unilateral facet fracture dislocations have lost the mechanical bony buttress that resists rotation and anterior translation. Reduction is usually easily performed, and consequently, redisplacement commonly occurs with attempted nonoperative treatment. Therefore, operative treatment is the recommended approach for these injuries. Before surgery, the patient should have MRI evaluation of the intervertebral disk. If posterior disk herniation is noted, then the treatment of choice is anterior diskectomy, fusion, and plating. If the disk does not appear to impinge on the cord, then the patient is treated with posterior fusion. Because of increased rotational stability, either the Edwards oblique wiring technique or lateral mass plate fixation is recommended.[8, 86, 91a] In a small percentage of patients, foraminal stenosis is present secondary to displacement of fracture fragments, and these may require a concomitant posterior foraminotomy in addition to the posterior fusion. In a unilateral facet dislocation without associated fracture, the rotational instability can be addressed more directly with an oblique wiring technique.

Oblique Facet Wire Fixation

Facet wire fixation was initially described by Robinson and Southwick as a treatment of kyphotic and swan-neck deformities associated with cervical laminectomies.[27, 82] In cases of rotational instability of the cervical spine, Edwards reported successful outcomes in 26 of 27 patients treated with the oblique wire.[45]

Surgical Technique: Oblique Wire

The patient is positioned prone. A posterior midline exposure is performed. Dissection is carried out to the far lateral edge of the lateral mass. Reduction of the dislocated facet, if not previously achieved by closed methods, is then carried out. The facet joint is opened, the joint cartilage is curetted, and a small flat elevator is placed in the facet joint. A 3-mm air drill is used with a bur to create a hole from the midpoint, or summit, of the lateral mass downward into the facet joint. The Penfield elevator placed in the joint acts as a stop to the bur. A 20-gauge wire or titanium cable is then passed down and through the hole and out of the joint. A small hemostat or needle driver is used to grasp the wire to pull it out of the joint; distraction of the joint by levering on the spinous process can facilitate wire passage. The wire or cable is then looped around the immediately caudad spinous process. Bone graft is packed in place, and the wire is tightened. A lateral x-ray is obtained to document proper alignment of the reduction. A Rogers interspinous wire or, alternatively, a Bohlman triple-wire procedure can be added after passage of the oblique wire (Fig. 12–12). The laminae, spinous processes, and facet joints are decorticated, and autologous cancellous bone graft is placed in the decorticated bed. Postoperatively, the patient is immobilized in a brace for 8 to 12 weeks.

Fracture Separation of the Lateral Mass

Roy-Camille identified a complex fracture of the lateral mass, characterized by two fracture lines in the pedicle and the lamina, creating a separation of the lateral mass from the vertebral body and posterior elements.[86] The lateral mass becomes a free-floating element. It rotates in a parasagittal plane, so that the facet joint can be seen almost end-on on an anteroposterior x-ray. This instability allows subluxation of both the cranial and caudad vertebral levels. This highly unstable injury is best treated with surgical stabilization, with the preferred method being lateral mass fixation of the two adjacent motion segments.

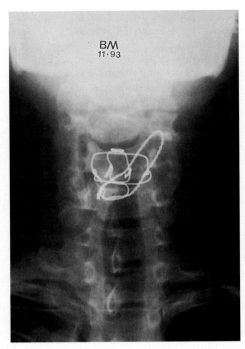

Figure 12–12. *Left Edwards oblique wiring of C4–C5 supplemented by the Bohlman triple-wire technique.*

Lateral Mass Fixation

Lateral mass fixation of the cervical spine was originally introduced by Roy-Camille, who described the use of Vitallium plates with 14-mm screws.[86] His screw placement technique was modified by Magerl to provide fixation for an atlanto-occipital hook plate.[32] These techniques gained popularity because of their increased rigidity, which subsequently lowered the incidence of lost reduction and decreased postoperative brace requirements.[8, 32] The other advantage of lateral mass fixation is its efficacy in cases of fractured or deficient laminar spinous processes, in multilevel instability, and to control rotational instability.

Lateral mass fixation is extensile and allows extension of fusion constructs across either the occipitocervical or cervicothoracic junctions. Studies have confirmed the biomechanical superiority of lateral mass plates and screws when compared with posterior wire fixation or anterior plate constructs.[1, 30, 86, 104] However, complications, including nerve root injury and plate/screw loosening, have been reported. Heller reported a 6% incidence of iatrogenic nerve injury and a 0.2% incidence of facet joint violation in a series of 654 lateral mass screws reviewed.[56] Additionally, loosening was observed in more than 1% of cases, and hardware failure was seen in 0.5% of cases. Clinical reports indicate that lateral mass fixation is highly effective.[8, 32] Anderson reported on a prospective study of 102 patients with unstable cervical spine injuries treated with lateral mass fixation using atlanto-occipital reconstruction plates.[7] At follow-up of 14 months, all patients exhibited healed fusions and maintained postoperative reductions, with only 1.5 degrees of increased kyphosis and 0.1 mm of increased translation noted at follow-up. Two patients had iatrogenic C7 radiculopathies secondary to drilling and screw placement. Heller additionally noted that C7 roots were at greater risk from screw placement in the often abnormally shaped C7 lateral mass.[3, 56] If clear lateral mass borders at C7 are not readily identified intraoperatively and preoperative imaging fails to document sufficient size of the lateral mass, then avoiding screw fixation at this level is advocated. Treatment alternatives would be to extend fixation to T1, to use the C7 pedicles, or to use a posterior wire fixation technique.

Surgical Technique: Lateral Mass Fixation

The patient is placed prone on a turning frame, with the neck in a neutral position. Gardner-Wells tongs are used to maintain intraoperative traction. A lateral x-ray is obtained, documenting reduction before exposure. A standard subperiosteal exposure is performed, with care taken to limit exposure to avoid spontaneous iatrogenic extension of the fusion.

The lateral masses are carefully identified. These should have a rectangular outline. The medial border is the valley of the junction of the lateral lamina and the medial edge of the lateral mass. The lateral border of the lateral mass is its edge as it abuts muscle. The superior and inferior borders of the lateral mass are defined by the superior and inferior facet joints. The vertebral artery is located directly anterior to the medial valley; therefore, all screws must start lateral to this point and be angled laterally. Several screw insertion techniques have been previously described, including the Roy-Camille, the Magerl, and the An approaches.[3, 32, 86] We recommend a modification of the Magerl technique.[7, 8] The starting point is 1 to 2 mm medial to the exact center of the lateral mass, and the screws are then oriented in a cephalad

and lateral direction with cephalad angulation of approximately 30 degrees (attempting to parallel the joint surface) and outward 10 to 15 degrees (Fig. 12–13). This generally is done with a 2-mm drill bit with an adjustable drill guide; alternatively, a 2-mm smooth K-wire with a diamond tip may be used, because this may decrease possible injury should the nerve root be inadvertently encountered. The initial length on the drill guide is set to 14 mm, and a step-drilling technique is used. The hole is assessed for perforation of the far cortex. This is facilitated with the blunt end of a 1.7-mm K-wire. The hole is deepened in 2-mm increments, or until a depth of 18 mm is reached. The hole is tapped, and a screw of appropriate length is used.

Several lateral mass plates are available. The atlanto-occipital titanium reconstruction plates (Synthes) come with 8-mm and 12-mm hole spacings in various lengths; a new version of this plate is now available that better accommodates the oblique screw head position of the lateral mass screws. The axis plates (Medtronic Sofamor Danek) are available in 11-mm, 13-mm, and 15-mm hole spacings and have two positions for screws in each hole. In a multilevel construct, the cephalad and caudad lateral masses are drilled initially, which facilitates safe screw placement. The plate can be contoured and positioned and, if necessary, the additional screw holes are drilled through the plate. An additional interspinous process wire can be placed from cephalad to caudad. This can be tightened to help adjust final positioning and increase cervical lordosis. Before the plate is placed, the posterior thirds of the facets are decorticated with a bur, and autologous iliac crest cancellous bone graft is packed into the facets. The plates are then placed over the lateral masses and affixed with appropriate 3.5-mm titanium screws. The screws are tightened in sequential fashion. As the plate is being

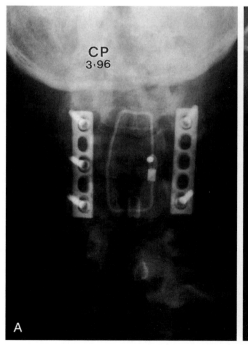 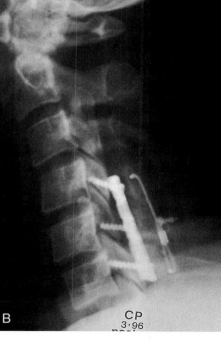

Figure 12–13. C4–C6 lateral mass plate and screw fixation supplemented by interspinous wiring with titanium cable. Note the superior and lateral angulation of the screws.

tightened, it is observed; if it begins to shift laterally, then the screws may be beginning to cut out. Postoperatively, the patient is mobilized in a hard collar or cervicothoracic brace for 8 to 12 weeks.

Bilateral Facet Dislocations

Bilateral facet dislocations are often among the most dramatic cervical injuries and are often associated with significant spinal cord injury. Unfortunately, many patients have been reported to be neurologically intact initially and subsequently deteriorated after reaching a medical facility.[19] Beatson and others have shown that complete rupture of all of the ligamentous structures, with the exception of the anterior longitudinal ligament (which is often stripped periosteally from the vertebral body), is present.[12, 108] Although prolonged treatment with bed rest or halo vest immobilization has been suggested, because of the high degree of instability and the ligamentous nature of the injury, most patients today should undergo surgical treatment and bony fusion.

Several important factors are considered in the treatment of patients with bilateral facet dislocations, including the status of the intervertebral disk and any associated disk herniation, the presence of fractures of the posterior elements, the timing and method of the reduction, the possibility of vertebral artery injury, and the timing and approach of surgical intervention. Occasionally patients will present neurologically intact, whether from the presence of a capacious spinal canal or from increased spinal diameter secondary to pedicular fractures or, less likely, from a slow onset of the dislocation.

The flexion-distraction forces needed to create a bilateral facet dislocation result in a tearing of the disk annulus and the possibility of an associated disk herniation into the spinal canal. This can result in further cord compression, which can prevent neurologic recovery even after reduction of the dislocation.[46] In a more unfortunate scenario, patients who are neurologically intact may have increased cord compression after successful bony reduction from the presence of a persistent disk herniation, and subsequently develop progressive neurologic deficits.[42, 103] Rizzolo identified acute disk disruptions in 42% of patients with cervical trauma.[79] In this series, 56% of patients with facet trauma had a herniated nucleus pulposus, although there was no correlation with the presence of disk herniation and neurologic outcome.

Doran identified nine patients with herniated nucleus pulposus and bilateral facet dislocations and recommended obtaining an MRI before undertaking any attempt at reduction.[42] Others disagree with this approach and recommend immediate closed reduction to effect indirect decompression of the spinal cord; this maximizes the likelihood of neurologic recovery by minimizing the time of decompression. Several case reports have noted reversal of complete spinal cord injury when reduction was performed within the first 2 to 3 hours after injury.[63] This correlates with observations in animal models.[38] The additional time needed to obtain an MRI can delay successful reduction, thus decreasing the patient's likelihood of optimal neurologic recovery. However, reduction of bilateral facet dislocations has resulted in neurologic deterioration in some cases. Eismont identified six patients treated surgically who had concomitant herniated disks.[46] Two patients deteriorated after open reduction via a posterior approach, whereas one worsened during attempted closed reduction. Robertson had three cases that worsened. One occurred 3 days after closed reduction, one occurred after a posterior open reduction, and one deteriorated during transport to the hospital.[81] Berrington reported on two patients who deteriorated secondary to displaced disk herniations, one after open reduction and one after a spontaneous reduction.[15]

From these reports, neurologic worsening from disk herniation was commonly associated with difficult reductions, failed attempts at closed reduction, and radiographic evidence of abnormal disk space narrowing. Neurologic deterioration is more likely after open posterior reduction and wire fixation. Also, most of the patients who worsened had minimal or no neurologic deficits on initial presentation.

The halo vest provides the greatest degree of external immobilization of the cervical spine. It is often successful in treating the upper cervical spine; however, results can be poor in patients with facet dislocations in the lower and mid-cervical spine. Whitehill reported six cases of loss of reduction in the halo vest.[109] Bucholz treated 125 patients with cervical trauma by halo vest immobilization; in this group, 9 of the 20 patients with bilateral facet dislocations or perched facets failed treatment and needed surgery.[26] Sears reported that only 44% of his patients in halo vests achieved stability and 50% had some degree of residual malalignment.[91] Anderson evaluated fracture site motion during a position change from supine to upright in 47 patients treated with a halo vest and noted that translation increased by 1.7 mm and angulation increased by 11 degrees.[6] The halo vest is poorly suited for unstable lower cervical injuries because of its inability to control intersegmental motion, although it effectively limits overall motion.[74] In patients who are not otherwise surgical candidates, however, the halo vest provides the best means of external immobilization either temporarily or definitively.

We propose the following treatment protocol for patients with bilateral facet dislocations. Patients who are neurologically intact should have strict cervical immobilization and prompt evaluation by MRI or CT myelography before any attempt at reduction is made. If these imaging modalities are not available, then a closed reduction should be attempted, using a strict protocol with an awake, cooperative patient. If the patient notes any increase in neurologic deficit during the closed reduction attempt, this should be discontinued and reduction postponed until preoperative imaging can be obtained documenting the canal status. In patients who show evidence of a disk herniation on MRI, an anterior diskectomy is performed before reduction; after diskectomy, reduction can often be obtained by traction or by the use of anterior cervical distractors (either Caspar pin types or intervertebral spreaders). Spinal cord monitoring should be used during attempts at reduction, especially when a general anesthetic is in effect. If a successful reduction is obtained, it can be stabilized with an anterior interbody bone graft fusion and anterior cervical plating. If the reduction attempt is not successful, then a posterior approach and subsequent open reduction and posterior fusion are performed. Before the anterior incision is closed, a Smith-Robinson graft can be placed between the vertebrae, although it may displace with posterior reduction, necessitating a third procedure to reposition the interbody graft (see Fig. 12–8).

Patients with bilateral facet dislocations who present with significant cord deficits should undergo an immediate attempt at closed reduction with tong traction. These patients should be alert, responsive, and carefully monitored with serial x-rays and serial neurologic exams. If the patient reports any increased neurologic symptoms, such as paresthesias or worsening sensory or motor loss, then prompt discontinuation of traction and immediate MRI screening are mandated. If reduction is achieved, then MRI should be done to evaluate the status of the disk. If the disk herniation is compressing the spinal cord, then an anterior cervical diskectomy and fusion with a plate should be performed. If the disk is normal and the posterior bony structures are adequate, then a simple posterior fusion can be done with an interspinous wire technique. If fractures are present, then a posterolateral mass fixation can be performed. Alternatively, if the anterior approach is required, then anterior stabilization can be performed using a cervical plate.

Careful analysis is required for severe bilateral facet dislocations with 100% translation or patients who present with distraction of the intervertebral space. We have noted vertebral artery injuries and higher levels of paralysis in these cases than in those with bony injury. Traction is especially dangerous, because all ligamentous structures have been torn. These patients are best treated with early open reduction and anterior and possibly posterior plate fixation.

Occasionally, bilateral facet dislocations are associated with bilateral pedicular fractures. This creates an increase in the spinal canal dimensions and thus decreases the risk of neurologic injury.[55] The proposed mechanism of injury is hyperextension, similar to the etiology of traumatic spondylolisthesis at C2 (the so-called hangman's fracture). These fractures in the subaxial spine are difficult to reduce and maintain by traction because of the pedicle fractures. Surgically, an anterior approach with bone graft and plate fixation is recommended.[72]

Anterior Column Injuries

Vertebral Body Compression Fractures

Simple wedge compression fractures may occur from axial loading, with fracture of the superior endplate and vertebral body wedging. Minimal kyphosis and no spinal canal compromise are present. These stable injuries can be treated with cervicothoracic bracing, as discussed earlier.

Vertebral Body Compression Fractures with Associated Posterior Ligament Injury

Webb identified flexion injuries that appear initially as benign wedge compression fractures.[106] These injuries are caused by hyperflexion forces and, along with the anterior vertebral fracture, have unappreciated posterior osteoliga-

mentous disruption. Because of both anterior compression fracture and, more importantly, the loss of the posterior ligamentous structures, this is a very unstable injury. On evaluation by the White and Panjabi rating scale, it will have a score above 5. The injury is notorious for a slowly progressive increasing kyphotic deformity until facet perching or dislocation occurs. Patients with vertebral body compression fractures should be carefully examined for disruption of the posterior interosseous ligament, including clinical clues such as tenderness along the spinous processes, gaps between the spinous processes, interspinous widening on the plain x-rays, or evidence of increased signal in the area of the interspinous ligaments on MRI. Compression fractures associated with posterior ligament injuries are treated definitively by surgical posterior fusion, either with interspinous wiring or posterior lateral mass plates, if necessary.

Discoligamentous Extension Injury

Stable extension injuries of the anterior column include rupture of the anterior longitudinal ligament and the disk annulus, and the extension teardrop fracture—all without vertebral body subluxation. Spinal alignment should always be evaluated, because small amounts of retrolisthesis are easily overlooked. Anterior longitudinal ligament ruptures can be identified radiographically by an increase in the disk space height anteriorly and by increased evidence of retropharyngeal soft tissue swelling. Occasionally, these patients will have increased lordotic angulation. These injuries reduce easily with neutral upright positioning. Treatment of ruptured anterior longitudinal ligament is orthotic immobilization for 6 to 8 weeks.

Extension Teardrop Fractures

The extension teardrop fracture is a small triangular bone fragment avulsed from the anteroinferior corner of the vertebral body. In some cases, the fracture may be an osteophyte or may be confused with an incomplete ossification of an osteophyte. This is a stable injury, but it must be differentiated from the unstable *flexion teardrop fracture* of Schneider, which has the associated fracture of the vertebral body, retropulsion into the spinal canal, and interspinous disruption. Treatment of the extension teardrop fracture is a collar or cervicothoracic brace for 6 to 8 weeks.

Traumatic Retrolisthesis

Extension injuries are frequently associated with small amounts of posterior vertebral subluxation (2 to 3 mm). This has been commonly called "traumatic retrolisthesis." These injuries are of intermediate instability. This degree of retrolisthesis may be difficult to differentiate from degenerative retrolisthesis. MRI with fat suppression can clearly identify acute traumatic discoligamentous injuries in questionable cases. The treatment of traumatic retrolisthesis is based on the nature of neurologic involvement. Patients who are neurologically intact may be treated with a collar or cervicothoracic brace. (It should be noted that the height of the collar should not be excessive anteriorly, to avoid neck extension.) Patients with transient or persistent neurologic deficit should be placed in tong traction and undergo MRI.

If neural deficits do not resolve with traction, then anterior cervical diskectomy, bone graft, and plate fixation are warranted in an attempt to restore vertebral column height.

Hyperextension can result in significant posterior translation of the vertebral body and resulting spinal cord injury. Because of injuries to the longitudinal ligaments and disk annulus, in this situation cranial traction can be ineffective in achieving or maintaining reduction. Posterior element fractures at multiple levels are common and may be displaced into the spinal canal. These patients should be treated with cranial tong traction and rapid neuroimaging. Definitive treatment is best accomplished with anterior decompression and fusion with anterior plate fixation. Forsyth,[50] Harris,[55] and Allen[2] have identified extension fractures that result in 50% posterior vertebral body translation and bilateral facet dislocations that can occur from hyperextension injury mechanisms. Severe comminution of the posterior elements is often present. Because of the loss of all spinal stability, the posterior dislocation can reduce spontaneously and, with further head flexion, continue forward to simulate bilateral facet dislocation. Merianos documented similar cases associated with bilateral pedicular fractures.[72] In these injuries, it is difficult to reduce or maintain the reduction because of the separation of the anterior and posterior spinal columns.

Patients with severe traumatic retrolisthesis are difficult to manage. Traction should be attempted and, if successful, anterior decompression with interbody fusion with a plate should be performed. If reduction cannot be achieved or maintained, then an anterior approach is warranted, with reduction followed by fusion and anterior plate fixation. These patients may also require posterior fixation with lateral mass plates to achieve alignment and spinal stability. In the presence of displaced laminar fractures, laminectomy is indicated when neurologic deficits are present.

Burst Fractures

Burst-type fractures in the cervical spine have a similar appearance to those at the thoracolumbar junction. Their stability and treatment depends on the stability of the posterior elements. The injury often occurs at C6 and C7 and can be missed on initial x-rays if vertebral bodies C1 through T1 are not visualized. CT scans and MRI should be done to fully evaluate the posterior osseoligamentous structures. The initial treatment of all burst-type fractures is reduction with tong traction. In most cases, the anterior and posterior longitudinal ligaments are spared; thus, large traction weights and ligamentotaxis can be safely used to effect indirect decompression of the canal. As noted earlier, small serial increases in the weight, with intervening documented serial neurologic examinations and radiographic evaluation, is required when using this technique. Weights can be applied up to approximately 70% of body weight to achieve a successful reduction.[35, 97]

Definitive treatment is based on fracture stability and neurologic function. Patients with stable fractures that do not involve the posterior elements can be considered for treatment with halo vest immobilization for approximately 3 months. It must be noted that the halo vest cannot maintain axial distraction; thus some loss of reduction is inevitable, unfortunately including some retrolisthesis of bone into the canal.

Patients with unstable burst fractures and injury to the posterior osseoligamentous complex are best treated with surgical stabilization. Before the development of effective and safe anterior cervical plates, these patients were treated successfully with posterior wire fixation, with or without halo vest immobilization. Lateral mass plate fixation is biomechanically more effective than the posterior wiring techniques in controlling the axial forces. Anderson reported successful outcomes in 12 patients with unstable burst fractures and flexion teardrop fractures treated with posterolateral mass plates.[9] But we now recommend the anterior approach, using rigidly locked cervical plates (see Fig. 12–9). This technique allows a direct approach to and removal of the fractured vertebral body and displaced disks, excellent anterior decompression, and subsequent reconstruction with a strut graft and plate spanning the two injured motion segments. Others have recommended a combined anterior and posterior approach sequentially for these highly unstable fractures. We have found that this approach is rarely necessary because of the effectiveness of the anterior cervical plate stabilization.[25]

Cervical burst fractures in patients with neurologic injury should be treated with anterior decompression and fusion with the anterior cervical plates. Anterior decompression directly removes displaced bone and disk fragments, which may allow injured but viable neural tissues to recover.

Flexion Teardrop Fractures

The flexion teardrop fracture described by Schneider unfortunately is commonly associated with significant spinal cord injury and often occurs in young patients (see Fig. 12–10).[90] The injury is similar in stability to unstable burst fractures and is best treated surgically. We recommend an anterior approach with an anterior corpectomy, reconstruction with autologous tricortical iliac crest bone graft, and stabilization with an anterior cervical plate. In patients without neurologic deficits and with satisfactory alignment following traction, posterior fusion with lateral mass plates and wire fixation can be considered.

Anterior Decompression and Fusion

Near or just proximal to the site of spinal cord injury, intact neuronal tissue may be impaired by displaced bone or disk fragments, thus preventing the return of function. Anterior decompression removes these offending agents, not only improving function of the exiting anterior horn cell function and the exiting nerve root, but also relieving pressure on the axonal tracts in the white matter. Because most patients have compression from the ventral side of the cord, anterior decompression makes biomechanical sense and offers the best chance for full recovery. Other advantages of anterior decompression include the simplicity of the approach and positioning, avoidance of soft tissue and muscle stripping that occurs with the posterior approach, and the ability to restore anterior column height. An anterior approach may minimize the number of levels that must be fused if there is extensive comminution in the posterior elements. Bohlman reviewed 57 patients with incomplete motor quadriplegia treated by anterior decompression and fusion at least 1 month after injury.[20] Of these, 29 patients became ambulatory after the procedure, and another 6 exhibited significantly improved ambulatory status. Moreover, 39 patients had objective improvement in upper extremity function. In another study, 52 patients with complete motor quadriplegia were similarly treated with late anterior decompression, with the goal of restoring upper extremity function.[5] Of these patients, 60% showed functional improvement in the upper extremities after decompression, whereas only one patient became ambulatory. In both groups, only one patient deteriorated neurologically after the procedure. The results in both groups were significantly better if decompression was done within 1 year of the injury. Unfortunately, the efficacy of decompression in the first few days following the injury is unknown.

The primary disadvantage of anterior decompression is the loss of stability. This is caused by removal of the anterior longitudinal ligament and the residual disk annulus. Several authors have reported recurrent neurologic deficits after anterior decompression secondary to progressive instability.[49, 98] This is more likely in patients with a concomitant posterior osteoligamentous injury. In addition, patients with complete quadriplegia with impaired ventilation may develop respiratory compromise secondary to the inability to overcome retropharyngeal soft tissue swelling that can occur following anterior decompression. This occurred in 10% of patients in Anderson's series. To avoid respiratory complications, Anderson recommends maintaining quadriplegic patients who have undergone anterior decompression and fusion on mechanical ventilation for 2 to 3 days after surgery.[5]

Anterior decompression and fusion is indicated in patients with persistent neurologic deficits and residual anterior cord or root compression. Preoperatively, the patient should be evaluated by MRI. The timing of anterior decompression remains controversial, with no literature supporting either aggressive early treatment or delayed treatment. Prophylactic decompression to prevent later neurologic injury in patients with residual spinal compromise is rarely warranted. In cases of trauma, we routinely perform anterior plate fixation after anterior decompression and fusion.

COMPLICATIONS

The complications of lower cervical injuries are those primarily associated with the medical problems relating to spinal cord injury and to the loss of fracture reduction. Medical problems are especially common in patients with associated quadriparesis or quadriplegia, and include gastrointestinal hemorrhage, pulmonary insufficiency, deep venous thrombosis, urinary tract infection, and decubitus ulcers. Occult intra-abdominal injuries can occur in approximately 4% of patients with traumatic quadriplegia; thus peritoneal lavage is indicated if there is any suspicion of abdominal injury.[95] The multidisciplinary management of

these multiple medical problems is best performed in a center dedicated to the treatment of spinal cord injuries.[13, 19] Gastrointestinal hemorrhage occurs in up to 6% of patients with spinal cord injuries who are given steroids.[22] This adverse effect can be mitigated by careful monitoring and correction of gastric acidity with antacids and administration of histamine-2 blockers. Pulmonary insufficiency may result from pulmonary edema, atelectasis, or pneumonia, all of which are secondary to poor respiratory excursion and prolonged recumbence.[14] Early death from spinal cord injury is usually secondary to a pulmonary complication. Deep venous thrombosis occurs in approximately 25% of quadriplegic patients after acute injury. Rapid mobilization of the patient after spinal stabilization will minimize this risk and thus is a primary goal of surgical treatment.[65] Prophylactic measures, such as sequential pneumatic devices and/or subcutaneous heparin, are indicated. Urinary tract infections are also very common and are often secondary to the prolonged use of indwelling catheters. Intermittent catheterization is thus the preferred technique during the immediate postoperative period. Decubitus ulcers are less common with early spinal stabilization, which allows mobilization of the patient. Excellent nursing care at a spinal cord injury center, with frequent repositioning to prevent prolonged cutaneous pressure, will also minimize this complication.

Neurologic deterioration occurs in 1% to 5% of patients after spinal injury.[9, 31, 48] In only approximately 50% of these cases is the cause of deterioration preventable or attributable to physician actions. Common etiologies include fractures occurring in patients with ankylosed spines, missed diagnoses, loss of reduction during turning, or during placement of a halo device. Other causes, such as timing of surgery and intervertebral disk extrusion, have been discussed earlier. To minimize the risk of neurologic deterioration, all patients should undergo external brace stabilization until the cervical spine has been "cleared," including a minimum of three x-ray views (anteroposterior, lateral, and open mouth). Early reduction and stabilization are advisable, except in patients with minimal neurologic injury and associated facet dislocation, in whom disk status should be determined before reduction.

Stabilization with rigid fixation is especially important for patients with ankylosing spondylitis. Patients exhibiting deterioration should undergo immediate imaging with x-rays and MRI; if an operative lesion is detected, the patient should undergo prompt surgery to decompress the cord and stabilize the spinal column.

Hemodynamic instability commonly occurs after spinal cord injury because of interruption of descending sympathetic tracts, resulting in vasodilation and hypotension. Vagal predominance causes bradycardia, further lowering cardiac output. A low pulse rate is helpful in identifying the associated hypotension as occurring from spinal cord injury rather than from hypovolemic shock. This condition of neurogenic shock should be treated with vasopressors or other agents that increase peripheral vascular resistance, rather than with fluid resuscitation. The bradycardia may necessitate treatment with atropine or, rarely, a pacemaker. Because of loss of autoregulation, spinal cord blood flow to the injured region is determined solely by blood pressure. Therefore, rapid correction of hypotension is required to restore cord profusion.

CONCLUSION

Lower cervical spine injuries are often associated with significant morbidity and mortality. Improvements have been made in prehospital, emergency, and rehabilitative care, resulting in a better prognosis for patients. The initial care requires meticulous screening of all trauma patients for spinal injury. Once a lower cervical spine injury has been identified, other fractures need to be excluded. The fracture type should be determined by CT and/or MRI. Patients with stable fractures may be treated in an orthosis and carefully monitored until healing is documented. Patients with unstable patterns and those with spinal cord injury are placed in traction to accomplish urgent fracture reduction and neural decompression. An exception, as mentioned, is the neurologically intact patient with a bilateral facet dislocation, who should have MRI evaluation before attempts are made at reduction to rule out disk herniation. Spinal cord-injured patients treated within 8 hours of injury are given high-dose methylprednisolone, according to the NASCIS II protocol. Definitive treatment is based on fracture patterns, residual neurologic compression, and the level of neurologic function. The timing of surgery remains controversial. Early surgery in animal models appears to promote recovery. In clinical studies, early surgery appears to decrease the morbidity and mortality of recumbence but may increase the risk of neurologic deterioration.

Newer surgical techniques are now available that provide more rigid fixation from either anterior or posterior approaches and allow for more rapid patient mobilization. Successful implementation of these techniques requires careful assessment of the fracture pathomechanics as they relate to the patient's deficient biomechanical elements, a detailed understanding of the patient's individual anatomy, strict attention to surgical technique, and meticulous bone grafting. Finally, routine postoperative mobilization as an adjunct to plate fixation is advocated. All of these factors are necessary to achieving a successful surgical outcome.

REFERENCES

1. Abitbol JJ, Zdeblick T, Kunz D, et al: A biomechanical analysis of modern anterior and posterior cervical stabilization techniques. Presented at the Annual Meeting of the Cervical Spine Research Society, December 2–4, 1992, Palm Springs, CA.
2. Allen BL, Ferguson RL, Lehmann R, O'Brian RP: A mechanistic classification of closed indirect fractures and dislocations of the lower cervical spine. Spine 7:1–27, 1982.
3. An HS, Gordin R, Renner K: Anatomic considerations for plate-screw fixation of the cervical spine. Spine 16(suppl): S548–S551, 1991.
4. Anderson PA: Personal communication, September 1995.
5. Anderson PA, Bohlman HH: Anterior decompression and arthrodesis of the cervical spine: Long-term motor improve-
6. ment. Part II—Improvement in complete traumatic quadriplegia. J Bone Joint Surg Am 74A:683–692, 1992.
6. Anderson PA, Budorick TE, Easton KB, et al: Failure of halo vest to prevent in vivo motion in patients with injured cervical spines. Spine 16(suppl):S501–S505, 1991.
7. Anderson PA, Grady MS: Posterior stabilization of the lower cervical spine with lateral mass plates and screws. In Albert T, Smith M (eds): Operative Techniques in Orthopaedics. Philadelphia, WB Saunders, 1996.
8. Anderson PA, Henley MB: Progressive neurologic deficit in spinal injured patients at a level I trauma center. Orthop Trans 14:603, 1990.
9. Anderson PA, Henley MB, Grady MS, et al: Posterior cervical arthrodesis with AO reconstruction plates and bone graft. Spine 16(suppl):S72–S79, 1991.
10. Anderson PA, Krengel WF: Early vs. delayed stabilization after cervical spinal cord injury. Presented at the Federation of Spine Association Annual Specialty Day, San Francisco, February 21, 1993.
11. Assenmacher DR, Ducker TB: Experimental traumatic paraplegia. The vascular and pathological changes seen in reversible and irreversible spinal-cord lesions. J Bone Joint Surg Am 53A:671–680, 1971.
12. Beatson TR: Fractures and dislocations of the cervical spine. J Bone Joint Surg Br 45B:21–35, 1963.
13. Bedbrook G: The Care and Management of Spinal Cord Injuries. New York, Springer-Verlag, 1981.
14. Bellamy R, Pitts FW, Stauffer ES: Respiratory complications in traumatic quadriplegia. Analysis of 20 years' experience. J Neurosurg 39:596–600, 1973.
15. Berrington NR, van Staden JF, Willers JG, van der Westhuizen J: Cervical intervertebral disc prolapse associated with traumatic facet dislocations. Surg Neurol 40:395–399, 1993.
16. Beyer CA, Cabanela ME: Unilateral facet dislocations and fracture-dislocations of the cervical spine: A review. Orthopedics 15:311–315, 1992.
17. Blumberg KD, Catalano JB, Cotler JM, Balderston RA: The pullout strength of titanium alloy MRI-compatible and stainless steel MRI-incompatible Gardner-Wells tongs. Spine 18:1985–1986, 1993.
18. Bohlman HH: The triple-wire technique for posterior stabilization of fractures and dislocations of the lower cervical spine. In Sherk HH (ed): The Cervical Spine. An Atlas of Surgical Procedures, vol 9. Philadelphia, Lippincott, 1994, pp 145–150.
19. Bohlman HH: Acute fractures and dislocations of the cervical spine. An analysis of 300 hospitalized patients and review of the literature. J Bone Joint Surg Am 61A:1119–1142, 1979.
20. Bolhman HH, Anderson PA: Anterior decompression and arthrodesis of the cervical spine: Long-term motor improvement. Part I—Improvement in incomplete traumatic quadriparesis. J Bone Joint Surg Am 74A:671–682, 1992.
21. Bohlman HH, Bahniuk E, Raskulinecz G, Field G: Mechanical factors affecting recovery from incomplete spinal cord injury: A preliminary report. Johns Hopkins Med J 145:115–125, 1979.
22. Bracken MB, Collins WF, Freeman DF, et al: Efficacy of methylprednisolone in acute spinal cord injury. JAMA 251:45–52, 1984.
23. Bracken MB, Shepard MJ, Collins WF, et al: A randomized, controlled trial of methylprednisolone or naloxone in the treatment of acute spinal cord injury. Results of the Second National Acute Spinal Cord Injury Study. N Engl J Med 322:1405–1411, 1990.
23a. Bracken MB, Shepard MJ, Holford TR, et al: Administra-

tion of methylprednisolone for 24 or 48 hours or tirilazad mesylate for 48 hours in the treatment of acute spinal cord injury: Results of the Third National Acute Spinal Cord Injury Randomized Controlled Trial. JAMA 277:1597–1604, 1997.

24. Breig A: The therapeutic possibilities of surgical bioengineering in incomplete spinal cord lesions. Paraplegia 9:173–182, 1972.

25. Brodke DS, Anderson PA, Newell D, et al: Anterior versus posterior stabilization of cervical spine fractures in spinal cord-injured patients. Presented at the Annual Meeting of the Cervical Spine Research Society, 1995.

26. Bucholz RD, Cheung KC: Halo vest versus spinal fusion for cervical injury: Evidence from an outcome study. J Neurosurg 70:884–892, 1989.

27. Callahan RA, Johnson RM, Margolis RN, et al: Cervical facet fusion for control of instability following laminectomy. J Bone Joint Surg Am 59A:991–1002, 1977.

28. Chang DG, Tencer AF, Ching RP, et al: Geometric changes in the cervical spinal canal during impact. Spine 19:973–980, 1994.

29. Chapman JR, Anderson PA: Internal fixation techniques for the treatment of lower cervical spine injuries. J Orthop Trauma 1:205–219, 1991.

30. Coe JD, Warden KE, Sutterlin CE III, McAfee PC: Biomechanical evaluation of cervical spine stabilization methods in a human cadaveric model. Spine 14:1122–1131, 1989.

31. Colterjohn NR, Bednar DA: Identifiable risk factors for secondary neurological deterioration in the cervical spine-injured patient. Spine 20:2293–2297, 1995.

32. Cooper PR, Cohen A, Rosiello A, Koslow M: Posterior stabilization of cervical spine fractures and subluxations using plates and screws. J Neurosurg 23:300–306, 1988.

33. Cotler HB, Kulkarni MV, Bondurant FJ: Magnetic resonance imaging of acute spinal cord trauma: Preliminary report. J Orthop Trauma 2:1–4, 1988.

34. Cotler JM: Personal communication, Philadelphia, 1988.

35. Cotler JM, Herbison GJ, Nasuti JF, et al: Closed reduction of traumatic cervical spine dislocation using traction weights up to 140 pounds. Spine 18:386–390, 1993.

36. Crockard A: Evaluation of spinal laminar fixation by a new, flexible stainless steel cable (Sof'wire): Early results. Neurosurgery 35:892–898, 1994.

37. Davis AG: Fractures of the spine. J Bone Joint Surg 11:133–156, 1929.

38. Delamarter RB, Sherman J, Carr JB: Pathophysiology of spinal cord injury. Recovery after immediate and delayed decompression. J Bone Joint Surg Am 77A:1042–1049, 1995.

39. DeVivo MJ, Stover SL: Long-term survival and causes of death in spinal cord injury. *In* Stover SL, Delisa JA, Whiteneck GG (eds): Clinical Outcomes from the Model Systems. Gaithersburg, MD, Aspen, 1995, pp 289–316.

40. Ditunno JF, Cohen ME, Formal C, Whiteneck GG: Functional outcomes in spinal cord injury. In Stover SL, Delisa JA, Whiteneck GG (eds): Clinical Outcomes from the Model Systems. Gaithersburg, MD, Aspen, 1995, pp 170–184.

41. Dolan EJ, Tator CH, Endrenyi L: The value of decompression for acute experimental spinal cord compression injury. J Neurosurg 53:749–755, 1980.

42. Doran SE, Papadopoulos SM, Ducker TB, Lillehei KO: Magnetic resonance imaging documentation of coexistent traumatic locked facets of the cervical spine and disk herniation. J Neurosurg 79:341–345, 1993.

43. Ducker TB, Kindt GW, Kempe LG: Pathological findings in acute experimental spinal cord trauma. J Neurosurg 35:700–708, 1971.

44. Ducker TB, Salcman M, Daniell HB: Experimental spinal cord trauma III: Therapeutic effect of immobilization and pharmacologic agents. Surg Neurol 10:71–76, 1978.

45. Edwards CC, Matz SO, Levine AM: The oblique wiring technique for rotational injuries of the cervical spine. Orthop Trans 10:455, 1986.

46. Eismont FJ, Arena MJ, Green BA: Extrusion of an intervertebral disc associated with traumatic subluxation or dislocation of cervical facets. Case report. J Bone Joint Surg Am 73A:1555–1560, 1991.

47. Eismont FJ, Clifford S, Goldberg M, Green B: Cervical sagittal canal size in spine injury. Spine 8:663–666, 1984.

47a. Emery SE, Pathria MN, Wilber RG, et al: Magnetic resonance imaging of posttraumatic spinal ligament injury. Spine 2:229–233, 1989.

48. Farmer J, Vacarro A, Albert TJ, et al: Neurologic progression following cervical spinal cord injury. Orthop Trans 19:308, 1995.

49. Flynn TB: Neurologic complications of anterior cervical interbody fusion. Spine 7:536–539, 1982.

50. Forsyth HF: Extension injuries of the cervical spine. J Bone Joint Surg Am 46A:1792–1797, 1964.

51. Fuentes JM, Bloncourt J, Vlahovitch B, Castan P: Tear drop fractures. Contribution to the study of its mechanism and of osteo-disco-ligamentous lesions. Neurochirurgie 29:129–134, 1983.

52. Go BK, DeVivo MJ, Richards JS: The epidemiology of spinal cord injury in spinal cord injury. In Stover SL, Delisa JA, Whiteneck GG (eds): Clinical Outcomes from the Model Systems. Gaithersburg, MD, Aspen, 1995, pp 21–55.

53. Grady MS, Anderson PA: Cervical spine injuries: Management. Contemp Neurosurg 13:1–6, 1991.

54. Hadley MN, Fitzpatrick BC, Sonntag VKH, Browner CM: Facet fracture-dislocation injuries of the cervical spine. Neurosurgery 30:661–666, 1992.

55. Harris JH, Yeakley JW: Hyperextension-dislocation of the cervical spine. Ligament injuries demonstrated by magnetic resonance imaging. J Bone Joint Surg Br 74B:567–570, 1992.

56. Heller JG, Silcox DH III, Sutterlin CE III: Complications of posterior cervical plating. Spine 20:2442–2448, 1995.

57. Holdsworth F: Fractures, dislocations and fracture-dislocations of the spine. J Bone Joint Surg Am 52A:1534–1551, 1970.

58. Ikata T, Iwasa K, Morimoto K, et al: Clinical considerations and biomechanical basis of prognosis of cervical spinal cord injury. Spine 14:1096–1101, 1989.

59. Jacobs RR, Asher MA, Snider RK: Thoracolumbar spinal injuries. A comparative study of recumbent and operative treatment in 100 patients. Spine 5:463–477, 1980.

60. Janssen L, Hansebout RR: Pathogenesis of spinal cord injury and newer treatments: A review. Spine 14:23–32, 1989.

61. Kang JD, Figgie MP, Bohlman HH: Sagittal measurements of the cervical spine in subaxial fractures and dislocations. An analysis of 288 patients with and without neurological deficits. J Bone Joint Surg Am 76A:1617–1628, 1994.

62. Keenen TL, Antony J, Benson DR: Noncontiguous spinal fractures. J Trauma 30:489–491, 1990.

62a. Klein GR, Vaccaro AR, Albert TJ, et al: Efficacy of magnetic resonance imaging in the evaluation of posterior cervical spine fractures. Spine 24:771–774, 1999.

63. Lee AS, MacLean JC, Newton DA: Rapid traction for

reduction of cervical spine dislocations. J Bone Joint Surg Br 76B:352–356, 1994.

64. Levine AM: Facet injuries in the cervical spine. In Camins MB, O'Leary PF (eds): Disorders of the Cervical Spine. Baltimore, Williams & Wilkins, 1992, pp 293–302.

65. Levine AM, Edwards CC: Complications in the treatment of acute spinal injury. Orthop Clin North Am 17:183–203, 1986.

66. Levine AM, Mazel C, Roy-Camille R: Management of fracture separations of the articular mass using posterior cervical plating. Spine 17(suppl):S447–S454, 1992.

67. MacDonald RL, Schwartz ML, Mirich D, Sharkey PW, Nelson WR: Diagnosis of cervical spine injury in motor vehicle crash victims: How many radiographs are enough? J Trauma 30:392–397, 1990.

68. Mackersie RC, Shackford SR, Garfin SR, Hoyt DB: Major skeletal injuries in the obtunded blunt trauma patient: A case for routine radiologic survey. J Trauma 28:1450–1454, 1988.

69. Marar BC: Hyperextension injuries of the cervical spine. The pathogenesis of damage to the spinal cord. J Bone Joint Surg Am 56A:1655–1662, 1974.

70. Marshall LF, Knowlton S, Garfin SR, et al: Deterioration following spinal cord injury: A multicenter study. J Neurosurg 66:400–404, 1987.

70a. Matar LD, Helms CA, Richardson WJ: "Spinolaminar breach": An important sign in cervical spinous process fractures. Skeletal Radiol 29:75–80, 2000.

71. Mazur JM, Stauffer ES: Unrecognized spinal instability associated with seemingly "simple" cervical compression fractures. Spine 8:687–692, 1983.

72. Merianos P, Manousidis D, Samsonas P, et al: Injuries of the lower cervical spine associated with widening of the spinal canal. Injury 25:645–648, 1994.

73. Merriam WF, Taylor TKF, Ruff SJ, McPhail MJ: A reappraisal of acute traumatic central cord syndrome. J Bone Joint Surg Br 68B:708–713, 1986.

74. Mirza S, Moquin R, Anderson PA, et al: Stabilizing properties of the halo vest. Orthop Trans 18:697, 1994.

75. Nicoll EA: Fractures of the dorso-lumbar spine. J Bone Joint Surg Br 31B:376–394, 1949.

76. Panjabi MM, Duranceau J, Goel V, et al: Cervical human vertebrae: Quantitative three-dimensional anatomy of the middle and lower regions. Spine 16:861–869, 1991.

77. Reid DC, Henderson R, Saboe L, Miller JD: Etiology and clinical course of missed spine fractures. J Trauma 27:980–986, 1987.

78. Rivlin AS, Tator CH: Effect of duration of acute spinal cord compression in a new acute cord injury model in the rat. Surg Neurol 10:38–43, 1978.

79. Rizzolo SJ, Piazza MR, Cotler JM, et al: Intervertebral disc injury complicating cervical spine trauma. Spine 16(suppl): S187–S189, 1991.

80. Roaf R: A study of the mechanics of spinal injury. J Bone Joint Surg Br 42B:810–823, 1960.

81. Robertson PA, Ryan MD: Neurologic deterioration after reduction of cervical subluxation: Mechanical compression by disc tissue. J Bone Joint Surg Br 74B:224–227, 1992.

82. Robinson RA, Southwick WO: Indications and techniques for early stabilization of the neck in some fracture dislocations of the cervical spine. South Med J 53:565–579, 1960.

83. Rogers WA: Fracture and dislocations of the cervical spine. An end result study. J Bone Joint Surg Am 39A:341–376, 1957.

84. Rorabeck CH, Rock MG, Hawkins RJ, Bourne RB: Unilateral facet dislocation of the cervical spine: An analysis of the results of treatment in 26 patients. Spine 12:23–27, 1987.

85. Ross SE, Schwab CW, David ET, et al: Clearing the cervical spine: Initial radiologic evaluation. J Trauma 27:1055–1060, 1987.

86. Roy-Camille R, Saillant G, Laville C, Benazet JP: Treatment of lower cervical spinal injuries: C3 to C7. Spine 17(suppl):S442–S446, 1992.

87. Schaefer DM, Flanders A, Northrup BE, et al: Magnetic resonance imaging of acute cervical spine trauma: Correlation with severity of neurologic injury. Spine 14:1090–1095, 1989.

88. Schlegel J, Bayley J, Yuan H, Fredericksen B: Timing of surgical decompression and fixation of acute spinal fractures. J Orthop Trauma 10:323–330, 1996.

89. Schneider RC, Crosby EC, Russo RH, Gosch HH: Traumatic spinal cord syndromes and their management (Chapter 32). Clin Neurosurg 20:424–492, 1973.

90. Schneider RC, Knighton R: Chronic neurological sequelae of acute trauma to the spine and spinal cord, the syndrome of chronic injury to the cervical spinal cord in the region of the central canal. J Bone Joint Surg Am 41A:905–919, 1959.

91. Sears W, Fazl M: Prediction of stability of cervical spine fracture managed in the halo vest and indications for surgical intervention. J Neurosurg 72:426–432, 1990.

91a. Shapiro S, Snyder W, Kaufman K, Abel T: Outcome of 51 cases of unilateral locked cervical facets: Interspinous braided cable for lateral mass plate fusion compared with interspinous wire and facet wiring with iliac crest. J Neurosurg 91(suppl):S19–S24, 1999.

92. Shono Y, McAfee PC, Cunningham BW: The pathomechanics of compression injuries in the cervical spine. Nondestructive and destructive investigative methods. Spine 18:2009–2019, 1993.

93. Slucky AV, Eismont FJ: Treatment of acute injury of the cervical spine. Instr Course Lect 44:67–80, 1995.

94. Smith MD, Emery SE, Dudley A, et al: Vertebral artery injury during anterior decompression of the cervical spine. A retrospective review of 10 patients. J Bone Joint Surg Br 75B:410–415, 1993.

95. Soderstrom CA, McArdle DQ, Ducker TB, Militello PR: The diagnosis of intra-abdominal injury in patients with cervical cord trauma. J Trauma 23:1061–1065, 1983.

96. Songer MN, Spencer DL, Meyer PR, Jayaraman G: The use of sublaminar cables to replace Luque wires. Spine 16(suppl): S418–S421, 1991.

97. Star AM, Jones AAM, Cotler JM, et al: Immediate closed reduction of cervical spine dislocations using traction. Spine 15:1068–1072, 1990.

98. Stauffer ES, Kelly EF: Fracture-dislocations of the cervical spine: Instability and recurrent deformity following treatment by anterior interbody fusion. J Bone Joint Surg Am 59A:45–48, 1977.

99. Sutterlin CE III, McAfee PC, Warden KE, et al: A biomechanical evaluation of cervical spinal stabilization methods in a bovine model. Static and cyclical loading. Spine 13:795–802, 1988.

99a. Tan E, Schweitzer ME, Vaccaro L, Spetell AC: Is computed tomography of nonvisualized C7-T1 cost-effective? J Spinal Disord 12:472–476, 1999.

100. Taylor AR, Blackwood W: Paraplegia in hyperextension cervical injuries with normal radiographic appearances. J Bone Joint Surg Br 30B:245–248, 1948.

101. Torg JS, Pavlov H, Genuario SE, et al: Neurapraxia of the cervical spinal cord with transient quadriplegia. J Bone Joint Surg Am 68A:1354–1370, 1986.

102. Torg JS, Sennett B, Vegso JJ, Pavlov H: Axial loading injuries to the middle cervical spine segment. An analysis and classification of 25 cases. Am J Sports Med 19:6–20, 1991.

103. Tribus CB: Cervical disk herniation in association with traumatic facet dislocation. Tech Orthop 9:5–7, 1994.

104. Ulrich C, Wörsdörfer O, Claes L, Magerl F: Comparative study of the stability of anterior and posterior cervical spine fixation procedures. Arch Orthop Trauma Surg 106:226–231, 1987.

105. Waters RL, Yoshida GM: Prognosis of spinal cord injuries. In Levine AM (ed): Orthopaedic Knowledge Update: Trauma. Rosemont, IL, American Academy of Orthopaedic Surgery, 1996, pp 303–310.

106. Webb JK, Broughton RB, McSweeney T, Park WM: Hidden flexion injury of the cervical spine. J Bone Joint Surg Br 58B:322–337, 1976.

107. Weiland DJ, McAfee PC: Posterior cervical fusion with triple wire strut graft technique: 100 consecutive patients. J Spine Disord 4:15–21, 1991.

108. White AA III, Panjabi MM: The problem of clinical instability in the human spine: A systematic approach. In White AA, Panjabi MM (eds): Clinical Biomechanics of the Spine, 2nd ed. Philadelphia, JB Lippincott, 1990, pp 277–378.

109. Whitehill R, Richman JA, Glaser JA: Failure of immobilization of the cervical spine by the halo vest. A report of five cases. J Bone Joint Surg Am 68A:326–332, 1986.

110. Willis BK, Greiner F, Orrison WW, Benzel Executive Committee: The incidence of vertebral artery injury after midcervical spine fracture or subluxation. Neurosurgery 34:435–442, 1994.

111. Yashon D: Pathogenesis of spinal cord injury. Orthop Clin North Am 9:247–261, 1978.

112. Young W: Secondary injury mechanisms in acute spinal cord injury. J Emerg Med 11:13–22, 1993.

Neoplasms of the Cervical Spine

13

PRIMARY AND METASTATIC BONE TUMORS OF THE CERVICAL SPINE

Sanford E. Emery, M.D.

*Be kind, for everyone you meet is fighting
a harder battle.*
— Plato

HISTORICAL PERSPECTIVE

The identification of tumors in the spine dates back to the Incas and Egyptian mummies with examples of disseminated neoplasms.[74, 80] Literature on metastatic tumors of the spine was based largely on autopsy studies in much of the early 20th century.[35, 58, 72] Information regarding primary tumors of the spine was limited because of the relatively low incidence of cases. A milestone in data collection of bone tumors in the United States was the establishment in 1922 of the Bone Sarcoma Registry of the American College of Surgeons. With Ernest Codman of Boston as its first director, this organization initiated the concept of pooling data on rare bone tumors that ultimately helped clarify diagnostic classification and treatment of these disorders.

GENERAL PRINCIPLES

Spinal tumors often present a formidable challenge for the surgeon, requiring thorough medical evaluation and preoperative planning as well as compassion for the patient and family. This area of spine surgery is anything but routine and demands application of biological and biomechanical principles on a case-by-case basis. Like patients with other musculoskeletal tumors, these patients usually require a multidisciplinary approach of surgeon, medical oncologist, radiation oncologist, and often the neuroradiologist to coordinate and optimize the treatment plan.[79]

PATHOPHYSIOLOGY

Primary tumors of bone can be found in the anterior or posterior elements, with certain predilection depending on the tumor type. Metastatic disease typically finds red marrow and thus is most common in the vertebral body. This can result in anterior spinal cord compression from direct tumor extension into the canal or from a pathologic fracture of the body. Tumor extension into the epidural space without fracture usually causes slow, chronic compression and is thus better tolerated by the spinal cord. Rapid onset of pain and paralysis may herald a pathologic fracture causing cord compression from tumor and/or bone fragments. The location of the lesion and its effect on the spinal canal play major roles in determining the surgical treatment of either benign or malignant cervical tumors.

CLINICAL PRESENTATION

Patients with tumors of the cervical spine usually present with neck pain regardless of the patient's age. Bone lesions typically produce axial pain, but root compression may cause radicular symptoms of pain, weakness, and/or sensory changes. Spinal cord compression may result from direct tumor spread into the canal or from a pathologic fracture with canal encroachment, as mentioned earlier. Depending on the severity of cord compression, weakness, numbness, or full-blown paralysis with sphincter dysfunction may be present.

DIAGNOSTIC EVALUATION

Though not usually diagnostic, plain x-rays should be obtained in these patients, looking for signs of bone destruction (or formation) as well as evidence of fracture, deformity, or instability. Magnetic resonance imaging (MRI) is usually the next radiologic procedure of choice, with the ability to image bone, disc, paraspinal soft tissue, and the spinal cord.[60] If better bony detail is needed, such as to evaluate the status of posterior element involvement, then computed tomography (CT) scanning provides additional information. Bone scans may help diagnose an osteoid osteoma or determine the spread of bony metastatic disease. Myelography and CT-myelography can also sometimes provide information not well visualized on MRI, such as root impingement or facet destruction. Angiography should be considered for localization of the vertebral arteries in selected cases; this allows for embolization of large tumors with predilection for brisk hemorrhage, such as metastatic renal cell carcinoma.

Laboratory investigation should not be forgotten in the workup of these patients. Routine complete blood count and chemistries, plus erythrocyte sedimentation rate and serum protein electrophoresis (SPEP), may lead to a specific diagnosis (e.g., myeloma) and directly affect the workup algorithm.

For most patients, tissue diagnosis is needed. If a needle biopsy is considered technically feasible, it should be done by an experienced radiologist or surgeon because of the adjacent structures at risk. In the absence of impending instability or neurologic deficit, a diagnostic biopsy may result in nonoperative treatment, such as radiation for a malignancy or antibiotics for vertebral osteomyelitis, thus avoiding an open procedure.

SURGICAL INDICATIONS

There are four main indications for surgical intervention in patients with bony neoplasms of the cervical spine:

1. Neurologic deficit
2. Instability (or impending pathologic fracture)
3. Pain unresponsive to nonoperative measures such as radiation or chemotherapy
4. Need for tissue diagnosis

One or all of these indications may be present. Some patients do not fit neatly into this list but, as stated earlier, require individualized, thoughtful recommendations by the spinal surgeon. Other factors that enter into the decision and/or timing of surgery include the tumor type (e.g., radiosensitive, such as myeloma), the patient's ability to tolerate general anesthesia, the rapidity of onset of paralysis (i.e., the slower the onset, the better the chance for recovery), or the need for embolization to help control

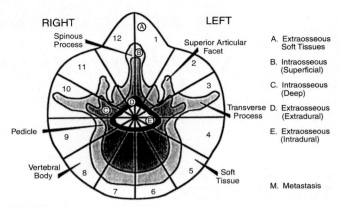

Figure 13–1. *The WBB (Weinstein, Boriani, Biagini) surgical staging system. The transverse extension of the vertebral tumor is described with reference to 12 radiating zones (numbered 1 to 12 in a clockwise order) and to 5 concentric layers (A to E), from the paravertebral extraosseous compartments to the dural involvement. The longitudinal extent of the tumor is recorded according to the levels involved. (From Boriani S, Weinstein JN, Biagini R: Primary bone tumors of the spine—Terminology and surgical staging. Spine 22:1036–1044, 1997.)*

intraoperative bleeding. High-dose steroid therapy can be helpful in the setting of early or impending neurologic compromise to allow some time for preoperative planning. Steroids are also recommended in patients with substantial spinal cord compression receiving radiation treatments, to help prevent the local swelling effects of irradiation that could tip the scales toward neural deficit.

PREOPERATIVE PLANNING

Once the decision to operate and timing of surgery are determined, preoperative planning is of paramount importance. The entire pathoanatomy must be considered in the context of the goals of the operation, usually decompression and stabilization. The location of the tumor, number of levels involved, direction of cord compression, and degree of bone destruction help determine whether an anterior, posterior, or combined approach is best.[4a, 22, 44] Metastatic tumors typically involve the vertebral body; if the posterior elements are intact, then anterior decompression and stabilization are indicated. Patients with metastatic disease causing instability without significant anterior involvement may need a posterior fusion followed by radiation therapy to aid local control.

The anatomy of the cervical spine makes it difficult to apply Enneking's staging classification[17, 18] for bone neoplasms. Prognostically, extension of tumor external to the canal may be very different than tumor in the canal, although both are considered to be extracompartmental spread. Similarly, descriptions of surgical margins such as wide or radical take on new consequences for the spine, given the location of the spinal cord and vertebral arteries. En bloc excision of cervical tumors has been described recently by Fujita and colleagues using Tomita's T-saw technique and ligation of one vertebral artery.[23a]

Boriani, Hart, and Weinstein have developed a clock-face–like model for classification of tumors based on location in the spine[7, 32] (Fig. 13–1). This model takes into account the location of the pathology from an anteroposterior or lateral direction, as well as with respect to the depth of penetration toward the spinal canal. Boriani used this as a guide to preoperative planning.[4a] Efforts such as this may help spine surgeons and oncologists communicate to optimize treatment strategies for patients in the future.

PRIMARY BENIGN CERVICAL TUMORS OF BONE

Osteochondroma

Osteochondroma is the most common benign tumor in the spine. Like most benign tumors, it is usually located in the posterior elements and occurs in younger patients.[25] Presenting symptoms are typically pain, but neurologic manifestations may occur because the underlying root or cord may be compressed by a large osteochondroma.[11, 13, 37, 49, 52, 56a] Often plain films will suggest the lesion, with CT scans providing the best anatomic detail (Fig. 13–2). MRI or CT-myelography may be needed to evaluate neural compression, and magnetic resonance angiography (MRA) can help locate the vertebral artery if necessary. Surgical excision is the treatment of choice for symptomatic lesions, usually involving an intralesional or marginal removal with a low recurrence rate. A posterior, anterior, or combined approach may be needed depending on the exact pathoanatomy. Fusion is commonly but not always indicated, again depending on the pathoanatomy and requirements for excision.[4] Malignant

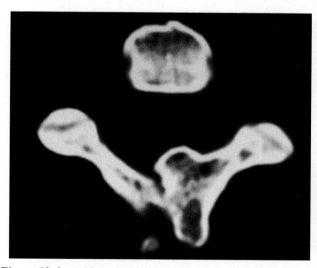

Figure 13–2. *A 15-year-old female with a history of multiple hereditary exostoses had an acute episode of neck pain without any trauma. Plain films suggested a lesion of the posterior elements of C6. This cross-sectional CT scan shows an osteochondroma at the junction of the lamina and spinous process of C6. There is no cord compression or instability. Her symptoms resolved with conservative measures, and thus no surgery was indicated.*

transformation to chondrosarcoma is believed to occur in 1% of patients with solitary osteochondromas and 1% to 25% of tumors in patients with hereditary multiple exostoses.[82a] In these patients, observation rather than prophylactic excision of osteochondromas of the spine seems prudent given the rarity of the problem and the lack of data specific to the spine.

Osteoblastoma and Osteoid Osteoma

Osteoblastomas of the spine constitute 10% to 20% of benign cervical spine tumors. Patients are usually under age 30, and there is a male:female ratio of 2:1.[26, 43] These lesions usually originate in the posterior elements, though they have been reported in the odontoid.[49a] Their locally aggressive, expansile behavior can lead to large lesions and ultimately spinal canal compromise with neural compression. The radiographic appearance is variable, ranging from lytic to blastic depending on the degree of mineralization. Histology demonstrates active osteoid formation with varying degrees of ossification, a fibrovascular stroma, and, in many cases, giant cells. A rim of reactive bone is usually present, but not to the degree of osteoid osteomas.

The treatment for osteoblastomas of the cervical spine is surgical excision. Wide or marginal resection is preferable to prevent recurrence,[5, 24, 77] but even intralesional curettage is successful in most cases.[43] Radiation treatment is controversial and has not been found to change the outcome;[43] thus its use is usually reserved for tumors that continue to grow or have recurred and are unresectable.[2a, 5]

Osteoid osteomas have a similar histologic appearance as osteoblastomas, and so are often considered a smaller manifestation of the same tumor. Typically these lesions cause pain that is responsive to salicylate treatment.[27, 36] Torticollis and occasionally scoliosis have been noted in osteoid osteomas of the cervical spine.[21, 56, 58a] A central nidus is the radiographic hallmark, which in the spine usually is detectable only on CT scans. Bone scans are also helpful as an initial screening test to help localize the lesion (Fig. 13–3). Reactive new bone formation surrounding the nidus is more evident in osteoid osteomas than in osteoblastomas. In long bones, data suggest that long-term anti-inflammatory medication therapy may be used to treat symptoms, with ultimate "healing" of the lesion.[40] To my knowledge, no data are available on this treatment for spine lesions. If symptoms are mild and no neural structures are threatened, then symptomatic treatment with observation seems reasonable. Pain may dictate surgical resection, which must include the nidus for symptom relief.

The need for surgical reconstruction after excision of osteoblastomas or osteoid osteomas depends on the location of the lesion and the amount of bone resected. A simple laminectomy may be all that is required for excision, with fusion unnecessary.[21, 36] Lesions involving the facet, pedicle, or the anterior structures require more extensive resection[34] (see Fig. 13–3). Posterior fusion alone or a combined anterior/posterior approach may be needed for successful removal and stabilization.[27]

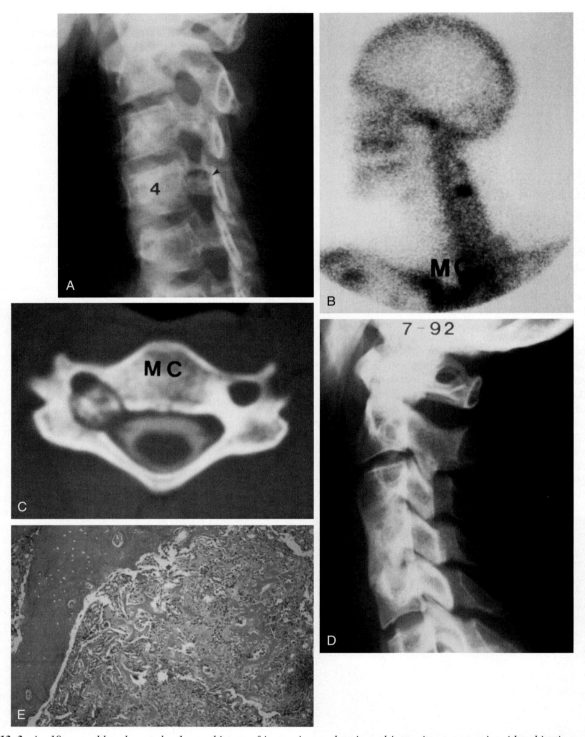

Figure 13–3. *An 18-year-old male noted a 1-year history of increasing neck pain and intermittent arm pain with subjective weakness. A, An oblique plain film shows an abnormality in the pedicle of C4. B, A bone scan shows increased uptake in the same location. C, A CT myeloaxial image demonstrates the right C4 pedicle lesion, suggestive of a nidus. D, An anterolateral resection and iliac crest fusion were performed. E, Histology revealed a nidus with hypercellularity and osteoid formation consistent with osteoid osteoma.*

Hemangiomas

Hemangiomas are a common finding in the spinal column, occurring in up to 10% of the population. These lesions are located in the vertebral body and are usually, although not always, asymptomatic.[23, 45] The diagnosis can usually be made by CT scan demonstrating the stippled pattern on cross-sectional imaging. If the anterior column is weakened, then trauma can cause a pathologic fracture with resultant pain and/or neurologic deficit. If this occurs, the patient most likely will need anterior decompression and strut fusion for stabilization. A study of intralesional injection of ethanol demonstrated good results for a small series of thoracic and lumbar symptomatic hemangiomas.[13b]

Aneurysmal Bone Cysts

This lesion is an expansile, benign tumor characterized by multiloculated, blood-filled cysts without an endothelial lining of the cavities. They typically occur in young people, with the highest incidence in the second decade of life.[12] The vast majority of aneurysmal bone cysts arise from the posterior elements, although local spread into the vertebral body is not uncommon. The differential diagnosis includes giant cell tumor, osteoblastoma, simple bone cysts, and osteogenic sarcoma. Other primary bone tumors, such as osteoblastomas and osteosarcomas, have been found within an aneurysmal bone cyst.[41] Treatment of these lesions is resection with stabilization if needed, depending on the amount and location of bony resection.[9, 10, 29, 51a, 54, 70, 73a] Wide resection is the treatment of choice in long bones and has been described for thoracic and lumbar lesions.[20, 68, 73] The regional anatomy of the cervical spine, particularly the vertebral arteries, make en bloc vertebrectomy problematic.[23a] Curettage or marginal excision is usually successful for aneurysmal bone cysts, however.[13a, 52a] Adjunct radiation is generally recommended only for recurrent lesions because of the risk of radiation-induced sarcomas. Preoperative embolization can be used to decrease surgical blood loss, although this must be done with caution around the cord. Percutaneous embolization with an alcoholic solution of zein (Ethiblok, Ethnor Laboratories/Ethicon, Norderstedt, Germany) has been described as definitive treatment in a series of 18 patients with aneurysmal bone cysts, 2 cases of which were in the cervical spine.[28a] Another case report described successful treatment of an aneurysmal bone cyst of the first cervical vertebrae with two percutaneous intralesional injections of calcitonin and methylprednisolone.[26a]

Giant Cell Tumors

Giant cell tumors in the cervical spine can be problematic because they are locally aggressive and tend to recur with incomplete excision.[31, 64] This entity is considered a benign tumor, but metastatic potential has been demonstrated in rare cases.[19, 76] They are lytic in appearance, and because of significant bone destruction, a pathologic fracture with neurologic sequelae can occur. Most cases involve the vertebral body or both anterior and posterior structures, although posterior element tumors have been described.[59] Complete excision results in a lower recurrence rate,[31] but en bloc spondylectomy in the cervical spine is difficult because of the local anatomy. Surgical treatment needs to address any cord or root compression as well as stability, and may require both anterior and posterior reconstruction (Fig. 13–4). Radiation has been used primarily in conjunction with excision,[38a] but because of the risk of radiation-induced sarcoma, most authors reserve radiotherapy for incompletely resected or recurrent tumors. One case report described the use of cryosurgery and irradiation for a large lesion of C2.[47]

Eosinophilic Granuloma (Langerhans Cell Histiocytosis)

This lesion is found primarily in children either as an isolated lesion of the vertebral body or as part of the systemic syndromes Hand-Schüller-Christian disease and Letterer-Siwe disease. It most commonly affects persons over age 21.[34b] Patients may present after vertebral collapse (vertebra plana), which sometimes produces neurologic symptoms.[28] Eosinophilic granuloma is generally a self-limiting disease, and in most children the height of the vertebral body will reconstitute slowly over time.[54a, 82b] Needle biopsy may be needed to rule out the other two conditions in the differential diagnosis, vertebral osteomyelitis or Ewing's sarcoma, but many patients with a typical presentation may be observed. Minor neurologic compromise from a pathologic fracture or soft tissue extension[28] may be successfully treated with irradiation and bracing. Major deficit or instability requires an anterior approach with decompression and arthrodesis.[62]

PRIMARY MALIGNANT CERVICAL TUMORS OF BONE
Plasmacytoma/Multiple Myeloma

The most common malignancy of the osseous skeleton in adults is multiple myeloma, and most spine surgeons in their career will need to surgically treat patients with axial disease. The typical age range is 40 to 70, but the disease should be considered in the differential diagnosis for anyone over 20. Solitary plasmacytoma is believed to be an early form of the disseminated disease, because nearly all patients with a solitary lesion ultimately develop myeloma.[81] The prognosis for solitary plasmacytoma is more favorable, however, with a 5-year survival of 60%.[46] Once multiple myeloma with spinal involvement was manifested, the 4-year survival was 0% in Valderrama and Bullough's study.[75] One report suggests that MRI of the entire spine in early myeloma may detect abnormal marrow changes that portend a more rapid progression of the disease.[42a]

Plasmacytoma or multiple myeloma usually involves the vertebral body, although both the anterior and posterior column can be involved in advanced cases. The radiographic pattern is lytic, and the lesion may be cold on bone scan. Because the tumor is radiosensitive, the mainstay of treatment is radiation therapy. Chemotherapy and bone

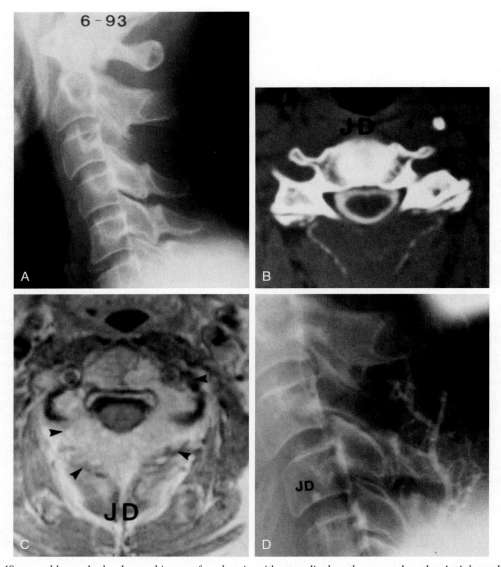

Figure 13–4. *A 48-year-old man had a 1-year history of neck pain without radiculopathy or myelopathy. A, A lateral plain film demonstrates missing posterior elements of C3. B, A CT myeloaxial image shows replacement of the C3 lamina without neural compression. C, MRI shows not only the posterior element involvement, but also the tumor within the pedicle and left side of the vertebral body, surrounding the vertebral artery. D, Arteriography was performed, and a large ascending feeder vessel was embolized.*

marrow transplantation are generally used in patients who have developed multiple myeloma. Particularly in the cervical spine, however, significant bone destruction or pathologic fracture may warrant surgical intervention in addition to medical management. Anterior decompression is usually indicated, followed by strut graft stabilization and internal fixation (Fig. 13–5). Surgical resection is typically intralesional by necessity, and adjuvant radiation is needed. Delaying irradiation for approximately 4 weeks is recommended, if possible, to achieve a higher rate of graft incorporation.[15, 69] Because these patients (particularly those with plasmacytomas) have an extended disease-free period, I prefer to use osseous grafts rather than spacers, such as polymethylmethacrylate (PMMA) for anterior support.

Chordoma

This malignancy arises from remnant notochord elements in the spine and often occurs in the sacrococcygeal or suboccipital regions.[50] The tumors are slow growing but commonly recur locally and metastasize. The ultimate prognosis is very poor, with only 28% survival at 10 years for all areas of the spine.[6, 61] Chordoma usually occurs in adults, particularly elderly men, and is the second most common primary malignancy of the spine after plasmacytomas.

The radiographic pattern is generally lytic with scattered calcifications. A large soft tissue mass is usually evident on further diagnostic imaging.[80a] Spinal cord compression commonly occurs because of the slow growth, size, and late

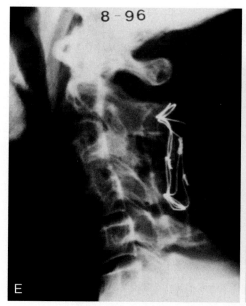
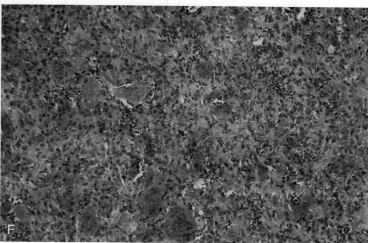

Figure 13–4 Continued. *E, This was approached posteriorly first, with resection followed by wiring and bone grafting. The patient was then turned over and an anterior resection of the vertebral body was followed by strut grafting. The patient remained neurologically intact and went on to a successful arthrodesis. F, Histology was consistent with a giant cell tumor of the C3 vertebra. He had no adjunct radiation. At 5-year follow-up he had no evidence of recurrence.*

presentation of these tumors. Because chordomas are relatively radioresistant and insensitive to chemotherapeutic agents, surgical excision is the treatment of choice. Intralesional excision, even combined with irradiation, is not effective for cure. Given the anatomy of the cervical spine, this is nearly always the only option open to the spine surgeon, although en bloc resection has been reported by Fujita and colleagues.[23a] Surgical efforts for cervical tumors are usually palliative but can improve the quality of life when treating cord compression or instability.[82] For these large tumors high in the cervical spine, an anterior/posterior resection and reconstruction are usually indicated.[41a] Adjuvant high-dose conventional radiation therapy or proton-beam treatments may prolong survival.[3, 42]

Osteosarcoma

Osteogenic sarcoma of the spine is a rare site for primary disease. These tumors can appear in almost any age group, although lesions arising from previously irradiated vertebrae[14] or from pagetoid bone will typically occur in the older population. Pain is the presenting symptom in virtually all patients, but the aggressive nature of the tumor often produces neurologic involvement as well. Radiographic presentation can be lytic or sclerotic, and is often a mixture of both. These tumors are usually in the vertebral body, but can be located in both the anterior and posterior elements or the posterior elements alone. Their lethal outcome warrants aggressive combined treatment modalities. Preoperative chemotherapy will yield a good tumor response in some patients. Aggressive surgical resection followed by radiation may improve the outlook,[38, 71] but the overall prognosis is still very poor.[48, 65] Unfortunately, in

the cervical spine en bloc excision of these large, expansile lesions is rarely an option.

Chondrosarcoma

Like osteosarcomas, chondrosarcomas are relatively rare in the cervical spine. These typically slow-growing lesions can become very large before symptoms occur. The tumors may arise de novo or from preexisting enchondromas or osteochondromas.[66, 82a] They may be found in the anterior elements, posterior elements, or both. Chondrosarcomas are notoriously resistant to radiation and chemotherapy. Surgical excision with wide margins offers the best chance for cure,[6a, 82c] but for anatomic reasons this is usually impossible in the cervical spine. Attempts at excision may require anterior, posterior, or combined approaches followed by the appropriate reconstruction. Radiation therapy is used as an adjunct for incomplete resection.[33] Proton-beam irradiation[34a] has more recently been used for these radioresistant tumors with some increase in survival rate.[3]

METASTATIC TUMORS OF THE CERVICAL SPINE

Metastatic disease is by far the most common type of spinal neoplasm presenting in the adult population. Treatment of these tumors is multidisciplinary and should focus on improving quality of life.[57] Five classic tumors often metastasize to bone: breast, prostate, lung, kidney, and thyroid. Typically metastatic deposits occur in the red marrow of the vertebral body rather than the posterior elements alone. Anterior lesions can result in bone

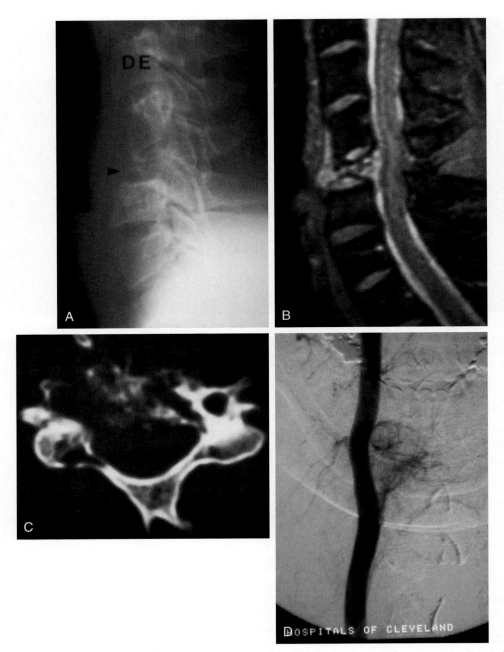

Figure 13–5. *A 36-year-old man presented with an acute onset of neck and right arm pain, with upper extremity weakness on physical examination. There was no known diagnosis. A, A lateral plain film shows a pathologic fracture of C5 with collapse. B, A sagittal MRI demonstrates increased signal intensity of C5 with collapse and mild canal encroachment. C, A transverse CT image shows anterior and some posterior involvement of a lytic process. D, An angiogram was performed to evaluate the path of the right vertebral artery through the lesion and possibly perform embolization. The tumor blush drained into the anterior spinal artery, so embolization was not performed due to the risk of causing cord ischemia.*

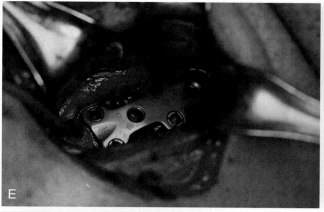

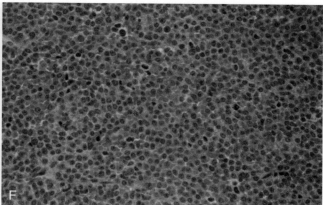

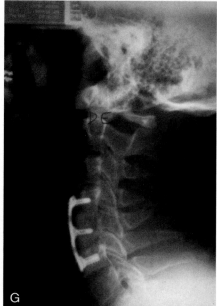

Figure 13–5 Continued. *E, The patient underwent open exploration where a biopsy and frozen section revealed plasma cells consistent with plasmacytoma. Subtotal vertebrectomy, anterior strut grafting with autogenous iliac crest, and anterior plating were performed. The vessel loop is around the vertebral artery below the level of the tumor, to establish control in case a different diagnosis had warranted a wider excision attempt. F, Histology of the specimen with multiple plasma cells. G, The patient was treated in a two-poster type brace and went on to successful arthrodesis, as shown in this lateral x-ray. He underwent perioperative radiation, chemotherapy, and later underwent bone marrow transplantation when he developed other sites indicative of multiple myeloma.*

destruction, pathologic fracture, kyphosis, and neural compression (Fig. 13–6).[67] Neurologic deficit can result from root impingement or frank cord compression. Compression can be from tumor mass, bone, or disk from a pathologic fracture. Kyphosis will cause the cord to drape over the anterior elements, or impingement may occur from subluxation because of instability. Combined anterior and posterior element involvement can occur and lead to a highly unstable cervical spine.

The decision regarding surgery or medical management of cervical spine metastases requires appropriate clinical and radiographic evaluation, plus judgment. Most patients with severe pain, neurologic compromise, or an unstable spine will obtain a better quality of life with operative intervention with an acceptable complication rate.[1a, 77a, 80b] Visible bone destruction on plain x-rays warrants earlier stabilization for cervical lesions compared with other regions of the spine that are inherently more stable, such as the thoracic spine. Harrington's description of five classes

of metastatic disease can be used as a guideline to surgical intervention.[30]

Class I: No significant neurologic involvement, no bone destruction

Class II: Some involvement of bone without collapse or instability

Class III: Major neurologic impairment without significant involvement of bone (e.g., epidural metastases alone)

Class IV: Vertebral collapse or instability with pain but no neurologic compromise

Class V: Vertebral collapse or instability with neurologic impairment

Generally, class I and II lesions are treated with systemic chemotherapy and local irradiation.[55] Temporary bracing with a collar may alleviate symptoms until the local tumor

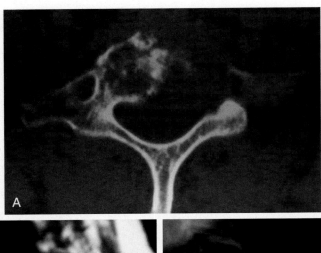

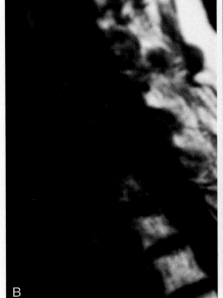

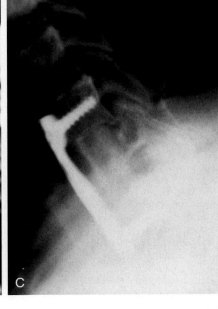

Figure 13–6. A 56-year-old woman with known metastatic breast carcinoma presented with a 1-month history of neck and left arm pain. She reported recent increased pain and demonstrable left arm weakness. A, A cross-sectional CT image shows lytic changes in the C7 vertebral body and pedicle. B, A sagittal MRI shows the pathologic fracture of C7 with mild cord compression. C, A lateral plain film taken after the patient underwent an anterior C7 corpectomy, fibula strut grafting, and anterior plating. She recovered her motor deficits and healed her graft, but succumbed to widespread metastatic disease approximately 1 year postoperatively.

is under control. Class III disease may require urgent decompression, unless the tumor type is very radiosensitive, such as lymphoma or multiple myeloma. Patients with class IV and V disease need decompression and/or stabilization procedures to prevent or treat spinal cord injury.[34c, 57a] Percutaneous vertebroplasty with injection of polymethylmethacrylate into vertebral bodies with metastases has been reported by Weill and colleagues.[78] These authors used this technique for painful metastatic segments or for impending fracture and had eight patients in their series with cervical lesions.

Special Considerations

With the exception of multiple myeloma and lymphoma, most metastatic tumors are of intermediate or low sensitivity to radiation. This means that for most tumors, progression may be slowed before cord impingement, but if epidural extension is already substantial, then radiation cannot be expected to melt the disease away. Renal cell carcinoma is known to be a highly vascular tumor, and preoperative embolization is generally recommended to cut

down on blood loss.[39] Tumor type is also important when attempting to predict the patient's life span. Breast and prostate carcinoma can be quite indolent. In these patients, I prefer bony arthrodesis rather than methylmethacrylate for reconstructive procedures. In more aggressive tumors, such as adenocarcinoma of the lung, a shorter life span may warrant using an anterior spacer such as PMMA rather than waiting for grafts to heal.[63]

The timing of perioperative irradiation has been a puzzle for spine surgeons and radiation oncologists. Early radiation for tumor control is often in direct conflict with optimization of bone graft healing. Radiation is known to be detrimental to both fracture healing and anterior strut graft incorporation.[16] Emery and colleagues[8] and Bouchard and colleagues[15] used a canine and rabbit model respectively for anterior graft healing and posterior graft healing in the face of irradiation. Delaying irradiation for 3 weeks postoperatively significantly improved the arthrodesis rate in these animal models. For patients with anterior strut grafts or posterior corticocancellous grafts, I prefer to wait at least 4 weeks, if possible, before beginning postoperative irradiation.

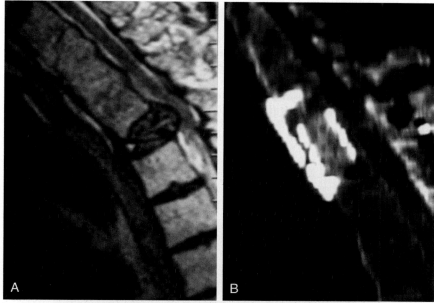

Figure 13–7. A 63-year-old man had a history of metastatic renal cell carcinoma for 8 years. He developed lower neck pain and slowly progressive paraparesis. A sagittal MRI (A) shows a pathologic fracture of T1 with frank cord compression. Note the three-level anterior fusion done years earlier to treat degenerative disease. He was treated with an anterior corpectomy of T1 through a low transverse neck incision, strut grafting with a titanium cage packed with allograft, anterior plating, and supplemented with posterior instrumentation and fusion from C4 to T3. A postoperative sagittal CT scan (B) and cross-section (C) demonstrates the anterior cage, anterior plate, and posterior instrumentation. Maximal stabilization is usually needed at the cervicothoracic junction due to the biomechanical forces involved.

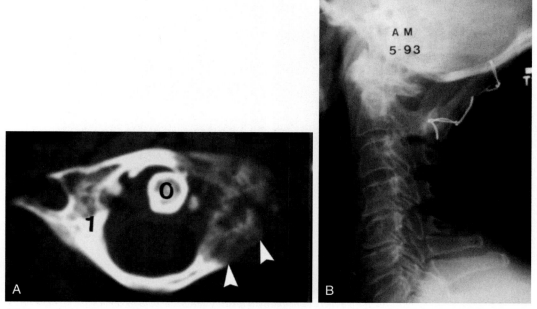

Figure 13–8. This transverse CT scan (A) shows destruction of the lateral mass of C1 from metastatic prostate carcinoma without cord compression. The patient had undergone radiotherapy but still had significant neck pain requiring constant use of a cervical collar. He underwent posterior occipitocervical fusion with autogenous iliac crest bone graft and wiring. He went on to a solid union (B) with resolution of his neck pain. Disease progression was controlled with hormonal therapy.

SURGICAL TECHNIQUES

Surgical treatment of many primary and most metastatic tumors of the cervical spine requires at least an anterior approach. The goal of this approach is to provide decompression of the canal and anterior stabilization. A single- or multilevel corpectomy is typically performed, as described in Chapter 4. Vertebral artery control may be prudent (see Figure 13–5) if the tumor is lateral and must be excised as completely as possible. Strut grafting can be done with autograft (ilium or fibula),[22] allograft fibula, PMMA,[2, 63] ceramics,[51] or titanium cage spacers (Fig. 13–7).[1c] I prefer true arthrodesis with autogenous bone grafts for patients with a projected life span of more than 6

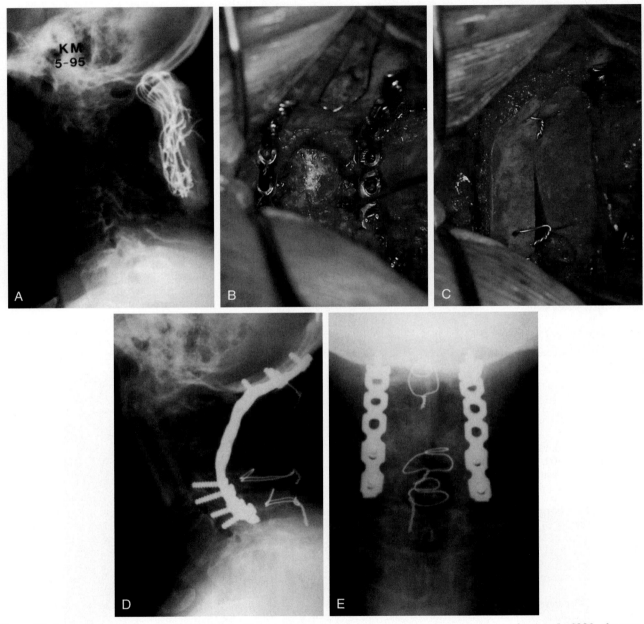

Figure 13–9. *A 51-year-old woman had a 6-year history of metastatic breast cancer to the upper cervical spine. In 1991, she was treated in an outside institution with a posterior fusion using cement and wiring from C1 to C5. She initially did well, but 4 years later continued tumor destruction of the anterior column led to cervical kyphosis (A) with severe neck pain. She underwent posterior exploration with the removal of the cement and wires followed by tumor excision to decompress her cord posteriorly. Her head was brought into neutral alignment utilizing gentle extension by adjusting the head holder, done with spinal cord monitoring under direct vision. Occipitocervical plating was carried out (B) with autogenous iliac crest bone grafting (C). She was then turned over, and an anterior decompression with tumor debulking and fibular strut grafting from the ring of C1 to C5 was performed to reconstruct the anterior column. Her anterior and posterior grafts (D and E) healed, and she was totally independent for another 3 years before succumbing to her disease.*

months. Internal fixation is essential to maximize healing and minimize postoperative external immobilization.[1b, 11a] If PMMA is used as an anterior strut, then maximum stability must be achieved before leaving the operating room, because no union can occur.

Posterior approaches to the cervical spine in this patient population are often effective for stabilization rather than decompression (Fig. 13–8). Laminectomy alone in the face of anterior column destruction from neoplasm is a destabilizing operation and must be avoided. Instrumentation techniques include simple wiring, lateral mass plating, and occipitocervical fixation with plates or rods. Fusion methods include autogenous corticocancellous bone grafting, allografting, and even PMMA wrapped around short K-wires placed through the spinous processes. The more rigid the internal fixation, the less bracing needed, which improves the patient's quality of life.

Combined anterior and posterior (circumferential) stabilization may be particularly helpful in patients with significant bony destruction.[44] This combined approach may indeed be necessary if anterior and posterior elements are destroyed, causing gross instability. Although most high cervical tumors at C1–C2 can be managed by posterior stabilization (see Fig. 13-8),[53] patients with cord compression or severe anterior and posterior involvement are good candidates for an anterior decompression, grafting, and posterior occipitocervical stabilization (Fig. 13–9).

REFERENCES

1a. Abdu WA, Provencher M: Primary bone and metastatic tumors of the cervical spine. Spine 23:2767–2777, 1998.

1b. Abumi K, Kaneda K: Pedicle screw fixation for nontraumatic lesions of the cervical spine. Spine 22:1853–1863, 1997.

1c. Ahlgren B, Morris G, Garfin S: Cervical spine tumors. State of the Art Reviews 10:123–144, 1996.

2. Atanasiu JP, Badatcheff F, Pidhorz L: Metastatic lesions of the cervical spine. A retrospective analysis of 20 cases. Spine 18:1279–1284, 1993.

2a. Berberoglu S, Oguz A, Aribal E, Ataoglu O: Osteoblastoma response to radiotherapy and chemotherapy. Med Pediatr Oncol 28:304–309, 1997.

3. Berson AM, Castro JR, Petti P, et al: Charged particle irradiation of chordoma and chondrosarcoma of the base of skull and cervical spine: The Lawrence Berkeley Laboratory experience. Int J Radiat Oncol Biol Phys 15:559–565, 1988.

4. Bohlman HH, Sachs BL, Carter JR, et al: Primary neoplasms of the cervical spine. Diagnosis and treatment of twenty-three patients. J Bone Joint Surg Am 68A:483–494, 1986.

4a. Boriani S, Biagini R, De Iure F, et al: Resection surgery in the treatment of vertebral tumors. Chir Organi Mov 83:53–64, 1998.

5. Boriani S, Capanna R, Donati D, et al: Osteoblastoma of the spine. Clin Orthop 278:37–45, 1992.

6. Boriani S, Chevalley F, Weinstein JN, et al: Chordoma of the spine above the sacrum. Treatment and outcome in 21 cases. Spine 21:1569–1577, 1996.

6a. Boriani S, De Iure F, Bandiera S, et al: Chondrosarcoma of the mobile spine: Report on 22 cases. Spine 25:804–812, 2000.

7. Boriani S, Weinstein JN, Biagini R: Primary bone tumors of the spine—Terminology and surgical staging. Spine 22:1036–1044, 1997.

8. Bouchard JA, Koka A, Bensusan JS, et al: Effects of irradiation on posterior spinal fusions. A rabbit model. Spine 19:1836–1841, 1994.

9. Bret P, Confavreux C, Thouard H, Pialat J: Aneurysmal bone cyst of the cervical spine: Report of a case investigated by computed tomographic scanning and treated by a two-stage surgical procedure. Neurosurgery 10:111–115, 1982.

10. Buck RE, Bailey RW. Replacement of a cervical vertebral body for aneurysmal cyst. A case report. J Bone Joint Surg Am 51A:1656–1659, 1969.

11. Calhoun JM, Chadduck WM, Smith JL: Single cervical exostosis: Report of a case and review of the literature. Surg Neurol 37:26–29, 1992.

11a. Caspar W, Pitzen T, Papavero L, et al: Anterior cervical plating for the treatment of neoplasms in the cervical vertebrae. J Neurosurg 90:27–34, 1999.

12. Cohen DM, Dahlin DC, MacCarty CS: Vertebral giant cell tumors and variants. Cancer 17:461–472, 1964.

13. Cooke RS, Cumming WJK, Cowie RA: Osteochondroma of the cervical spine: Case report and review of the literature. Br J Neurosurg 8:359–363, 1994.

13a. de Kleuver M, van der Heul RO, Veraart BE: Aneurysmal bone cyst of the spine: 31 cases and the importance of the surgical approach. J Pediatr Orthop 7B:286–292, 1998.

13b. Doppman JL, Oldfield EH, Heiss JD: Symptomatic vertebral hemangiomas: Treatment by means of direct intralesional injection of ethanol. Radiology 214:341–348, 2000.

14. Dowdle JA Jr, Winter RB, Dehner LP: Postradiation osteosarcoma of the cervical spine in childhood. A case report. J Bone Joint Surg Am 59A:696–971, 1977.

15. Emery SE, Brazinski MS, Koka A, et al: The biological and biomechanical effects of irradiation on anterior spinal bone grafts in a canine model. J Bone Joint Surg Am 76A:540–548, 1994.

16. Emery SE, Hughes SS, Junglas WA, et al: The fate of anterior vertebral bone grafts in patients irradiated for neoplasm. Clin Orthop 300:207–212, 1994.

17. Enneking WF: A system of staging musculoskeletal neoplasms. Clin Orthop 204:9–24, 1986.

18. Enneking WF, Spanier SS, Goodman MA: A system for the surgical staging of musculoskeletal sarcoma. Clin Orthop 153:106–120, 1980.

19. Fabiani A, Brignolio F, Favero M, et al: Benign and malignant cranio-spinal giant cell tumours. Report of four cases. Acta Neurochir 64:133–150, 1982.

20. Fidler MW: Radical resection of vertebral body tumours: A surgical technique used in ten cases. J Bone Joint Surg Br 76B:765–772, 1994.

21. Fielding JW, Keim HA, Hawkins RJ, Gabrielian JC: Osteoid osteoma of the cervical spine. Clin Orthop 128:163–164, 1977.

22. Fielding JW, Pyle RN Jr, Fietti VG Jr: Anterior cervical vertebral body resection and bone-grafting for benign and malignant tumors. A survey under the auspices of the Cervical Spine Research Society. J Bone Joint Surg Am 61A:251–253, 1979.

23. Friedman DP: Symptomatic vertebral hemangiomas: MR findings. Am J Roentgenol 167:359–364, 1996.

23a. Fujita T, Kawahara N, Matsumoto T, Tomita K: Chordoma in the cervical spine managed with en bloc excision. Spine 24:1848–1851, 1999.

24. Gelberman RH, Olson CO: Benign osteoblastoma of the atlas. A case report. J Bone Joint Surg Am 56A:809–810, 1974.

25. Glasauer FE: Benign lesions of the cervical spine. Acta Neurochir 42:161–175, 1978.

26. Glasauer FE: Benign osteoblastoma of cervical spine. NY State J Med, August 1979, pp 1424–1427.

26a. Gladden ML Jr, Gillingham BL, Hennrikus W, Vaughan LM: Aneurysmal bone cyst of the first cervical vertebrae in a child treated with percutaneous intralesional injection of calcitonin and methylprednisolone: a case report. Spine 25:527–530, 2000.

27. Goldstein GS, Dawson EG, Batzdorf U: Cervical osteoid osteoma: A cause of chronic upper back pain. Clin Orthop 129:177–180, 1977.

28. Green NE, Robertson WW Jr, Kilroy AW: Eosinophilic granuloma of the spine with associated neural deficit. Report of three cases. J Bone Joint Surg Am 62A:1198–1202, 1980.

28a. Guibaud L, Herbreteau D, Dubois J, et al: Aneurysmal bone cysts: Percutaneous embolization with an alcoholic solution of zein—series of 18 cases. Radiology 208:369–373, 1998.

29. Gupta VK, Gupta SK, Khosla VK, et al: Aneurysmal bone cysts of the spine. Surg Neurol 42:428–432, 1994.

30. Harrington KD: Metastatic disease of the spine: Current concepts review. J Bone Joint Surg Am 68A:1110–1115, 1986.

31. Hart RA, Boriani S, Biagini R, et al: A system for surgical staging and management of spine tumors: A clinical outcome study of giant cell tumors of the spine. Spine 22:1773–1783, 1997.

32. Hart R, Weinstein J: Primary benign and malignant musculo-skeletal tumors of the spine. Semin Spine Surg 7:288–303, 1995.

33. Harwood AR, Krajbich JI, Fornasier VL: Radiotherapy of chondrosarcoma of bone. Cancer 45:2769–2777, 1980.

34. Hershman E, Bjorkengren AJ, Fielding JW, Allen SC: Osteoid osteoma in a cervical pedicle. Resection via transpillar approach. Clin Orthop 213:115–117, 1986.

34a. Isacsson U, Hagberg H, Johansson KA, et al: Potential advantages of protons over conventional radiation beams for paraspinal tumours. Radiother Oncol 45:63–70, 1997.

34b. Islinger RB, Kuklo TR, Owens BD, et al: Langerhans' cell histiocytosis in patients older than 21 years. Clin Orthop 379:231–235, 2000.

34c. Jenis LG, Dunn EJ, An HS: Metastatic disease of the cervical spine: A review. Clin Orthop 359:89–103, 1999.

35. Joll CA: Metastatic tumors of bone. Br J Surg 11:38–72, 1923.

36. Jones DA: Osteoid osteoma of the atlas. J Bone Joint Surg Br 69B:149, 1987.

37. Kak VK, Prabhakar S, Khosla VK, Banerjee AK: Solitary osteochondroma of spine causing spinal cord compression. Clin Neurol Neurosurg 87:135–138, 1985.

38. Kebudi R, Ayan I, Darendeliler E, et al: Primary osteosarcoma of the cervical spine: A pediatric case report and review of the literature. Med Pediatr Oncol 23:162–165, 1994.

38a. Khan DC, Malhotra S, Stevens RE, Steinfeld AD: Radiotherapy for the treatment of giant cell tumor of the spine: A report of six cases and review of the literature. Cancer Invest 17:110–113, 1999.

39. King GJ, Kostuik JP, McBroom RJ, Richardson W: Surgical management of metastatic renal carcinoma of the spine. Spine 16:265–271, 1991.

40. Kneisl JS, Simon MA: Medical management compared with operative treatment for osteoid-osteoma. J Bone Joint Surg Am 74A:179–185, 1992.

41. Levy WM, Miller AS, Bonakdarpour A, Aegerter E. Aneurysmal bone cyst secondary to other osseous lesions. Report of 57 cases. Am J Clin Pathol 63:1–8, 1975.

41a. Logroscino CA, Astolfi S, Sacchettoni G: Chordoma: Long-term evaluation of 15 cases treated surgically. Chir Organi Mov 83:87–103, 1998.

42. Lybeert MLM, Meerwaldt JH: Chordoma: Report of treatment results in eighteen cases. Acta Radiol Oncol 25:41–43, 1986.

42a. Mariette X, Zagdanski AM, Guermazi A, et al: Prognostic value of vertebral lesions detected by magnetic resonance imaging in patients with stage I multiple myeloma. Br J Haematol 104:723–729, 1999.

43. Marsh BW, Bonfiglio M, Brady LP, Enneking WF: Benign osteoblastoma: Range of manifestations. J Bone Joint Surg Am 57A:1–9, 1975.

44. McAfee PC, Bohlman HH, Ducker TB, et al: One-stage anterior cervical decompression and posterior stabilization. A study of one hundred patients with a minimum of two years of follow-up. J Bone Joint Surg Am 77A:1791–1800, 1995.

45. McAllister VL, Kendall BE, Bull JWD: Symptomatic vertebral hemangiomas. Brain 98:71–80, 1995.

46. McLain RF, Weinstein JN: Solitary plasmacytomas of the spine: A review of 84 cases. J Spinal Disord 2:69–74, 1989.

47. Mirra JM, Rand F, Rand R, et al: Giant-cell tumor of the second cervical vertebra treated by cryosurgery and irradiation. Clin Orthop 154:228–233, 1981.

48. Mnaymneh W, Brown M, Tejada F, Morrison G: Primary osteogenic sarcoma of the second cervical vertebra. Case report. J Bone Joint Surg Am 61A:460–462, 1979.

49. Morard M, de Preux J: Solitary osteochondroma presenting as a neck mass with spinal cord compression syndrome. Surg Neurol 37:402–405, 1992.

49a. Mori Y, Takayasu M, Saito K, et al: Benign osteoblastoma of the odontoid process of the axis: A case report. Surg Neurol 49:274–277, 1998.

50. Murali R, Rovit RL, Benjamin MV: Chordoma of the cervical spine. Neurosurgery 9:253–256, 1981.

51. Ono K, Yonenobu K, Ebara S, et al: Prosthetic replacement surgery for cervical spine metastasis. Spine 13:817–822, 1988.

51a. Ozaki T, Halm H, Hillmann A, et al: Aneurysmal bone cysts of the spine. Arch Orthop Trauma Surg 119:159–162, 1999.

52. Palmer FJ, Blum PW: Osteochondroma with spinal cord compression: Report of three cases. J Neurosurg 52:842–845, 1980.

52a. Papagelopoulos PJ, Currier BL, Shaughnessy WJ, et al: Aneurysmal bone cyst of the spine: Management and outcome. Spine 23:621–628, 1998.

53. Phillips E, Levine AM: Metastatic lesions of the upper cervical spine. Spine 14:1071–1077, 1989.

54. Poolos PN, White RJ: Aneurysmal bone cyst of the cervical spine: A twelve-year follow-up after surgical treatment. Surg Neurol 14:259–362, 1980.

54a. Raab P, Hohmann F, Kühl J, Krauspe R: Vertebral remodeling in eosinophilic granuloma of the spine: A long-term follow-up. Spine 23:1351–1354, 1998.

55. Rao S, Badani K, Schildhauer T, Borges M: Metastatic malignancy of the cervical spine—A nonoperative history. Spine 17(suppl):S407–S412, 1992.

56. Raskas DS, Graziano GP, Herzenberg JE, et al: Osteoid osteoma and osteoblastoma of the spine. J Spinal Disord 5:204–211, 1992.

56a. Ratliff J, Voorhies R: Osteochondroma of the C5 lamina with cord compression: Case report and review of the literature. Spine 25:1293–1295, 2000.

57. Raycroft JF, Hockman RP, Southwick WO: Metastatic tumors involving the cervical vertebrae: Surgical palliation. J Bone Joint Surg Am 60A:763–768, 1978.

57a. Riley LH III, Frassica DA, Kostuik JP, Frassica FJ: Metastatic disease to the spine: Diagnosis and treatment. AAOS Instr Course Lect 49:471–477, 2000.

58. Rix RR, Geschickter CF: Tumors of the spine. With a consideration of Ewing's sarcoma. Arch Surg 36:899–948, 1938.

58a. Saifuddin A, White J, Sherazi Z, et al: Osteoid osteoma and osteoblastoma of the spine: Factors associated with the presence of scoliosis. Spine 23:47–53, 1998.

59. Sanjay BKS, Sim FH, Unni KK, et al: Giant-cell tumors of the spine. J Bone Joint Surg Br 75B:148–154, 1993.
60. Sevick RJ: Cervical spine tumors. Neuroimaging Clin N Am 5:385–400, 1995.
61. Shallat RF, Taekman MS, Nagle RC: Unusual presentation of cervical chordoma with long-term survival: Case report. J Neurosurg 57:716–718, 1982.
62. Sherk HH, Nicholson JT, Nixon JE: Vertebra plana and eosinophilic granuloma of the cervical spine in children. Spine 3:116–121, 1978.
63. Sherk HH, Nolan JP Jr, Mooar PA: Treatment of tumors of the cervical spine. Clin Orthop 233:163–167, 1988.
64. Shikata J, Yamamuro T, Shimizu K, et al: Surgical treatment of giant-cell tumors of the spine. Clin Orthop 278:29–36, 1992.
65. Shives TC, Dahlin DC, Sim FH, et al: Osteosarcoma of the spine. J Bone Joint Surg Am 68A:660–668, 1986.
66. Shives TC, McLeod RA, Unni KK, Schray MF: Chondrosarcoma of the spine. J Bone Joint Surg Am 71A:1158–1165, 1989.
67. Siegal T, Tiqva P, Siegal T: Vertebral body resection for epidural compression by malignant tumors. Results of forty-seven consecutive operative procedures. J Bone Joint Surg Am 67A:375–382, 1985.
68. Stener B, Johnsen OE: Complete removal of three vertebrae for giant cell tumour. J Bone Joint Surg Br 53B:278–287, 1971.
69. Stevenson S, Emery SE, Goldberg VM: Factors affecting bone graft incorporation. Clin Orthop 324:66–74, 1996.
70. Stillwell WT, Fielding JW: Aneurysmal bone cyst of the cervicodorsal spine. Clin Orthop 187:144–146, 1984.
71. Sundaresan N, Rosen G, Huvos AG, Krol G: Combined treatment of osteosarcoma of the spine. Neurosurgery 23:714–719, 1988.
72. Symmers D: The metastasis of tumors: A study of 298 cases of malignant growth exhibited among 5155 autopsies at Bellevue Hospital. Am J Med Sci 154:225–240, 1917.
73. Tomita K, Kawahara N, Baba H, et al: Total en bloc spondylectomy—A new surgical technique for primary malignant vertebral tumors. Spine 22:324–333, 1997.
73a. Turker RJ, Mardjetko S, Lubicky J: Aneurysmal bone cysts of the spine: Excision and stabilization. J Pediatr Orthop 18:209–213, 1998.
74. Urteaga B, Pack GT: On the antiquity of melanoma. Cancer 19:607–610, 1966.
75. Valderrama JAF, Bullough PG: Solitary myeloma of the spine. J Bone Joint Surg Br 50B:82–90, 1968.
76. Verbiest H: Giant cell tumours and aneurysmal bone cysts of the spine. J Bone Joint Surg Br 47B:699–713, 1965.
77. Weatherly CR, Jaffray D, O'Brien JP: Radical excision of an osteoblastoma of the cervical spine. A combined anterior and posterior approach. J Bone Joint Surg Br 68B:325–328, 1986.
77a. Weigel B, Maghsudi M, Neumann C, et al: Surgical management of symptomatic spinal metastases: Postoperative outcome and quality of life. Spine 24:2240–2246, 1999.
78. Weill A, Chiras J, Simon JM, et al: Spinal metastases: Indications for and results of percutaneous injection of acrylic surgical cement. Radiology 199:241–247, 1996.
79. Weinstein J, McLain R: Primary tumors of the spine. Spine 12:843–851, 1987.
80. Wells C: Ancient Egyptian pathology. J Laryngol Otol 77:261–265, 1963.
80a. Wippold FJ II, Koeller KK, Smirniotopoulos JG: Clinical and imaging features of cervical chordoma. Am J Roentgenol 172:1423–1426, 1999.
80b. Wise JJ, Fischgrund JS, Herkowitz HN, et al: Complication, survival rates, and risk factors of surgery for metastatic disease of the spine. Spine 24:1943–1951, 1999.
81. Wright CJ: Long survival in solitary plasmacytoma of bone. J Bone Joint Surg Br 48B:767–771, 1961.
82. Wu KK, Mitchell DC, Guise ER: Chordoma of the atlas. J Bone Joint Surg Am 61A:140–141, 1979.
82a. Wuisman PIJM, Jutte PC, Ozaki T: Secondary chondrosarcoma in osteochondromas: Medullary extension in 15 of 45 cases. Acta Orthop Scand 68:396–400, 1997.
82b. Yeom JS, Lee CK, Shin HY, et al: Langerhans' cell histiocytosis of the spine: Analysis of twenty-three cases. Spine 24:1740–1749, 1999.
82c. York JE, Berk RH, Fuller GN, et al: Chondrosarcoma of the spine: 1954 to 1997. J Neurosurg 90:73–78, 1999.

14

SPINAL CORD TUMORS

Thomas A. Becherer, M.D.
Deborah A. Blades, M.D.

*Though a good deal is too strange to be believed,
nothing is too strange to have happened.*
— Thomas Hardy

HISTORICAL PERSPECTIVE

The recognition of spinal cord tumors as a surgical disease began more than a century ago. In 1887, the first successful excision of a spinal cord tumor was achieved by Sir Victor Horsley.[37] Subsequently, Horsely performed 20 similar procedures without any mortality.[1] Cushing, Elsberg, and Fraser expanded Horsley's experience in the early 20th century by popularizing surgical treatment of spinal cord lesions.[23] In the modern era, James Greenwood reviewed these pioneering works and added microsurgical techniques, bipolar electrocautery, and magnifying loupes, all of which added to the viable option of surgical resectability in the treatment of these clinically challenging lesions.[19, 32]

INCIDENCE

Spinal cord tumors are rare, with an incidence of approximately 3 to 10 per 100,000 population.[52] Intraspinal neoplasms account for 15% of all primary tumors of the central nervous system (CNS) in adults[88] and 10% of those in children.[96] Spinal cord tumors are generally classified by their location; most arise primarily from the spinal cord tissue, nerve roots, or meninges. This chapter describes intradural tumors, which are divided into two groups, intramedullary and extramedullary. Extradural tumors, chiefly metastatic lesions,[5] are discussed in Chapter 13.

Intradural intramedullary tumors, 80% of which are primary gliomas, arise within the cord substance. They represent one-third of all adult spinal cord tumors and nearly one-half of pediatric spinal cord tumors.[36, 94] Intradural extramedullary tumors, most of which are neurilemmomas and meningiomas, arise extrinsic to the cord and constitute two-thirds of adult spinal cord tumors and the remainder of pediatric spinal cord tumors.

CLINICAL PRESENTATION

Clinically, spinal cord tumors vary widely in their symptoms and signs. The clinical manifestations are determined by the tumor's specific location. Generally these tumors are characterized by a delayed presentation of 2 to 3 years or longer. Moreover, the symptoms overlap those of multiple sclerosis, syringomyelia, pernicious anemia, and herniated disks, often complicating rapid diagnosis.[53] Interestingly, patients usually attribute the initial symptoms to minor trauma.[7]

The most common complaint, occurring in 60% to 70% of patients,[63] is pain around the spinal axis.[6] Radicular pain is reported less often than generalized back and neck pain. Many patients describe pain at night that awakens them from sleep;[74, 94] pain may also be exacerbated by Valsalva's maneuver.[4, 93] Pain and other symptoms can present without objective findings.

Objective findings, when they occur, are often subtle. Sensory disturbances are generally paresthesias and/or painful dysesthetic pain syndromes. Cervical spine involvement can be identified by motor findings generally in the upper extremities, ranging from mild weakness to atrophy of the hands. Long-tract signs with upper and lower extremity involvement with associated gait disturbance are also common. Many lesions are positioned asymmetrically within the dura mater. This asymmetry can manifest clinically as a Brown-Sequard–type syndrome, with ipsilateral motor findings and contralateral sensory disturbances predominating. Urinary frequency can occur, signifying micturation pathway involvement. When the sympathetic system is disrupted in the cervical spine, symptoms can manifest in the form of dysfunctional sweating below the level of tumor involvement, in addition to a full-blown Horner's syndrome.

Uncommonly, spinal cord tumors can present with increased intracranial pressure. This is rare in adults, but an incidence of 15% has been reported in children.[9] In upper cervical lesions, hydrocephalus is more common, and papilledema may be evident. The presumed reason for hydrocephalus is increased protein in the cerebrospinal fluid (CSF) with or without myelographic block.[103] Aseptic arachnoiditis from an inflammatory reaction in response to the tumor also has been proposed by some authors.[84, 96] In malignant tumors, hydrocephalus can represent meningeal infiltration with tumor (Fig. 14–1).[25]

The clinical course of cervical spinal cord tumors differs between children and adults in several ways. The time to diagnosis is generally shorter in children than in adults, by an average of 1-1/2 years. A clinical presentation dominated by pain is less common in children than in adults.[44] Typically an objective complaint, such as weakness or ataxia, is more common in children.[67, 94] Most importantly

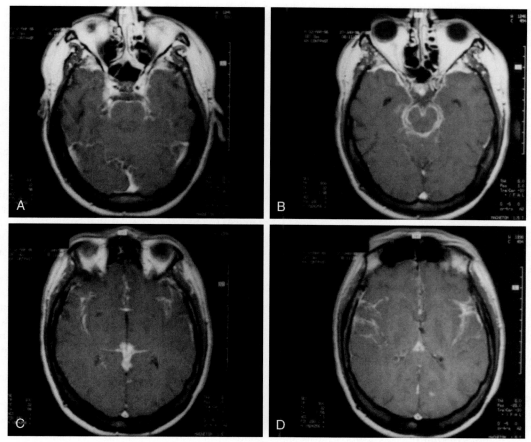

Figure 14–1. *A, Axial postcontrast T1-weighted image shows linear enhancement of the gyri of the occipital lobe. B, Dense enhancement around the midbrain. C and D, Linear enhancement of the sylvian fissures bilaterally, indicating leptomeningeal spread of malignant astrocytoma.*

for orthopedic surgeons and primary clinicians alike, the identification of a musculoskeletal anomaly such as torticollis,[73] scoliosis,[107] or kyphosis[97] in a child should prompt investigation for a spinal cord tumor.[101]

DIAGNOSTIC EVALUATION

Radiographic localization is the primary modality used to diagnose spinal cord tumors. Regardless of the type of radiologic procedure used, a specific presumptive diagnosis should be avoided until definitive biopsy specimens are evaluated.[94] Today, magnetic resonance imaging (MRI) has emerged as the primary diagnostic tool for evaluating spinal cord tumors.[99]

Plain x-rays are not routinely used to diagnose spinal cord tumors, because the yield is low.[44] Despite this generalization, plain film abnormalities are found in 26% of ependymomas,[76] 19% of meningiomas,[53] 50% of neurilemmomas,[54] and 37% of hemangioblastomas.[9] These abnormalities include widening of the interpedicular distance, erosion of the posterior element, scalloping of the vertebral body, thinning of the laminae,[63] widening of the neural foramina, scoliosis,[29] and kyphosis.[4]

Both myelography and computed tomography (CT)-

myelography, although more invasive, can also be useful diagnostic tools for patients who are otherwise unable to undergo MRI. The typical findings that suggest a spinal cord lesion are widening of the spinal cord, a tapered spread of contrast or block, and cysts that sometimes fill with contrast medium within 12 to 24 hours.

Along with the radiographic findings from myelography, CSF can be sent for laboratory investigation.[38] CSF analysis was once an integral part of the workup for an intraspinal mass, but with the advanced imaging techniques of MRI, this has largely been abandoned. The CSF findings consistent with spinal cord tumor are elevated protein level[78] and a manometric block during compression of the jugular veins (Queckenstedt's maneuver[44]).

Angiography is generally not very useful in diagnosing spinal cord tumors. The vessels supplying spinal cord tumors are beyond the resolution of angiography, making identification of vascular supply futile.[58] (However, in the case of intraspinal vascular malformations, spinal angiography is a mandatory diagnostic tool.[86])

MRI has emerged as the procedure of choice for assisting in the diagnosis and treatment of intraspinal lesions.[43, 94, 99] Axial and sagittal views permit precise localization of the levels involved, especially when using the T2-weighted spin echo or gradient recalled echo pulse sequences.[49, 61, 96] The multiple modes of accessing images provide useful information about tissue expansion, cystic degeneration, necrosis, hemorrhage, and edema.[55] Administration of gadolinium as a contrast agent helps delineate areas of tumor involvement for surgical planning, because most tumors of the cervical spine enhance to variable degrees.[98, 99] The evolution from CT-myelography to MRI has been compared with the change from pneumoencephalography to cranial CT, and the techniques for producing images with MRI continue to improve.[86] Nevertheless, when planning treatment one must realize that although MRI is very sensitive, its specificity is limited.

METASTASIS

Approximately 2% of all patients with systemic cancer develop spinal cord metastasis.[18, 70] Intramedullary spinal cord metastasis constitutes 1% to 5% of all spinal axis metastases.[43] With the advent of increasing survival times in patients with systemic disease, the frequency of CNS metastasis is also increasing.[18] The signs and symptoms of intramedullary spinal cord metastasis cannot be distinguished from those of external spinal cord compression on clinical examination.[43] When a patient with a presumed metastasis to the intradural space is evaluated, the intracranial compartment also must be evaluated for metastasis.[71, 74] Radiographically, the general appearance of metastatic lesions makes them indistinguishable from primary intramedullary spinal cord tumors.[55] The treatment of choice usually is radiation; however, surgical removal may be indicated in cases of controlled systemic disease and isolated spinal cord metastasis.[105]

Metastases reach the intradural compartment in two distinct ways.[5] The first way is hematogenously, as in lung, breast, and colorectal cancers; melanoma; lymphoma; leukemia; and fibrosarcoma.[22, 75] The second way is from leptomeningeal spread, as in medulloblastomas, ependymomas, glioblastomas, pineal region tumors, and intracranial metastasis.[11, 60, 61]

PATHOPHYSIOLOGY
Intramedullary Tumors
Gliomas

Gliomas represent 80% of the intradural intramedullary neoplasms. The overwhelming majority of the gliomas are astrocytomas and ependymomas, distributed in relation to age. Astrocytomas predominate in patients age 30 or younger, whereas ependymomas are more common in patients older than 30. Other, less common gliomas are oligodendrogliomas, gangliogliomas, and subependymomas.

Astrocytomas. Cervical spine astrocytomas are intramedullary neoplasms that occur at all ages but more frequently in patients under age 30 and slightly more often in males.[103] Approximately 1% of all CNS tumors and 6% to 8% of all spinal tumors are cervical astrocytomas. They are generally histologically benign (Kernohan grade I or II[10]), with an

average 10-year survival.[3] The more malignant forms (Kernohan grade III and IV) are less common than their intracranial counterparts, with 10% occurring in children and 25% in adults.[94] The malignant variety carries a dismal prognosis, with a median survival of 6 months in adults and up to 1 year in children.[13, 15, 96] Unfortunately, despite all of the advances in treatment for intramedullary neoplasms, the outcome in malignant astrocytomas has not been altered, and the most important prognostic factor is the histologic grade.[57]

Radiographically, the astrocytoma's classic appearance is spinal cord widening with an asymmetrical intra-axial location within the spinal cord (Fig. 14–2). The average sagittal span is five or six spinal segments. These neoplasms are occasionally cystic, and the cysts can take up myelographic dye on a delayed basis.[103] Contrast enhancement is present regardless of histologic grade; however, it is generally patchy (Fig 14–3). A syringomyelic cavity is identified in 38% of astrocytomas.

The gross appearance of an astrocytoma at surgery is a grayish, indiscrete, relatively avascular tumor.[94] When the astrocytoma is malignant, the vascularity is more grossly apparent.[15] Most astrocytomas are fibrillary and infiltrative in nature, making resection difficult. Epstein reported that nonneoplastic neurons can be found in surgical specimens of low-grade astrocytomas, but radical resection is not associated with increased morbidity or long-term dysfunction.[27] Pilocytic astrocytomas also occur in the cervical spine; these may be more amenable to resection secondary to the presence of a well-circumscribed margin, although its location may preclude surgical extirpation (Fig. 14–4).[103]

The extent of resection for "benign" astrocytomas is an unsettled issue.[83] Based on early reports,[32] there has been a reluctance to attempt complete resection of cervical spine astrocytomas that has prevailed into the modern era.[58]

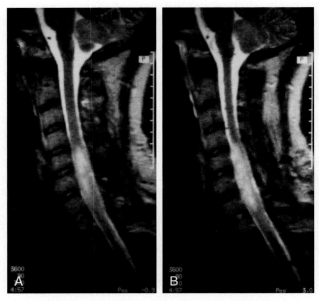

Figure 14–2. Sagittal T2-weighted image showing widening of the cervical spinal cord by a heterogeneous hyperintense mass that proved to be a malignant astrocytoma.

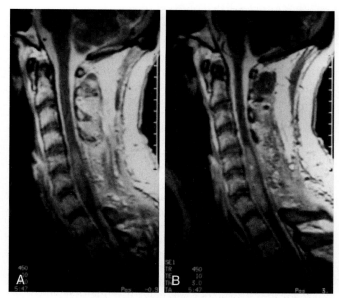

Figure 14–3. Sagittal T1-weighted contrast enhanced image of the cervical spine showing widening of the cervical cord by an enhancing mass in addition to diffuse enhancement of the subarachnoid space extending intracranially due to a malignant astrocytoma.

Performing laminectomy and myelotomy without an aggressive attempt at tumor removal has been advocated, because radical debulking offers no significant improvement in long-term outcome.[20] Some authors have advocated radical resection in pediatric patients using microsurgical technique versus decompressive laminectomy and biopsy alone; they found mean survival times of 173.5 months in the radical group and 66.6 months in the decompressive group.[77] Even in cases of recurrence or residual tumor, favorable results have been reported after radical resection in children.[26] Cervical spinal cord astrocytoma appears to be more amenable to radical resection in children; in records where

up to 95% of the cases were resected, minimal morbidity was incurred, and favorable results of 70% remission at 5 years were noted.[2] In contrast, some authors have concluded that survival is not affected by the extent of resection.[45] Their judgment may reflect a different situation in adults, where astrocytomas tend to infiltrate more and thus are less amenable to resection.[17] Certainly, if a clear plane is identified grossly, then radical resection should be attempted in a patient of any age.

Of course, malignant astrocytomas are not amenable to complete resection. In fact, attempts at aggressive resection have been met with dismal outcomes. The dissemination rate of malignant astrocytomas throughout the spinal axis as well as intracranially may be as high as 58%.[15]

Ependymomas. Cervical spine ependymomas are the most common intramedullary neoplasms in the adult population and are less common in children. Unlinked to gender,[63, 68, 91, 104] ependymomas constitute 2% of all CNS tumors.[7, 87] These tumors have a defined grading system; however, with the exception of ependymoblastomas, the grade of neoplasm is not associated with the overall prognosis.[68, 80] The rare ependymoblastomas behave in a more aggressive and malignant fashion: the overall 5- and 10-year survival rates are 68% and 50%, respectively.[81] The primary goal of treatment is complete surgical excision.[31, 36, 40, 58]

Radiographically, a cervical ependymoma typically appears as a centrally located mass with uniform contrast uptake. Syringomyelic cavities are noted in 46% of ependymomas (Fig. 14–5).[61] Cysts can also be identified at the rostral or caudal poles of the lesion.[33] With knowledge of the location of cysts, surgical excision occasionally can be facilitated by aspirating the cysts.[29]

On surgery, an ependymoma appears as a fleshy, well-circumscribed, vascular mass.[63] Significantly, although the tumor is well defined, the walls may be quite friable, making surgical excision complicated. The hallmark of histologic diagnosis is the presence of perivascular

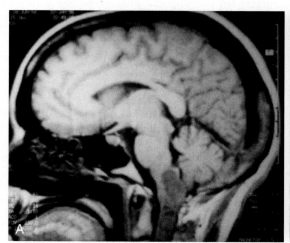
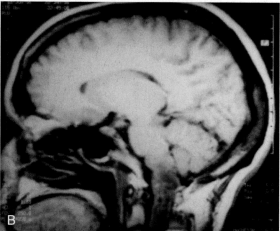

Figure 14–4. Sagittal T1-weighted contrast enhanced image of the craniocervical junction showing expansion of the cervico-medullary substance by a pilocytic astrocytoma.

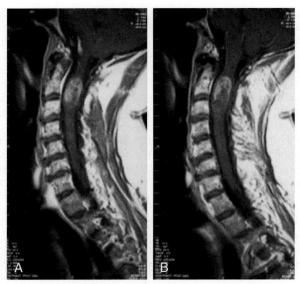

Figure 14–5. Sagittal T1-weighted contrast-enhanced image of the cervical spine showing widening of the upper cervical cord by an enhancing multicystic lesion that proved to be an ependymoma.

pseudorosettes or true ependymal rosettes.[68] The various pathologic subtypes are cellular, papillary, myxopapillary, tanycytic, and anaplastic.[33]

The importance of complete surgical excision of ependymomas has been well documented. The histologic features have not been prognostically significant. It does appear that younger patients have a more aggressive variety of ependymoma, the opposite of the situation seen in patients with astrocytomas.

Other Gliomas. Oligodendrogliomas do occur in the cervical spine, though rarely.[3] This neoplasm is biologically identical to its intracranial counterpart, except that it typically does not have calcifications grossly or histopathologically.[5] Oligodendrogliomas are treated in the same fashion as astrocytomas of the cervical spine. The mean survival time is 2.4 years.[96]

Other reported gliomas in the cervical spine are subependymomas and gangliogliomas.[96] These tumors are known for their indolent behavior and well-circumscribed margins at the time of surgical resection.

Hemangioblastomas

Tumors of the vascular epithelial cell, hemangioblastomas represent 1.6% to 5.8% of all intramedullary spinal cord tumors.[90] They rarely occur in the cervical spine except when associated with von Hipple-Lindau syndrome. In fact, 20% to 33% of cervical spine patients with hemangioblastomas have von Hipple-Lindau syndrome.[19, 43, 70, 94]

The von Hipple-Lindau syndrome is described as a multiplicity of hemangioblastomas as well as other tumors. It is an autosomal dominant disorder with incomplete (70%) penetrance and variable expression. Along with the CNS hemangioblastomas, patients suffer from retinal angiomato-

sis, congenital cysts of visceral organs, pheochromocytomas, and renal cell carcinoma.[12] A screening program has been suggested for patients with hemangioblastomas and for families with von Hipple-Lindau syndrome that includes family history, physical examination, ophthalmologic examination, abdominal ultrasonography, complete blood count, urinalysis, cranial CT or MRI, abdominal CT or MRI, and MIBG scintigraphy of the adrenals.[70]

The typical radiographic presentation is a cystic mass with a vascular nodule.[43, 61] The tumor generally abuts the pial surface by a pedicle or a broad base. Vascular flow voids are readily apparent on MRI,[61] and a syringomyelic cavity is seen in 63% of cervical hemangioblastomas.[9] This tumor can also have associated marked vasogenic edema, but the etiology of this edema has not been established. These tumors may secrete a "vasogenic edemic" factor or have a vascular shunt.[94] Some have suggested that a vascular shunt does not explain the edema, because spinal arteriovenous malformations do not exhibit this edema.[90]

These lesions are amenable to complete surgical resection.[9, 41] Given the vascularity of the mass, directly incising or debulking the mass is not recommended; rather, a plane is developed around the mass, and it is removed en bloc. Another helpful surgical technique is to keep the venous pedicle intact until the mass has been prepared for removal, to allow for venous drainage during resection.[94]

Extramedullary Tumors
Nerve Sheath Tumors

The nerve sheath tumors generally arise from sensory roots and constitute 30% of all intraspinal neoplasms.[78] Most are intradural extramedullary tumors; however, extradural involvement has been reported.[61] The strict intramedullary nerve sheath tumor has also been reported and is considered to either arise from the plexus of nerves associated with blood vessels entering the cord or grow centripetally from the dorsal root entry zone or from a displaced neural crest during development. The radiographic appearance is of a soft tissue mass that occasionally exits the foramen in a "dumbbell" fashion. When such a "dumbbell" lesion is encountered, the neural foramen can be widened (Fig. 14–6).[43]

Neurofibromas. These tumors of Schwann cells and fibroblasts[61] present 80% to 85% of the time as an intradural lesion, and the remainder of the time as extradural. This is the lesion associated with neurofibromatosis 1 (NF-1).

NF-1 is an autosomal dominant disorder with 100% penetrance and its locus located on chromosome 17. This disorder occurs in 1 in 3000 live births, and one-half of new cases arise from spontaneous mutations.[100] The disorder is characterized by café-au-lait spots, neurofibromas, axillary freckling, iris hematomas, Lisch nodules, optic gliomas, and sphenoid dysplasia. The neurofibromas associated with NF-1 can undergo malignant degeneration, thereby increasing the challenge of definitive treatment.[21, 54, 56, 59, 66]

Schwannomas. The schwannoma is a nerve sheath tumor comprised solely of Schwann cells. Schwannomas constitute 95% of all solitary, sporadic, and benign spinal nerve sheath tumors. Schwannomas are associated with neurofibromatosis 2 (NF-2), an autosomal dominant syndrome characterized by bilateral acoustic schwannomas or a unilateral acoustic schwannoma with a neurofibroma, meningioma, glioma, schwannoma, or a juvenile posterior subcapsular lenticular opacity. The frequency of this disorder is 1:50,000, and at least 60% of tumors related to NF-2 that present sporadically can exhibit deletions or rearrangements in chromosome 22.[43, 56, 59, 66] These nerve sheath tumors usually can be shelled out of normal nerve tissue. Depending on the amount of bone resection for exposure, posterior stabilization may be needed after resection (see Fig. 14–6).

Meningiomas

This benign tumor of the arachnoidal cap cells is the second most common intradural spinal tumor.[89, 92] The typical patient is female (the female-to-male ratio is 4:1) and over age 40.[53, 61, 94] NF-2 is a predisposing factor for this tumor.[8] Meningiomas have a slow, indolent course that reflects the specific location and the specific areas of the neural elements compressed or involved.[92] Intramedullary meningiomas are extremely rare but have been reported, with all cases in the cervical spine.[82] Extradural meningiomas in the cervical spine constitute 5% of the total and tend

to recur following resection.[53, 89] The treatment is generally surgical. According to Harvey Cushing, "successful operation for a spinal meningioma represents one of the most gratifying of all operative procedures."[19]

The radiographic appearance of cervical spinal meningiomas is quite variable, but they generally appear as soft tissue masses that are isointense compared with cord tissue on T1- and T2-weighted MRI imaging with marked enhancement.[61] In the cervical spine, meningiomas typically take a ventral position. Calcification is rarely (0.6%) seen on plain x-rays.[89, 92] Similar to neurofibromas but much less commonly, meningiomas can widen the neural foramina.

Other Extramedullary Tumors

Intraspinal lipomas constitute 1% of all spinal tumors.[102] These are rarely cervical tumors. The tumor itself is a non–DNA-producing tumor and has no documented clinical recurrence in this region. Lipomas are classified as one of the group of inclusion tumors that also includes dermoids, epidermoids, cysts, and teratomas.[5, 31, 58]

Cavernous malformations and arteriovenous malformations (AVMs) are also in the differential diagnosis of cervical spinal tumors. In fact, AVMs make up 3% to 4% of spinal cord masses.[14] MRI typically shows a reticulated

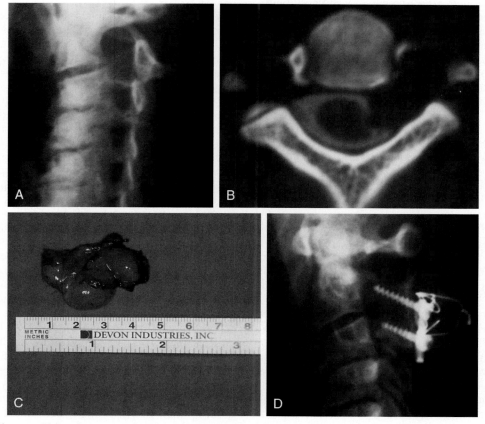

Figure 14–6. A 50-year-old female presented with neck and shoulder pain. An oblique plain film (A) shows an enlarged C2–C3 foramen. A CT/myelogram (B) shows a mass in the foramen. Surgical resection via a posterior approach was done and retrieved this schwannoma (C), followed by posterior instrumentation and fusion (D).

mass with a hypointense rim. Surgical excision is recommended for symptomatic lesions.[62] Foix-Alajouanine syndrome is a subacute necrotizing myelopathy usually associated with an AVM. Foix-Alajouanine syndrome occurring in the absence of an AVM is radiographically and clinically indistinguishable from an intramedullary spinal cord tumor.[43]

The following masses are rarely reported in the cervical spinal cord: myxomas, sarcomas, abcesses, hemangiopericytomas, meningeal cysts, and inclusion tumors.[5, 21, 47, 48, 51, 69, 73]

TREATMENT

Surgery

Surgical excision of spinal cord tumors has continued to evolve since its infancy in the late 1800s; however, the three main indications have remained constant. First, operative diagnosis and exploration is the primary goal in surgical decision making.[58] Second, after the gross characteristics are explored, the goal of a surgical cure is approached microsurgically.[95] Finally, in patients with a progressive neurologic deterioration, surgical intervention is undertaken to preserve neurologic function and provide pain relief.[16, 67]

The surgical approach for intramedullary cervical spinal cord tumors begins with proper preparation and positioning. The patients are given general anesthesia in a routine fashion, including a standard endotracheal intubation. Perioperative steroids and antibiotics are recommended.[96]

Although some surgeons report performing this surgery with the patient in a sitting position, the prone position with a perpendicular orientation is ideal. The patient's head can be fixed in place using the Mayfield three-point fixation device.[42, 58, 95, 107]

Intraoperative monitoring, in the form of somatosensory evoked potentials, is generally used as an investigative tool.[96] It also provides rapid assessment of integrity, but no evaluation of anterior cord function can be extrapolated.[17] Some have reported the use of motor evoked potentials (MEP) with subtotal neuromuscular blockade, using epidural or subarachnoid electrodes; MEP are recorded in the quadriceps and tibialis anterior musculature. Neither mode of monitoring has been adopted for routine use.[1]

A standard cervical laminectomy is performed for exposure in most cases. We commonly perform a laminoplasty in children to prevent postoperative and late kyphotic deformity.[44, 96, 107]

Before the midline durotomy is performed, intraoperative ultrasonography is used to determine the extent of the mass.[16, 28, 96] Next, the dura is incised in the midline along the rostral-caudal extent of the mass, and the microscope is brought into the operative field. The dorsal median raphe of the spinal cord must be accurately identified, which can be difficult in the presence of significant expansion of the cord.[29] The midline can be identified between the dorsal root entry zones, or occasionally the posterior median septum is visible. The region of maximal cord swelling is chosen to initiate the myelotomy. First, the pial vessels are cauterized in the midline; then, using sharp dissection, the pia is incised.[58, 64] An alternative to the sharp incision is the use of a carbon dioxide laser set at 5 to 10 watts.[16, 46]

Once the myelotomy has been defined, dissectors are used to follow vessels and the anatomical plane to the mass. The plated bayonet is a tool developed specifically to dissect in the plane between the tumor and normal cord. This tool helps maintain the integrity of neural structures.[24] Once a sufficient plane is developed, 7-0 or 8-0 monofilament nylon sutures are used to retract the pial edges.[96]

The tumor is generally identified approximately 2 mm below the myelotomy incision. Next, the length of the tumor should be defined rostrally and caudally. Every attempt at total excision should be made, based on the gross intraoperative findings.[16, 96]

The treatment of infiltrative lesions is controversial. Some authors have suggested that the intraoperative identification of an astrocytoma precludes further resection, because these tumors are rarely resectable.[42] Others have suggested that infiltrative lesions should be debulked with a cavitronic ultrasonic aspirator (CUSA) or laser.[16, 25, 30, 46] Some have suggested that even infiltrative lesions can be safely resected aggressively as a definitive treatment.[2, 25, 26, 96]

When the mass is well demarcated, it should be resected entirely. A plane is usually developed, and fibrous adhesions are lysed. As feeding vessels are encountered, they are cauterized as well. Once the posterior extent has been identified, the mass should be debulked. CUSA is an excellent tool for debulking, because it enables rapid tumor reduction with very little heat generation and minimal tissue displacement.[95] As the dissection proceeds anteriorly, traction becomes more difficult, and the anterior spinal artery may be encountered.

Once the tumor has been removed, the resection bed must be examined carefully to ensure proper and complete hemostasis. A series of warm irrigations will usually suffice to stimulate hemostasis.[64] The pial sutures are removed, and the edges are not reapproximated. The dura is then closed in a watertight fashion.[16] If necessary, a dural patch graft may be used to avoid tension or, in the case of recurrent tumor, to better reapproximate the dural edges.

Special attention should be paid to closure of the posterior cervical wound. At minimum, a three-layer closure is recommended, with at least one watertight layer, preferably the fascial layer. Colored sutures are used to aid location of the midline in the event of tumor recurrence. Subcutaneous drainage can enhance wound integrity in the early postoperative period. Occasionally, fascial-relaxing incisions are performed to help reduce tension on the midline suture line. Meticulous care taken in wound closure will help prevent wound problems in light of possible postoperative radiation and recurrence.[108, 109]

Initially following surgery, the patient will experience an increased neurologic deficit, especially in regard to posterior column function. Immediately postoperatively, the patient should remain intubated for 24 to 48 hours, anticipating pulmonary problems with regard to cervical spinal cord function.[36] The initial neurologic compromise is usually transient, resolving within 3 months.[95] Permanent refractory neurologic worsening is encountered in less than

5% of cases.[96] Earlier we discussed the controversy surrounding the resection of infiltrative astrocytomas; however, it has been well established that complete excision of ependymomas provides for the best overall outcome. Several preoperative factors affect the outcome of resection, including age, degree of preoperative neurologic deficit, location (with cervical carrying an increased risk), histology, and surgical technique.[42, 94]

Because several possible operative complications are well documented, vigilant postoperative assessment is essential. The first of these, CSF leakage, can be treated or prevented by avoiding excess tension or pressure at the operative site. Lumbar drainage can help treat this complication. When a CSF leak is persistent, the suspicion of hydrocephalus must be addressed; a ventriculoperitoneal shunt may be necessary in such cases. A spinal deformity is a concern. Some have addressed this problem prophylactically with laminoplasty; when identified postoperatively, bracing can help treat this problem.[96] Finally, herniation and incarceration of the spinal cord can be prevented with a meticulous and watertight dural closure.[27]

The special cases of intradural and extramedullary tumor surgery must be addressed. The same principles described earlier are maintained, with some additions. A curvilinear incision is generally required to gain lateral exposure. In fact, a unilateral foraminotomy or facetectomy may be necessary to expose the most lateral extent of the mass.[92, 95] The dura is incised lateral to midline, and debulking the tumor will help minimize manipulation of the spinal cord.[54] Because many of these lesions involve the dorsal root, the dorsal root may need to be sacrificed; however, less than 23% of patients develop a recognizable neurologic deficit when this method is applied.[50, 95] A favorable outcome is predictable; in fact, 85% of patients are intact or improved at 6 months.[54, 92] Several factors are related to a poorer outcome, including advanced age, preoperative neurologic deficits, long duration of symptoms, subtotal tumor removal, extradural tumor extension, and increased calcification.[53, 54]

Meningiomas also present a difficult surgical problem with their typical extensive dural involvement and risk of recurrence. Overall recurrence has been estimated as negligible at 5 years and 13% at 10 years. Surgeons have addressed this problem in various ways. The rate of recurrence with dural resection has been estimated at 4% to 8%, versus 0% to 5.6% for coagulation of the dural margins presumed to be affected by tumor.[53, 65, 89]

Periodic postoperative follow-up is recommended with serial neurologic and MRI examinations. The typical appearance of the postoperative cervical spinal cord is notable atrophy above and below the level of surgery, dorsal tethering, and usually a residual smaller syrinx.[94] Postoperative plain films should also be obtained on follow-up to identify instability during the postoperative period. Reoperation should be considered for symptomatic recurrences.[95]

Surgical Alternatives

The use of radiation therapy is a much-debated issue. Of course, for tumors generally considered to be radioresistant, such as meningiomas, radiotherapy is not recommended.[8]

However, malignant astrocytomas should be aggressively radiated to include the entire spinal axis. The issue becomes more controversial with the low-grade gliomas. Some believe that because many patients improve with surgical treatment and because gliomas are indolent tumors, radiotherapy is not necessarily efficacious.[36] But in some series of primary spinal cord tumors, radiation therapy has increased tumor control and survival.[34] It has been well established that with complete resection of an intraspinal ependymoma, no further adjuvant treatment is recommended.[96] Some have advocated adjuvant radiotherapy in cases of astrocytoma or incomplete resection of ependymoma.[17, 35, 85, 106] The usual suggested dosage is 5500 cGy as a localized treatment. Epstein has suggested that with total removal of low-grade astrocytoma, radiotherapy appears to be unnecessary.[27] For hemangioblastomas, radiotherapy has not been proven curative; however, there are isolated reports of symptomatic relief.[9]

For recurrent meningiomas, an innovative treatment using the progesterone receptor antagonist Ru486 also may have a role. This and other potentially useful hormonal treatments may be available in the future.[8]

SUMMARY

Neoplasms of the cervical spinal cord represent daunting clinical and surgical challenges to the surgeon. Early diagnosis and treatment is paramount, with the primary goal of preserving neurologic function. The efficacy of surgery in managing intramedullary spinal cord lesions in particular is well established. With the use of microsurgical techniques and specially designed microinstruments, these lesions are no longer out of our surgical reach. Long-term tumor control and preservation of neurologic function are no longer mutually exclusive, but can be achieved as a result of the pioneering efforts of our predecessors. More information and experience are needed to completely define the role of surgery in the treatment of so-called benign astrocytomas (pilocytic astrocytomas) and the role of adjuvant radiotherapy in the treatment of high-grade lesions after surgical management.

REFERENCES

1. Adams DC, Emerson RG, Heyer EJ, et al: Monitoring of intraoperative motor-evoked potentials under conditions of controlled neuromuscular blockade. Anesth Analg 77:913–918, 1993.
2. Allen JC, Lassoff SJ: Outcome after surgery for intramedullary spinal cord tumors [letter]. Neurosurgery 26:1091, 1990.
3. Alvisi C, Cerisoli M, Giuliani M: Intramedullary spinal gliomas: Long-term results of surgical treatments. Acta Neurochir 70:169–179, 1984.
4. Anderson FM, Carson MJ: Spinal cord tumors in children: A review of the subject and presentation of 21 subjects. J Pediatr 43:190–207, 1953.
5. Anzil AP: Spinal cord pathology. Neurosurg Clin N Am 5:147–174, 1994.
6. Austin GM: The significance and nature of pain in tumors of the spinal cord. Surg Forum 10:782–785, 1959.
7. Barone BM, Elvidge AR: Ependymomas: A clinical survey. J Neurosurg 33:428–438, 1970.

8. Black PM: Meningiomas. Neurosurgery 32:643–657, 1993.

9. Browne TR, Adams RD, Roberson GH: Hemangioblastoma of the spinal cord: Review and report of five cases. Arch Neurol 33:435–441, 1976.

10. Bruner JM: Neuropathology of malignant gliomas. Semin Oncol 21:126–138, 1994.

11. Calvo FA, Hornedo J, de la Torre A, et al: Intracranial tumors with risk of dissemination in neuroaxis. Int J Radiat Oncol Biol Phys 9:1297–1301, 1983.

12. Christoferson LA, Gustafson MB, Petersen AG, et al: Von Hippel-Lindau's Disease. JAMA 178:280–282, 1961.

13. Ciappetta P, Salvati M, Capoccia G, et al: Spinal glioblastomas: Report of seven cases and review of the literature. Neurosurgery 28:302–306, 1991.

14. Cogen P, Stein BM: Spinal cord arteriovenous malformations with significant intramedullary components. J Neurosurg 59:471–478, 1983.

15. Cohen AR, Wisoff JH, Allen JC, Epstein F: Malignant astrocytomas of the spinal cord. J Neurosurg 70:50–54, 1989.

16. Cooper PR, Epstein F: Radical resection of intramedullary spinal cord tumors in adults. J Neurosurg 63:492–499, 1985.

17. Cooper PR: Outcome after operative treatment of intramedullary spinal cord tumors in adults: Intermediate and long-term results in 51 patients. Neurosurgery 25:855–859, 1989.

18. Costigan DA, Winkelman MD: Intramedullary spinal cord metastasis: A clinicopathological study of 13 cases. J Neurosurg 62:227–233, 1985.

19. Cushing H, Eisenhardt L: Meningiomas: Their Classification Regional Behavior, Life History and Surgical End Results. Springfield, IL, Charles C Thomas, 1969.

20. DeSousa AL, Kalsbeck JE, Mealey J, et al: Intraspinal tumors in children: A review of 81 cases. J Neurosurg 51:437–445, 1979.

21. Ducatman BS, Scheithauer BW, Piepgras DG, et al: Malignant peripheral nerve sheath tumors: A clinicopathologic study of 120 cases. Cancer 57:2006–2021, 1986.

22. Edelson RN, Deck MD, Posner JB: Intramedullary spinal cord metastasis: Clinical and radiographic findings in nine cases. Neurology 22:1222–1231, 1972.

23. Elsberg C: Diagnosis and Treatment of Surgical Diseases of the Spinal Cord and its Membranes. Philadelphia, WB Saunders, 1916.

24. Epstein FJ, Ozek M: The plated bayonet: A new instrument to facilitate surgery for intra-axial neoplasms of the spinal cord and brain stem. J Neurosurg 78:505, 1993.

25. Epstein FJ, Wisoff JH: Spinal cord astrocytoma of children and young adults. In Long DL (ed): Current Therapy in Neurological Surgery. New York, Marcel Dekker, 1985, pp 159–161.

26. Epstein FJ, Epstein N: Surgical treatment of spinal cord astrocytomas of childhood: A series of 19 patients. J Neurosurg 57:685–689, 1982.

27. Epstein FJ, Farmer JP, Freed D: Adult intramedullary astrocytomas of the spinal cord. J Neurosurg 77:355–359, 1992.

28. Epstein FJ, Farmer JP, Schneider SJ: Intraoperative ultrasonography: An important surgical adjunct for intramedullary tumors. J Neurosurg 74:729–733, 1991.

29. Fischer G, Mansuy L: Total removal of intramedullary ependymomas: Follow-up study of 16 cases. Surg Neurol 14:243–249, 1980.

30. Flamm ES, Ransohoff J, Wuchinich D, et al: Preliminary experience with ultrasonic aspiration in neurosurgery. Neurosurgery 2:240–245, 1978.

31. Fornari M, Pluchino F, Solero CL, et al: Microsurgical treatment of intramedullary spinal cord tumors. Acta Neurochir Suppl 43:3–8, 1988.

32. Frazier C: Surgery of the Spine and Spinal Cord. New York, Appleton, 1918.

33. Friede RL, Pollack A: The cytogenetic basis for classifying ependymomas. J Neuropathol Exp Neurol 37:103–118, 1978.

34. Garcia DM: Primary spinal cord tumors treated with surgery and postoperative irradiation. Int J Radiat Oncol Biol Phys 11:1933–1939, 1985.

35. Garrett PG, Simpson WJK: Ependymomas: Results of radiation treatment. Int J Radiat Oncol Biol Phys 9:1121–1124, 1983.

36. Garrido E, Stein BM: Microsurgical removal of intramedullary spinal cord tumors. Surg Neurol 7:215–219, 1977.

37. Gowers W, Horsley V: A case of tumor of the spinal cord. Removal. Recovery. Med Chir Trans 71:377–428, 1888.

38. Grant FC, Austin GM: The diagnosis, treatment, and prognosis of tumors affecting the spinal cord in children. J Neurosurg 13:535–545, 1956.

39. Greenwood J Jr: Surgical removal of intramedullary tumors. J Neurosurg 26:276–282, 1967.

40. Greenwood J Jr: Intramedullary tumors of spinal cord: A follow-up study after total surgical removal. J Neurosurg 20:665–668, 1963.

41. Guidetti B, Fortuna A: Surgical treatment of intramedullary hemangioblastoma of the spinal cord: Report of six cases. J Neurosurg 27:530–540, 1967.

42. Guidetti B, Mercuri S, Vagnozzi R: Long-term results of the surgical treatment of 129 intramedullary spinal gliomas. J Neurosurg 54:323–330, 1981.

43. Hackney DB: Neoplasms and related disorders. Top Magn Reson Imaging 4(2):37–61, 1992.

44. Haft H, Ransohoff J, Carter S: Spinal cord tumors in children. Pediatrics 23:1152–1159, 1954.

45. Hardison HH, Packer RJ, Rorke LB, et al: Outcome of children with primary intramedullary spinal cord tumors. Child's Nerv Syst 3:89–92, 1987.

46. Herrmann H, Neuss M, Winkler D: Intramedullary spinal cord tumors resected with CO_2 laser microsurgical technique: Recent experience in fifteen patients. Neurosurgery 22:518–522, 1988.

47. Hitchon PW, Haque AU, Olson JJ, et al: Sarcoidosis presenting as an intramedullary spinal cord mass. Neurosurgery 15:86–90, 1984.

48. Holtzman RN, Hughes JE, Sachdev RK, et al: Intramedullary cysticercosis. Surg Neurol 26:187–191, 1986.

49. Katz BH, Quencer RM, Hinks RS: Comparison of gradient-recalled-echo and T2-weighted spin-echo pulse sequences in intramedullary spinal lesions. Am J Neuroradiol 10:815–822, 1989.

50. Kim P, Ebersold MJ, Onofrio BM, et al: Surgery of spinal nerve schwannoma: Risk of neurological deficit after resection of involved root. J Neurosurg 71:810–814, 1989.

51. Koppel BS, Daras M, Duffy KR: Intramedullary spinal cord abscess. Neurosurgery 26:145–146, 1990.

52. Kurland LT: The frequency of intracranial and intraspinal neoplasms in the resident population of Rochester, Minnesota. J Neurosurg 15:627–641, 1958.

53. Levy WJ, Bay J, Dohn D: Spinal cord meningioma. J Neurosurg 57:804–812, 1982.

54. Levy WJ, Latchaw J, Hahn JF, et al: Spinal neurofibromas: A report of 66 cases and a comparison with menigiomas. Neurosurgery 18:331–334, 1986.

55. Li MH, Holtas S: MR imaging of spinal intramedullary tumors. Acta Radiol 32:505–513, 1991.

56. Listernick R, Charrow J: Neurofibromatosis type 1 in childhood. J Pediatr 116:845–853, 1990.

57. Liu HC, De Armond SJ, Edwards MSB: An unusual spinal meningioma in a child: Case report. Neurosurgery 17:313–316, 1985.

58. Malis LI: Intramedullary spinal cord tumors. Clin Neurosurg 25:512–540, 1978.

59. Mapstone TB: Neurofibromatosis and central nervous system tumors in childhood. Neurosurg Clin N Am 3:771–779, 1992.

60. Marks JE, Adler SJ: A comparative study of ependymomas by site of origin. Int J Radiat Oncol Biol Phys 8:37–43, 1982.

61. Masaryk TJ: Neoplastic disease of the spine. Radiol Clin N Am 29:829–845, 1991.

62. McCormick PC, Michelsen WJ, Post KD, et al: Cavernous malformations of the spinal cord. Neurosurgery 23:459–463, 1988.

63. McCormick PC, Torres R, Post KD, et al: Intramedullary ependymoma of the spinal cord. J Neurosurg 72:523–532, 1990.

64. McCormick PC: Anatomic principles of intradural spinal surgery. Clin Neurosurg 41:204–223, 1994.

65. Mirimanoff RO, Dosoretz DE, Linggood RM, et al: Meningioma: analysis of recurrence and progression following neurosurgical resection. J Neurosurg 62:18–24, 1985.

66. Mulvihill JJ, Parry DM, Sherman JL, et al: Neurofibromatosis 1 (Recklinghausen disease) and neurofibromatosis 2 (bilateral acoustic neurofibromatosis): An update. Ann Intern Med 113:39–52, 1990.

67. Murovic J, Sundaresan N: Pediatric spinal axis tumors. Neurosurg Clin N Am 3:947–958, 1992.

68. Mork SJ, Loken AC: Ependymoma: A follow-up study of 101 cases. Cancer 40:907–915, 1977.

69. Nabors MW, Pait TG, Byrd EB, et al: Updated assessment and current classification of spinal meningeal cysts. J Neurosurg 68:366–377, 1988.

70. Neumann HP, Eggert HR, Weigel K, et al: Hemangioblastomas of the central nervous system: A 10-year study with special reference to von Hippel-Lindau syndrome. J Neurosurg 70:24–30, 1989.

71. Olson ME, Chernik NL, Posner JB: Infiltration of the leptomeninges by systemic cancer: A clinical and pathologic study. Arch Neurol 30:122–137, 1974.

72. Onofrio BM: Intradural extramedullary spinal cord tumors. Clin Neurosurg 25:540–555, 1978.

73. Pasaoglu A, Patiroglu TE, Orhon C, et al: Cervical spinal intramedullary myxoma in childhood: Case report. J Neurosurg 69:772–774, 1988.

74. Perrin RG, Livingston KE, Aarabi B: Intradural extramedullary spinal metastasis: A report of 10 cases. J Neurosurg 56:835–837, 1982.

75. Post MJ, Quencer RM, Green BA, et al: Intramedullary spinal cord metastases, mainly of nonneurogenic origin. Am J Roentgenol 148:1015–1022, 1987.

76. Rawlings CE, Giangaspero F, Burger PC, et al: Ependymomas: A clinicopathologic study. Surg Neurol 29:271–281, 1988.

77. Reimer R, Onofrio BM: Astrocytomas of the spinal cord in children and adolescents. J Neurosurg 63:669–675, 1985.

78. Ross AT, Bailey OT: Tumors arising within the spinal canal in children. Neurology 3:922–930, 1953.

79. Ross DA, Edwards MS, Wilson CB: Intramedullary neurilemomas of the spinal cord: Report of two cases and review of the literature. Neurosurgery 19:458–464, 1986.

80. Ross GW, Rubinstein LJ: Lack of histopathological correlation of malignant ependymomas with postoperative survival. J Neurosurg 70:31–36, 1989.

81. Salazar OM, Rubin P, Bassano D, et al: Improved survival of patients with intracranial ependymomas by irradiation: Dose selection and field extension. Cancer 35:1563–1573, 1975.

82. Salvati M, Artico M, Lunardi P, et al: Intramedullary meningioma: Case report and review of the literature. Surg Neurol 37:42–45, 1992.

83. Sandler HM, Papadopoulos SM, Thornton AF, et al: Spinal cord astrocytomas: Results of therapy. Neurosurgery 30:490–493, 1992.

84. Schijman E, Zuccaro G, Monges JA: Spinal tumors and hydrocephalus. Child's Brain 8:401–405, 1981.

85. Schwade JG, Wara WM, Sheline GE, et al: Management of primary spinal cord tumors. Int J Radiat Oncol Biol Phys 4:389–393, 1978.

86. Scotti G, Scialfa G, Colombo N, et al: Magnetic resonance diagnosis of intramedullary tumors of the spinal cord. Neuroradiology 29:130–135, 1987.

87. Shaw EG, Evans RG, Scheithauer BW, et al: Radiotherapeutic management of adult intraspinal ependymomas. Int J Radiat Oncol Biol Phys 12:323–327, 1986.

88. Sloof JL, Kernohan JW, MacCarty CS: Primary Intramedullary Tumors of the Spinal Cord and Filum Terminale. Philadelphia, WB Saunders, 1964.

89. Solero CL, Fornari M, Giombini S, et al: Spinal meningiomas: Review of 174 operated cases. Neurosurgery 25:153–160, 1989.

90. Solomon RA, Stein BM: Unusual spinal cord enlargement related to intramedullary hemangioblastoma. J Neurosurg 68:550–553, 1988.

91. Sonneland PR, Scheithauer BW, Onofrio BM: Myxopapillary ependymoma: A clinicopathologic and immunocytochemical study of 77 cases. Cancer 56:883–893, 1985.

92. Souweidane MM, Benjamin V: Spinal cord meningiomas. Neurosurg Clin N Am 5:283–291, 1994.

93. Spurling RG, Mayfield FH: Neoplasms of the spinal cord: A review of forty-two surgical cases. JAMA 107:924–929, 1936.

94. Stein BM, McCormick PC: Intramedullary neoplasms and vascular malformations. Clin Neurosurg 39:361–387, 1992.

95. Stein BM: Surgery of intramedullary spinal cord tumors. Clin Neurosurg 26:529–542, 1979.

96. Steinbok P, Cochrane DD, Poskitt K: Intramedullary spinal cord tumors in children. Neurosurg Clin N Am 3:931–945, 1992.

97. Svien HJ, Thelen EP, Keith HM: Intraspinal tumors in children. JAMA 155:959–961, 1954.

98. Sze G, Krol G, Zimmerman RD, et al: Intramedullary disease of the spine: Diagnosis using gadolinium-DTPA-enhanced MR imaging. Am J Roentgenol 151:1193–1204, 1988.

99. Sze G: Magnetic resonance imaging in the evaluation of spinal tumors. Cancer 67:1229–1240, 1991.

100. Sørensen SA, Mulvihill JJ, Nielsen A: Long-term follow-up of von Recklinghausen neurofibromatosis: Survival and malignant neoplasms. N Engl J Med 314:1010–1015, 1986.

101. Tachdjian MO, Matson DD: Orthopaedic aspects of intraspinal tumors in infants and children. J Bone Joint Surg Am 47A:223–248, 1965.

102. Thomas JE, Miller RH: Lipomatous tumors of the spinal canal: A study of their clinical range. Mayo Clin Proc 48:393–400, 1973.

103. Warf BC, Scott RM: Spinal cord astrocytomas. In Black PM, Schoene WC, Lampson LA (eds): Contemporary Issues in Neurological Surgery: Astrocytomas: Diagnosis, Treatment,

and Biology. Boston: Blackwell Scientific, 1993, pp 202–208.

104. West CR, Bruce DA, Duffner PK: Ependymomas: Factors in clinical and diagnostic staging. Cancer 56:1812–1816, 1985.

105. Winkelman MD, Adelstein DJ, Karlins NL: Intramedullary spinal cord metastasis: Diagnostic and therapeutic considerations. Arch Neurol 44:526–531, 1987.

106. Wood EH, Berne AS, Taveras JM: The value of radiation therapy in the management of intrinsic tumors of the spinal cord. Radiology 63:11–24, 1954.

107. Yasui T, Hakuba A, Katsuyama J, et al: Microsurgical removal of intramedullary spinal cord tumours: Report of 22 cases. Acta Neurochir Suppl 43:9–12, 1988.

108. Zide BM, Wisoff JH, Epstein FJ: Closure of extensive and complicated laminectomy wounds: Operative technique. J Neurosurg 67:59–64, 1987.

109. Zide BM: How to reduce the morbidity of wound closure following extensive and complicated laminectomy and tethered cord surgery. Pediatr Neurosurg 18:157–166, 1992.

Inflammatory Disorders

15

RHEUMATOID ARTHRITIS OF THE CERVICAL SPINE

Sanford E. Emery, M.D.
Scott D. Boden, M.D.

*One thought driven home is better
than three left on base.*
— James Liter

HISTORICAL PERSPECTIVE

For many years, rheumatoid arthritis was believed to have developed as a disease around 1800 (with a description by Landré-Beauvais, a French medical student, in his doctoral thesis),[50] which is quite recent from a historical perspective. This viewpoint was supported by the lack of confirmed rheumatoid findings in ancient archeologic specimens, which is in contradistinction to skeletal remains from Egyptian mummies that are definitive for ankylosing spondylitis.[4, 46] More recently, however, some authors have found descriptions that they believe to be consistent with rheumatoid arthritis dating back to the 17th and 18th centuries.[23, 48]

Although perhaps recognized as early as 1890 by Garrod in his *Treatise on Rheumatism and Rheumatoid Arthritis,*[18] rheumatoid cervical spine instability was first specifically addressed in the spine literature by several authors in the 1950s and 1960s.[29, 38, 39, 52, 55] Most of these papers focused on the description of atlantoaxial instability. The surgical treatment of this problem followed closely, with several series published in the 1960s and 1970s.[5, 14, 22, 33, 40] For decades, Gallie-type wiring with bone grafting or cement has been used for posterior stabilization.[17] The Brooks wiring plus bone graft technique, first reported in 1978, has also been a popular fusion method for C1–C2.[6] More recently, interlaminar clamps and especially the transarticular screw technique of Magerl have provided better fixation for atlantoaxial stability.[21]

Occipitocervical procedures were first reported by Foerster in 1927 in the German literature.[16] The first paper describing the use of an iliac crest bone graft for occipitocervical fusion was that of Kahn and Yglesias in 1935.[26] Early small series of patients undergoing this procedure for diagnoses including congenital anomalies and posttraumatic instability began to appear in the 1950s.[28, 37] Hamblen used wire plus iliac crest bone grafting for occipitocervical fusion in 13 patients.[22] Four of these patients had upper cervical spine instability from rheumatoid arthritis. Brattström and Granholm described this procedure with wire fixation and methylmethacrylate in 1976.[5] Subsequent reports using wiring and graft techniques include those of Wertheim and Bohlman in 1987[53] and Clark and colleagues in 1989.[8] The addition of internal fixation to bone grafting appeared in the late 1980s, with reports of an occipitocervical looped rod wired into place by Ransford and coworkers[42] and a similar construct described by Flint et al.[15] Occipitocervical plating has become popular after descriptions by Grob et al[20] and Smith et al.[49] Many of these techniques were not initially described for patients with rheumatoid arthritis, but have been adapted to treat upper cervical spine instability in these patients.

PATHOPHYSIOLOGY

The pathophysiologic hallmark of rheumatoid arthritis includes synovial inflammation, pannus formation, and erosions of the joint and periarticular soft tissue structures. The cervical spine relies heavily on soft tissue integrity for stability; thus inflammation of the ligament and capsular structures can result in various types of instability, more so than in the thoracic or lumbar spine. Instability can cause root impingement, leading to radiculopathy, or, more commonly, spinal cord compression, resulting in myelopathy. The atlanto-dens articulation is a synovial joint, and pannus formation here can destroy the transverse ligament or erode the dens itself. Either problem can result in atlantoaxial instability. Destruction of the lateral masses of C1 resulting in bone loss allows vertical migration of C2 up into the skull. Termed *basilar invagination,* this complication can produce brain stem compression. In the subaxial spine, all facet joints are true synovial joints, and the same inflammatory destructive processes can result in subaxial subluxation at one level or multiple levels. Although rheumatoid arthritis does not specifically affect the disks because they are not synovial joints, affected patients can have concomitant cervical spondylosis in the subaxial spine, which may contribute to pain, neural compression, or instability.

CLINICAL PRESENTATION

Neck pain is usually present in patients developing instability from rheumatoid disease. Suboccipital pain suggests atlantoaxial pathology or basilar invagination. Middle or lower cervical spine pain is typically from subaxial subluxation, although pain localization in any given patient may be poor. Arm pain consistent with radiculopathy or nerve root compression may also be present from subaxial instability or routine spondylosis. Symptoms and signs of cervical myelopathy may be straightforward, but more often than not are subtle in this patient population. Rather than manifesting gait imbalance, loss of fine motor control in the upper extremities, or global numbness of the hands, the patient with rheumatoid disease may simply exhibit slow deterioration in independence and become wheelchair-bound. Often, hand deformities mask motor deficits in the distal upper extremities. A patient who becomes increasingly dependent on a cane, then a walker, and then a wheelchair may be misdiagnosed as having increasing arthritic symptoms in the major joints when he or she actually has myelopathy manifesting as a decreasing ability to ambulate. A high index of suspicion for cervical myelopathy must be maintained by physicians caring for this patient population. Brain stem compression from basilar invagination or C1–C2 instability may produce respiratory or cranial nerve symptoms including dysphagia and nystagmus, although one study suggested that this is uncommon.[45]

Neurologic examination of the patient with severe rheumatoid arthritis can be difficult. Motor testing can be complicated by joint destruction or contractures in both the upper and lower extremities. Previous surgical procedures, such as wrist or ankle fusion, may obviate the usual testing of certain muscle groups. Every effort should be made to patiently test motor, sensory, and reflex function, looking mainly for long-tract signs, such as hyperreflexia, Babinski's sign, Hoffmann's sign, and clonus, that may suggest cervical myelopathy.

DIAGNOSTIC EVALUATION

Three main diagnoses result from rheumatoid disease in the neck: (1) C1–C2 instability, (2) basilar invagination, and (3) subaxial subluxation. All three of these diagnoses can usually be made or at least suspected with plain x-rays. The lateral cervical spine view, including flexion and extension views, is the most helpful. This can detect static and/or dynamic instability in the upper or lower cervical spine. It is important to determine whether a subluxation is fixed or dynamic. If cord compression exists with a fixed deformity, then anterior decompression may be necessary to relieve the neurologic compromise. If neural compression is present only in flexion, as in dynamic instability, then a simpler posterior fusion in extension when the subluxation is reduced can reestablish the canal, eliminate the cord impingement, and successfully treat the patient. Open-mouth odontoid views may show erosive changes of the C1–C2 articulations or even erosion of the dens. Plain tomography is an excellent way to examine the patho-anatomy of the upper cervical spine, but this has largely been replaced by computed tomography (CT) scans with coronal and sagittal reconstruction techniques.

Atlantoaxial instability is usually well seen on plain flexion-extension lateral x-rays. Measurements of the anterior atlanto-dens interval (AADI) and the posterior atlanto-dens interval (PADI) can be obtained. The AADI, the distance from the anterior ring of the atlas to the anterior cortex of the odontoid, should be no more than 3.5 mm in adults. The PADI is measured from the posterior cortex of the odontoid to the inner cortex of the posterior ring of the atlas. This represents the space available for the cord as defined by the bony elements. A PADI of 14 mm or less indicates increased risk of cord compression and myelopathy.[3] One must keep in mind that soft tissue pannus behind the odontoid may contribute to cord compression; thus the space available for the cord may actually be less than is evident on plain films. Neuroradiologic investigation, such as magnetic resonance imaging (MRI), is needed to more accurately define the pathoanatomy.

Several measurements have been described using lateral plain x-rays to define basilar invagination (Fig. 15–1). These measurements generally involve the relationship of the odontoid and the base of the skull or some anatomic landmark in the C2 body in relationship to the foramen magnum. If the dens can be visualized on plain x-ray, then we prefer the simplicity of McGregor's line, a line drawn from the hard palate to the posterior base of the skull. If the dens is above this line, then basilar invagination exists. The measurement of Redlund-Johnell[43] is useful if the dens cannot be visualized due to overlapping shadows. Riew and colleagues suggested that no single radiographic method has a high sensitivity and specificity and only a combination of

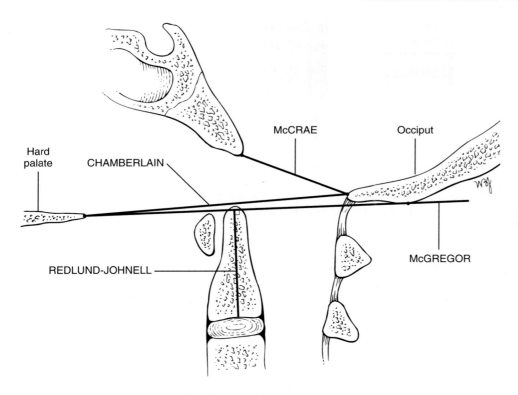

Figure 15–1. *Drawing of lines for measurements of basilar invagination. Chamberlain's line: odontoid tip > 6 mm above the line. McCrae's line: odontoid tip above this line. McGregor's line: males, odontoid tip > 8 mm above the line; females, odontoid tip > 9.7 mm above the line. Redlund–Johnell distance: males, < 34 mm; females, < 29 mm.*

three methods is highly predictive.[43a] If plain x-rays cannot rule out the diagnosis, then CT imaging with sagittal reconstructions or MRI scanning are in order. MRI is also important for visualization of the brain stem, because severe invagination can result in anterior brain stem compression.[10] A cervical-medullary angle, which can be measured from the sagittal MRI scan, is obtained by drawing a line along the brain stem longitudinally and a second line along the cervical cord. An angle of these intersecting lines of less than 135 degrees (i.e., the brain stem is draped over the odontoid) indicates increased risk of neurologic symptoms.[7] If MRI is not possible, CT-myelography will provide satisfactory evaluation of neural compression.

Plain lateral x-rays along with flexion-extension views can be useful in determining the bony space available for the spinal cord in the subaxial spine. Measurements from the back of the vertebral body to the interlaminar line define the spinal canal. Subluxations in rheumatoid disease decrease the canal size and can cause cord compression with myelopathy, as discussed earlier. A subaxial cervical spinal canal diameter of 12 mm or less often heralds cord compression and myelopathy in patients with cervical spondylosis;[12] in patients with rheumatoid disease, 14 mm is a better warning level, because of the possible presence of soft tissue pannus.

INDICATIONS FOR SURGERY

Reasons for recommending surgery in this patient population generally can be categorized as (1) pain, (2) neurologic dysfunction, and (3) abnormal radiographic parameters. Any one of these categories can be a sound indication for surgical intervention, but in most patients two or more are present. Pain not associated with instability usually can be managed nonoperatively. Treatment includes intermittent use of a soft collar for immobilization, administration of nonsteroidal anti-inflammatory drugs, and trials of physical therapy. If instability exists, then surgical stabilization may be indicated to successfully treat the painful motion segment. Significant pain without neurologic deficit most commonly occurs in atlantoaxial instability.

Although neural compression can present as radicular symptoms in the arm with pain, weakness, or numbness, more typically these patients have spinal cord compression and myelopathy because of the instability patterns noted earlier. Clinical evidence of cervical myelopathy generally is an indication for operative intervention. Because spinal cord compression in the upper cervical spine with true instability can result in sudden death, appropriate intervention is very important.[34] Ranawat's classification of neurologic deficit in the rheumatoid population is still used and has some predictive value regarding the outcome after surgery (Table 15–1).[41] The preoperative severity of myelopathy is one of the better predictors of recovery in other patient populations,[12] and this holds true for the patients with rheumatoid disease as well. Ranawat class III patients tend to have less recovery and more morbidity after operative treatment. Thus, early myelopathy evident on clinical examination with gait imbalance, long-tract signs, or frank weakness with corroborative cord compression on radiographic studies are indications for operative intervention to halt the neurologic deterioration and promote recovery.

Boden et al. analyzed radiographic parameters associated with increased risk of paralysis in 42 patients with

Table 15–1. *Ranawat Classification for Patients with Rheumatoid Arthritis Involving the Cervical Spine*

Class	Definition
I	No neural deficits
II	Subjective findings of weakness with hyperreflexia and dysesthesia
IIIA	Objective findings of weakness and long tract signs Able to ambulate
IIIB	Objective findings of weakness and long tract signs Not able to ambulate

rheumatoid arthritis.[3] Radiographic measurements of C1–C2 instability were performed and compared with postoperative neurologic recovery. For C1–C2 instability, AADI was traditionally the measurement of interest, to quantify the degree of instability present. But Boden's study showed that the more useful radiographic measurement is the PADI. Because patients have different-sized C1 rings, the PADI is a more accurate representation of space available for the spinal cord. A PADI of 14 mm demarcates neurologically intact patients from those in whom paralysis has developed (Fig. 15–2). It should again be emphasized that neuroradiologic imaging should be performed to identify pannus behind the odontoid that may contribute to cord compression not identifiable on plain x-ray, but the PADI is a straightforward screening measurement on flexion-extension lateral plain x-rays that can be quite helpful.

Indications for operative treatment of basilar invagination usually fall under the categories of pain and/or paralysis, as noted earlier. One radiographic measurement on sagittal MRI, the cervical medullary angle, has been correlated with an increased risk of paralysis in one study. An angle between the brain stem and the upper cervical cord of less than 135 degrees connotes brain stem compression by the dens. We consider this measurement to be a relative indication for surgical intervention, and it needs to be considered with the entire clinical picture for that particular patient.

OPERATIVE TREATMENT
Atlantoaxial (C1–C2) Instability

Posterior C1–C2 arthrodesis techniques can be categorized as (1) wiring techniques, (2) hook–claw constructs, and (3) transarticular screws. Bone graft plus wiring has been performed for decades with satisfactory results, although it does require more rigid postoperative immobilization. Claw-type instrumentation constructs, such as the Halifax clamp, have been used successfully by some authors but have not gained wide acceptance. This type of fixation may provide resistance to flexion but does not do as well in resisting translation or extension. More recently, transarticular screw fixation has been described for rigid C1–C2 fixation and is becoming increasingly popular for rheumatoid as well as nonrheumatoid populations. Here we describe two common wiring techniques, along with transarticular screw fixation.

Modified Gallie-Type Wiring Plus Bone Graft

The basis of this technique was described in 1939 for cervical spine fractures (Fig. 15–3).[17] It provides stable, though not rigid, fixation and is fairly straightforward to perform. Wire fixation is obtained on the ring of C1 and at the base of the spinous process of C2. Corticocancellous blocks of iliac crest–bone graft are wired into place in direct contact with C1 and C2 laminae. We have seen loss of reduction using this technique plus a two-poster–type brace. Thus, if maintaining an adequate PADI by reduction of C1 were critical, then we would recommend a halo vest postoperatively. In the unusual case in which the ring of C1 subluxes in a posterior direction, then one must be careful when tightening the wires in the modified Gallie technique, because this will tend to draw the ring of C1 posteriorly; a

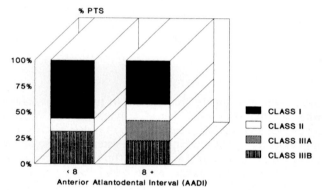

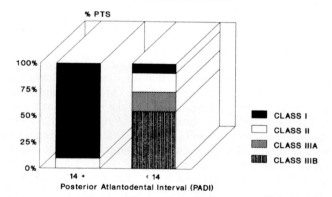

Figure 15–2. *Prediction of the development of paralysis in 73 patients who had rheumatoid arthritis. Although the anterior atlanto-odontoid interval (AADI) did not correlate well with paralysis (p > 0.10), a posterior atlanto-odontoid interval (PADI) of 14 mm clearly demarcated neurologically intact patients (Class I) from those in whom paralysis developed (Classes II and III) (p = 0.000001). (From Boden SD, Dodge LD, Bohlman HH, Rechtine GR: Rheumatoid arthritis of the cervical spine: A long-term analysis with predictors of paralysis and recovery. J Bone Joint Surg Am 75A:1288, 1993, Fig. 2.)*

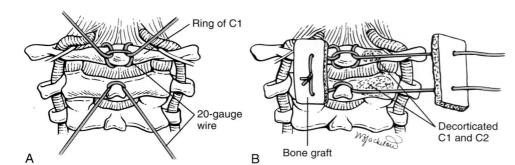

Figure 15–3. *Modified Gallie-type wiring for a posterior C1–C2 arthrodesis.*

Ring of C1

20-gauge wire

Bone graft

Decorticated C1 and C2

A

B

Brooks wiring technique may be more appropriate in this situation.[6]

In the rheumatoid population dealing with instability and neural compression, careful induction of anesthesia and positioning of the head on the operating table are particularly important. A tong-type head holder is helpful to rigidly fix the skull and neck. The amount of flexion or extension can be adjusted to obtain reduction of the atlantoaxial instability. Tucking of the chin to open the occiput–C1 ring interspace is an important step; this space is needed to facilitate passing the sublaminar wire under the ring of C1. Note that if sufficient reduction of the C1 ring to provide an adequate posterior space available for the cord cannot be achieved, or if sufficient room to allow safe wire passage is not obtained, then a C1 laminectomy should be performed and the procedure changed to an occipitocervical arthrodesis.

A posterior exposure is used with careful adherence to the midline to minimize bleeding. Exposure of the base of the skull, the ring of C1, and the lamina of C2 using Cobb elevators is the minimum field needed. C1 should be exposed only 1½ to 2 cm to each side of the midline, to avoid brisk bleeding from lateral veins and the underlying vertebral arteries. Small curettes are used to develop the plane under the ring of C1 for wire passage. A 20-gauge wire is looped and the tip contoured so as to safely pass it under the ring. The loop is hooked with a small nerve hook, and pulled through by approximately 2 cm. The free ends of the 20-gauge wire are then fed through the loop, and the wire is cinched down tightly onto the ring of C1 in the midline. The ends of this wire are then tagged to hold them out of the field. A bur hole is made at the base of the spinous

process of C2, and a second 20-gauge wire is passed through this hole and looped on itself to provide some stress distribution.

Two rectangular corticocancellous bone blocks are then harvested from the iliac crest. We prefer autogenous bone graft to provide the best chance of successful arthrodesis. Near–full-thickness crest blocks enable tightening of the wires over the cortical surface to provide good bony contact as well as stability. The wires are twisted down on each side in a vertical fashion so they begin cutting through the cortical surface of the graft. Cancellous chips can be placed in the crevices, with particular care taken to ensure bony contact onto the ring of C1, because nonunions tend to occur here. A drain is typically used, and the wound is closed in layers. Postoperative immobilization can be in a rigid brace or halo vest, depending on the degree of instability, as noted earlier.

Brooks-Type Fusion

This wiring technique differs from the modified Gallie technique in that it uses left-sided and right-sided sublaminar wires passing under C2 as well as C1 (Fig. 15–4).[6] Positioning and exposure is as described for the modified Gallie technique. A laminotomy is needed between C2 and C3; 20-gauge sublaminar wires are fed under C2 and C1 first on one side, then on the other. A suture passer can help facilitate this technique, because the distance is greater than that under C1 alone. Typically, the 20-gauge wire is left doubled on each side. Corticocancellous bone blocks are fashioned from the iliac crest so as to lie on top of the C1 and C2 laminae. Careful carpentering of the bone block is

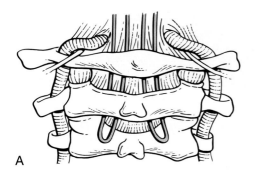

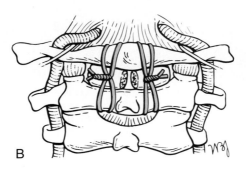

Figure 15–4. *Brooks-type wiring for a posterior C1–C2 arthrodesis. Sublaminar wires are passed under both C1 and C2 (A) and are tightened down over wedge-shaped, sculpted corticocancellous grafts (B). The shaping of the grafts minimizes the chance of graft displacement into the canal.*

A

B

needed to avoid graft slippage into the C1–C2 interspace. The wires are then tightened down in a longitudinal fashion over the bone block without actually passing through the block. This is also done on the opposite side and should provide stable fixation and good bony contact. This provides slightly more rotational stability than the modified Gallie technique because of the left- and right-sided wire fixation. As noted before, if maintenance of reduction is critical, then we recommend concomitant use of a halo vest postoperatively.

Transarticular C1–C2 Screws

This technique involves bilateral screws traversing the C2 isthmus from a posterior to anterior direction and crossing the C1–C2 joint, exiting in front of the C1 ring (Fig. 15–5).[21] It provides more rigid fixation of the C1–C2 motion segment and can be combined with the previously described wiring techniques. It is a more demanding operative technique that requires thorough knowledge of the pertinent anatomy and high-quality intraoperative biplanar fluoroscopy. An anomalous vertebral artery resulting in an isthmus too narrow for a 3.5- or 4.0-mm screw precludes the use of this fixation method; patients need to be screened preoperatively with a sagittal CT scan to identify this situation. Unreducible subluxations, obscure anatomic landmarks, or severe upper thoracic kyphosis may also preclude the use of this technique.

Positioning of the patient's head and neck is the same as in the previously described wiring techniques; however, the arm attachment from the tongs to the operating table is ideally radiolucent, to facilitate anteroposterior fluoroscopic imaging. A longer incision may be needed than used in simple wiring techniques to obtain a correct angle for drilling and screw placement. A percutaneous stab wound can also be made in the distal cervical region with long drill guides to help achieve the appropriate angle. The starting point for K-wire insertion is the junction of the lamina and the facet joint of C2 in the mediolateral direction and the inferior edge of the lamina–facet junction in the cephalad-caudad direction. The proposed starting point should be checked with fluoroscopy in two planes to ensure its appropriateness. A small indentation or hole can be made with a tiny bur. A thin guidewire is then driven under x-ray guidance across the C2 isthmus. This guidewire should hug the superior cortex of the isthmus, to minimize the risk of cutting out inferiorly into the area of the vertebral artery. The guidewire should aim at the anterior central prominence of the ring of C1 evident on the lateral view. On the anteroposterior view, the guidewire should be parallel to the cord or angled slightly laterally. Visualization of the facets, such as is seen with a standard open-mouth odontoid view, is needed to ensure safe placement. Some authors recommend performing a laminotomy between C1 and C2 and palpating the C2 pedicle to localize the medial wall; this is helpful if anteroposterior x-ray views are less than ideal. The guidewire is driven just into the anterior cortex of C1, which, because of the convexity of the anterior C1 ring, is short of the midline prominence evident on the lateral x-ray view. The surgeon can do this initial step with a drill rather than a guide pin; however, the newer cannulated instrumentation greatly facilitates this technique and is recommended. Sequential drilling, tapping, and placing a 3.5- or 4-mm

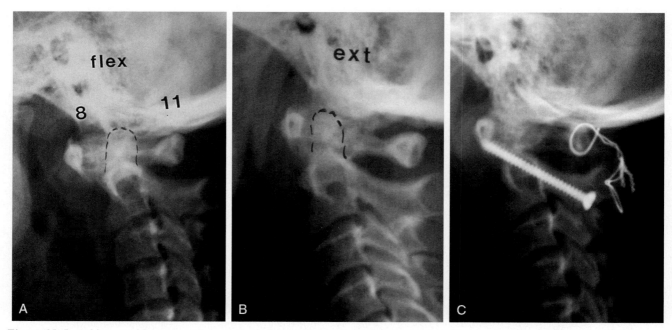

Figure 15–5. *A 23-year-old female with juvenile rheumatoid arthritis had a history of neck pain without neurologic deficit. A lateral cervical spine flexion view (A) shows C1–C2 instability with an anterior AADI of 8 mm and a PADI of 11 mm. Extension (B) results in satisfactory reduction. The patient was treated operatively with transarticular screws, wiring, and autogenous bone grafting (C). A soft collar was used postoperatively because of her body habitus and excellent intraoperative fixation. She healed uneventfully with resolution of her neck pain.*

cannulated screw, usually 40 to 44 mm in length, are performed sequentially with x-ray supervision. Care must be taken to avoid driving the guide pin into the soft tissues of the oropharynx. The technique is repeated on the opposite side. We prefer autogenous bone grafting with a modified Gallie technique to provide good bony contact and added stability for the construct. Because this is a more rigid technique, less rigid postoperative external immobilization is usually needed, depending on the surgeon's assessment of the fixation and bone quality. Where excellent fixation has been achieved, a soft collar may be sufficient.

Occipital-Cervical Fusion

This technique involves arthrodesis of the skull to the cervical spine, typically C2 or lower. It is the principal surgical option for the treatment of basilar invagination in the rheumatoid population, because it arrests any further vertical migration of the cervical spine into the foramen magnum. It is also used in patients who have a fixed atlantoaxial subluxation causing dorsal cord impingement from the posterior ring of C1; in these patients, a C1 laminectomy followed by occipitocervical fusion is usually the procedure of choice. Long corticocancellous rectangles of autogenous iliac crest bone graft can be wired into place and, with orthotic postoperative immobilization such as a halo vest, good results have been obtained.[32, 53]

The use of instrumentation has been increasing. This provides increased stability and can decrease the need for halo vest immobilization postoperatively. We prefer occipitocervical plating done bilaterally,[19, 25, 47, 49] though other authors have used rod-loop plus wiring constructs with reported success.[13, 29a, 35, 42] Regardless of the specific type of instrumentation used, occipitocervical arthrodesis requires thorough knowledge of the anatomy and experience with these procedures, particularly when using instrumentation.

Technique of Occipitocervical Fusion. Typically, the patient is placed in a three-prong head holder for rigid immobilization. Intraoperative traction may be needed in severe cases of basilar invagination. For a patient with all levels of the subaxial cervical spine included in the arthrodesis, care should be taken to ensure the patient is looking straight ahead, because he or she will be in that fixed position postoperatively. In this situation, a halo vest can be placed to allow for minor adjustments to ensure a straight-ahead gaze, followed by a pancervical arthrodesis while the patient is still in the anterior shell of the halo vest. The posterior shell is replaced immediately after the operation at which time the head–neck relationship will not have changed.

A midline exposure is performed to expose the base of the skull and as many levels in the cervical spine as needed. The occiput is exposed up to the external occipital protuberance, which is the bony prominence in the midline approximately 5 to 7 cm from the base of the occiput. This protuberance is the site for wire purchase. A unicortical tunnel with a bridge of superficial cortical bone is made using a bur to initiate the tunnel from each side, followed by a towel clamp to complete the tunnel within the tables of the skull. A 20-gauge wire is passed through this tunnel and fed through again so as to loop around this cortical bony bridge. Another wire can be passed under the ring of C1 and looped onto itself and cinched around the ring, providing that the posterior arch of C1 has not been removed for decompression purposes. A wire is then fed through the base of the spinous process of C2, looped onto itself to distribute this stress, and pulled tightly. Other wires can be used more distally as needed at the base of the spinous processes.

Long corticocancellous rectangles of near–full-thickness iliac crests are then harvested from the patient's pelvis. Typically these are 9 to 10 cm long and 1.5 cm wide. A small (1.5-mm) drill bit is used to place holes in these corticocancellous grafts. The wires are passed through these holes, with the cancellous side of the graft facing downward onto the skull and the lamina. The opposite-side corticocancellous rectangle is then placed in a similar fashion. The grafts are carefully and firmly pressed down onto the base of the skull and the laminae of C2, or more distally if a longer graft has been used. The left and right ends of the occipital wire are then twisted together to secure the grafts to the base of the skull. The natural concavity of the iliac crest provides for excellent contact with the occiput and the cervical lamina. The two wires on the left from C1 and C2 are twisted together, and then the two wires on the right are twisted together in a vertical fashion. This construct provides stable fixation, particularly in patients with good-quality iliac bone. Extra cancellous bone can be packed in the crevices. The wound is then closed in layers, typically over a small suction drain. For this technique of wiring plus bone graft, some patients can be successfully placed in a two-poster brace, but most will require halo vest immobilization for maximum stability.

Technique of Occipitocervical Plating. Internal fixation for occipitocervical fusion is a useful adjunct in the rheumatoid population (Fig. 15–6). Even in patients with significant osteoporosis, excellent fixation can be obtained in the occiput, with the limitations of fixation depending on the distal cervical levels.

Originally, occipitocervical platings were performed using acetabular reconstruction-type plates, which allowed for contouring.[49] Several manufacturers have developed plating systems, and plate-rod hybrid implants are also available. Contouring of the implant is important and requires a large bend near the base of the skull. If a long plate or rod construct is used, then fixation into C2 and the lower vertebrae first, followed by skull fixation, is recommended, because these more distal points of fixation require more precise anatomic location. If possible, a C1–C2 transarticular screw can be placed at this level to provide maximum purchase. However, C2 pedicle screws can also provide excellent C2 fixation. The technique of transarticular screw fixation was described earlier, and lateral mass fixation for the distal cervical levels is described for subaxial fusion techniques later in this chapter. A C2 pedicle screw is similar to a transarticular screw placement, but requires a more superior and lateral starting point, slight medial angulation, and less cephalad direction for the screw.

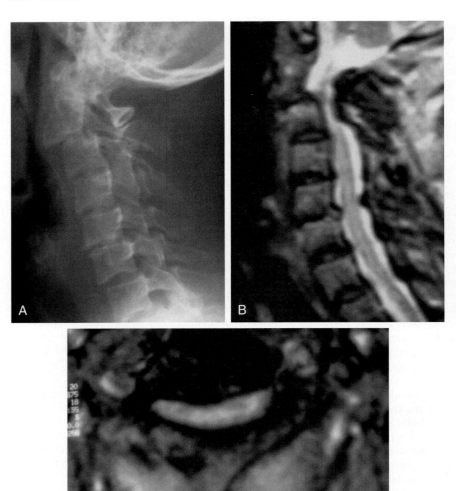

Figure 15–6. This 46-year-old female had a long history of rheumatoid arthritis since she was a young girl. She has had chronic neck pain but developed worsening pain over the past 6 weeks with increasing numbness of her arms and some truncal numbness. Some weakness of her upper extremities was evident on physical examination. Her plain lateral x-ray (A) shows C2–C3 subluxation with a fixed C1–C2 deformity. She had multiple levels of subluxation on flexion-extension views, including C7–T1. Her MRI (B and C) showed severe cord compression at the C2–C3 level.

Fixation to the skull requires knowledge of the venous sinus anatomy to prevent bleeding complications. The transverse sinuses lie at the level of the external occipital protuberance; all screws should be placed distal to this region. The thickness of the skull decreases farther from the midline and closer to the foramen magnum.[44] Thicker areas of the skull can support unicortical fixation well, but we prefer bicortical fixation for increased strength. Two to three screws per side should be used. We prefer to make the holes in the occiput using a 2-mm diamond bur. This minimizes the chance of a cerebrospinal fluid leak, because the inner cortex can be better palpated with the diamond bur. These holes can be tapped and followed by 3.5- or 4.0-mm screws of appropriate length. Each hole should be measured, but typical lengths run from 6 to 12 mm for bicortical purchase. If a spinal fluid leak is encountered, a hole can be bone-waxed or the screw simply placed to stop the leak. Any leaks should be avoided if possible; however, to our knowledge there have been no adverse clinical sequelae from this occurrence.

Postoperative immobilization using internal fixation techniques typically allows for immobilization in a two-poster brace. Patients with poor bone stock or highly unstable conditions may require concomitant use of a halo vest. Eight weeks of immobilization is adequate for most patients, followed by a soft collar for comfort for a couple of weeks. Radiographic follow-up is required to help avoid complications and monitor bone graft healing.

Resection of the Odontoid

Chronic anterior brain stem compression can result from fixed atlantoaxial subluxation. This impingement can be caused by the odontoid itself or by associated pannus material. In severe cases, preoperative traction or operative C1 laminectomy will not adequately decompress the spinal cord, and anterior resection of the odontoid may be necessary.[9, 26a] This can be done through a transoral approach, although this approach carries an increased risk of infection because of mouth flora. The high retropharyngeal approach to the upper cervical spine described by

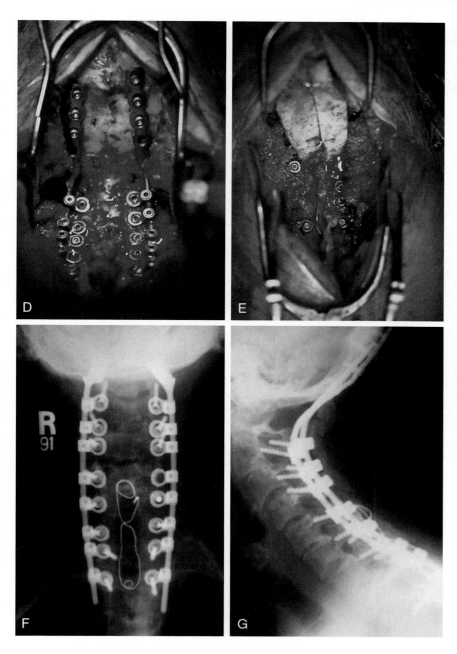

Figure 15–6 Continued. *She underwent posterior decompression with laminectomies of C1 through C3 and posterior occiput-to-T2 instrumentation (D) and iliac bone grafting (E). Her anteroposterior (F) and lateral (G) postoperative follow-up films show the long instrumentation with multiple points of fixation including upper thoracic pedicle screw fixation for a maximum purchase in osteoporotic bone.*

Whitesides[54] and later by McAfee and colleagues[30] is an alternative approach that we prefer.

Most patients with mild to moderate impingement on the brain stem from the odontoid can be successfully treated with posterior C1 laminectomy and occipitocervical stabilization. This approach eliminates dynamic compression of the cord, and if the myelopathy resolves, no further intervention is necessary. Note that pannus material can slowly resorb after successful fusion.[56] If symptoms persist, then anterior odontoid resection is necessary. If a solid posterior occipitocervical arthrodesis exists, then resection of the odontoid without any grafting will suffice. If there is no previous solid arthrodesis, then anterior grafting from C2 or C3 up to the clivus is performed using an iliac or fibula

strut. We follow with a posterior occipitocervical fusion for maximal stabilization.

Subaxial Subluxation

Subaxial subluxation refers to instability below the level of C2. This nearly always manifests as forward slippage of the superior vertebral body in relation to the vertebra below. This can be dynamic instability, as determined by motion on lateral flexion and extension views, or secondary structural changes, which can stiffen the abnormal segment into a fixed subluxation. Fixed subaxial anterolisthesis can result in spinal cord compression, typically at the posterior-superior corner of the lower vertebral body. This may require anterior corpectomy and strut grafting to adequately decompress the spinal canal and stabilize the segment. If the subluxed level is not fixed and can be reduced in extension, then the patient's head and neck can be placed in the reduced position in the operating room and a simple posterior fusion performed. This reestablishes the diameter of the spinal canal and also provides stability. A patient with mild to moderate cord compression after partial reduction and mild signs and symptoms of myelopathy may be satisfactorily treated with a posterior fusion in situ that will stop dynamic impingement on the cord and thus relieve symptoms.

Posterior Cervical Arthrodesis Technique

Posterior wiring and bone grafting can provide stable fixation at a very high union rate. The triple-wire technique described by Bohlman[31] (see Fig. 5–13 in Chapter 5) uses a 20-gauge wire woven in a figure-eight fashion through the base of the spinous processes of the involved vertebrae. This is the midline tethering wire. The wire is typically looped on itself through the superior spinous process and inferior spinous process to help distribute stress, which can be very important in osteoporotic bone in the rheumatoid patient. Then 22-gauge wires can be individually passed and again looped back through the same hole of the spinous process at each segment being fused. These ends are then passed up through holes placed in rectangular corticocancellous grafts. These rectangular blocks are near–full-thickness grafts harvested from the patient's iliac crest. These 22-gauge wires are then twisted down on themselves in a vertical fashion to pull the bone graft slabs down onto the lamina surfaces. Decortication may be performed before this, but it does not seem to be necessary for successful posterior cervical fusion. Small cancellous chips can be packed in crevices. A small drain is usually preferred, and the wound is closed in layers. A two-poster orthosis is usually sufficient for 6 to 8 weeks. Although usually osteoporotic, a patient with rheumatoid disease typically will heal well if adequate stability and bone graft material are provided.

Technique of Lateral Mass Plating

Internal fixation with lateral mass plating can achieve more rigid fixation for posterior cervical arthrodesis. There are minor variations on this procedure; here we describe the technique reported by Magerl.[1, 2, 24] The lateral masses must be well exposed and hemostasis achieved. The lateral mass is usually bisected in both the superoinferior and mediolateral directions. A starting point 1 mm medial to this crosshair location is chosen for the screws. A 1.5-mm bur can be used to make a dent in the cortical bone, followed by a 2-mm drill bit. Screw direction is 25 to 30 degrees lateral and 30 to 40 degrees superior. These angles will prevent penetration into the foramen with subsequent root impingement and avoid injury to the vertebral artery, which lies directly anterior to the lateral mass. The holes are drilled and tapped typically in a unicortical fashion to provide satisfactory

fixation; bicortical fixation can be used with care. Depending on the size of the patient, 14- to 18-mm screws are typically used. These facet joints usually provide satisfactory fixation even in patients with osteoporosis, because mainly cortical bone is used. The C7 lateral mass is usually transitional anatomy and thus is thinner, so there is a greater risk in placing the screw into the C7–T1 facet joint. Many authors will opt for a C7 pedicle screw to avoid this problem. This starting point is in the midpoint of the superior C7 facet from a mediolateral direction and the inferior edge of the superior facet from a superoinferior direction. The screw is angled approximately 40 degrees medially and perpendicular to the vertebral body in the sagittal plane. We have used this type of fixation and have found fluoroscopy to be very useful. An experienced x-ray technician is also helpful, because visualization in the lateral view through the patient's shoulders may require manipulation of the imaging technique.

SUMMARY

Success rates of radiographic union for posterior procedures in the rheumatoid cervical spine should be extremely high. This is particularly true for subaxial fusions.[51] Atlantoaxial procedures have a small surface area of C1 for bone grafting and are often significantly unstable; thus, historically, the nonunion rate has been 10% or higher for these procedures.[8] However, with more modern internal fixation techniques, such as transarticular screws, the rate of arthrodesis has improved.[11, 21]

Occipitocervical arthrodesis is a more demanding technique, but with good bone grafting technique[32, 53] and the use of internal fixation, a high rate of union can be expected.[47] All of these stabilization procedures can provide significant pain relief. With adequate decompression of the neural elements, neurologic recovery can also be expected.[36] As shown in other populations with myelopathy, the outcome is determined largely by the degree of myelopathy present preoperatively. Patients with severe quadriparesis before surgery may improve postoperatively, but the results are not as predictable.

Perioperative complications include wound healing problems, general nutritional problems, and potential loss of fixation because of poor bone stock or poor surgical technique. Late complications include pseudarthrosis and adjacent segment instability. Kraus et al. documented a higher incidence of subaxial subluxation after occipitocervical arthrodesis compared with C1–C2 procedures.[27] This is probably related to the increased weight of the head transferring stress to already-diseased segments in the subaxial cervical spine. Matsunaga and colleagues documented a higher incidence of subaxial subluxation after occipitocervical arthrodesis when the skull was fused in kyphosis relative to C2.[29b] We recommend including any levels with evidence of preoperative instability in the index operation, to help prevent subsequent breakdown at these levels.

REFERENCES

1. An HS, Gordin R, Renner K: Anatomic considerations for plate-screw fixation of the cervical spine. Spine 16(suppl): S548–S551, 1991.

2. Anderson PA, Henley MB, Grady MS, et al: Posterior cervical arthrodesis with AO reconstruction plates and bone graft. Spine 16(suppl):S72–S79, 1991.

3. Boden SD, Dodge LD, Bohlman HH, Rechtine GR: Rheumatoid arthritis of the cervical spine: A long-term analysis with predictors of paralysis and recovery. J Bone Joint Surg Am 75A:1282–1297, 1993.

4. Bourke JB: A review of the paleopathology of arthritic diseases. In Brothwell D, Sandison AT (eds): Diseases in Antiquity. Springfield, IL, Charles C Thomas, 1967, pp 352–369.

5. Brattström H, Granholm L: Atlanto-axial fusion in rheumatoid arthritis: A new method of fixation with wire and bone cement. Acta Orthop Scand 47:619–628, 1976.

6. Brooks AL, Jenkins EB: Atlanto-axial arthrodesis by the wedge compression method. J Bone Joint Surg Am 60A:279–284, 1978.

7. Bundschuh C, Modic MT, Kearney F, et al: Rheumatoid arthritis of the cervical spine: Surface coil MR imaging. Am J Roentgenol 151:181–187, 1988.

8. Clark CR, Goetz DD, Menezes AH: Arthrodesis of the cervical spine in rheumatoid arthritis. J Bone Joint Surg Am 71A:381–392, 1989.

9. Crockard HA, Calder I, Ransford AO: One-stage transoral decompression and posterior fixation in rheumatoid atlanto-axial subluxation. J Bone Joint Surg Br 72B:682–685, 1990.

10. Dvorak J, Grob D, Baumgartner H, et at: Functional evaluation of the spinal cord by magnetic resonance imaging in patients with rheumatoid arthritis and instability of upper cervical spine. Spine 14:1057–1064, 1989.

11. Eleraky MA, Masferrer R, Sonntag VK: Posterior atlantoaxial facet screw fixation in rheumatoid arthritis. J Neurosurg 89:8–12, 1998.

12. Emery SE, Bohlman HH, Bolesta MJ, Jones PK: Anterior cervical decompression and arthrodesis for the treatment of cervical spondylotic myelopathy. Two to seventeen-year follow-up. J Bone Joint Surg Am 80A:941–951, 1998.

13. Fehlings MG, Errico T, Cooper P, et al: Occipitocervical fusion with a five-millimeter malleable rod and segmental fixation. Neurosurgery 32:198–207, 1993.

14. Ferlic DC, Clayton ML, Leidholt JD, Gamble WE: Surgical treatment of the symptomatic unstable cervical spine in rheumatoid arthritis. J Bone Joint Surg 57A:349–354, 1975.

15. Flint GA, Hockley AD, McMillan JJ, Thompson AG: A new method of occipitocervical fusion using internal fixation. Neurosurgery 21:947–950, 1987.

16. Foerster O: Die Leitungsbahnen des Schmerzgefühls. Berlin und Wien, Urban und Schwarzenburg, 1927, p 266.

17. Gallie WE: Fractures and dislocations of the cervical spine. Am J Surg 46:495–499, 1939.

18. Garrod AC: A Treatise on Rheumatism and Rheumatoid Arthritis. London, Charles Griffin, 1890.

19. Grob D, Dvorak J, Panjabi MM, Antinnes JA: The role of plate and screw fixation in occipitocervical fusion in rheumatoid arthritis. Spine 19:2545–2551, 1994.

20. Grob D, Dvorak J, Panjabi M, et al: Posterior occipitocervical fusion: A preliminary report of a new technique. Spine 16(suppl):S17–S24, 1991.

21. Grob D, Jeanneret B, Aebi M, Markwalder TM: Atlanto-axial fusion with transarticular screw fixation. J Bone Joint Surg Br 73B:972–976, 1991.

22. Hamblen DL: Occipito-cervical fusion: Indications, technique and results. J Bone Joint Surg Br 49B:33–45, 1967.

23. Hansen SE: The recognition of rheumatoid arthritis in the eighteenth century. The contribution of Linné and Boissier de la Croix de Sauvages. Scand J Rheumatol 22:178–182, 1993.

24. Heller JG, Carlson GD, Abitbol JJ, Garfin SR: Anatomic comparison of the Roy-Camille and Magerl techniques for screw placement in the lower cervical spine. Spine 16(suppl): S552–S557, 1991.

25. Huckell CB, Buchowski JM, Richardson WJ, et al: Functional outcome of plate fusions for disorders of the occipitocervical junction. Clin Orthop 359:136–145, 1999.

26. Kahn EA, Yglesias L: Progressive atlanto-axial dislocation. JAMA 105:348–352, 1935.

26a. Kerschbaumer F, Kandziora F, Klein C, et al: Transoral decompression, anterior plate fixation, and posterior wire fusion for irreducible atlantoaxial kyphosis in rheumatoid arthritis. Spine 25:2708–2715, 2000.

27. Kraus DR, Peppelman WC, Agarwal AK, et al: Incidence of subaxial subluxation in patients with generalized rheumatoid arthritis who have had previous occipital cervical fusions. Spine 16(suppl): S486–S489, 1991.

28. Lipscomb PR: Cervico-occipital fusion for congenital and posttraumatic anomalies of the atlas and axis. J Bone Joint Surg Am 39A:1289–1301, 1957.

29. Lourie H, Stewart WA: Spontaneous atlantoaxial dislocation: A complication of rheumatoid disease. N Engl J Med 265:677–681, 1961.

29a. Matsunaga S, Ijiri K, Koga H: Results of a longer than 10-year follow-up of patients with rheumatoid arthritis treated by occipitocervical fusion. Spine 25:1749–1753, 2000.

29b. Matsunaga S, Onishi T, Sakou T: Significance of occipito-axial angle in subaxial lesion after occipitocervical fusion. Spine 26:161–165, 2001.

30. McAfee PC, Bohlman HH, Riley LH Jr, et al: The anterior retropharyngeal approach to the upper part of the cervical spine. J Bone Joint Surg Am 69A:1371–1383, 1987.

31. McAfee PC, Bohlman HH: One-stage anterior cervical decompression and posterior stabilization with circumferential arthrodesis: A study of twenty-four patients who had a traumatic or a neoplastic lesion. J Bone Joint Surg Am 71A:78–88, 1989.

32. McAfee PC, Cassidy JR, Davis RF, et al: Fusion of the occiput to the upper cervical spine: A review of 37 cases. Spine 16(suppl):S490–S494, 1991.

33. McGraw RW, Rusch RM: Atlanto-axial arthrodesis. J Bone Joint Surg Br 55B:482–489, 1973.

34. Mikulowski P, Wollheim FA, Rotmil P, Olsen I: Sudden death in rheumatoid arthritis with atlanto-axial dislocation. Acta Med Scand 198:445–451, 1975.

35. Moskovich R, Crockard HA, Shott S, Ransford AO: Occipitocervical stabilization for myelopathy in patients with rheumatoid arthritis. Implications of not bone-grafting. J Bone Joint Surg Am 82A:349–365, 2000.

36. Peppelman WC, Kraus DR, Donaldson WF III, Agarwal A: Cervical spine surgery in rheumatoid arthritis: Improvement of neurologic deficit after cervical spine fusion. Spine 18:2375–2379, 1993.

37. Perry J, Nickel VL: Total cervical-spine fusion for neck paralysis. J Bone Joint Surg Am 41A:37–60, 1959.

38. Pratt TLC: Spontaneous dislocation of the atlanto-axial articulation occurring in ankylosing spondylitis and rheumatoid arthritis. J Fac Radiol 10:40–43, 1959.

39. Purser DW, Sharp J: Spontaneous atlanto-axial dislocation: A complication of spondylitis. J Bone Joint Surg Br 39B:582, 1957.

40. Rana NA, Hancock DO, Taylor AR, Hill AGS: Atlanto-axial subluxation in rheumatoid arthritis. J Bone Joint Surg Br 55B:458–470, 1973.

41. Ranawat CS, O'Leary P, Pellicci P, et al: Cervical spine fusion in rheumatoid arthritis. J Bone Joint Surg Am 61A:1003–1010, 1979.

42. Ransford AO, Crockard HA, Pozo JL, et al: Craniocervical instability treated by contoured loop fixation. J Bone Joint Surg Br 68B:173–177, 1986.

43. Redlund-Johnell I, Pettersson H: Radiographic measurements of the cranio-vertebral region. Designed for evaluation of abnormalities in rheumatoid arthritis. Acta Radiol Diag 25:23–28, 1984.

43a. Riew KD, Hilibrand AS, Palumbo MA, et al: Diagnosing basilar invagination in the rheumatoid patient: The reliability of radiographic criteria. J Bone Joint Surg Am 83A:194-200, 2001.

44. Roberts DA, Doherty BJ, Heggeness MH: Quantitative anatomy of the occiput and the biomechanics of occipital screw fixation. Spine 23:1100–1107, 1998.

45. Rogers MA, Crockard HA, Moskovich R, et al: Nystagmus and joint position sensation: Their importance in posterior occipitocervical fusion in rheumatoid arthritis. Spine 19:16–20, 1994.

46. Ruffer MA, Rietti A: On osseous lesions in ancient Egyptians. J Pathol Bacteriol 16:439–465, 1912.

47. Sasso RC, Jeanneret B, Fischer K, Magerl F: Occipitocervical fusion with posterior plate and screw instrumentation. A long-term follow-up study. Spine 19:2364–2368, 1994.

48. Short CL: The antiquity of rheumatoid arthritis. Arthritis Rheum 17:193–205, 1974.

49. Smith MD, Anderson P, Grady MS: Occipitocervical arthrodesis using contoured plate fixation: An early report on a versatile fixation technique. Spine 18:1984–1990, 1993.

50. Snorrason E: Landré-Beauvais and his Goutte asthénique primitive. Acta Med Scand 142(suppl 266):115–118, 1952.

51. Weiland DJ, McAfee PC: Posterior cervical fusion with triple-wire strut graft technique: One hundred consecutive patients. J Spinal Disord 4:15–21, 1991.

52. Werne S: Spontaneous dislocation of the atlas (as a complication of rheumatoid arthritis). Acta Rheumatol Scand 3:101–107, 1957.

53. Wertheim SB, Bohlman HH: Occipitocervical fusion: Indications, technique, and long-term results in thirteen patients. J Bone Joint Surg Am 69A:833–836, 1987.

54. Whitesides TE: Extrapharyngeal approach to the upper cervical spine. In Evarts CM (ed): Surgery of the Musculoskeletal System, vol 4. New York, Churchill Livingstone, 1983, pp 13–18.

55. Wilson PD Jr, Dangelmajer RC: The problem of atlanto-axial dislocation in rheumatoid arthritis. J Bone Joint Surg Am 45A:1780, 1963.

56. Zygmunt S, Saveland H, Brattstrom H, et al: Reduction of rheumatoid periodontoid pannus following posterior occipitocervical fusion visualised by magnetic resonance imaging. Br J Neurosurg 2:315–320, 1988.

16

CERVICAL SPINE IN ANKYLOSING SPONDYLITIS

Henry H. Bohlman, M.D.
Sanford E. Emery, M.D.

HISTORICAL PERSPECTIVE

Ankylosing spondylitis (AS), one of the spondyloar-thropathies, has been clinically recognized for thousands of years, dating back to Egyptian times.[11] Clinical descriptions were provided by Marie and Strumpel in the late 19th century.[6] The association of AS and the major histocompat-ibility antigen, HLA-B27, was recognized by Brewerton et al.[5] and Schlosstein et al.[12] in 1973.

The HLA system comprises a set of proteins encoded by genes on chromosome 6; these HLA antigens are involved with the immune recognition of foreign molecules to oneself. Some sort of alteration within the HLA system leads to immunologic attack against one's own cells, which is the basis for autoimmunity.[1] HLA-B27 is found in only 8% of American whites but is in more than 87% of those individuals with AS.[8] The exact role of HLA-B27 is still unknown. The fact that HLA-B27 is linked to the genes on chromosome 6 indicates a strong genetic predisposition. Indeed, clinically it is well known that various family members can have the same disease.

The pathophysiologic mechanisms of the disease process in AS include inflammation, bone erosion, and ultimately ankylosis. The inflammatory infiltrate is mainly lympho-cytic; involved musculoskeletal sites include joints and entheses (the sites where ligaments and tendons attach), as well as the axial skeleton including the sacroiliac, apophyseal, and costovertebral joints, which are usually involved to varying degrees. Progression of the inflamma-tory process produces ossification of the annulus and bridging syndesmophytes, ultimately producing the charac-teristic "bamboo" spine, which is completely ankylosed.

CLINICAL PRESENTATION

The typical patient with AS is a young adult male who presents with the insidious onset of low back pain and stiffness. The pain may radiate into the buttocks and the legs and can mimic sciatica, although the pain rarely radiates past the knees. Symptoms, as in other arthritides, are usually worse in the morning and improve with increased activity.

Over time, the inflammatory process leads to progressive ankylosis of the spine, and the patient may develop kyphosis of the cervical, thoracic, or lumbar spine, or all three. This results clinically in a stooped posture, pain, and great difficulty and work expenditure with ambulation and activities of daily living. An additional problem is the loss of intercostal breathing function and chest expansion because of ankylosis of the costovertebral joints, leading to restrictive lung disease. The patient then becomes an abdominal breather.

A clinical history is extremely important in diagnosing AS and distinguishing it from mechanical back pain. Calin et al. described five main clinical features of AS: (1) onset of back discomfort before age 40; (2) insidious onset; (3) persistence for at least 3 months; (4) associ-ation with morning stiffness; and (5) improvement with exercise.[2, 6]

Physical examination findings are not very specific in the early stages of AS, although disease progression leads to loss of cervical and other spinal motion, loss of chest expansion, and decreasing height. Laboratory results include positive tests for HLA-B27 as well as elevated erythrocyte sedimen-tation rate and C-reactive protein level, but these do not necessarily correlate with the level of disease activity.

One of the earliest radiographic manifestations of AS is sacroiliitis, manifested by erosions and sclerosis of the subchondral bone of the sacroiliac joints. Eventually these joints become ankylosed, as does the spine.

COMPLICATIONS

One major complication of AS that may occur at any age is a severe kyphotic (or "chin-on-chest") deformity, which may be progressive once kyphosis reaches approximately 50 degrees. This deformity is always accentuated by a thoracic kyphotic deformity. The patient with AS can also develop spondylodiscitis at any level of the spine, which erodes the disc space and causes severe pain. Once spondylodiscitis runs its course, the disc space usually becomes ankylosed, although pseudarthrosis may occur. This inflammatory process is quite painful and necessitates treatment with analgesics and anti-inflammatory agents and immobilization.

As the cervical spine becomes ankylosed, the inflamma-tory process of the disease may produce atlantoaxial dislocation and rotatory deformities, with resultant atlanto-axial instability and pain with or without spinal cord compression. Finally, with minor trauma or falls, a fracture may occur in the ankylosed cervical spine, usually at the lower segments, producing increased deformity, pain, and/or neurologic deficit.

Atlantoaxial Instability

Progressive ankylosis of the subaxial cervical spine may lead to atlantoaxial instability and erosion of the C1-C2 joints secondary to the inflammatory process of AS. The patient may present with a rotatory subluxation and accentuation of kyphosis, along with cervico-occipital pain and/or neurologic deficit. This problem necessitates application of a halo cast and gentle traction and reduction of the deformity, followed by posterior arthrodesis (Fig. 16-1A to E).

Fractures of the Ankylosed Spine

In patients with AS, cervical spine fracture may occur with even minor trauma or fall. The fracture often goes unnoticed, particularly if it occurs at the cervicothoracic junction, which is very difficult to visualize radiologically with plain x-rays. Surely, acute fracture should be suspected and investigated in every patient who has sustained a neck injury (even a seemingly minor injury) and who demonstrates increased pain in the cervical spine after the episode.[7] In this situation, the examiner needs to go to any length to make an appropriate diagnosis or rule out significant trauma. This is best done with plain cervical x-rays, taken with the patient holding weights and pulling the shoulders down to provide complete visualization of C7

and T1. If this is not possible (which it may not be, especially in a stocky patient), then computed tomography (CT) scan reconstruction or magnetic resonance imaging (MRI) should be done to rule out fracture.

In more chronic cases of AS, some patients have sustained what they interpreted as a minor injury and did not initially seek the advice of a physician or emergency room staff. After a number of months with neck pain and increasing deformity, these patients present with increasing cervical kyphosis and pseudarthrosis at the fracture level due to improper immobilization. A patient diagnosed early with acute fracture may be repositioned into the preinjury state of the spine and immobilized with a halo vest for 8 to 12 weeks or until CT reconstruction demonstrates fracture healing. A patient with chronic AS with an established pseudarthrosis usually requires an extension cervical osteotomy and posterior arthrodesis for stabilization and healing, ideally followed by a halo cast for 3 months and then a rigid two-poster orthosis for 2 more months (Fig. 16-2A to F).[9, 14]

More severe trauma (e.g., a fall from a roof) may cause an acute fracture-dislocation of the cervical spine, producing incomplete or complete spinal cord injury. Acute fracture of the ankylosed spine from major trauma is a very unstable injury that calls for surgical stabilization to avoid morbidity and mortality, which is high, especially when associated with paralysis. In the ankylosed spine, the surrounding ligamentous structures are calcified or ossified, and thus the fracture is grossly unstable without the usual surrounding structure of ligaments to protect the spine from subluxation or dislocation. Immobilization and establish-

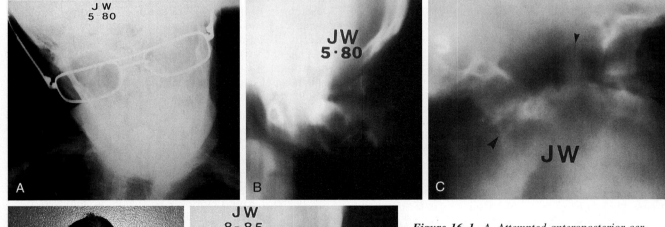

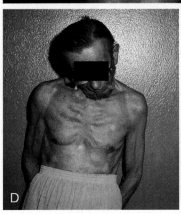
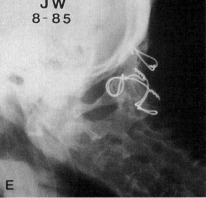

Figure 16–1. *A, Attempted anteroposterior cervical spine radiograph of a 68-year-old physician with a fixed atlantoaxial rotatory subluxation. B, Lateral tomogram of atlantoaxial dislocation. Note erosion of the odontoid. C, Anteroposterior tomogram of the atlantoaxial joint. Note the erosion of both the odontoid and the atlantoaxial joint, producing the rotatory subluxation. D, Photograph of the patient with the rotatory and flexion deformity. E, Lateral radiograph of the patient 5 years after reduction of the C1-C2 dislocation and cervico-occipital fusion, which is now completely arthrodesed.*

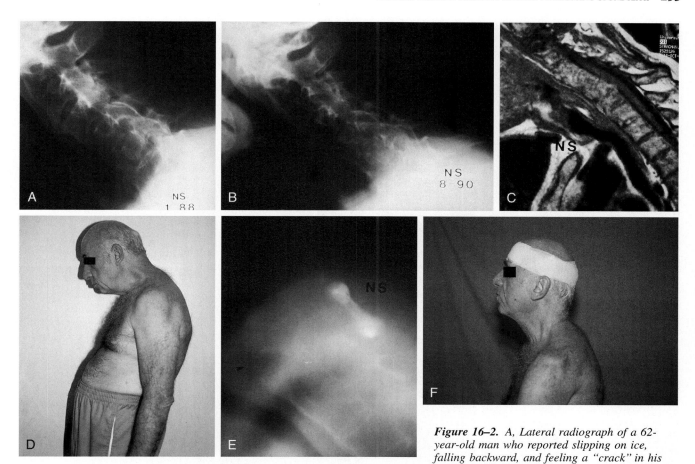

Figure 16–2. *A, Lateral radiograph of a 62-year-old man who reported slipping on ice, falling backward, and feeling a "crack" in his neck. Five days later, an x-ray was taken, a fracture was not appreciated, and he was treated with a collar. There appears to be an angular kyphotic deformity at C6-C7. B, Two years and 8 months after the original injury, the patient had developed progressive kyphotic deformity of the cervical spine. This lateral radiograph shows the progressive deformity. C, Sagittal MRI reveals the remote fracture site and some element of bone protrusion into the spinal canal. D, Lateral photograph of the patient demonstrating the cervicothoracic kyphosis. E, The patient underwent a cervical extension osteotomy with posterior arthrodesis and wiring. This lateral radiograph demonstrates the anterior osteotomy and the posterior arthrodesis. F, Note the corrected kyphotic deformity in the photograph after removal of the halo cast. (From Boden SD, Dodge LD, et al: J Bone Joint Surg 75A:1288, 1993.)*

ment of stability are extremely important to protect the spinal cord. In this situation, the patient should be immediately immobilized in the premorbid spinal-deformed state, which may be kyphotic, with no attempt made to correct the spine into a more neutral position. (Such correction will cause posterior subluxation of the upper cervical vertebrae on the lower cervical vertebrae, exacerbating the neurologic deficit secondary to spinal cord and nerve root compression.) As documented by Bohlman,[3] failure to immediately immobilize and stabilize the patient increases the risk of massive epidural hemorrhage. Surgical stabilization may be done by anterior plate fixation, if the patient does not have a severe preexisting kyphotic deformity, or by posterior plate or wire fixation with iliac bone graft (Fig. 16-3A to G).

After surgical stabilization, these patients need prompt mobilization. AS is associated with a very high incidence of pulmonary compromise and death due to restrictive lung disease and paralysis. A tracheostomy may be needed to control pulmonary secretions.

MANAGEMENT OF CHRONIC DEFORMITY

Nonoperative Chronic Management

Once a patient has been diagnosed with AS, it is important that he or she be followed by a rheumatologist and treated with appropriate medication. This may include various forms of nonsteroidal anti-inflammatory drugs or the new cyclooxygenase-2 drugs, which are less likely to produce gastric irritation. We recommend an exercise program and postural training (e.g., sleeping without a pillow, sleeping on one's back) for patients with progressive ankylosis of the spine in an effort to prevent kyphosis. These measures are not always sufficient to prevent chronic deformity, however. In cases of spondylodiscitis at various levels, bracing and analgesics usually suffice until the level spontaneously fuses. If fusion does not occur spontaneously, it may have to be done operatively at a later date.

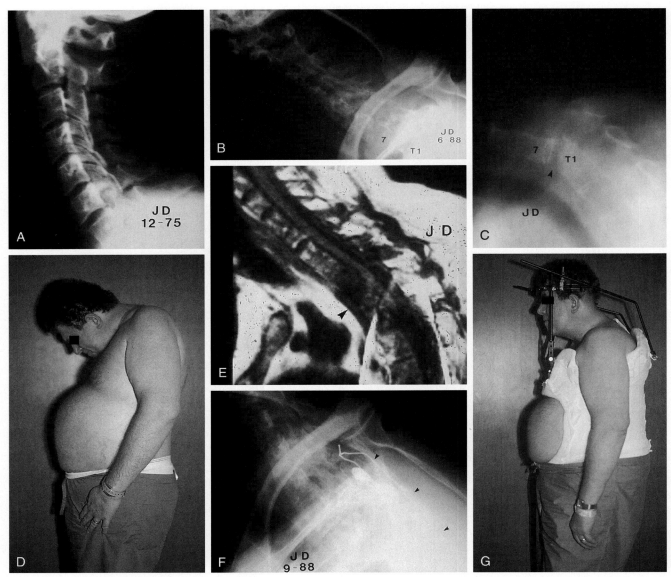

Figure 16–3. *A, Lateral radiograph of a patient with AS at age 26, before his injury, demonstrating no kyphotic deformity. B, Lateral radiograph of the patient 17 months after a fall on the ice when he landed backward on his shoulders and his back. He initially had neck pain, but no x-rays were taken. After the injury, the patient developed progressive chin-on-chest deformity. C, Lateral tomogram of the cervical spine demonstrating an unhealed fracture at C7-T1. D, Photograph of the patient with chin-on-chest deformity. The patient had been ambulatory with the unhealed fracture for 17 months without paralysis. E, Lateral MRI of the cervical spine demonstrating the fracture site with the spine in a more neutral position. F, The patient was treated with reduction of the fracture to the original kyphotic position by a posterior arthrodesis and wiring. This lateral radiograph demonstrates the posterior fusion mass and wire fixation. G, Photograph of the patient in his halo cast postoperatively with correction of the deformity.*

Treatment of patients with AS requires a team approach for long-term care. This includes the rheumatologist as well as the orthopaedic surgeon and primary care medical physician, along with, in the event of surgical correction, an anesthesiologist well versed in the techniques of anesthesia for cervical osteotomy.

Surgical Management

Patients with AS may develop, even without trauma, chronic kyphotic deformity that becomes extremely dis-

abling, incapacitating, and painful. Once the deformity develops approximately 50 degrees in conjunction with a thoracic kyphosis, the mere weight of the head pulls the cervical spine into increasing kyphosis. The bone, although ankylosed, is a living organ, and as such remodels progressively into the kyphotic position until, in the most extreme circumstance, the chin comes to rest on the sternum. This extremely disabling deformity hinders the patient's ability to shave, eat solid foods, and perform other routine activities, and produces dysphagia (Fig. 16-4A to C). The patient may find it difficult to look forward when walking, sleep in anything but a side-lying position, and drink out of a glass. As the deformity becomes more severe, muscle pain increases from trying to hold the neck in a more correct position.

Indications for surgical correction of a cervical spine deformity depend on the extent of the deformity, the degree of disability, and the patient's age and general medical condition.[13, 14] The degree of deformity of the cervical and thoracolumbar spine is measured using the chin–brow angle technique. This involves drawing a line from the patient's brow to chin and intersecting it with a vertical line from the chin to occiput to the floor. The chin–brow-to-vertical angle provides an excellent prediction of the amount of deformity present and the amount of correction needed.[15] As mentioned earlier, once 50 to 60 degrees of cervical kyphosis has developed, the deformity will continue to progress. Correcting the deformity before it progresses to the chin-on-chest stage is highly desirable.

Preoperatively, we evaluate the spinal canal using MRI to ensure no spinal cord compression in areas where the osteotomy is to be performed. We occasionally do a CT scan reconstruction of the cervical spine, as well as plain x-ray, to assess and measure the deformity.

The patient is admitted to the hospital 1 day before the operation, and under local anesthesia, a halo vest and a molded Risser jacket are applied.[4, 16] (A halo vest is not stable enough to immobilize a cervical osteotomy; a well-molded jacket allows for good fixation around the pelvic area.) A large abdominal window must be provided, because these patients are abdominal breathers. Sufficient room also must be provided to enable a posterior approach to the lower cervical spine and upper thoracic area. A complete medical workup with pulmonary function studies and blood gas analysis is indicated because of restrictive lung disease. Smoking further complicates this problem, interfering with postoperative pulmonary recovery.

On the day after admission, the patient is brought to the operating room. The patient is then lightly sedated and placed in a sitting position with the halo attached to overhead traction of approximately 10 pounds. The patient is carefully padded and securely strapped to the operating table, with the head and neck in a vertical position, to keep the torso from sliding forward on the operating table as the correction forces are applied posteriorly to the head and neck (Fig. 16-5A to C). The cervical spine and occiput are prepped and draped in the usual manner. A 1:2 solution of 0.75% Marcaine with epinephrine in saline is administered, allowing sufficient volume of anesthetic to infiltrate the entire area involved in the osteotomy. The anesthetic is injected down to the periosteum from approximately C4 to T1.

Once the local anesthetic has taken effect, the midline incision is made over the same length of the spine. Bleeders are clamped and cauterized, and dissection is carried down to the periosteum (which is elevated). Self-retaining retractors are placed. An x-ray is taken to identify the pertinent spinal levels. The spinous processes of C6 and C7 are then removed. Once the ligamentum flavum is separated, the spinal canal is entered through the inferior lamina of C7 with rongeurs and Kerrison punches. If the periosteum has been infiltrated with local anesthetic, the patient should feel no pain throughout the laminectomy procedure. A complete laminectomy of C6 and C7 and the superior portion of T1 is performed. At this point, epidural bleeders are controlled with bipolar coagulation, Gelfoam, and cotton patties.

Once the laminectomy has been completed, the surgeon can explore laterally and identify the C7 pedicle and the exiting C8 nerve root. A Leksell rongeur and Kerrison punches are used to perform wide foraminotomies at C7-T1, the level at which the osteotomy is to be performed. (This level is selected because it is inferior to the entrance of the vertebral artery at the C6 level and thus avoids the risk of damaging that structure.) Once the foraminotomies are completed all the way out into the lateral soft tissue and no bone remains to compress the C8 nerve root, the inferior one-third of the pedicle at C7 is removed with a diamond power burr. At this point, if the patient feels uncomfortable

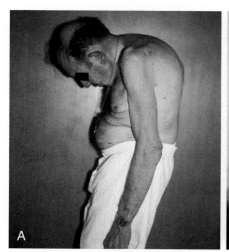
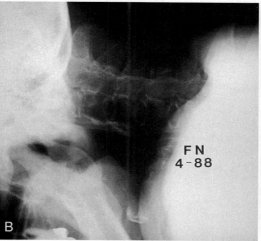
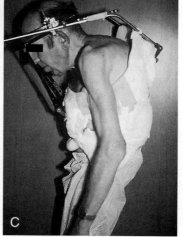

Figure 16–4. *A, Photograph of a lateral view of a 58-year-old accountant with a 37-year history of AS and progressive chin-on-chest deformity. B, Standing lateral radiograph of the same patient showing his chin-on-chest deformity. This required a cervical osteotomy for correction. C, Postoperative correction of the patient in his halo cast.*

paresthesias of the C8 nerve, a small cotton patty soaked with 2% xylocaine can be placed on the C8 nerve roots to alleviate this symptom (Fig. 16-5D). Throughout the procedure, the anesthesiologist and surgeon can talk to the patient and observe motor function and sensation.[4]

After the laminectomy and foraminotomies are complete, the bone that has been removed is saved for bone grafting. Holes are drilled through the base of the spinous processes of C5 and T1, and malleable 18-gauge wires with buttons are placed through the spinous processes for attachment of a Luque rectangle, which is bent to adapt to the deformity correction and thus stabilize the spine once the osteotomy is completed. The posterior surfaces of C6, C7, and T1 are slightly decorticated with a burr in preparation for spinal correction and bone grafting (Fig. 16-5E).

At this point, a surgical assistant goes to the front of the patient and stabilizes the halo ring. The patient is then given a brief general anesthetic. Once the patient anesthetized,

gentle extension of the skull and cervical spine is done. The correction can be easily visualized as it occurs by noting a slight buckling of the dura as the correction is made. Kyphosis along with some rotation can be corrected until the patient is in the neutral position looking forward. The operating surgeon can easily walk around to the front of the drapes and observe the desired correction. The C8 nerve roots must be viewed bilaterally to ensure no impingement once the correction is completed. At this point, the patient is awakened and asked to move all four extremities; the Luque rectangle is then wired into place on the spinous processes from C5 to below T1. Gelfoam is placed over the dura, and the bone graft is inserted into the lateral gutters. The wound is irrigated with antibiotic solution and closed over a suction drain, and a dressing is applied. Then the halo ring is hooked with vertical rods to the cast and locked into place. The patient is taken to the recovery room and then, once stable, to the floor.

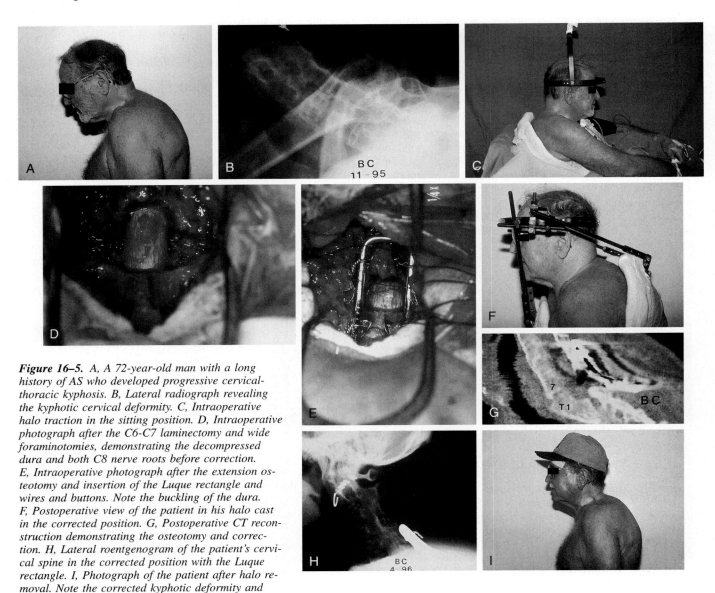

Figure 16–5. *A, A 72-year-old man with a long history of AS who developed progressive cervical-thoracic kyphosis. B, Lateral radiograph revealing the kyphotic cervical deformity. C, Intraoperative halo traction in the sitting position. D, Intraoperative photograph after the C6-C7 laminectomy and wide foraminotomies, demonstrating the decompressed dura and both C8 nerve roots before correction. E, Intraoperative photograph after the extension osteotomy and insertion of the Luque rectangle and wires and buttons. Note the buckling of the dura. F, Postoperative view of the patient in his halo cast in the corrected position. G, Postoperative CT reconstruction demonstrating the osteotomy and correction. H, Lateral roentgenogram of the patient's cervical spine in the corrected position with the Luque rectangle. I, Photograph of the patient after halo removal. Note the corrected kyphotic deformity and the patient looking straight ahead.*

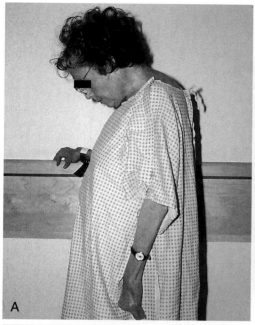

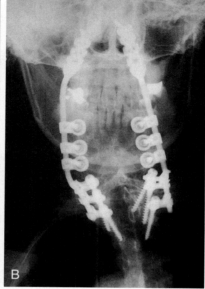

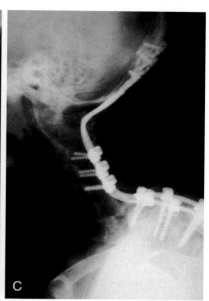

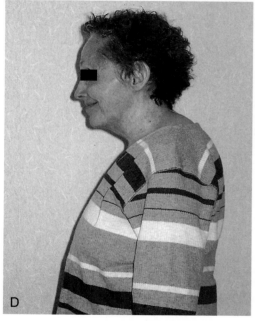

Figure 16–6. A, Preoperative photo of a 58-year-old woman with a fixed chin-on-chest deformity secondary to rheumatoid arthritis. B and C, Postoperative anteroposterior and lateral radiographs after cervical osteotomy performed using general anesthesia with the patient in the prone position. An occipital-to-thoracic fusion was performed because of poor bone stock and severe exfoliative psoriasis, necessitating maximal internal fixation if a halo vest was not tolerated postoperatively. Internal fixation such as this requires general anesthesia. D, Postoperative photograph showing clinical correction.

The patient may be ambulated the same day with a walker and the aid of a physical therapist. Occasionally a patient will experience dysphagia from the correction osteotomy and impingement of the esophagus. This usually resolves with administration of intravenous fluids over several days. However, a patient who has undergone correction of a severe deformity may need a gastrostomy tube or hyperalimentation for a time (Fig. 16-5F to I).

After the patient is discharged, follow-up CT scan reconstructions are scheduled at 6 weeks and then 6 weeks thereafter. The patient is maintained in the halo cast for 3 months and then in a two-poster rigid brace for another 2 months. At that point, another CT scan reconstruction is performed to determine the solidity of the bone graft.

This technique has proved quite successful over the years. We have performed it in approximately 26 patients since 1976. Patients are extremely grateful for the correction of the deformity and the resultant improved ability to perform activities of daily living.

An alternative technique is to use fiberoptic intubation and take a posterior approach with the patient in the prone position, using intraoperative spinal cord monitoring with cortical evoked potentials. Once the laminectomy is completed with the foraminotomies, the osteotomy is performed with some extension of the head and neck in the prone position. Then lateral mass screws with islets are attached to a malleable rod[10] to prevent translation of the osteotomy site and offer another form of stabilization.

Internal fixation over many levels can be performed using this technique, because it is done under general anesthesia (Fig. 16-6A). We believe that this technique is feasible, but it does not provide as much leverage to do the osteotomy as is afforded in the sitting position, and the patient is not awake for monitoring of spinal cord function.

Possible pulmonary complications of cervical osteotomy include restrictive lung disease, resulting in pneumonia or atelectasis. Nonunion of the osteotomy site is possible, but has not occurred in our experience in 26 years. In our earlier years, when we did not have a good means of providing internal fixation, subluxation of the osteotomy in the halo was a possibility. We have experienced one neurologic complication, in a patient who underwent a 90-degree correction of a chin-on-chest deformity of 5 years' duration. The correction was probably excessive and led to spinal subluxation, compressing the cord, causing quadriplegia and ultimately death from pulmonary complications due to the paralysis. Although neurologic injury is always a possibility, today's methods of internal fixation should prevent it. In general, the procedure has been very successful.

REFERENCES

1. Arnett FC: Serogenegative spondyloarthropathies. Bull Rheum Dis 37:1–12, 1987.
2. Blackburn WD Jr, Alarcon GS, Ball GV: Evaluation of patients with back pain of suspected inflammatory nature. Am J Med 85:766–770, 1988.
3. Bohlman HH: Acute fractures and dislocations of the cervical spine: An analysis of three hundred hospitalized patients and review of the literature. J Bone Joint Surg Am 61:1119–1142, 1979.
4. Bohlman HH, Dabb B: Anterior and posterior cervical osteotomy. In Bradford DS (ed): Master Techniques in Orthopaedic Surgery: The Spine. Philadelphia, Lippincott-Raven, 1997, pp 75–88.
5. Brewerton DA, Hart FD, Nicholls A, et al.: Ankylosing spondylitis and HL-A 27. Lancet 1:904–907, 1973.
6. Calin A, Porta J, Fries JF, Schurman DJ: Clinical history as a screening test for ankylosing spondylitis. JAMA 237:2613–2614, 1977.
7. Graham B, Van Peteghem PK: Fractures of the spine in ankylosing spondylitis. Diagnosis, treatment, and complications. Spine 14:803–807, 1989.
8. Hochberg M: Epidemiology. In Calin A (ed): Spondyloarthropathies. Orlando, FL, Grune & Stratton, 1984, pp 21–42.
9. McMaster MJ: Osteotomy of the cervical spine in ankylosing spondylitis. J Bone Joint Surg Br 79:197–203, 1997.
10. Mehdian SMH, Freeman BJC, Licina P: Cervical osteotomy for ankylosing spondylitis: An innovative variation on an existing technique. Eur Spine J 8:505–509, 1999.
11. Ruffer MA, Rietti A: On osseous lesions in ancient Egyptians. J Pathol Bacteriol 16:439–465, 1912.
12. Schlosstein L, Terasaki PI, Bluestone R, Pearsom CM: High association of an HL-A antigen, W27, with ankylosing spondylitis. N Engl J Med 288:704–706, 1973.
13. Simmons EH: Ankylosing spondylitis: Surgical considerations. In Herkowitz H, Garfin SR, Balderston RA, et al. (eds): The Spine, 3rd ed. Philadelphia, WB Saunders, 1992, pp 1447–1511.
14. Simmons EH: Kyphotic deformity of the spine in ankylosing spondylitis. Clin Orthop 128: 65–77, 1977.
15. Simmons EH: The cervical spine in ankylosing spondylitis. In Bridwell KH, DeWald RL (eds): The Textbook of Spinal Surgery. Philadelphia, Lippincott-Raven, 1997, pp 1129–1158.
16. Urist MR: Osteotomy of the cervical spine: Report of a case of ankylosing rheumatoid spondylitis. J Bone Joint Surg Am 40:833–843, 1958.

17

CERVICAL SPINE INFECTIONS

Muzaffar Hussain, M.D.
Donald P.K. Chan, M.D.

To know what you know and to know what you don't know is a characteristic of one who knows.
— Confucius

HISTORICAL PERSPECTIVE

Spine infections have been recognized since the Greek and Egyptian civilizations of 3000 B.C. The earliest recorded cases of spine infection can be traced in the archives of Hippocrates on a tuberculous spine documented between 400 B.C. and 100 A.D.[44]

Pott's paraplegia was described by Percivall Pott (1779) in the 18th century.[57] For the next 150 years, tuberculosis of the spine remained a disease that was difficult to treat until the emergence of the antibiotic era.

Lannelongue in 1897 gave the first descriptive account of pyogenic spondylitis.[43] For a long time, spine infections had remained a catastrophic disease with a very high death rate, between 40% and 70%.[35, 42] Previously, treatment of spinal tuberculosis had been by a plaster cast, bed rest, and admission to a sanitarium. Posterior decompression was frequently done until the late 19th century and early 20th century and later was discredited by Seddon[65] because it failed to eradicate the disease anteriorly and instead often led to instability of the spine.[40] Albee and Hibbs are independently credited for popularizing the posterior spine fusion in 1911 using autogenous tibial bone grafts[1, 36] to treat spinal tuberculosis, although this was later abandoned because it failed to prevent progressive kyphosis and smoldering infection.

Although Ito and associates are credited with the first description of the anterior approach to the spine in 1934,[38] it was Hodgson and Stock in 1956 who popularized decompression of the spinal canal for tuberculosis through an anterior approach.[37] They recommended wide excision, aggressive debridement, and strut bone grafting, which is often called the "Hong Kong operation."

The outcome of spine infections has improved significantly over the last several decades, because of better diagnostic and imaging techniques and treatment methods, particularly antibiotic therapy. The natural history has been dramatically altered, and overall mortality rate has been lowered from 40% to 70% to 1% to 20%, with an average of 5%.[9, 34]

EPIDEMIOLOGY

The overall incidence of tuberculous infections of the spine has decreased considerably over the last 5 decades. The incidence of pyogenic spondylitis has increased slightly.[14, 66] Infection of the spine occurs in 2% to 7% of all skeletal infections.[42, 60] The cervical spine is involved in 3% to 6% of these skeletal infections,[25, 47] although this incidence is reportedly as high as 27% in intravenous drug abusers.[33, 63] Waldvogel and colleagues showed that 19% of cases of nonvertebral osteomyelitis later spread to the spine.[70] Nagel and associates reported that 8% of their patients admitted with back pain were later found to have spinal infections.[53] Some 52% of cases of vertebral osteomyelitis occur in patients over age 50; the disorder has a predilection for males, with a 2:1 male-to-female ratio.[62] The literature suggests that diabetics, intravenous drug abusers, patients on steroids, alcoholics, immunocompromised patients, patients with rheumatoid arthritis, and the elderly are at increased risk for vertebral osteomyelitis.

The incidence of postsurgical spine infection is less than 1% to 3%, depending on the type and nature of surgery.[23, 46, 69] Spinal instrumentation is associated with the highest rate of postsurgical infection, ranging from 0.5% to 15%.[68] Diabetics, alcoholics, and immunocompromised patients seem to be at greater risk of developing postoperative spine infection.

The incidence of tuberculous spondylitis has decreased considerably over the last 5 decades in developed countries but remains very high in a number of developing countries. Up to 5% of patients with tuberculosis exhibit signs of spine involvement.[13] Tuberculous spondylitis is also associated with a neurologic deficit in up to 40% of cases. Cervical spine involvement is rare in tuberculosis, occurring in only 3% to 5% of all cases.[48] A case report of concomitant tuberculous and pyogenic infection in the cervical spine has been described.[28a]

Epidural abscess not associated with vertebral osteomyelitis or diskitis is a disease more common in adults over age 50 and in medically debilitated patients. The overall incidence of epidural abscess is 0.2 to 1.2 per 10,000 hospital admissions.[4] The disease rarely occurs in children under age 12.[3] Epidural abscess is reported to occur in the cervical spine in 14% of cases.[18] The risk factors are diabetes mellitus, immunocompromised status, and certain invasive procedures, including diskography, epidural catheterization, and spinal surgery. Patients with true vertebral osteomyelitis or diskitis may have increased risk of a concomitant epidural abscess in the cervical spine relative to the thoracic or lumbar regions.[31a]

ETIOLOGY

A hematogenous source of infection is the most important and most frequently implicated cause of vertebral osteomyelitis. Urinary tract infection and bacteremia of genitourinary instrumentation are the main sources of infection.[27] However, the primary source can be identified in only approximately two-thirds of cases.[62] The main documented sources of infection are urinary tract (29%), skin (13%), and respiratory tract (11%).[62] Other infections and invasive procedures–including typhoid fever, ear infection, bacteremia of dental extraction, hemodialysis, and endocarditis—occasionally may lead to vertebral osteomyelitis.[8, 11, 45, 56, 62]

Infections may also occur by direct extension in gunshot and other penetrating wounds.[64] Spinal surgery, diskography, and chemonucleolysis are other uncommon sources of direct inoculation of organisms.[6, 16, 20, 46, 64] Cervical angiography, pharyngeal resection, and foreign bodies in a hypopharynx have reportedly caused cervical spine infections on rare occasions.[7, 12, 32]

In cases of tuberculous spondylitis, the source may be hematogenous spread from other foci or spread along lymphatics or by direct extension from adjacent lymph nodes or visceral lesions. In developed countries, including North America, the incidence of tuberculous spondylitis is on the rise as the number of AIDS and immunocompromised cases increase.[33] The respiratory tract and the urinary tract are the most common sources of tuberculous spondylitis, but it also may spread from other skeletal foci of tuberculosis.[15, 28, 44]

Fungal infections of the cervical spine are relatively rare but occur more frequently in immunocompromised patients. Thus, a high index of suspicion is mandated in these patients to ensure early detection of disease.

ANATOMICAL FEATURES OF SPINAL BLOOD SUPPLY

Knowledge of the vascular supply and architecture of the spine is essential to understanding the pathogenesis and spread of spine infections. The arterial and venous supply of the spine has been extensively studied for more than a century. In 1940, Batson showed free communication between the pelvic venous plexus and the vertebral venous system.[5] He demonstrated the communication by radio-opaque dye injected in cadavers and live animals in which raising the intra-abdominal pressure obstructed the flow in the abdominal vena caval system but not the vertebral system. In 1959, Wiley and Trueta refuted Batson's theory of venous spread of infection and showed that the vertebral venous system can be filled only in a retrograde fashion at very high injection pressures compared with the ease of injections to the metaphyseal arterioles.[73] Their work showed that at each spinal segment, the vertebral artery

gives a nutrient vessel that enters the body. The posterior spinal arteries enter the spinal canal through each neural foramen. Subsequently, these arteries divide into ascending and descending branches, which anastomose with similar branches at each level. This posterior network of arterial vessels joins near the center of the vertebral body and enters in a large posterior nutrient foramen. Wiley and Trueta concluded that the richer arterial blood supply in the vicinity of cartilaginous endplates of the vertebral body was a more likely route of microorganism spread than retrograde venous flow as suggested by Batson. They also demonstrated how organisms can easily spread hematogenously to the metaphyseal areas of the adjacent vertebrae through rich arteriolar anastomoses.

Whalen and associates carried out extensive studies on the microvasculature of the vertebral endplates of fetal cadavers and rabbits.[71] They concluded that intervertebral disks are avascular, even in the very young. They saw no change in this pattern of vasculature with age. The cartilaginous endplates of the vertebral bodies showed a pattern of endarterial circulation.

The upper cervical spine has an unusual blood supply. A venous plexus around the odontoid called the pharyngeal vertebral vein usually has lymphovenous anastomosis.[55] This peculiar venous plexus may be the hematogenous route of spread to this area of the cervical spine.

MICROBIOLOGY

A host of organisms can infect the spine in both primary and postsurgical cases of vertebral osteomyelitis. Until a few decades ago, *Staphylococcus aureus* was the predominant organism isolated in cases of vertebral pyogenic osteomyelitis. *S. aureus* was the most common causative organism (60%) in a series reported by Waldvogel and associates,[70] but trends show a drop in *S. aureus* vertebral osteomyelitis cases and a rise in gram-negative bacillary infections. The other cases are caused by a wide spectrum of organisms. As antibiotic use becomes more widespread, the incidence of resistant *S. aureus* infections has been rising. Studies show that about 50% of the *S. aureus* organisms are now penicillin resistant and about 33% are also resistant to methicillin. The most common gram-negative bacteria are *Escherichia coli, Pseudomonas aeruginosa,* and proteus, which are common in urinary tract infections. There is a higher rate of pseudomonas infections in intravenous drug abusers. Vertebral osteomyelitis of the cervical spine caused by salmonella is relatively rare and can occur after an acute intestinal salmonella infection. However, in some cases of salmonella osteomyelitis, no evidence of previous infection can be found.[51] These organisms also have a strong tendency to lodge in diseased or unhealthy tissues. Occasionally, pyogenic infections may superinfect an underlying granulomatous infection following repeated attempts at biopsy. Infections with mixed organisms or anaerobic bacteria are uncommon and are usually associated with open fractures, foreign bodies, and gunshot wounds. Occasionally, coagulase-negative staphylococci or other low-virulence organisms such as diphtheroids may lead to slow-smoldering infection, which can further delay the diagnosis. Other organisms occasionally found in cervical spine infections include pneumococcus, gonococcus, meningococcus, *Serratia, Brucella, Eikenella,* and actinomycosis. Fungal organisms, most commonly *Blastomyces* and *Coccidioides*, may cause vertebral osteomyelitis, particularly in immunocompromised patients. Tuberculous spondylitis of the cervical spine is most commonly caused by *Mycobacterium tuberculosis,* although any other species of mycobacterium may be responsible.

PATHOPHYSIOLOGY

At one time, the intervertebral disk was considered the main focus in spine infections. Today, however, new evidence suggests that cartilaginous endplates and metaphyses are the initial foci in hematogenous infections.

Pyogenic Vertebral Osteomyelitis/ Diskitis

The infection is usually hematogenous in origin. The bacteria or other microorganisms are lodged in the low-pressure, low-flow capillary loops of endarticular circulation in the metaphyseal region of the vertebral body, through either the arterial (Wiley and Trueta[73]) or venous route (Batson[5]). The next series of events depends on the interplay between the host defenses and virulence of the offending organism. If the body's defenses are good, the organism may be localized and destroyed. But if the organism overcomes the body's defense mechanisms, it may proliferate and subsequently release various chemical toxins that obliterate the capillaries by thrombosis and can lead to local necrosis and microabscess formation. This initial stage of infection in the metaphyses impairs the nutritional requirements of the intervertebral disk. The disk undergoes a process of breakdown from loss of solutes and lack of water content, resulting in loss of height. Bacteria also release powerful proteolytic enzymes, which digest the disk rapidly in pyogenic infections, leading to reduced intervertebral disk space. The poor vascularity of the disks also inhibits penetration of antibiotics during treatment. If the infection is not detected or treated at this stage, this process continues unabated, and the architecture of the vertebral body is progressively destroyed, leading to erosions of the vertebral endplates. Granulation tissue or frank pus may collect in the canal, producing anterior cord compression. Later, the vertebral bodies may collapse, causing a kyphotic deformity with or without cord impingement. Abscesses can track anteriorly in the paravertebral region, and retropharyngeal abscesses may track down the mediastinum, causing fatal mediastinitis. Rarely, retropharyngeal abscess in cervical osteomyelitis may obstruct the airway or track into the posterior triangle of the neck or into the supraclavicular fossa. Sometimes abscesses caused by virulent microorganisms do not follow anatomical fascial planes and may extend into the viscera. Rarely, the infective process may penetrate through the dura, leading to development of subdural abscess or meningitis.[26] Rarely,

infection of the odontoid peg can lead to meningitis or an abscess of medulla oblongata or to significant instability in the atlantoaxial region.[59]

Tuberculous Spondylitis

Tuberculous osteomyelitis of the cervical spine usually results from hematogenous spread. The genitourinary and pulmonary systems are the most common primary foci, although occasionally spinal tuberculosis can result from other skeletal foci.[15, 28, 44]

Rarely, infection may result from direct extension of the disease locally, particularly from lymph nodes in the cervical spine. The infective process starts in the metaphyseal area and extends under the anterior longitudinal ligament to involve the adjacent vertebral bodies. In tuberculous spondylitis, the disk is relatively resistant to infection—in contrast to pyogenic infections, in which the disk rapidly disintegrates because of bacterial enzymes.[15, 58] The decreased disk space height in tuberculous spondylitis may result from either extension of the disease or dehydration of the disk material from impaired nutritional function of the endplate.[44] In cases of tuberculous spondylitis involving the central part of the vertebral body, the infective process may remain within the central part, isolated to one vertebra. This type of infection may be mistaken for a neoplastic bone lesion. The disease frequently leads to vertebral body collapse and so is more likely to result in considerable spinal deformity.[19] Tuberculosis most commonly involves the anterior elements of the spine, with the posterior elements involved only rarely. In children, there is more extensive and diffuse involvement of the spine with formation of large abscesses. The thick prevertebral fascia usually allows pus to collect in the retropharyngeal space. If the retropharyngeal abscess enlarges, it can compress the pharynx, trachea, or esophagus and result in respiratory distress or dysphagia. In adults, increased immune response of the host from previous subclinical exposure to tuberculosis makes the infective process more localized and abscesses usually are small at the time of diagnosis.

Histopathologically, tuberculous spondylitis is characterized by acid-fast–positive granuloma. The hallmark of the disease is caseating granuloma, consisting of tubercles composed of monocytes and epithelioid cells with central caseation. Langerhans-type giant cells are typical in the tubercle. Acid-fast stains easily identify *M. tuberculosis;* however, immunofluorescent techniques are more sensitive.

Generally, the degree and extent of destruction of the vertebral body are greater in tuberculosis than in pyogenic osteomyelitis. Infection usually destroys one-third to one-half of the vertebral body, but in some cases complete destruction of one or even two or more vertebral bodies may occur. Similarly, the resulting deformity is usually greater in tuberculosis than in pyogenic infections, because of greater bone destruction. Abscess formation is also more common in tuberculosis than in pyogenic osteomyelitis. In cases of continued infection, the granulation material or caseation tissue may compress the neural structures directly or secondary to collapse of the vertebral body. Similarly, the cord rootlets may incur ischemic necrosis because of blood vessel thrombosis from the inflammatory process or toxins.[41, 62]

Epidural Abscess

Much of the current understanding of the anatomy of the epidural space stems from the excellent work done by Dandy on cadavers.[17] Usually, the epidural space contains fat and epidural veins enclosed in loose areolar tissue. In the cervical region of the spine, the epidural space is a potential space with almost no fat between the vertebral body and dura. The epidural space is present only dorsal to the commencement of the spinal nerve rootlets. Anteriorly, the dura is closely applied to the spinal canal from C1 to the sacrum. Dorsally, the epidural space begins at about the C7 level and gradually increases in depth along the vertebral column.

Because of these anatomic features of the epidural space, most epidural abscesses occur in the lumbar and thoracic regions of the vertebral column. Epidural abscesses of the cervical spine account for only 14% of all epidural abscesses.[18] The vast majority of the epidural abscesses are located dorsally. In epidural abscesses, the infective process may initiate from direct spread from a foci of vertebral osteomyelitis, from hematogenous seeding from a distant source, or from iatrogenic causes. Primary infection of the epidural space is uncommon. Rarely, the epidural abscess may develop without evidence of vertebral osteomyelitis; a literature review has shown that about 10% of cases of epidural abscesses resulted from direct inoculation of organisms during surgery or after other surgical or diagnostic procedures.[18] The epidural abscess commonly leads to deficits possibly from compression by granulation tissue, pus, or impaired spinal cord blood supply (Fig. 17–1). Some researchers have identified thrombosis or thrombophlebitis of the veins of the cord, and others have also identified thrombosis of the arterioles along with veins in cases of epidural space infection.[9, 61]

CLINICAL PRESENTATION

The most striking characteristic of the cervical spine infections is a considerable delay in diagnosis. This delay is up to 2 to 3 months in more than 50% of cases.[31, 62] Up to 50% of cases may involve a history of recent urinary tract infection or urinary instrumentation, particularly in males.

The symptoms are usually subtle, and the onset is insidious. Neck pain is the most common and consistent feature. This may be the presenting symptom in up to 90% of patients. The severity of the pain is usually out of proportion to the patient's activity. This may be associated with torticollis or neck stiffness from muscle spasm, and neck movement may be painful and restricted. Night pain is common. Patients with vertebral osteomyelitis may exhibit low-grade fever, malaise, anorexia, nausea, and weight loss in subacute or chronic cases. Up to 1% of patients may have some signs of meningeal irritation. Cervical spine infections may be associated with varying degrees of neurologic compromise ranging from radiculopathy to myelopathy.

Patients with tuberculous spondylitis may have prolonged low-grade pyrexia, night sweats, anorexia, anemia, weight loss, and signs of pulmonary or renal involvement. A cold abscess or discharging sinus in the neck may be a late presentation. Neurologic symptoms may be present in up to 10% to 40% of cases. Rarely, a retropharyngeal abscess (either pyogenic or tuberculous) may compress the trachea or esophagus, causing respiratory distress or dysphagia.[39a] The patient may also have deformity along with the neurologic deficit. Usually there is a long delay in diagnosis of tuberculous spondylitis, varying from a few months to up to 2 years.

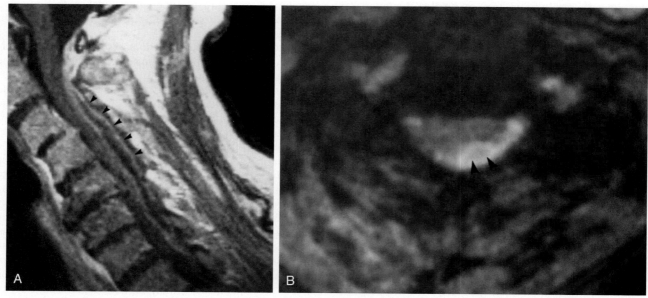

Figure 17–1. *Sagittal (A) and transverse (B) MRI images of a true epidural abscess show the dorsal location with spinal cord compression. Frank pus was found at the time of surgical decompression.*

Intravenous (IV) drug abusers have a more fulminant and acute course of disease. They may have high-grade pyrexia. They seldom show signs of neurologic deficits; interestingly, the incidence of neurologic deficit is much lower in IV drug abusers compared with the general population. Sudden onset of neck pain in IV drug users should raise suspicion of early spine infection.

In some cases of cervical spine infection, early in the course of disease, neck pain may be difficult to distinguish from pain of other more common spinal disorders. Sometimes neck pain may radiate to the interscapular region or to the shoulder, similar to the radiating pain in cervical spondylosis. Disease progression and spread to the surrounding tissues, cord, or spinal nerve rootlets may produce signs of nerve root irritation or long-tract signs with myelopathy and progressive neck deformity. Some patients may have bladder or bowel dysfunction. In one series of 18 patients with cervical spine infection, 13 had radiculopathy or myelopathy at presentation.[67]

Cervical spine infections are associated with increased incidence of neurologic deficits. Various risk factors predispose some patient populations to paralysis. These factors include rheumatoid arthritis, diabetes, steroid use, advanced age, and a more cephalad site of infection. Patients with *S. aureus* infections are more prone to significant neurologic deficits than patients with *Pseudomonas* infections.[21, 39]

On physical examination, most patients have localized neck tenderness around the diseased area, and some may also show a fluctuating mass or fullness of the neck. Usually there is muscle spasm, and neck movements are painful and restricted. In patients with neurologic involvement, the examiner may be able to elicit signs of nerve root irritation, myelopathy, or long-tract signs.

The clinical manifestations of tuberculous spondylitis of the cervical spine vary with age. Children usually have extensive damage with large abscesses but a relatively lower rate of neurologic deficit. In the older population, the tuberculous process may be more localized with less abscess formation but a higher incidence of neurologic deficits.

DIAGNOSTIC EVALUATION

The routine workup to diagnose cervical spine infections should include a detailed history and complete physical and neurologic examination. Laboratory studies include white blood cell (WBC) count, erythrocyte sedimentation rate (ESR), C-reactive protein, and blood, urine, and sputum cultures. Imaging studies include plain x-rays, magnetic resonance imaging (MRI), nuclear bone scanning, and computed tomography (CT) scanning.

Laboratory Studies

ESR is the most predictive test laboratory study for cervical spine infection. Up to 92% of affected patients have considerably elevated ESR values.[62] In unusual cases of occult infections from microorganisms of low virulence, the ESR may be normal. It has been documented that the ESR is decreased to 33% of the original value after successful treatment with antibiotics in all patients and decreased to 50% of the original value in most patients.[62] Persistent elevated ESR may suggest failure or inadequacy of treatment.

WBC count is less reliable in the diagnosis of cervical spine infections, and the absence of leukocytosis should not exclude the possibility of spine infection. If the organism cannot be grown on cultures, then serologic tests may be used in certain infections. A rising antistaphylococcal titer on sequential testing may suggest the presence of *S. aureus* infection; a rising antistreptolysin O titer may suggest streptococcal infections; and elevated agglutination test results may point to *Brucella* and salmonella infections. In suspected gonococcal infections, specific complement fixation tests may be used. The diagnosis of tuberculosis and fungal infections of the spine may be aided by specific skin tests, although false-negative tuberculin skin test results occur in up to 30% of cases.

Cultures

Appropriate cultures must be done before antibiotic therapy is started for cervical spine infections. Blood and urine cultures should be obtained particularly when the patient has an acute temperature elevation. Swabs from any suspected primary site of infection (e.g., skin lesion, sputum, urine, discharging sinus) should be taken for culture of both aerobic and anaerobic organisms. Routine cerebrospinal fluid (CSF) culture is not recommended in the diagnosis of cervical spine infection, but certainly has a role in patients exhibiting signs of meningeal irritation.

Diagnostic Biopsy

Accurate microbiologic diagnosis is essential to determine the infectious organism and guide proper treatment in cases of cervical spine infection. Because blood cultures are positive in less than 25% of all cases of cervical spine infection, closed or open biopsy is strongly recommended to confirm the diagnosis. Closed needle aspiration biopsy can be safely performed under x-ray control or CT-guided needle biopsy for exact localization. Definitive diagnosis can be obtained in up to 68% to 86% of cases.[2, 30, 54, 62] Open biopsy is indicated if the closed biopsy techniques fail to yield organisms. Open biopsy has a higher yield because of direct localization of the infected area and the availability of a large volume of specimens.

Needle biopsy may yield false-negative results in certain cases in which either the patient already received antibiotic therapy or biopsy material failed to include infected tissue. If a needle biopsy is negative in a patient who is already receiving antibiotics, the antibiotics should be stopped for 48 to 72 hours and another biopsy specimen obtained. If the second biopsy also fails to yield organisms, then open biopsy should be considered. Even then, biopsy may not be positive if there has been earlier administration of antibiotics or there has been a long interval between the onset of infection and the biopsy. Closed or needle biopsy is especially useful in early cases in which there is no evidence of spinal instability or neurologic deficit and surgery may not be required. In other cases with more advanced disease and where decompression and stabilization is required, open biopsy with definitive surgical debridement is preferred. All biopsy samples should be submitted for histopathologic tests to exclude malignancy, and the staining techniques should include gram staining, acid-fast staining, and staining for fungi.

Radiologic Evaluation
Plain X-rays

Plain x-rays are not very helpful in the earlier stages of the disease. In most cases, plain x-rays do not reveal changes for 3 to 4 weeks after the onset of infection. The most consistent and earliest radiographic findings are narrowing of the intervertebral disk space and blurring of endplates with endplate erosion.[15b] These findings may be difficult to differentiate from degenerative cervical disk disease in elderly patients. The retropharyngeal space may appear widened. Before changes become apparent on plain x-rays, as early as 10 to 14 days after the onset of infection, tomograms may suggest infection by revealing localized osteopenic areas near the vertebral body endplates.[29] In later stages, bone rarefaction and subchondral reactive bone formation are seen. Continued disease progression may cause extensive destruction and vertebral collapse, segmental kyphosis, and abscess formation. Postinfection sclerosis and reactive new bone formation may continue to progress and in some cases may lead to spontaneous spinal fusion. In tuberculous spondylitis, disk space narrowing may not

occur for up to 2 to 3 years, but diffuse and intense osteopenia and a large prevertebral mass with fine calcification in the paravertebral soft tissue spaces are relatively pathognomonic of tuberculosis (Fig. 17–2). Central body involvement resembles a tumor; chest x-rays may help detect a pulmonary focus.

Infection of the upper cervical spine may present as a retropharyngeal abscess with subluxation of C1–C2 (Fig. 17–3). In epidural abscess, plain x-rays are commonly negative, except where vertebral osteomyelitis or disk space infection is concurrent.

Other Imaging Modalities
Radionuclide Scans

Radionuclide scans are relatively accurate in identifying and localizing cervical spine infections before plain radiographs become positive. These studies include technetium 99m (Tc 99m) bone scan, gallium (Ga 67) scan, and indium 111 labeled leukocyte (In 111 WBC) scan.

The TC 99m bone scan reveals diffusely increased uptake or increased activity in the area of infection on the early blood pool images and more focal activity on delayed static images. Its relative accuracy is 86%, with specificity of 78% and sensitivity of 90%.[52]

A useful adjunct to the Tc 99m scan for the diagnosis of spine infection, the Ga-67 scan shows increased uptake in a more localized fashion at the infection site. The Ga 67 scan has an accuracy rate similar to that of the Tc 99m scan, with accuracy of 85% and sensitivity of 89%.[10] Unlike the

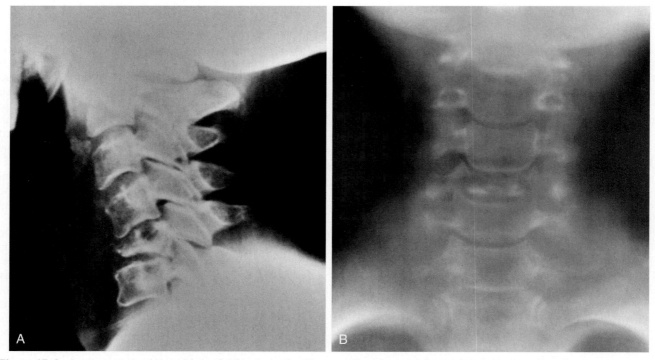

Figure 17–2. Anteroposterior (A) and lateral (B) x-rays of a 52-year-old patient with history of chronic myelogenous leukemia who presented with neck pain and interscapular pain. The x-rays show a destructive lesion of the body of C5 with disc space narrowing and kyphotic deformity and rarefaction suggestive of tuberculosis. Note the anterior soft tissue swelling. Open biopsy and cultures confirmed the diagnosis of tuberculosis.

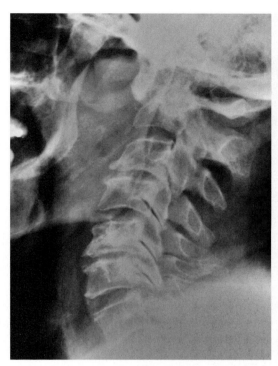

Figure 17–3. Lateral x-ray of a patient with a large prevertebral or retropharyngeal abscess. A large soft tissue shadow is displacing the pharynx and trachea anteriorly. There is also destruction of odontoid peg with settling of the atlantoaxial joint.

Tc 99m scan, the Ga 67 scan shows normal activity during resolution of infection and thus is useful in monitoring the response to treatment. When these two scans are combined, they are 94% accurate in determining the infection of the spine.[52]

The In 111 labeled WBC scan is only 31% accurate in diagnosing spine infections[72] and thus is not recommended for this application.

Magnetic Resonance Imaging

MRI is now the imaging modality of choice for evaluating cervical spine infections. Good-quality MRI is highly accurate and is a method of quickly identifying early spine infections and recognizing intraspinal and paravertebral abscesses. With an accuracy of 94% (specificity of 93% and sensitivity of 96%), MRI compares favorably with the combined accuracy of Tc 99m and Ga 67 scans.[52] MRI provides much more anatomical information than can be provided by a combination of radionuclide scans. MRI is also excellent in localizing dural compression on both sagittal and axial planes and helpful in assessing the spread of infection into the epidural space or toward adjoining soft tissues.

MRI shows very characteristic changes in the disk space and subchondral bone in spine infections. T1-weighted images show confluent hypointensity of signal of the vertebral endplates and adjacent disks with loss of normal anatomic outline of the vertebral endplates and nucleus pulposus (Fig. 17–4). The complementary T2-weighted sequences show hyperintensity of the intervertebral disk and vertebral body and, in most cases, loss of the intranuclear cleft of the nucleus pulposus normally present in the adult disk.[4] These signal changes are thought to result from initial ischemia and increased water content because of inflammatory exudate in the infected area. These characteristic changes cannot differentiate between pyogenic and granulomatous infections of the spine; thus MRI does not eliminate the role of diagnostic biopsy. The false-negative rate of MRI may be reduced with the addition of gadolinium-labeled diethylenetriaminepentaacetic acid (G-DTPA). This also enhances the delineation of epidural abscesses and much better defines the extent of infection.[52]

Subsequent studies have better defined the MRI changes of vertebral osteomyelitis.[15a] The classic findings are as described earlier, with confluent decreased signal changes of the disk and adjacent vertebral bodies on T1 images and increased signal changes in the disk space on T2 images. However, a certain percentage of patients with diskitis do not exhibit classic T2 changes and may show isointense or decreased signal intensity.[15b] Clinical judgment is essential in determining the diagnosis not only in those patients with unusual MRI findings, but in all cases of suspected vertebral osteomyelitis.

Computed Tomography

CT provides additional useful information regarding bony destruction and degree of neural compression and has an important role in the diagnosis of spine infections. CT scanning also commonly reveals abscesses and paravertebral soft tissue swellings. CT findings may include lytic lesions in the subchondral bone, irregularity and multiple holes in endplates visible in cross-sectional views, reactive sclerosis around lytic defects, and disintegration of the circumferential bony ring near the periphery of the disk. CT also provides good detail of uninvolved surrounding bony anatomy, which can help the surgeon plan reconstructive procedures. CT-guided needle biopsies of the cervical spine are being used more often and have proven very safe at all levels of the spinal column (Fig. 17–5). The procedure facilitates proper needle placement in the vertebral body and disk in both adults and children.

Myelography is a confirmatory investigation for diagnosis of epidural abscesses. This should be done at a level away from the abscess, and both caudal and cranial sides of the abscess must be delineated. Postmyelography CT provides information about the spinal column; it clearly defines neural compression by bony impingement or by abscesses and further helps determine whether the infection extends into the neural tissue. In addition, a CSF sample can be obtained concomitantly for testing for meningitis. Myelography used in conjunction with CT carries a small risk of possible intrathecal dissemination of infection.

MANAGEMENT/TREATMENT

Before the advent of antibiotics, the mainstay of treating spine infections was abscess drainage and bed rest. Mortality with this course of treatment was unacceptably high, up to 70%.[35, 42] The advent of antibiotics has totally

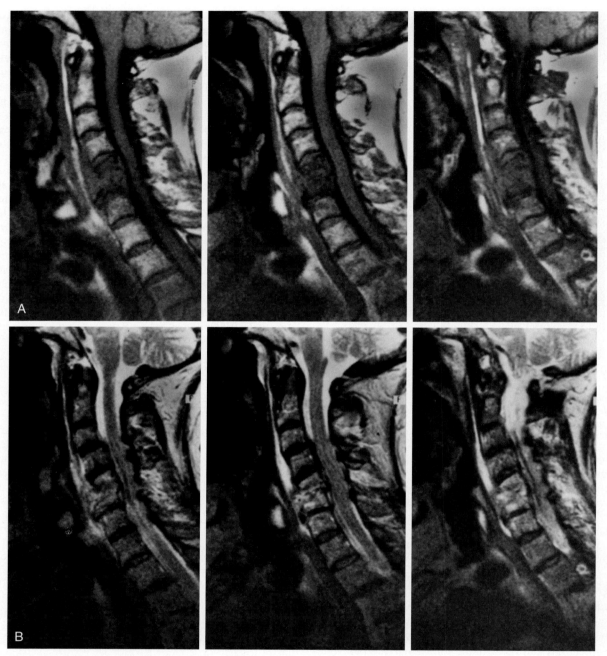

Figure 17–4. *A, Sagittal T1-weighted MRI image of the cervical spine showing decreased signal intensity of the disk space and adjoining bone and loss of normal anatomical details of the disk and endplates consistent with vertebral osteomyelitis. Mild kyphosis with impression of the spinal cord is also evident. B, Sagittal T2-weighted MRI image of cervical spine of same patient showing increased signal intensity due to edema in the anterior soft tissues as well as in the posterior longitudinal ligaments. Retropulsion of a vertebral fragment with compression is also visible.*

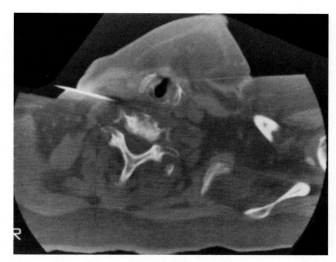

Figure 17–5. CT-guided aspiration biopsy. The tip of the needle is being directed toward the anterior part of the body of C5.

modified the natural history of spine infections; today the mortality rate of cervical spine infections is around 5%.

Nonoperative Management

The basic goals of treatment of cervical spine infections are to:

1. Identify pathogens by culture/biopsies.
2. Eradicate the spine infection and prevent recurrence.
3. Maintain or restore neurologic status.
4. Relieve pain.
5. Ensure spinal stability.

Along with the proper use of antibiotics, general supportive measures, and immobilization of the cervical spine, associated medical issues also must be addressed. Any systemic illness, including diabetes, should be vigorously controlled. Attention should be given to adequate nutrition. If there is another focus of infection in the body, such as the skin or genitourinary tract, it must be adequately treated. Biopsy, either closed or open, is mandatory in most cases, with the exception of pediatric diskitis.

It is generally recommended that antibiotics be withheld until pathogens are identified, except in cases where patients are extremely toxic with systemic illness. In these particular cases, broad-spectrum antibiotics should be commenced at heavy doses soon after the biopsy specimen is collected. Other patients who show a clinical picture of cervical spine infection but have an unrevealing biopsy and culture should be treated with systemic broad-spectrum antibiotics along with immobilization in a halo vest or orthosis for a period of 3 to 4 months.

When biopsy and culture are positive for a pathogen, antibiotics should be selected according to the sensitivity test results. Currently recommendations include systemic antibiotic therapy at maximal doses for 6 weeks followed by oral antibiotics for 3 months or until the infection completely resolves. Serum antibiotic levels should be monitored regularly to ensure that adequate serum concentrations are available for tissue penetration. Most aminoglycosides, including gentamicin, tobramycin, and clindamycin, penetrate the disk very well.[22] Systemic antibiotic therapy for less than 28 days is associated with a high relapse rate.[62]

The patient's clinical progress and neurologic status should be monitored regularly during the course of parenteral antibiotic treatment. The ESR should be checked periodically; it should start to fall by the third week or so and may be expected to fall by 50% to 70% at the completion of antibiotic therapy. Serum levels of aminoglycosides and other nephrotoxic antibiotics should be monitored to avoid toxicity, particularly in elderly and diabetic patients, who may already have renal impairment or may develop it during treatment.

This approach to medical management is successful in most patients with early pyogenic osteomyelitis of the cervical spine. In successfully treated patients, it can lead to spontaneous osseous fusion of the adjacent vertebral bodies. In cases where the patient fails to demonstrate clinical improvement and the ESR fails to drop within 1 to 2 weeks or the patient shows progression of neurologic deficit, medical treatment should be abandoned and surgical intervention considered without delay.[24, 24a, 31a]

The use of antitubercular drugs has greatly improved the success of treatment for tuberculous spondylitis of the cervical spine.[49] Surgery is indicated in cases of vertebral collapse, spinal instability, neurologic deficit, abscess formation, and segmental kyphosis. Chemotherapy along with general supportive measures and immobilization of the cervical spine have produced good results in up to 96% of patients with a minimal increase in kyphosis.[28] Currently used antitubercular drugs include isoniazid, rifampin, streptomycin, pyrazinamide, and ethambutol in 6- and 9-month courses.

Epidural abscess is considered both a medical and a surgical emergency. The goals of treatment are similar to those for other spine infections. Medical treatment with antibiotics alone is recommended for only a small group of patients who have abscesses involving a significant length of vertebral canal and for those patients without neurologic deficit who are considered poor surgical risks. In most patients, the treatment of choice is surgical drainage of abscesses and specific antibiotic treatment.

Surgical Management

If the disease has resulted in neurologic compromise, patients should be treated urgently with surgical debridement, decompression of the spinal cord, and fusion.

Indications for Surgery

Indications for surgery to treat cervical spine infection include:

1. The need for open biopsy to obtain microbiologic diagnosis in cases where needle biopsy is negative
2. Failure of medical treatment

3. Epidural or paravertebral/retropharyngeal abscesses

4. Evidence of spinal cord compression or deterioration in neurologic status

5. Spinal instability with significant vertebral body destruction and spinal deformity.

The principal objectives of surgery include radical anterior debridement with excision of all infected material, sequestra, and granulation tissue; drainage of abscesses; and decompression of the spinal cord and spinal nerve roots. After debridement, the spine should be stabilized with autogenous bone grafting (Fig. 17–6) and external immobilization.[24, 24A] The debrided tissue and pus are sent for histopathology and culture and sensitivity. Surgery should be done as soon as possible in patients with neural deficit, to prevent irreversible damage and maximize recovery.[21, 31a] Laminectomy is strongly contraindicated in the vast majority of cases, except in patients with epidural spinal abscesses, where the pathology is mostly posterior or dorsal. Laminectomy for vertebral body disease is contraindicated, because it results in increased spinal instability and neurologic deterioration.[40] In selected cases, supplemental segmental posterior stabilization and fusion may be considered after single-level or multilevel corpectomy to provide immediate mechanical stability and protection for neural tissues. This may obviate the need for a halo vest postoperatively, which is recommended if anterior debridement and reconstruction alone is performed.

After reconstructive surgery, antibiotic therapy should be continued as recommended. In early cases of cervical spine infection in which no appreciable bone loss has occurred, bone grafting may not be required after debridement. In 1976, Messer and Litvinoff reported on 12 patients with

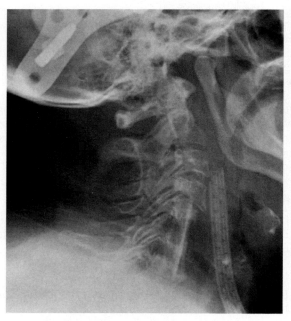

Figure 17–6. *Postoperative x-ray of same patient as shown in Figures 17–3 and 17–4. The patient underwent a C5–C6 corpectomy and autogenous fibular grafting. The fibular graft is in place, and the Penrose drain is visible.*

pyogenic spondylitis of the cervical spine.[50] They successfully treated 11 patients with simple drainage at the time of open biopsy along with parenteral antibiotics and immobilization without bone grafting. All 11 patients progressed to osseous fusion of vertebral bodies. In our experience, however, most cases require substantial debridement, and iliac strut grafting is highly recommended.[24] Several reports have documented immediate posterior instrumentation of the infected, unstable spine with successful results in the thoracic and lumbar spine.[10a, 61a] Anterior plating after debridement of cervical vertebral osteomyelitis has been successful in a small series.[58a] Immediate concomitant posterior stabilization after anterior debridement and strut grafting will provide excellent stability and carries a minimal risk of persistent infection.

Because most epidural abscesses are located dorsally, laminectomy is recommended. However, care should be taken to preserve the facet joints as much as possible to enhance spinal stability. When epidural abscesses are associated with vertebral body osteomyelitis, anterior and posterior decompression is usually required. In these cases, spinal stability is significantly compromised, and spinal fusion is also necessary.

AUTHORS' PREFERRED METHOD

We believe that a high index of suspicion is necessary for the early detection of suspected cervical spine infection. This will help avoid a long delay in diagnosis, the hallmark of cervical spine infections.

Along with routine laboratory and imaging studies, we recommend CT-guided aspiration/biopsy in almost all cases. Medical treatment is usually instituted in cases detected early in the course of disease without neurologic deficit. This includes hospitalization with bed rest and parenteral antibiotics according to the results of culture and sensitivity tests. The cervical spine is immobilized externally with an orthosis or halo vest. Patients who do not respond to medical treatment or those who present late in the course of the disease require surgical treatment, as discussed earlier.

The extrapharyngeal or extraoral approach is useful in infections of the upper cervical spine, C1–C2. This gives sufficient exposure and permits decompression and debridement. A transoral approach runs the risk of contamination with oral flora. If instability rather than neural deficit is present at C1–C2, then another option is posterior stabilization (typically an instrumented occipitocervical fusion) and intravenous antibiotics (Fig. 17–7).[73a]

For infections of the lower cervical spine, C3–C7, we prefer the traditional anterior approach of Southwick and Smith Robinson. After adequate debridement, strut grafting with autogenous tricortical iliac crest graft is done in all cases. Autogenous fibula can be used if necessary, but iliac struts are preferred because they have less cortical bone to revascularize and thus may be more resistant to persistent infection. After surgery, systemic antibiotics are continued for a total of 6 weeks, followed by oral antibiotics for another 3 months. The preoperatively applied halo vest is worn for 2 to 3 months. Alternatively, concomitant posterior

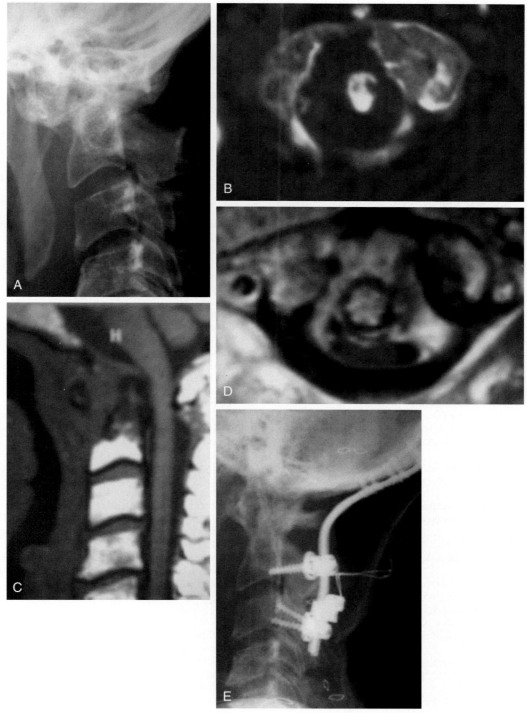

Figure 17–7. *A 60-year-old male presented with a 3-month history of increasing upper cervical spine pain. Examination demonstrated severe pain on neck rotation and hyperreflexia, but no motor or sensory findings. A, This lateral plain x-ray shows C1–C2 instability with a suggestion of bone destruction. B, A CT scan shows some bony changes in the C1–C2 facet joints and subluxation of the dens. C, The T1-weighted sagittal MRI demonstrates signal changes within the odontoid and soft tissue in the atlanto-dens interval. D, The T2-weighted transverse MRI cut shows asymmetric increased signal change in the facets plus severe cord compression due to the subluxation. E, After a posterolateral needle biopsy documented inflammatory cells and no neoplasm, the patient underwent a C1 laminectomy and posterior occipitocervical stabilization with instrumentation and autogenous bone grafting. An organism was never successfully cultured, and he was treated with 6 weeks of intravenous antibiotics followed by 3 months of oral antibiotics until resolution of his symptoms.*

instrumentation and fusion will stabilize most patients and allow for a rigid orthosis rather than a halo postoperatively. Anterior plating in the setting of pyogenic vertebral osteomyelitis has been used successfully with no evidence of persistent infection.[58a]

In cases of tuberculous spondylitis, we prefer to start antitubercular antibiotics a few days before anterior debridement and fusion. In cases of epidural abscess, if anterior debridement and fusion are needed along with posterior decompressive laminectomy, then we strongly consider internal fixation of the spine plus a halo vest to treat this grossly unstable situation.

REFERENCES

1. Albee FH: Transplantation of a portion of the tibia into the spine for Pott's disease: A preliminary report. JAMA 57:885–886, 1911.
2. Armstrong P, Green G, Irving JD: Needle aspiration/biopsy of the spine in suspected disc infection. Br J Radiol 51:333–337, 1978.
3. Baker CJ: Primary epidural abscess. Am J Dis Child 121:337–339, 1971.
4. Baker AS, Ojemann RG, Swartz MN, Richardson EP Jr: Spinal epidural abscess. N Engl J Med 293:463–468, 1975.
5. Batson OV: The function of the vertebral veins and their role in the spread of metastasis. Ann Surg 112:138–149, 1940.
6. Bergman I, Wald ER, Meyer JD, Painter MJ: Epidural abscess and the vertebral osteomyelitis following serial lumbar punctures. Pediatrics 72:476–480, 1983.
7. Biller HF, Ogura JH, Rontal M, Ehrlich C: Cervical osteomyelitis complicating pharyngeal resection. Arch Otolaryngol 94:165–168, 1971.
8. Bonfiglo M, Lange TA, Kim YM: Pyogenic vertebral osteomyelitis: Disk space infections. Clin Orthop 96:234–247, 1973.
9. Browder J, Meyers R: Infections of the spinal epidural space. An aspect of vertebral osteomyelitis. Am J Surg 37:4–26, 1937.
10. Bruschwein DA, Brown ML, McLeod RA: Gallium scintigraphy in the evaluation of disk-space infections. J Nucl Med 21:925–927, 1980.
10a. Carragee EJ: Instrumentation of the infected and unstable spine: A review of 17 cases from the thoracic and lumbar spine with pyogenic infections. J Spinal Disord 10:317–324, 1997.
11. Carvell JE, Maclarnon JC: Chronic osteomyelitis of the thoracic spine due to Salmonella typhi: A case report. Spine 6:527–530, 1981.
12. Cashion EL: Cervical intervertebral disc space infection following cerebral angiography. Neuroradiology 2:176–178, 1971.
13. Cleveland M: Tuberculosis of the spine. A clinical study of 203 patients from Sea View and St. Luke's Hospital. Am Rev Tuberculosis 41:215–231, 1940.
14. Collert S: Osteomyelitis of the spine. Acta Orthop Scand 48:283–290, 1977.
15. Compere EL, Garrison M: Correlation of pathologic and roentgenologic findings in tuberculosis and pyogenic infections of the vertebra: The fate of the intervertebral disk. Ann Surg 104:1038–1067, 1936.
15a. Dagirmanjian A, Schils J, McHenry M, Modic MT: MR imaging of vertebral osteomyelitis revisited. Am J Roentgenol 167:1539–1543, 1996.
15b. Dagirmanjian A, Schils J, McHenry M, Modic MT: Spinal osteomyelitis. Semin Spine Surg 9:38–50, 1997.
16. Connor PM, Darden BV: Cervical discography complications and clinical efficacy. Spine 18:2035–2038, 1993.
17. Dandy WE: Abscesses and inflammatory tumors in the spinal epidural space (so-called pachymeningitis external). Arch Surg 13:477–494, 1926.
18. Danner RL, Hartman BJ: Update on spinal epidural abscess: 35 cases and review of literature. Rev Infect Dis 9:265–274, 1987.
19. Doub HP, Badgley CE: The roentgen signs of tuberculosis of the vertebral body. Am J Roentgenol 27:827–837, 1932.
20. Dripps RD, Vandam LD: Hazards of lumbar puncture. JAMA 147:1118–1121, 1951.
21. Eismont FJ, Bohlman HH, Soni PL, et al: Pyogenic and fungal vertebral osteomyelitis with paralysis. J Bone Joint Surg Am 65A:19–29, 1983.
22. Eismont FJ, Weisel SW, Brighton CT, Rothman RH: Antibiotic penetration into rabbit nucleus pulposus. Spine 12:254–256, 1987.
23. El Gindi S, Aref S, Salama M, Andrew J: Infection of intervertebral discs after operation. J Bone Joint Surg Br 58B:114–116, 1976.
24. Emery SE, Chan DPK, Woodward HR: Treatment of hematogenous pyogenic vertebral osteomyelitis with anterior debridement and primary bone grafting. Spine 14:284–291, 1989.
24a. Fang D, Cheung KMC, Dos Remedios IDM, et al: Pyogenic vertebral osteomyelitis: Treatment by anterior spinal debridement and fusion. J Spinal Disord 7:173–180, 1994.
25. Forsythe M, Rothman RH: New concepts in the diagnosis and treatment of infections of the cervical spine. Orthop Clin N Am 9:1039–1051, 1978.
26. Fraser RAR, Ratzan K, Wolpert SM, Weinstein L: Spinal subdural empyema. Arch Neurol 28:235–238, 1973.
27. Frederickson B, Yuan H, Orlans R: Management and outcome of pyogenic vertebral osteomyelitis. Clin Orthop 131:160–167, 1978.
28. Friedman B: Chemotherapy of tuberculosis of the spine. J Bone Joint Surg Am 48A:451–474, 1966.
28a. Fu WK, Wu WC, Ip FK: Concomitant tuberculosis and pyogenic infection of the cervical spine: A case report. Spine 23:139–143, 1998.
29. Garcia A Jr, Grantham SA: Hematogenous pyogenic vertebral osteomyelitis. J Bone Joint Surg Am 42A:429–436, 1960.
30. Ghelman B, Lospinuso MF, Levine DB, et al: Percutaneous CT guided biopsy of the thoracic and lumbar spine. Spine 16:736–739, 1991.
31. Griffiths HED, Jones PM: Pyogenic infection of the spine: A review of twenty-eight cases. J Bone Joint Surg Br 53B:383–391, 1971.
31a. Hadjipavlou AG, Mader JT, Necessary JT, Muffoletto AJ: Hematogenous pyogenic spinal infections and their surgical management. Spine 25:1668–1679, 2000.
32. Hagadorn B, Smith HW, Rosnagle RS: Cervical spine osteomyelitis secondary to a foreign body in the hypopharynx. Arch Otolaryngol 95:578–580, 1972.
33. Hanley EN, Phillip EO: Profile of patients who get spine infections and the type of infections that have a predilection for the spine. Semin Spine Surg 2:257, 1990.
34. Hatch, ES: Acute osteomyelitis of the spine. N Orleans Med Surg J 83:801, 1931.
35. Hatch ES: Acute osteomyelitis of the spine. Report of case with review of the literature. N Orleans Med Surg J 83:861–873, 1931.

36. Hibbs RA: An operation for progressive spinal deformities. NY State Med J 93:1013–1016, 1911.

37. Hodgson AR, Stock FE: Anterior spinal fusion: A preliminary communication on the radical treatment of Pott's disease and Pott's paraplegia. Br J Surg 44:266–275, 1956.

38. Ito H, Tsuchiya J, Asami G: A new radical operation for Pott's disease: Report of the ten cases. J Bone Joint Surg 16A:499–515, 1934.

39. Jabbari B, Pierce JF: Spinal cord compression due to pseudomonas in a heroin addict. Case report. Neurology 27:1034–1037, 1977.

39a. Jang YJ, Rhee CK: Retropharyngeal abscess associated with vertebral osteomyelitis and spinal epidural abscess. Otolaryngol Head Neck Surg 119:705–708, 1998.

40. Kemp HBS, Jackson JW, Shaw NC: Laminectomy in paraplegia due to infective spondylosis. Br J Surg 61:66–72, 1974.

41. Kemp HBS, Jackson JW, Jeremiah JD, Hall AJ: Pyogenic infections occurring primarily in intervertebral discs. J Bone Joint Surg Br 55B:698–714, 1973.

42. Kulowski J: Pyogenic osteomyelitis of the spine. An analysis and discussion of 102 cases. J Bone Joint Surg 18A:343–364, 1936.

43. Lannelongue OM: On acute osteomyelitis. Miscellaneous, Pathological, and Practical Medicine Tracts. Paris, 1879.

44. La Rocca H: Spinal sepsis. In Rothman RH, Simeone FA (eds): The Spine, 2nd ed. Philadelphia, WB Saunders, 1982, pp 757–774.

45. Leonard A, Comty CM, Shapiro FL, Raij L: Osteomyelitis in hemodialysis patients. Ann Intern Med 78:651–658, 1973.

46. Lindholm TS, Pylkkanen P: Discitis following removal of intervertebral disc. Spine 7:618–622, 1982.

47. Malawski SK, Lukawski S: Pyogenic infection of the spine. Clin Orthop 272:58–66, 1991.

48. Martin NS: Tuberculosis of the spine: A study of the results of treatment during the last twenty-five years. J Bone Joint Surg Br 52B:613–628, 1970.

49. Medical Research Council Working Party on Tuberculosis of the Spine: A controlled trial of six-month and nine-month regimens of chemotherapy in patients undergoing radical surgery for tuberculosis of the spine in Hong Kong. Tubercle 67:243–259, 1986.

50. Messer HD, Litvinoff J: Pyogenic cervical osteomyelitis. Chondro-osteomyelitis of the cervical spine frequently associated with parenteral drug use. Arch Neurol 33:571–576, 1976.

51. Miller ME, Fogel GR, Dunham WK: Salmonella spondylitis: A review and report of two immunologically normal patients. J Bone Joint Surg Am 70A:463–466, 1988.

52. Modic MT, Feiglin DH, Piraino DW, et al: Vertebral osteomyelitis: Assessment using MR. Radiology 157:157–166, 1985.

53. Nagel DA, Albright JA, Keggi KJ, Southwick WO: Closer look at spinal lesions: Open biopsy of vertebral lesions. JAMA 191:975–978, 1965.

54. Ottolenghi CE, Schajowicz F, De Schant FA: Aspiration biopsy of the cervical spine: Technique and results in thirty-four cases. J Bone Joint Surg Am 46A:715–733, 1964.

55. Parke WW, Rothman RH, Brown MD: The pharyngovertebral veins: An anatomical rationale for Grisel's syndrome. J Bone Joint Surg Am 66A:568–574, 1984.

56. Pinckney LE, Currarino G, Highgenboten CL: Osteomyelitis of the cervical spine following dental extraction. Radiology 135:335–337, 1980.

57. Pott P: Remarks on that Kind of Palsy of the Lower Limbs Which is Frequently Found to Accompany a Curvature of the Spine and is Supposed to be Caused by It, Together with Its Method of Cure. London, Johnson, 1779, pp 1–84.

58. Resnick D, Niwayama G: Osteomyelitis, septic arthritis and soft tissue infection: The axial skeleton. In Resnick D (ed): Diagnosis of Bone and Joint Disorders with Emphasis on Articular Abnormalities. Philadelphia, WB Saunders, 1981, pp 2130–2153.

58a. Rezai AR, Woo HH, Errico TJ, Cooper PR: Contemporary management of spinal osteomyelitis. Neurosurgery 44:1018–1025, 1999.

59. Rimalovski AB, Aronson SM: Abscess of medulla oblongata associated with osteomyelitis of odontoid process. Case report. J Neurosurg 29:97–101, 1968.

60. Robinson BHB, Lessof MH: Osteomyelitis of the spine. Guys Hospital Reports 110:303–318, 1961.

61. Russell NA, Vaughan R, Morley TP: Spinal epidural infection. Can J Neurol Sci 6:325–328, 1979.

61a. Safran O, Rand N, Kaplan L, et al: Sequential or simultaneous, same-day anterior decompression and posterior stabilization in the management of vertebral osteomyelitis of the lumbar spine. Spine 23:1885–1890, 1998.

62. Sapico FL, Montgomerie JZ: Pyogenic vertebral osteomyelitis: Report of nine cases and review of the literature. Rev Infect Dis 1:754–776, 1979.

63. Sapico FL, Montgomerie JZ: Vertebral osteomyelitis in intravenous drug abusers. Report of three cases and review of literature. Rev Infect Dis 2:196–206, 1980.

64. Schaefer SD, Bucholz RW, Jones RE, Carder HM: The management of transpharyngeal gunshot wounds to the cervical spine. Surg Gynecol Obstet 152:27–29, 1981.

65. Seddon HJ: Pott's paraplegia: Prognosis and treatment. Br J Surg 22:769–799, 1934/1935.

66. Stone DB, Bonfiglio M: Pyogenic vertebral osteomyelitis: A diagnostic pitfall for the internist. Arch Intern Med 112:491–500, 1963.

67. Stone JL, Cybulski GR, Rodriquez J, et al: Anterior cervical debridement and strut grafting for osteomyelitis of the cervical spine. J Neurosurg 70:879–883, 1989.

68. Thalgott JS, Cotler HB, Sasso RC, et al: Postoperative infections in spinal implants: Classification and analysis–A multi-center study. Spine 16:981–984, 1991.

69. Thibodeau AA: Closed space infection following removal of lumbar intervertebral disc. J Bone Joint Surg Am 50A:400–410, 1968.

70. Waldvogel FA, Medoff G, Swartz MN: Osteomyelitis: A review of clinical features, therapeutic considerations and unusual aspects. N Engl J Med 282:198–206, 260–266, 316–322, 1970.

71. Whalen JL, Parke WW, Mazur JM, Stauffer ES: The intrinsic vasculature of developing vertebral end plates and its nutritive significance to the intervertebral discs. J Pediatr Orthop 5:403–410, 1985.

72. Whalen JL, Brown ML, McLeod R, Fitzgerald RH Jr: Limitations of indium leukocyte imaging for diagnosis of spine infections. Spine 16:193–197, 1991.

73. Wiley AM, Trueta J: The vascular anatomy of the spine and its relationship to pyogenic vertebral osteomyelitis. J Bone Joint Surg Br 41B:796–809, 1959.

73a. Zigler J, Bohlman HH, Riley L, et al: Pyogenic osteomyelitis of the occiput, the atlas, and the axis: A report of five cases. J Bone Joint Surg Am 69A:1069–1073, 1987.

Postoperative Considerations

18

SURGICAL COMPLICATIONS

Michael J. Bolesta, M.D.
Robert G. Viere, M.D.

Show me a surgeon who has no complications and I will show you a surgeon who does not operate.
— Anonymous

If plan A fails, do not repeat plan A.
— Anonymous

Surgeons pride themselves on their skill and expertise. It must be recognized that confidence is needed by all who work with the delicate tissues around the human spine. As careful as we are, however, the results of our efforts sometimes disappoint patient and physician alike. This does not deter us in our quest to alleviate pain and suffering, and we cling to an ideal of excellence. To learn from failure and imperfect outcomes, both personal and collegial, is a sign of maturity and wisdom.

INFECTION

Infection is uncommon in cervical surgery. The most common sites are outside of the operative fields, in the pulmonary and urinary tracts. In the literature reviewed for this chapter, the rate of wound infection ranged from 0 to 4.5%.[15, 24, 55] For posterior cervical plating, a procedure that is gaining widespread acceptance, the incidence in two series was 1.5% in 78 cases[24] and 4.5% in 44 cases.[15] The etiology is uncertain but may reflect early experience with the technique with longer operative times.

Infection is uncommon in part because the neck is a clean area. The field can be contaminated by breaks in technique. When recognized intraoperatively, the wound may be irrigated copiously. With anterior approaches, infection is common when the esophagus is violated occultly.[36, 70] Prompt recognition will reduce the morbidity of this complication.[70] The surgeon who suspects transmural esophageal injury can have the anesthesiologist place a catheter in the proximal esophagus and inject an ampule of indigo carmine. This dye may leak through the hole, staining the field. Entry of dye into the gastrointestinal system is confirmed by excretion of dye in the urine. A recognized injury should be repaired and protected with a nasogastric tube, delayed oral nutrition, and antibiotics to cover oral organisms.[45] Delayed presentation will generally require abscess drainage, debridement, antibiotics, and salivary diversion.[51, 70] If the infection spreads to the mediastinum, the morbidity and mortality greatly increase. Generally such an infection presents early in the postoperative period, although Kuriloff and colleagues reported two cases that manifested 2 and 4 months later with abscess and pharyngocutaneous fistulae.[36] Both cases had bone infection that required debridement.

In the transoral approach to the upper cervical spine, the pharynx is entered intentionally. Fang and Ong noted pharyngeal infection in four of their six transoral cases.[14] Modern proponents discount this early report, reporting infection incidence of 0 to 3%.[37, 44] Careful handling of the soft tissues and administration of prophylactic antibiotics will reduce the incidence of infection, but lingering concern about deep contamination has prompted some surgeons to favor an extrapharyngeal approach.[35, 40, 73]

The harvest of autogenous bone puts another region at risk for infection. Hemostasis and the use of drains in cases of persistent oozing can minimize the size of the hematoma,

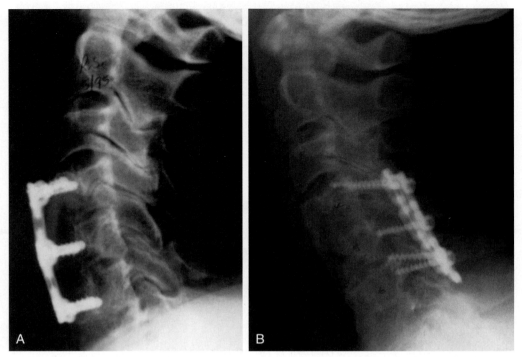

Figure 18–1. *A, A lateral x-ray of a 56-year-old man who underwent anterior C4–C5 and C5–C6 diskectomy and fusion with iliac strut fusion and plating from C4 to C6 1 year before this x-ray was taken; he had a distant anterior C6–C7 fusion as well. There is an area of radiolucency underneath the plate with erosion of the vertebral bodies. He complained of persistent neck pain and radicular symptoms but nothing else to suggest infection. The plate was removed along with abundant granulation tissue, and a pseudarthrosis was identified. Cultures grew a subspecies of* Propionibacterium. *B, Another x-ray taken 6 months after anterior debridement and posterior plating and fusion. The infection was eradicated, and all symptoms resolved.*

which can serve as an avascular media that supports bacterial growth. Irrigation before closure will dilute contaminants and may facilitate identification of small bleeding vessels. Careful handling of tissues will limit the amount of tissue necrosis and thus impair bacterial proliferation. Meticulous closure in layers will reduce dead space and minimize the hematoma. These techniques also apply to cervical wounds.

Other surgeons prefer allograft to avoid donor site morbidity. Transmission of viral and bacterial disease remains a concern to surgeons and the public. HIV infection from bone allograft has been reported in only four cases, and as of this writing has not occurred since the introduction of routine testing.[4, 57, 58] The risk is probably greatest with fresh frozen grafts, which depend solely on the freezing for sterilization.[9, 58] Prophylactic antibiotic therapy is not uniformly used by cervical surgeons and has not been proven necessary, but would seem reasonable when allograft or another foreign implant is used.

Once recognized, infection mandates prompt drainage of the abscess, debridement of devitalized tissue, and appropriate antibiotics. Metallic implants should be removed; biologic implants may need to be removed if loose or involved in the infection (Fig. 18–1). The antimicrobial agent chosen should be effective against the suspected organism and modified as needed based on results of deep wound culture. When a hollow viscus is involved, repair and diversion are necessary. Adequate nutrition is essential,

especially in debilitated patients. Though rarely needed, regional muscle flaps can be useful in closing posterior infections complicated by dehiscence.[56]

VASCULAR PROBLEMS

Many cervical procedures are associated with minor blood loss and mild anemia, which generally are well tolerated by most patients. The more extensive procedures can produce anemia of sufficient severity to require some form of transfusion. For elective procedures, the surgeon may consider collecting autogenous blood or using a cell saver, unless there is a contraindication, such as an infection or neoplasm being treated by the procedure. Other blood-conserving measures include controlled intraoperative hemodilution and hypotension. We reserve transfusion for those patients whose anemia is significantly symptomatic or who have serious comorbid disease that would be exacerbated by diminished oxygen transport.

The carotid artery and jugular vein border the anterior approaches to the cervical spine but are rarely injured unless the tissues are abnormally involved by scarring, inflammation, or neoplasm. If such abnormal involvement is anticipated preoperatively, angiography (conventional or magnetic resonance) may be quite useful. Branches of these major vessels, such as the superior thyroid artery, may need to be ligated or may be injured by anterior approaches and generally can be ligated. A pseudoaneurysm of this vessel after anterior diskectomy and grafting has been reported.[28] The patient presented 9 days after surgery, and was managed with embolization.

Of greater concern in most cases is the vertebral artery. Destructive inflammatory and neoplastic processes can encase, displace, or occlude this vessel and its associated venous plexus.[78] Preoperative angiography will determine the status of the vessel and whether or not it should be salvaged or bypassed. In the case of neoplasm, the angiographer may be able to occlude major feeder vessels to reduce operative hemorrhage. To be effective, this procedure should be done within 1 day of the resection.

The vertebral artery is at risk during an anterior approach if reflection of the longus colli is taken too far posterolaterally. More often, it is injured medially while decompression is being performed within the disk space or during corpectomy.[61] Taking care to identify the midline at the initial exposure and preserving the lateral cortex during corpectomy will reduce the risk of this complication. Preoperative computed tomography (CT) scanning and magnetic resonance imaging (MRI) can alert the surgeon to an anomalous medial course or ectasia of the vessel. In general, the vessel is more medial at the cephalad levels.[69] If the artery is injured, pressure is applied to control the hemorrhage. The artery is exposed proximally and distally by reflecting the longus colli laterally. A portion of the muscle may be resected as needed. By initially dissecting in the superolateral portion of the vertebral body, the transverse process is encountered. This affords some protection to the vessel and aids orientation. The anterior portion of the transverse process may subsequently be removed to expose the artery. Once proximal and distal control is achieved, the injury is inspected and the vessel either repaired or ligated,[21, 61] depending on the extent of injury and on the surgeon's assessment of the contralateral artery's ability to sustain brain stem perfusion. Consultation with a vascular surgeon may be helpful. The reported incidence is low, 0.3% of 1215 cases reviewed by Golfinos and colleagues.[21]

Posteriorly, the vertebral artery may be injured during exposure of the upper cervical spine. In the adult, limiting exposure of the posterior arch of the atlas to 15 mm to either side of midline will usually avoid the vessel. The venous plexus is usually encountered medial to the artery. The artery itself may have a relatively thin wall and be vulnerable to laceration. The increasing popularity of screw fixation puts the artery and veins at risk. The vessels lie just lateral to the lateral atlantoaxial joints and may be lacerated during exposure and decortication of those articulations during transarticular screw fixation and arthrodesis. Some individuals have an abnormally large vertebral artery groove, which thins the isthmus to a height of 2.1 mm or less. This abnormality can be found only by sophisticated imaging, such as CT with sagittal reconstructions. Madawi and colleagues found this anomaly in 11 of 50 (22%) dried axis specimens.[62] This type of fixation is not suitable for such individuals.

Lateral mass or pedicle screw fixation in the subaxial cervical spine can lead to vessel injury by wire, drill bit, tap or screw if the chosen trajectory takes the instrument into the transverse foramen. The risk of this problem may be minimized by thorough knowledge of the anatomy, careful study of the patient's images for variations from average, and attention to the intraoperative position of the instrumentation relative to the patient's position.[2, 3] Of the two types of fixation, lateral mass fixation poses less risk to the vertebral artery. At C7, below the usual entry of the vessel, many surgeons prefer superior fixation of the pedicle screw, because the lateral mass tends to be relatively thin at that level.[2] The advent of frameless stereotaxy may reduce the incidence of vascular injury in both anterior and posterior approaches, as well as improve placement of implants.[17] The current equipment does not sufficiently improve the accuracy of pedicle screws above C7 to warrant routine pedicle fixation, as reported by Ludwig and colleagues.[34]

NEURAL DYSFUNCTION

The recurrent laryngeal nerve usually runs in the tracheoesophageal groove. This is more constant on the left side, because the nerve enters the neck after circling the aortic arch. On the right side, the nerve takes a more variable course after encircling the subclavian artery; only rarely does it leave the carotid sheath and cross the operative field at the level of the thyroid gland. For this reason, many surgeons prefer to routinely approach the anterior cervical spine from a left anterolateral incision. Other surgeons choose the side of the incision based on their own handedness or the side opposite the most severe posterolateral compression to facilitate exposure. We have found that unless the neck is quite thick, both sides can be well visualized from either side. The recurrent laryngeal nerve is usually not seen. Most commonly, the injury, manifested as a weak voice of altered timbre, represents traction neurapraxia. The prognosis for recovery in these cases is good. Transection obviously leads to poor recovery. The incidence is difficult to determine, because symptoms may be mild and self-limiting. Tippets and Apfelbaum noted recurrent laryngeal nerve palsies in 16 of 220 (7%) Caspar platings, but all were transient.[67] Flynn's survey found 52 palsies among 82,114 (0.06%) anterior fusions; the lower incidence is explained in part by the methodology of using questionnaires.[16]

If an anterior approach is needed in an individual whose voice was altered by previous anterior cervical surgery, then this should be performed on the same side as the initial approach. If there is reason to favor the contralateral side, then preoperative laryngoscopy to assess vocal cord function would be prudent. Unilateral paralysis is a relative contraindication to a contralateral approach to avoid the severe morbidity of bilateral vocal cord dysfunction.

The superior laryngeal nerve runs initially posterior to, then medial to the internal carotid artery, dividing into internal and external branches. It is vulnerable during mobilization of the pharynx to expose the upper anterior cervical spine. This can produce anesthesia of the upper larynx, inhibiting protective reflexes and allowing foreign bodies to enter. The cricothyroid muscle is weakened, producing a deep, hoarse voice. Neurapraxia tends to resolve, but more severe injuries carry a poorer prognosis.

The spinal root is often the focus of cervical surgery, because radiculopathy is a common indication for intervention. The root may be inflamed and dysfunctional, and surgical manipulation may further traumatize it or its branches. Laminotomy and foraminotomy allow direct visualization of the root, but the root may be injured by retraction or by instruments used to address the pathology, which is generally anterior. Adequate exposure and careful technique minimize the risk of this problem. During laminectomy or laminoplasty for myelopathy, decompression depends on the dura and its contents shifting posteriorly away from the anterior osteophytes and ossified ligament, if present. Tethering of the nerve roots can produce root dysfunction; the C5 motor rootlets are particularly vulnerable. Concomitant foraminotomy may be contemplated if significant foraminal stenosis is present, especially if the patient has preoperative radicular symptoms in addition to myelopathy. Significant root weakness in the postoperative myelopathy patient should be evaluated with imaging and consideration given to decompression of the affected root. C5 root dysfunction after multilevel corpectomy also has been described and is prevented by limiting the width of decompression.[53] Spondylosis without myelopathy may present with dissociated motor loss and is managed with root decompression.[39]

Although the roots are not visualized in anterior approaches, decompression and symptom relief generally occur. Soft herniations usually can be removed easily. In the case of osteophytes, total resection is not necessary, because distraction by the bone graft increases the size of the foramen. The anterior approach can miss far lateral disk protrusions and necessitate a second, posterior approach. The optimal approach should be based on symptoms and location of the pathology on preoperative imaging studies.

The most dreaded complication of cervical surgery, feared by patient and physician alike, is tetraplegia. The incidence is low but depends to some degree on the preoperative state of the cervical spinal cord. Certainly, mild myelopathy has a better prognosis than advanced cases.[8] Flynn identified 311 significant neural injuries out of 82,114 anterior cervical fusions performed by 704 surgeons; most of the surgeons whose patients experienced myelopathic complications were unable to determine the etiology.[16] The cord may suffer direct trauma from operative manipulation; this is particularly critical when the canal is stenotic. Another cause of loss of cord function is vascular. Laminectomy is known to diminish cord flow, in some cases to a degree sufficient to jeopardize a compromised cord. Paradoxically, decompression of a chronically ischemic cord may lead to cord infarction, possibly because of the "no reflow" phenomenon. Described in experimental myocardial and brain injuries, this phenomenon is recognized as a problem in major extremity replantation. Evoked potential monitoring may allow early recognition of this devastating complication, but unless it is a correctable condition (e.g., extrinsic cord compression), the prognosis remains guarded. Corticosteroid therapy is often used, but outcome likely depends more on the nature and extent of spinal cord involvement than on this pharmacologic intervention.

If cord infarction is suspected intraoperatively, the surgeon should inspect the field for any correctable compression. In the presence of significant canal stenosis or myelopathy, distraction, if used at all, must be applied in small increments. Evoked potentials may be monitored in such cases. If distraction is applied, it should be eased if any significant change in potentials is noted. Any bone grafts or instrumentation inserted must be inspected carefully and removed if necessary. X-rays may be useful. Somatosensory evoked potential monitoring is widely available to detect perturbation of posterior column function. Motor evoked potential monitoring has not seen widespread adoption, probably because of technical factors; results correlate directly with motor function.[32]

If cord dysfunction is noted postoperatively, then plain x-rays should be obtained to check the position of grafts and implants. The surgeon may elect to perform wound exploration or to order further imaging, depending on the nature of the index procedure, examination findings, and x-ray results. MRI allows direct visualization of the spinal cord, which may aid prognostication. Perioperative MRI tends to provide poorer definition than elective studies for various reasons, including the patient's intolerance to lengthy sequences and inability to lay still. CT yields better bone detail but may miss soft tissue compression unless intrathecal contrast medium is used. Wound exploration is merited if demonstrable neural compression is noted. Even late decompression may induce some improvement.[46] An unusual cause of cord dysfunction after laminoplasty is entrapment of the cord within the split laminae at the apex of the lordosis.[31]

Yonenobu and colleagues analyzed neurologic deterioration in patients with myelopathy treated surgically.[76, 77] Causes of this deterioration include direct trauma to neural tissue during surgery, instability of the spine, progression of spondylotic changes above or below the level of fusion, nonunion, malunion, tethering of roots when the spinal cord shifts, and accidental trauma unrelated to surgery.

DURA

Although ossification of the posterior longitudinal ligament is uncommon, it may be associated with ectasia or absence of the dura mater.[60] This may result from chronic compression or may be part of the pathologic process producing the ossification. The latter cause seems more likely, because to the best of our knowledge, chronic compression from spondylosis has not been associated with this entity. One might expect a destructive neoplasm to also produce this entity, but the dura seems relatively resistant. The dura may also be disrupted by trauma, and of course the surgeon may injure the dura with various instruments. Cutting burs are useful for rapidly resecting bone, avoiding the need to insert part of a manual cutting instrument into the spinal canal. However, it may also injure soft tissue, such as blood vessels, nerve roots, dura, and spinal cord. For this reason, many surgeons use a diamond bur when working close to delicate soft tissue structures. Although it is safer, a diamond bur can still erode the dura. Kerrison rongeurs, curettes, and probes may also penetrate the dura. If the subarachnoid membrane remains intact, then the cerebrospinal fluid (CSF) is contained. More commonly, however, this delicate structure is also injured.

Prevention obviously depends on careful surgical technique. Even the most skilled surgeon occasionally produces an incidental durotomy. The surgeon should also recognize the increased possibility of a dural defect in ossification of the posterior longitudinal ligament and be prepared to manage it.

If durotomy is produced during an anterior diskectomy and fusion, then suturing the defect may not be technically possible. If the durotomy is small and lateral, then it may be possible to tamponade the CSF leak with a collagen sponge soaked in thrombin to produce a clot. The patient must be carefully monitored for evidence of a pseudomeningocele leading to a durocutaneous fistula or neural compression. Rarely, the collagen sponge itself can compress neural tissue as it swells in a confined space.[1]

The risk of dural injury increases after corpectomy, particularly if the posterior longitudinal ligament is attenuated or absent or has been resected during the procedure. During such extensive procedures, the dural defect may be visualized and repaired. Small holes may be closed primarily using sutures. Stapling devices have been approved for this use by the FDA. The staples come in various sizes and are MRI compatible. Larger defects may require a patch. Simply placing collagen sponges over such a defect has been ineffective in our experience. Fascia may be harvested from the bone donor site if bone graft has been harvested. Fascia lata makes an excellent patch if the thigh has been sterilely prepared beforehand. Lyophilized dura and processed bovine pericardium are other alternatives that avoid the morbidity associated with harvesting tissue from the patient. The risk of disease transmission is theoretically possible but to our knowledge has not been reported. These patch grafts may be applied as an onlay or secured with sutures, depending on the size of the defect and accessibility of the defect edges. We prefer to augment such repairs and seal the edges with fibrin glue. We have used allogeneic fibrinogen, but this carries a risk of disease transmission. Bovine fibrinogen does not expose the patient to human pathogens, but like the allogeneic product presents foreign proteins that could elicit an immune response. A device has been developed that allows the anesthesiologist to harvest autogenous platelet-rich plasma from the patient intraoperatively and produce autogenous fibrin.[48, 49] This may prove to be the best adhesive.

In cases requiring patching, we also decrease intrathecal pressure by placing the patient on strict, horizontal bed rest and inserting a percutaneous lumbar shunt.[33] This is left in place for 4 days if the patient will tolerate it and if no signs of meningitis occur. The patient is followed clinically, and daily CSF samples are analyzed for white blood cell count with differential. Some surgeons also send daily samples for culture. Antibiotics are used at the surgeon's discretion. The drain must be pulled if there is evidence of infection. The CSF is drained at a rate of 8 to 12 ml/hr, with the rate adjusted to minimize headache. Bed rest is continued for 24 hours after drain removal. Some believe that caffeine can constrict the puncture site and reduce the severity of headache.

Posterior durotomies tend to be more accessible and may be repaired primarily or patched, with the patch secured with sutures or staples. After a good, watertight repair, we mobilize the patient immediately. With more tenuous repairs or patches, we insert a percutaneous lumbar shunt, following the protocol described earlier.

After durotomy repair, the patient is examined and monitored. Occurrence of a postural headache should prompt a trial of bed rest and hydration. If the symptoms persist or recur, then wound exploration should be considered. Alternatively, a lumbar shunt may be used, unless a new neurologic deficit occurs. A deficit should prompt imaging or wound exploration for the pseudomeningocele presumed to be producing neural compression.

Leakage of CSF from the wound may also be treated by a lumbar shunt. Kitchel and colleagues reported on successful treatment of 15 of 19 patients with CSF leak in all regions of the spine using this technique.[33] If an associated neurologic deficit is seen, then the wound should be explored, the dura repaired or patched, and the shunting protocol followed. In the absence of a new or worsened neurologic deficit, simple draining may suffice. The surgeon may prefer to explore the wound and repair the defect if it is deemed to be accessible.

CSF leakage is not always obvious. The differential diagnosis includes hematoma, seroma, and abscess. CT without intrathecal contrast and MRI may be suggestive, but not definitive. Myelography, especially when followed by CT, is both sensitive and specific. A less commonly used alternative is nuclear myelography. In this technique, a radiopharmaceutical agent is instilled into the subarachnoid space, from where it diffuses through the dural defect into the surrounding tissues.

Peridural fibrosis has been implicated as a cause of failed back syndrome in the lumbar spine. This is not uniformly accepted in the spine community, but it may play a role in multiply-operated spinal columns with repeated surgical trauma to individual nerve roots, tethering, and compromise of the blood supply. To our knowledge, an analogous situation has not been seen in the cervical spine. Theoretically, an exuberant scar could produce root or cord compression, but we have no experience with this.

Another potential complication of large dural defects is herniation of the spinal cord or nerve rootlets. This can produce a significant neurologic deficit. Advanced imaging demonstrates the problem, which is managed by reducing the eventration and patching the dura.

ESOPHAGUS

The esophagus and pharynx are vulnerable during anterior approaches to the cervical spine. Although these structures are delicate, injury is uncommon. The risk is increased in patients who have undergone previous surgery in the area that included mobilization of those structures. Previous radiation treatment may lead to fibrosis of the esophagus or pharynx. If an anterior wound needs to be explored within the first few months of anterior surgery, the inflammatory component of the healing process may hinder identification of tissue planes and mobilization of these structures. Similarly, an anterior approach in the face of an active infection will obliterate the normal fascial planes. The surgeon usually can anticipate these challenges and exercise extra care during the dissection. If a rent in the viscus is identified, then a nasogastric tube should be placed and the rent repaired. Depending on the extent of the injury,

salivary diversion may be considered. Antibiotics are administered for at least 5 to 7 days, until the repair is stable.

Esophageal injury has also been reported with anterior instrumentation. Early plate designs were associated with screw backout. Esophageal motion over the protruding screw can lead to erosion and penetration.[59] Complaints of worsening dysphagia after anterior plating should prompt x-rays and revision, preferably before the entire esophageal

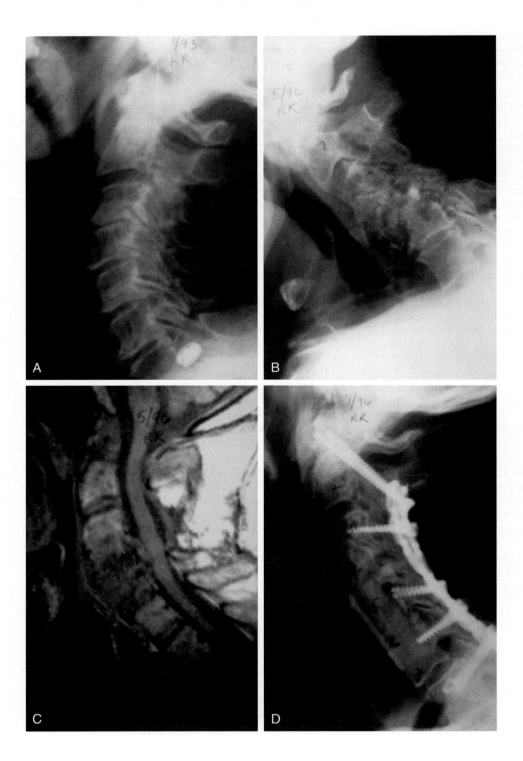

Figure 18–2. A, A lateral x-ray of a 71-year-old male with rheumatoid arthritis and cervical spondylotic myelopathy. Spinal cord compression was primarily posterior from C3 through C5. The myelopathy improved after laminectomy. B, A lateral x-ray taken 3 years later. The patient complained of severe neck and arm pain, and his myelopathy had worsened. C, An MRI showing destruction of the C4, C5, and C6 bodies. Histologically, this proved to be a large rheumatoid nodule. D, A lateral x-ray taken 2 months after resection, anterior fibular strut, and posterior plating and bone grafting from C1 to T1. The upper cervical spine was included to address concomitant atlantoaxial instability associated with the patient's rheumatoid disease. Lordosis was restored, but postoperatively the patient experienced severe esophageal dysmotility and dysphagia and needed a gastric tube for nutrition. His swallowing gradually improved over a period of 6 months.

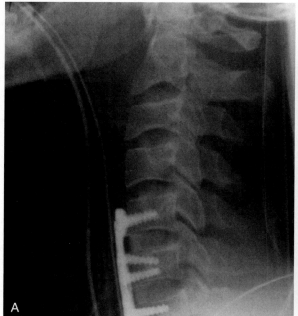 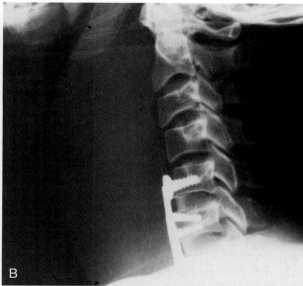

Figure 18–3. A, A lateral x-ray taken immediately after a two-level anterior cervical diskectomy, grafting, and plating. B, A lateral x-ray taken 24 hours later showing massive anterior swelling from a retropharyngeal hematoma. The patient complained of difficulty swallowing, and open drainage was performed.

wall is damaged. Newer plate designs include a locking mechanism to reduce the risk of this complication. Yee and Terry reported an unusual case of a screw backing out, penetrating the esophagus, traversing the alimentary tract, and being eliminated in the stool without any apparent adverse effect.[75]

At times, recognizing an esophageal disruption is difficult. The surgeon may instruct the anesthesiologist to place a nasogastric tube in the hypopharynx and instill indigo carmine dye. Visualization of dye in the wound indicates a transmural injury. It may be possible to identify the site of injury early, before excessive tissue staining occurs. Passage of dye is confirmed by its subsequent appearance in the urine. Transmural injuries are managed as described earlier. Hypopharyngeal diverticulum formation may also occur with retraction.[20]

It is also important to recognize the symptoms of esophageal perforation that may occur after cervical surgery.[19a] The most common symptoms are neck and throat pain, dysphagia, hoarseness, and aspiration. The most common findings are elevated temperature, localized induration or neck tenderness, crepitus or subcutaneous air in the neck or chest wall, unexplained tachycardia, and blood in the nasogastric tube.

Esophageal dysmotility is common after anterior approaches to the cervical spine. This is usually self-limiting and is managed by patient education. Use of small food boluses, thorough chewing, and, occasionally, a mechanically soft diet will generally suffice. The perceived difficulty in swallowing is likely due to the trauma of mobilization and retraction. If the symptoms are severe or persistent, a speech pathologist may be able to teach the patient techniques to reduce symptoms. In more severe cases, a

contrast swallow may be needed in consultation with an otorhinolaryngologist. Consideration should be given to placing a small-diameter feeding tube to administer nutrition and medication while the swelling is resolving (Fig. 18–2). Occasionally, a large hematoma can cause dysphagia (Fig. 18–3).

Dysphagia may also be associated with certain neck positions. In a patient with halo fixation, excessive flexion can obstruct the airway,[65] whereas extension can lead to difficulty swallowing. Depending on the condition being treated, adjusting the halo may obviate the problem. If a long instrumented fusion is anticipated, care must be taken to select a functional position for the neck, particularly if a chronic kyphotic deformity is being corrected. Overcorrection may make it difficult, if not impossible, for a patient to swallow, necessitating revision of the fusion.

FUSION

Placement of anterior bone grafts after diskectomy or corpectomy mandates confirmation of position radiographically before wound closure. This may be difficult, particularly in large individuals and in reconstructions involving the lower cervical spine. New or worsened neurologic deficit recognized in the recovery room will prompt radiographic study and wound exploration for posterior graft displacement. The risk of posterior graft displacement may be reduced through careful preparation of the recipient graft site. We prefer to leave a posterior lip of bone at both ends to act as a mechanical block to posterior graft dislodgment. When placing a graft with a bow (iliac crest), the surgeon must ensure that the apex does not protrude into the spinal canal. Advanced osteopenia may place the patient at risk for fracture of the graft, fracture of the anchor site, and displacement of graft material into the canal (Fig. 18–4). Halo immobilization may reduce this risk.

Anterior graft displacement is a more common problem, particularly after multilevel corpectomy. When there is normal lordosis and a relatively straight fibular graft is used, anterior displacement can readily occur. The risk of this complication may be reduced by countersinking the graft, fashioning anterior lips of bone at the receptor sites, and applying some form of external orthosis, perhaps a halo. Many surgeons use anterior plates in these situations. Placing these plates may be difficult in long reconstructions, and their efficacy in preventing displacement and promoting fusion remains unproven (Fig. 18–5). Nonetheless, conceptually they make sense if the patient's bone is of sufficient quality to hold the screws. Another, simpler approach is to fasten a short plate onto the distal body through the distal holes; the proximal holes are not used. The proximal plate acts as a block to anterior graft displacement. By not fixing the plate to the graft, some settling is permitted, which may be beneficial to healing. Anterior graft dislodgment often presents with dysphagia and odynophagia. Unrecognized, it can lead to delayed esophageal injury, resulting in fistula or abscess formation.[30] In one unusual case, the extruded Cloward graft was expectorated.[47] Interference screw fixation has been proposed as a simple means to prevent interbody graft displacement, and biomechanically this increases pullout strength.[71] We have no clinical experience with this technique, however.

Fibrous union of anterior interbody grafts can occur in up to 12% of anterior reconstructions.[5, 11] Risk factors include multilevel anterior cervical diskectomy and fusion, the use of allograft in multilevel diskectomy and fusion, and cigarette smoking. It has been our practice to decorticate the vertebral endplates to improve the chance of anterior interbody fusion and in corpectomy reconstruction, removing sclerotic bone with a high-speed bur and leaving lips of bone anteriorly and posteriorly to secure the graft in the desired location.[11] Care is taken to obtain healthy, bleeding bone without resecting the good-quality cancellous bone generally found immediately deep to the endplate. This is a modification of the original technique proposed by Robinson and Smith, who merely perforated the endplates with curettes.[50] That technique led to an unacceptably high fibrous union rate in a retrospective review of anterior cervical diskectomy and fusion. Theoretically, this modification could lead to graft subsidence and secondary kyphosis. A retrospective review of our early experience with this technique did not bear this out, however—the fusion rate was higher.[11] Patients with severe osteopenia probably should be immobilized for longer periods to ensure healing.

Anterior plates have been proposed as a means of increasing the union rate for diskectomy and fusion. But reported series to date, although promising, have not provided controlled, prospective, long-term data proving the efficacy of this approach.[55, 66]

Another strategy to reduce the risk of anterior interbody nonunion when multiple levels must be addressed is to

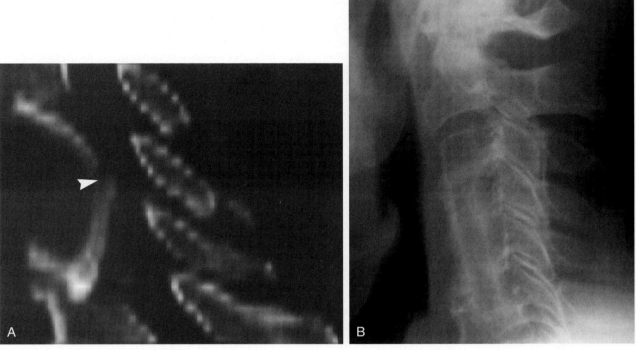

Figure 18–4. A, A CT scan sagittal reconstruction of a patient 1 week after a two-level cervical corpectomy and iliac strut fusion. The graft fractured and displaced into the spinal canal. It was replaced with a fibular strut. B, A lateral x-ray showing a mature fusion. The myelopathy resolved.

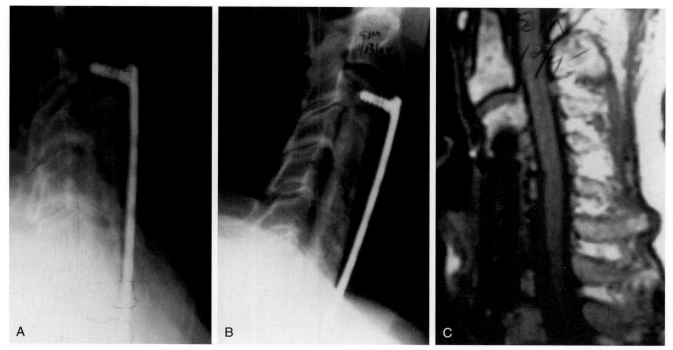

Figure 18–5. *A, A lateral x-ray of a 62-year-old man after a three-level corpectomy, fibular strut graft, and plating for severe myelopathy. Screws were placed in the cranial and caudal vertebrae. B, A lateral x-ray taken 2 weeks later, showing mild anterior displacement of the inferior graft and plate; the anterior inferior aspect of the C7 body had fractured. The patient was immobilized in an orthosis. C, A sagittal MRI taken 1 year later showing the anterior and inferior position of the fibular strut relative to C7. The myelopathy improved, and the arthrodesis was solid.*

perform subtotal corpectomy, preserving the posterior cortex and using one long graft to fuse three or more interspaces. This reduces the number of graft interfaces that must heal to two. The potential benefit of this reduction must be weighed against the increased complexity of the procedure, the requirement for a larger graft, and the increased risk of graft displacement associated with longer grafts.

A provocative report by Fuji and colleagues advocates treatment of a delayed anterior interbody union with simple posterior spinous process wiring unless the nonunion is long-standing.[19] In another clinical setting, lateral mass plating without bone graft was also sufficient to achieve fusion.[15] Generally, if we must subject the patient to another procedure, we combine the internal fixation with bone grafting (Fig. 18–6). In the future, bone growth factors and substitutes may be an alternative, but these are not available for clinical use at this time.

One approach to treating a pseudarthrosis after anterior cervical diskectomy and fusion involves anterior resection and iliac crest bone grafting with anterior cervical plating.[68a] Several series have demonstrated the superiority of posterior arthrodesis in treating symptomatic anterior interbody nonunions, except in cases of persistent anterior neural compression.[6, 38] The fusion rate after these procedures is much higher posteriorly and is often associated with conversion of the fibrous union to bony ankylosis anteriorly. Posterior constructs combine graft and internal fixation and are associated with high union rates. Malunions, generally

kyphosis, usually necessitate combined anterior and posterior procedures, including posterior osteotomy, traction, and anterior strut grafting, as well as revision posterior fixation and bone grafting.

The most common anterior malunion is kyphosis. This may lead to chronic neck pain, but a more ominous problem is chronic compression and possible ischemia of the cord leading to myelopathy (Fig. 18–7). Capen and colleagues noted a progressive kyphotic deformity, with a mean of 22 degrees, in 36 of 88 trauma cases managed with anterior decompression and strut grafting.[7] When an anterior approach is indicated for trauma, these authors recommend either halo immobilization or concomitant posterior wiring and fusion. Anterior plating is another alternative. Kyphosis is a recognized complication of laminectomy; close follow-up will allow for early recognition and treatment before severe deformity and neurologic dysfunction develop.[54] This is a particularly serious problem after laminectomy for tumor in pediatric patients. Titanium implants facilitate stable fusion and prevent deformity and neurologic deterioration, yet permit surveillance MRI studies.[68]

An established, fixed deformity is best treated by corpectomy through the kyphotic segments, in effect producing an osteotomy. The corpectomy decompresses the spinal cord and generally allows correction of the deformity, which is facilitated with halo traction. In severe cases, posterior osteotomy also may be necessary. Combined anterior strut and posterior arthrodesis complete the

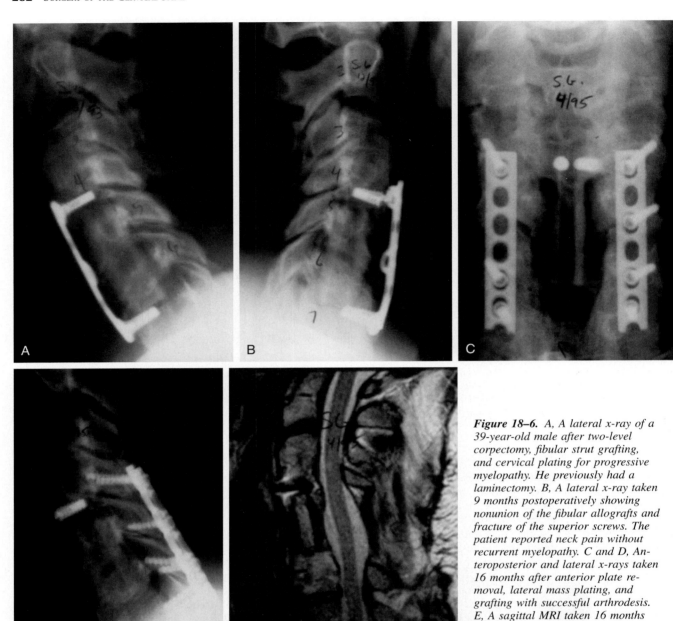

Figure 18–6. A, A lateral x-ray of a 39-year-old male after two-level corpectomy, fibular strut grafting, and cervical plating for progressive myelopathy. He previously had a laminectomy. B, A lateral x-ray taken 9 months postoperatively showing nonunion of the fibular allografts and fracture of the superior screws. The patient reported neck pain without recurrent myelopathy. C and D, Anteroposterior and lateral x-rays taken 16 months after anterior plate removal, lateral mass plating, and grafting with successful arthrodesis. E, A sagittal MRI taken 16 months after the last procedure showing complete decompression of the spinal cord.

reconstruction (Fig. 18–8). As a general rule, we prefer autograft for anterior interbody fusions and corpectomy reconstruction.

Another complication of bone nonunion and malunion is graft fracture (Fig. 18–9). The incidence of anterior graft failure can be reduced by using a saw instead of osteotomes to harvest the graft. Jones and colleagues nicely demonstrated that grafts harvested with a saw were biomechanically superior to those harvested with osteotomes, likely because of the microfractures created by the latter technique.[29]

Donor site morbidity has driven many surgeons and patients to opt for allograft. Zdeblick and Ducker found that for single-level interbody fusions, the rate of anterior fibrous union was 5% with both allograft and autograft, but healing was slower with allograft.[79] In that retrospective study, the incidence of fibrous union was 17% in two-level autograft patients and 63% in two-level allograft patients. At multiple levels, the rate of fibrous union with allograft alone is, in our opinion, unacceptably high. Addition of an anterior plate seems to improve outcomes with fibular allograft.[55] One of 48 autograft patients went on to a nonunion, compared with none of the allograft and plate patients. Among the autograft group, one patient had graft osteomyelitis, two patients had collapse, and two more than 75%; none of these problems occurred in the allograft patients. In another series, results

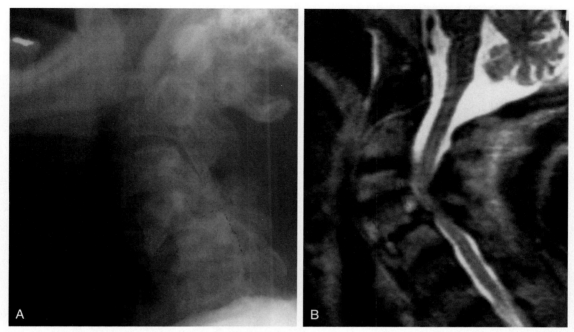

Figure 18–7. *A, A lateral x-ray of a 62-year-old male taken 3 years after cervical laminectomy for cervical canal stenosis. The patient's myelopathy progressed over 1 year, and he was wheelchair-bound for 4 months. There was significant postoperative instability with spondylolisthesis of C4–C5. B, A sagittal MRI showing the spondylolisthesis and severe spinal cord compression. The patient was managed with anterior decompression and strut grafting with posterior plating and bone grafting, and was ambulatory with a cane 3 months later.*

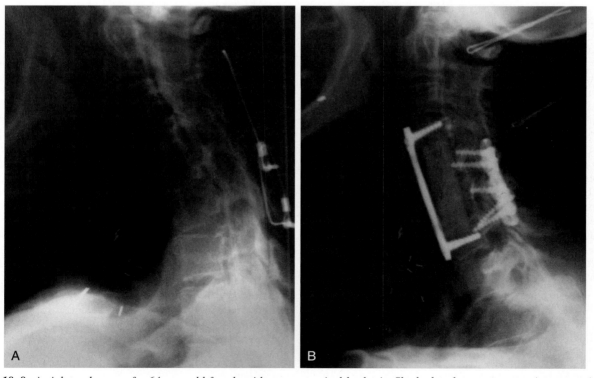

Figure 18–8. *A, A lateral x-ray of a 64-year-old female with severe cervical kyphosis. She had undergone two previous posterior fusions, initially from C4 to C6 with subsequent extension to C2. She complained of severe neck pain. Anterior migration of the posterior cervical muscles and early myelopathy were noted clinically. B, A lateral x-ray taken after anterior osteotomy and corpectomy followed by posterior osteotomy, correction of kyphosis and posterior plating, and then anterior fibular strut fusion and plating. The patient's neck pain improved, and her myelopathy resolved.*

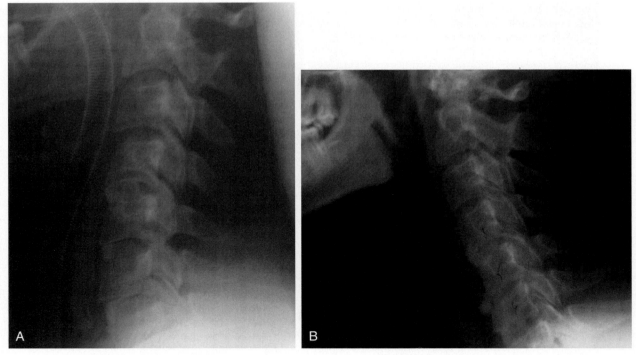

Figure 18–9. *A, A lateral x-ray of a 52-year-old man taken shortly after three-level anterior cervical diskectomy and fusion for radiculopathy. B, A lateral x-ray taken 6 weeks postoperatively showing fracture and fragmentation of the C5–C6 graft. The patient was asymptomatic.*

of allograft use in posterior arthrodesis were disappointing, even in children.[63]

Until bone growth factors and bone substitutes become available (and assuming that these prove clinically efficacious), autograft remains the substance of choice for posterior fusion. Thus, the patient and surgeon must accept a certain amount of donor site morbidity. The most common complaint is discomfort from the muscle stripping. When kept to a minimum and performed gently, this is self-limited and well tolerated. Cutaneous nerves, including the cluneal nerves, are difficult to discern and are usually transected during the approach. The resulting neuromata are annoying but only rarely necessitate injection. Exploration and resection have not been necessary in our practice.

The sural nerve may be at risk during fibular harvest. The peroneal nerve may be injured during the deep dissection. Careful subperiosteal exposure and protection of the soft tissues while using the saw will minimize this risk. Dissection near the fibular neck should be avoided.

A more vexing problem is injury to the lateral femoral cutaneous nerve after anterior graft harvest. This nerve can be injured outside of the pelvis; taking care to place the incision and dissection posterior to the anterior superior iliac spine will prevent this. More commonly, the nerve is injured inside the pelvis. The risk of this may be minimized through careful subperiosteal dissection of the iliacus muscle and retraction of the soft tissues when using a saw to cut the graft. Infection is an uncommon complication of bone graft harvest. The risk can be reduced by maintaining good hemostasis and using prophylactic antibiotics. An established infection is treated by irrigation and debride-

ment, closure over drains, and appropriate antibiotic therapy.

All bone graft harvest is associated with some degree of hemorrhage because of the exposed bony surfaces as well as the muscle stripping. Although careful technique may reduce this problem, patients who have taken an anti-inflammatory medication may ooze significantly. Bone wax and collagen sponges, with or without thrombin, may be used. In cases where persistent oozing cannot be controlled with thrombogenic agents and cauterization, a drain should be used. Hematoma usually is not a problem if kept to a minimum. A large hematoma can be uncomfortable and may become secondarily infected. Theoretically, a large hematoma can cause compartment syndrome, but we are unaware of any reports of this. Our practice is to not close leg fascia after a fibular harvest. A bleeding diathesis should be corrected if possible. Large hematomas may require drainage.

The ileum may be fractured either by the instruments or, more commonly, by propagation of the crack and contraction of the muscles (Fig. 18–10). The risk of this is diminished by placing the osteotomies at least 30 mm from the anterior superior iliac spine, using the saw for anterior iliac grafts, and maintaining careful osteotome technique.[25, 29] Most of these pelvic fractures may be treated symptomatically.[26] Ambulation is facilitated with a walker or crutches.

Ankle instability is a potential complication of distal fibula resection. This can be prevented by making the distal osteotomy 8 to 10 cm proximal to the ankle. Fibular harvest is associated with some weakness of the peroneal muscles.

This weakness is not functionally significant in most persons, but persistent gait abnormalities are discernible by gait analysis. Strengthening exercises are occasionally needed.

Stress fracture of the tibia is an uncommon result of fibular harvest and occurs many months after the harvest.[12] Diagnosis may be difficult. If plain x-rays are nondiagnostic, a technetium bone scan may be helpful. The stress fracture may be treated in a cast or an orthosis.

Instrumentation

Internal fixation in the cervical spine provides stability, allowing bone healing. When this biologic process fails, the device tends to fail from fracture or loosening. Although arthrodesis can occur after implant loosening or fracture, the presence of a fibrous union should be investigated. The differential diagnosis of loosening also includes infection. Constitutional symptoms may not be present. Concomitant infection should be suspected when constitutional symptoms are present or if there is a progressive destruction of bone about the implant.

Depending on the nature of the device and its location, a number of structures may be at risk. Here we consider each class of device and the structures at risk separately.

Posterior wires are usually placed between the spinous processes. Potential problems include fracture of the spinous processes or the wires with loss of fixation. If the hole at the base of the spinous process is placed too ventral, the canal can be violated. Careful hole selection and wire contouring will minimize this risk. The wire should never be forced through the hole. Careful handling of the wire and bone will reduce the risk of a fracture. The hole must be large enough to accommodate the wire without compromising the integrity of the bone. If fracture does occur, then alternate sites of wire fixation or a different method of fixation should be used.

Facet wiring was a useful technique when a posterior arthrodesis was necessary after laminectomy. Today, this has been largely supplanted by lateral mass plating. The risks are similar to those of lateral mass plating and are discussed in that section. Wires are also placed from the inferior spinous process to the lateral mass of the superior vertebra in cases of unilateral fracture dislocation of the facets. This technique also has been superseded by plate fixation. Most commonly, sublaminar wires are used to secure fixation of the posterior atlas. The surgeon must make sure that sufficient subarachnoid space is available to perform this maneuver without injuring the spinal cord. The technique is contraindicated when there is a fixed anterior subluxation or dislocation of the atlantoaxial complex. The Brooke technique of atlantoaxial arthrodesis requires passage of sublaminar wires at the atlas. This is technically demanding but yields a stable biomechanical construct. It is contraindicated when the canal is narrow at either of these levels. We generally use other means of fixation. Preoperative studies are essential in assessing the safety of sublaminar techniques. An uncommon but disturbing complication of sublaminar fixation is wire breakage, followed by intramedullary migration of a wire fragment.[18]

Halifax clamps were designed to provide stability without sublaminar manipulation. Results at the atlantoaxial

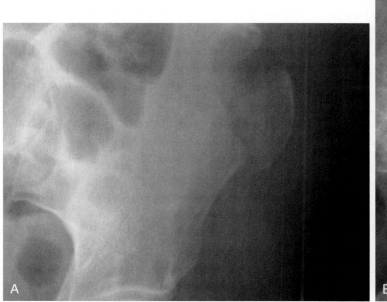
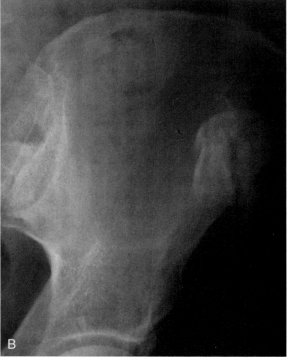

Figure 18–10. *A, A left iliac oblique x-ray showing a displaced fracture of the anterior superior iliac spine 2 days after anterior cervical diskectomy and fusion. The patient felt a pop and worsened graft site pain while walking. B, An x-ray taken 3 months later. There was no residual donor site pain.*

level have been disappointing, but they are better in the subaxial cervical spine.[64] Complications include screw loosening, clamp dislodgment, and nonunion.

More commonly, we use a modification of the Gallie technique. When more stability is necessary, we favor the transarticular screw technique described by Jeanneret and Magerl.[27] This requires reduction of the lateral atlantoaxial articulations and is technically demanding. One potential complication is failure to achieve good fixation. The pharynx can be injured if the drill is inserted too far anterior. Similarly, excessively long screws can injure this structure. Directing the drill or screw too far medial puts the spinal cord at risk. Lateral angulation can injure the vertebral artery. The isthmus of the axis may be injured by large instrumentation or improper trajectory, compromising the fixation. As noted in the discussion of vascular problems, approximately 20% of individuals may have an isthmus less than 2 mm thick, making vascular injury virtually inevitable.[62] The entry point is close to the C2–C3 articulation, which may be damaged. As originally described, the atlantoaxial articulations are not fused if the procedure is combined with midline fusion. We like to expose the joint and graft it, but care must be taken in preparing the posterior joint before grafting, because these maneuvers put the vertebral artery and accompanying veins at risk laterally and the cord medially.

Anterior screw fixation of odontoid fractures and fibrous unions has become more popular. Prerequisites include adequate bone quality and reduction of the fracture. Anterior screw fixation is greatly facilitated by biplane x-rays. Structures at risk include the esophagus and spinal cord. It is performed through an anterior approach based at the C5 or C6 level to allow proper trajectory of the drill, tap, and screw. This procedure was initially described with a two-screw technique, which proved technically very demanding. In some individuals, the odontoid is too small to accommodate two screws without fragmentation, violation of the odontoid cortex, or inadequate fixation. These difficulties led to the development a single-screw technique. Biomechanical studies have demonstrated that fixation is similar in the one-screw and two-screw techniques.[22, 41, 52] Complications include loss of fixation and nonunion. The salvage procedure for failure is a posterior atlantoaxial arthrodesis.

Both odontoid screw fixation and posterior atlantoaxial arthrodesis with transarticular screws depend heavily on technique augmented by intraoperative fluoroscopy. Cannulated screws and corresponding insertion equipment facilitate accurate screw placement.[10] Frameless stereotaxy also is available.[17] Current systems can be used for the transarticular screws but not for odontoid fixation.

As noted previously, the indications for and efficacy of anterior plate fixation in the cervical spine continue to evolve. This technique is clearly useful in trauma and may also have a role in treating degenerative disease. Early designs were plagued by loosening and screw backout, but current designs use locking screws to avoid this problem. Complications are minimized by accurate plate and screw fixation confirmed radiographically. This is very important, because it is fairly easy to misalign the long axis of the plate relative to the long axis of the cervical spine, and it is also

easy to place the plate off midline. These malalignments increase the risk of inadvertently entering the spinal canal or injuring the vertebral artery. Late complications include hardware fracture, loosening, and impingement on the esophagus. In cases of a fibrous nonunion but no impingement on the esophagus, a posterior arthrodesis is the treatment of choice. Symptomatic hardware prominence mandates removal.

The most serious complication of occipital fixation is damage to the transverse sinus, which can lead to fatal hemorrhage. This is best avoided by staying caudal to the inion, in the thickest portion of the occiput. The bone adjacent to the foramen magnum itself is thin, leaving the dura and epidural veins vulnerable during instrumentation. Similar risk with transosseous wire placement has led some to place their wires within the occipital bone, leaving the inner table intact.

In the subaxial spine, lateral mass fixation is a technically demanding procedure.[2, 3] The spinal cord is theoretically at risk, but this risk appears to be low. At greater risk are the nerve root, along with the vertebral artery and accompanying veins. Attention to detail will reduce this risk. In the future, frameless stereotaxy may be useful, particularly in cases involving previous posterior surgery and severe deformity.[17] Currently, fluoroscopy and plain x-rays are used in these complex cases. Unicortical screw fixation reduces the risk of neurovascular injury but is biomechanically inferior to bicortical fixation. A study by Heller and colleagues demonstrated the superiority of 3.2-, 3.5-, and 4.0-mm bicortical screws over 2.7-mm bicortical screws, all unicortical screws, and self-tapping screws.[23] Vertebral artery repair through the posterior approach is difficult but can be accomplished by resection of the lateral masses. Alternatively, an urgent anterior approach may be considered. Angiography and balloon occlusion may be options in cases in which the artery is deemed to be expendable. Nerve root injury should be assessed by CT. A misdirected or long screw can be replaced surgically. If no impingement occurred, the injury would have to be observed expectantly, because the dysfunction presumably would be due to the drill or tap. Heller and colleagues analyzed 78 consecutive patients, inserting 654 screws. Complication rates as a function of the number of screws inserted were nerve root injury, 0.6%; facet violations, 0.2%; vertebral artery injury, 0%; broken screw, 0.3%; screw avulsion, 0.2%; and screw loosening 1.1%. Complications as a percentage of the number of cases performed were spinal cord injury, 2.6%; iatrogenic foraminal stenosis, 2.6%; broken plate, 1.3%; lost reduction, 2.6%; adjacent segment degeneration, 3.8%; infection, 1.3%; and pseudarthrosis, 1.4%.[24]

Nonunion of a posterior arthrodesis may be approached by revision posterior bone grafting and revision instrumentation, or anterior fusion may be considered. Although we routinely use autogenous cancellous bone graft, Fehlings and coworkers reported 93% fusion using posterior plates without graft in 37 of 44 cases of instability.[15]

Rod constructs are less commonly used. Hooks and sublaminar wires may injure the dura or spinal cord or narrow the canal. Spinous process wires are safer but provide less secure fixation than plates. An unusual complication of Harrington instrumentation in the cervical spine is rod migration through the foramen magnum and into the cerebellum.[74]

INSTABILITY

Arthrodesis may fail to achieve stability. This is a particular problem in an unstable fracture or dislocation. Fibrous union, hardware failure with loss of reduction, failure of external immobilization, loss of reduction, and malunion of the fracture or attempted arthrodesis can occur. Adequate reduction, good fixation, and meticulous bone grafting with appropriate external immobilization will minimize the risks; but severe pathology, comorbid factors, and noncompliance with the surgeon's instruction can lead to failure. The resulting instability may produce pain, nerve root dysfunction, or myelopathy. The goals of treatment are to restore more anatomic alignment, to reduce the deformity sufficiently to achieve stability, and to decompress the neural elements.

MISCELLANEOUS

The posterior approach to the cervical spine may be taken with the patient seated or prone. The prone position does not give the anesthesiologist a good view of the patient's face, however. During muscle stripping, the patient's head may shift, and the supporting pads may place pressure on the globe. Ischemia after a lengthy procedure may be sufficient to produce retinal blindness.[43] We prefer to use Mayfield tongs rather than a horseshoe or other external pad to support the patient's head. Another possible cause of blindness is the ischemia associated with hypotension; this also may injure other organs.

The seated position, which allows blood to drain away from the surgical field, is favored by many surgeons. The unique complication associated with this position is air embolism. When using the seated position for multilevel laminectomy or laminoplasty, the surgeon may wish to monitor for embolism with transesophageal echocardiography and end-expiratory carbon dioxide monitoring. A central line allows the anesthesiologist to aspirate the air from an embolism.[42]

Airway obstruction is a rare complication of cervical surgery. It can occur with lengthy, multilevel corpectomy procedures, probably as a result of dissection, manipulation, and retraction of the trachea and larynx. In airway obstruction, the postoperative orthosis and laryngeal edema combine to make oroendotracheal intubation difficult, if not impossible. Even cricothyroidotomy can be challenging. Heavy cigarette smokers with myelopathy are particularly vulnerable, so we defer extubation for 24 to 72 hours to allow swelling to subside.[13] Protracted posterior procedures are also associated with airway problems. This is especially true with rheumatoid arthritis, likely reflecting the poor condition of patients with cervical instability. The risk of this complication can be decreased by obtaining the airway with fiberoptic-assisted intubation.[72] In severely deformed or neurologically impaired patients requiring halo immobilization or long posterior arthrodeses, we consider elective tracheostomy in both the anesthetic and early recovery periods.

REFERENCES

1. Alander DH, Stauffer ES: Gelfoam-induced acute quadriparesis after cervical decompression and fusion. Spine 20:970–971, 1995.
2. An HS, Gordin R, Renner K: Anatomic considerations for plate-screw fixation of the cervical spine. Spine 16(suppl): S548–S551, 1991.
3. Anderson PA, Henley MB, Grady MS, et al: Posterior cervical arthrodesis with AO reconstruction plates and bone graft. Spine 16(suppl):S72–S79, 1991.
4. Asselmeier MA, Caspari RB, Bottenfield S: A review of allograft processing and sterilization techniques and their role in transmission of the human immunodeficiency virus. Am J Sports Med 21:170–175, 1993.
5. Bohlman HH, Emery SE, Goodfellow DB, Jones PK: Robinson anterior cervical discectomy and arthrodesis for cervical radiculopathy. Long-term follow-up of one hundred and twenty-two patients. J Bone Joint Surg Am 75A:1298–1307, 1993.
6. Brodsky AE, Khalil MA, Sassard WR, Newman BP: Repair of symptomatic pseudoarthrosis of anterior cervical fusion. Posterior versus anterior repair. Spine 17:1137–1143, 1992.
7. Capen DA, Garland DE, Waters RL: Surgical stabilization of the cervical spine. A comparative analysis of anterior and posterior spine fusions. Clin Orthop 196:229–237, 1985.
8. Casey AT, Crockard HA, Bland JM, et al: Surgery on the rheumatoid cervical spine for the non-ambulant myelopathic patient—Too much, too late? Lancet 347:1004–1007, 1996.
9. Cook SD, Salkeld SL, Prewett AB: Simian immunodeficiency virus (human HIV-II) transmission in allograft bone procedures. Spine 20:1338–1342, 1995.
10. Dickman CA, Foley KT, Sonntag VK, Smith MM: Cannulated screws for odontoid screw fixation and atlantoaxial transarticular screw fixation. Technical note. J Neurosurg 83:1095–1100, 1995.
11. Emery SE, Bolesta MJ, Banks MA, Jones PK: Robinson anterior cervical fusion: Comparison of the standard and modified techniques. Spine 19:660–663, 1994.
12. Emery SE, Heller JG, Petersilge CA, et al: Tibial stress fracture after a graft has been obtained from the fibula. A report of five cases. J Bone Joint Surg Am 78A:1248–1251, 1996.
13. Emery SE, Smith MD, Bohlman HH: Upper-airway obstruction after multilevel cervical corpectomy for myelopathy. J Bone Joint Surg Am 73A:544–551, 1991.
14. Fang HSY, Ong GB: Direct anterior approach to the upper cervical spine. J Bone Joint Surg Am 44A:1588–1604, 1962.
15. Fehlings MG, Cooper PR, Errico TJ: Posterior plates in the management of cervical instability: Long-term results in 44 patients. J Neurosurg 81:341–349, 1994.
16. Flynn TB: Neurologic complications of anterior cervical interbody fusion. Spine 7:536–539, 1982.
17. Foley KT, Smith MM: Image-guided spine surgery. Neurosurg Clin N Am 7:171–186, 1996.
18. Fraser AB, Sen C, Casden AM, et al: Cervical transdural intramedullary migration of a sublaminar wire. A complication of cervical fixation. Spine 19:456–459, 1994.
19. Fuji T, Yonenobu K, Fujiwara K, et al: Interspinous wiring without bone grafting for nonunion or delayed union following anterior spinal fusion of the cervical spine. Spine 11:982–987, 1986.
19a. Gaudinez RF, English GM, Beghard JS, et al: Esophageal

perforations after anterior cervical surgery. J Spin Disord 13:77–84, 2000.

20. Goffart Y, Moreau P, Lenelle J, Boverie J (1991): Traction diverticulum of the hypopharynx following anterior cervical spine surgery. Case report and review. Ann Otol Rhinol Laryngol 100:852–855, 1991.

21. Golfinos JG, Dickman CA, Zabramski JM, et al: Repair of vertebral artery injury during anterior cervical decompression. Spine 19:2552–2556, 1994.

22. Graziano G, Jaggers C, Lee M, Lynch W: A comparative study of fixation techniques for type II fractures of the odontoid process. Spine 18:2383–2387, 1993.

23. Heller JG, Estes BT, Zaouali M, Diop A: Biomechanical study of screws in the lateral masses: Variables affecting pull-out resistance. J Bone Joint Surg Am 78A:1315–1321, 1996.

24. Heller JG, Silcox DHI, Sutterlin CEI: Complications of posterior cervical plating. Spine 20:2442–2448, 1995.

25. Hu R, Hearn T, Yang J: Bone graft harvest site as a determinant of iliac crest strength. Clin Orthop 310:252–256, 1995.

26. Hu RW, Bohlman HH: Fracture at the iliac bone graft harvest site after fusion of the spine. Clin Orthop 309:208–213, 1994.

27. Jeanneret B, Magerl F: Primary posterior fusion C1/2 in odontoid fractures: Indications, technique, and results of transarticular screw fixation. J Spine Disord 5:464–475, 1992.

28. Jenis LG, Leclair WJ: Late vascular complication with anterior cervical discectomy and fusion. Spine 19:1291–1293, 1994.

29. Jones AA, Dougherty PJ, Sharkey NA, Benson DR: Iliac crest bone graft. Osteotome versus saw. Spine 18:2048–2052, 1993.

30. Kelly MF, Spiegel J, Rizzo KA, Zwillenberg D (1991): Delayed pharyngoesophageal perforation: A complication of anterior spine surgery. Ann Otol Rhinol Laryngol 100:201–205, 1991.

31. Kimura S, Homma T, Uchiyama S, et al: Posterior migration of cervical spinal cord between split laminae as a complication of laminoplasty. Spine 20:1284–1288, 1995.

32. Kitagawa H, Itoh T, Takano H, et al: Motor evoked potential monitoring during upper cervical spine surgery. Spine 14:1078–1783, 1989.

33. Kitchel SH, Eismont FJ, Green BA: Closed subarachnoid drainage for management of cerebrospinal fluid leakage after an operation on the spine. J Bone Joint Surg Am 71A:984–987, 1989.

34. Ludwig SC, Kramer DL, Balderston RA, et al: Placement of pedicle screws in the human cadaveric cervical spine: Comparative accuracy of three techniques. Spine 25:1655–1667, 2000.

35. Kratimenos GP, Crockard HA: The far lateral approach for ventrally placed foramen magnum and upper cervical spine tumours. Br J Neurosurg 7:129–140, 1993.

36. Kuriloff DB, Blaugrund S, Ryan J, O'Leary P: Delayed neck infection following anterior spine surgery. Laryngoscope 97:1094–1098, 1987.

37. Louis R: Anterior surgery of the upper cervical spine. Chir Organi Mov 77:75–80, 1992.

38. Lowery GL, Swank ML, McDonough RF: Surgical revision for failed anterior cervical fusions. Articular pillar plating or anterior revision? Spine 20:2436–2441, 1995.

39. Matsunaga S, Sakou T, Imamura T, Morimoto N: Dissociated motor loss in the upper extremities. Clinical features and pathophysiology. Spine 18:1964–1967, 1993.

40. McAfee PC, Bohlman HH, Riley LH, et al: The anterior retropharyngeal approach to the upper part of the cervical spine. J Bone Joint Surg Am 69A:1371–1383, 1987.

41. McBride AD, Mukherjee DP, Kruse RN, Albright JA: Anterior screw fixation of type II odontoid fractures. A biomechanical study. Spine 20:1855–1859, 1995.

42. McCarthy RE, Lonstein JE, Mertz JD, Kuslich SD: Air embolism in spinal surgery. J Spinal Disord 3:1–5, 1990.

43. Merle H, Delattre O, Trode M, Catonne Y: Central retinal artery occlusion in surgery of the cervical vertebrae. J Franc Ophtalmol 17:603–607, 1994.

44. Merwin GE, Post JC, Sypert GW: Transoral approach to the upper cervical spine. Laryngoscope 101:780–784, 1991.

45. Newhouse KE, Lindsey RW, Clark CR, et al: Esophageal perforation following anterior cervical spine surgery. Spine 14:1051–1053, 1989.

46. Nikkhah G, Schonmayr R, Volkening D, Samii M: Chronic compression of the cervical myelon as complication of anterior interbody fusion (AIF): Neurological improvement after late anterior decompression. Case report. Neurosurg Rev 16:61–66, 1993.

47. Ogle K, Palsingh J, Hewitt C, Anderson M: Osteoptysis: A complication of cervical spine surgery. Br J Neurosurg 6:607–609, 1992.

48. Oz MC, Jeevanandam V, Smith CR, et al: Autologous fibrin glue from intraoperatively collected platelet-rich plasma. Ann Thorac Surg 53:530–531, 1992.

49. Reiss RF, Oz MC (1996): Autologous fibrin glue: Production and clinical use. Transfus Med Rev 10:85–92, 1996.

50. Robinson RA, Smith GW: Anterolateral cervical disc removal and interbody fusion for cervical disc syndrome. Bull Johns Hopkins Hosp 96:223–224, 1955.

51. Roche M, Gilly F, Carret JP, et al: Perforation of the cervical esophagus and hypopharynx complicating surgery by an anterior approach to the cervical spine. Ann Chir 43:343–347, 1989.

52. Sasso R, Doherty BJ, Crawford MJ, Heggeness MH: Biomechanics of odontoid fracture fixation. Comparison of the one- and two-screw technique. Spine 18:1950–1953, 1993.

53. Saunders RL: On the pathogenesis of the radiculopathy complicating multilevel corpectomy. Neurosurgery 37:408–412, 1995.

54. Seki K, Shimizu K, Matsushita M, et al (1994): Postlaminectomy kyphosis of the cervical spine complicating spinal cord tumor in the foramen magnum. No Shinkei Geka 22:481–484, 1994.

55. Shapiro S: Banked fibula and the locking anterior cervical plate in anterior cervical fusions following cervical discectomy. J Neurosurg 84:161–165, 1996.

56. Shektman A, Granick MS, Solomon MP, et al: Management of infected laminectomy wounds. Neurosurgery 35:307–309, 1994.

57. Simonds RJ: HIV transmission by organ and tissue transplantation. AIDS 7:S35–S38, 1993.

58. Simonds RJ, Holmberg SD, Hurwitz RL, et al: Transmission of human immunodeficiency virus type 1 from a seronegative organ and tissue donor. N Engl J Med 326:726–732, 1992.

59. Smith MD, Bolesta MJ: Esophageal perforation after anterior cervical plate fixation: A report of two cases. J Spine Disord 5:357–562, 1992.

60. Smith MD, Bolesta MJ, Leventhal M, Bohlman HH: Postoperative cerebrospinal-fluid fistula associated with erosion of the dura. Findings after anterior resection of ossification of the posterior longitudinal ligament in the cervical spine. J Bone Joint Surg Am 74A:270–277, 1992.

61. Smith MD, Emery SE, Dudley A, et al: Vertebral artery injury during anterior decompression of the cervical spine. A retrospective review of ten patients. J Bone Joint Surg Br 75B:410–415, 1993.

62. Madawi AA, Solanki G, Casey ATH, Crockard HA: Variation of the groove in the axis vertebra for the vertebral artery. Implications for instrumentation. J Bone Joint Surg Br 79B:820–823, 1997.

63. Stabler CL, Eismont FJ, Brown MD, et al: Failure of posterior cervical fusions using cadaveric bone graft in children. J Bone Joint Surg Am 67A:371–375, 1985.

64. Statham P, O'Sullivan M, Russell T: The Halifax interlaminar clamp for posterior cervical fusion: Initial experience in the United Kingdom. Neurosurgery 32:396–398, 1993.

65. Szabo MD, Crosby G: Excessive atlanto-occipital flexion as a cause of complete airway obstruction following anterior cervical spine fusion. J Clin Anesth 4:328–330, 1992.

66. Tippets RH, Apfelbaum RI: Anterior cervical fusion with the Caspar instrumentation system. Neurosurgery 22:1008–1013, 1988.

67. Tippets RH, Apfelbaum RI: Technical and clinical complications with Caspar plating. In Proceedings of the Cervical Spine Research Society Annual Meeting. Desert Palm, FL, Cervical Spine Research Society, 1992, pp 74–75.

68. Torpey BM, Dormans JP, Drummond DS: The use of MRI-compatible titanium segmental spinal instrumentation in pediatric patients with intraspinal tumor. J Spine Disord 8:76–81, 1995.

68a. Tribus CB, Corteen DP, Zdeblick TA: The efficacy of anterior cervical plating in the management of symptomatic pseudarthrosis of the cervical spine. Spine 24:860–864, 1999.

69. Vaccaro AR, Ring D, Scuderi G, Garfin SR: Vertebral artery location in relation to the vertebral body as determined by two-dimensional computed tomography evaluation. Spine 19:2637–2641, 1994.

70. van Berge Henegouwen DP, Roukema JA, de Nie JC, van Werken C: Esophageal perforation during surgery on the cervical spine. Neurosurgery 29:766–768, 1991.

71. Vazquez-Seoane P, Yoo J, Zou D, et al: Interference screw fixation of cervical grafts. A combined in vitro biomechanical and in vivo animal study. Spine 18:946–954, 1993.

72. Wattenmaker I, Concepcion M, Hibberd P, Lipson S (1994): Upper-airway obstruction and perioperative management of the airway in patients managed with posterior operations on the cervical spine for rheumatoid arthritis. J Bone Joint Surg Am 76A:360–365, 1994.

73. Whitesides TE Jr, Kelly RP: Lateral approach to the upper cervical spine for anterior fusion. South Med J 59:879–883, 1966.

74. Yablon IG, Cowan S, Mortara R: The migration of a Harrington rod after cervical fusion. Spine 18:356–358, 1993.

75. Yee GK, Terry AF: Esophageal penetration by an anterior cervical fixation device. A case report. Spine 18:522–527, 1993.

76. Yonenobu K, Hosono N, Iwasaki M, et al: Neurologic complications of surgery for cervical compression myelopathy. Spine 16:1277–1282, 1991.

77. Yonenobu K, Okada K, Fuji T, et al: Causes of neurologic deterioration following surgical treatment of cervical myelopathy. Spine 11:818–823, 1986.

78. Zambelli PY, Lechevallier J, Bracq H, Carlioz H: Osteoid osteoma or osteoblastoma of the cervical spine in relation to the vertebral artery. J Pediatr Orthop 14:788–792, 1994.

79. Zdeblick TA, Ducker TB: The use of freeze-dried allograft bone for anterior cervical fusions. Spine 16:726–729, 1991.

INDEX

Note: Page numbers followed by f indicate figures; those followed by t indicate tables.

291